Thieme

Operative Approaches in Orthopedic Surgery and Traumatology

2nd Edition

Fridun Kerschbaumer, MD
Professor
Head of the Orthopaedic Surgery and Rheumatology Department
Red Cross Hospital
Frankfurt, Germany

Kuno Weise, MD
Professor
Formerly Head of the BG Trauma Hospital Tübingen
University of Tübingen
Tübingen, Germany

Carl Joachim Wirth, MD
Professor
Formerly Head of the Department of Orthopaedic Surgery
Hannover Medical School
Hannover, Germany

Alexander R. Vaccaro, MD, PhD
Richard H. Rothman Professor and Chairman of Orthopaedic Surgery
Professor of Neurosurgery
Co-Director of the Delaware Valley Spinal Cord Injury Center
Co-Chief of Spine Surgery
Co-Director of the Spine Fellowship Program
President of the Rothman Institute
Thomas Jefferson University
Philadelphia, Pennsylvania, USA

747 illustrations

Thieme
Stuttgart · New York · Delhi · Rio de Janeiro

Library of Congress Cataloging-in-Publication Data
Kerschbaumer, F. (Fridun), author.
[Operative Zugangswege in Orthopädie und Traumatologie. English]
Operative approaches in orthopedic surgery and traumatology / Fridun Kerschbaumer, Kuno Weise, Carl Joachim Wirth, Alexander R. Vaccaro. – 2nd edition.
p. ; cm.
Authorized translation of the 4th German edition published and copyrighted 2013 by Georg Thieme Verlag, Stuttgart, Germany; title of the German edition: Operative Zugangswege in Orthopädie und Traumatologie.
Preceded by Operative approaches in orthopedic surgery and traumatology / R. Bauer, F. Kerschbaumer, and S. Poisel. 1987.
Includes bibliographical references and index.
ISBN 978-3-13-705502-0 (alk. paper) –
ISBN 978-3-13-173452-5 (e-book)
I. Weise, K. (Kuno), author. II. Wirth, Carl Joachim, author. III. Vaccaro, Alexander R., author. IV. Bauer, Rudolf, 1937 – Operative Zugangswege in Orthopädie und Traumatologie. English. Preceded by work: V. Title.
[DNLM: 1. Orthopedic Procedures–methods–Atlases. 2. Bone and Bones–surgery–Atlases. 3. Wounds and Injuries–surgery–Atlases. WE 17]
RD733.2
617.4'71–dc23
2015003532

Translator: Geraldine O'Sullivan, Dublin, Ireland

Illustrators: Gerhard Spitzer †
Holger Vanselow, Stuttgart
Reinhold Henkel †

Thieme Publishers Stuttgart
Rüdigerstrasse 14, 70469 Stuttgart, Germany
+49 [0]711 8931 421, customerservice@thieme.de

Thieme Publishers New York
333 Seventh Avenue, New York, NY 10001 USA
+1 800 782 3488, customerservice@thieme.com

Thieme Publishers Delhi
A-12, Second Floor, Sector-2, Noida-201301
Uttar Pradesh, India
+91 120 45 566 00, customerservice@thieme.in

Thieme Publishers Rio, Thieme Publicações Ltda.
Argentina Building 16th floor, Ala A, 228 Praia do Botafogo
Rio de Janeiro 22250-040 Brazil
+55 21 3736-3651

Cover design: Thieme Publishing Group
Typesetting by Druckhaus Götz GmbH, Ludwigsburg, Germany
Printed in China by Everbest Printing Ltd., Hong Kong

ISBN 978-3-13-705502-0 5 4 3 2 1

Also available as an e-book:
eISBN 978-3-13-173452-5

Important note: Medicine is an ever-changing science undergoing continual development. Research and clinical experience are continually expanding our knowledge, in particular our knowledge of proper treatment and drug therapy. Insofar as this book mentions any dosage or application, readers may rest assured that the authors, editors, and publishers have made every effort to ensure that such references are in accordance with **the state of knowledge at the time of production of the book.**

Nevertheless, this does not involve, imply, or express any guarantee or responsibility on the part of the publishers in respect to any dosage instructions and forms of applications stated in the book. **Every user is requested to examine carefully** the manufacturers' leaflets accompanying each drug and to check, if necessary in consultation with a physician or specialist, whether the dosage schedules mentioned therein or the contraindications stated by the manufacturers differ from the statements made in the present book. Such examination is particularly important with drugs that are either rarely used or have been newly released on the market. Every dosage schedule or every form of application used is entirely at the user's own risk and responsibility. The authors and publishers request every user to report to the publishers any discrepancies or inaccuracies noticed. If errors in this work are found after publication, errata will be posted at www.thieme.com on the product description page.

Some of the product names, patents, and registered designs referred to in this book are in fact registered trademarks or proprietary names even though specific reference to this fact is not always made in the text. Therefore, the appearance of a name without designation as proprietary is not to be construed as a representation by the publisher that it is in the public domain.

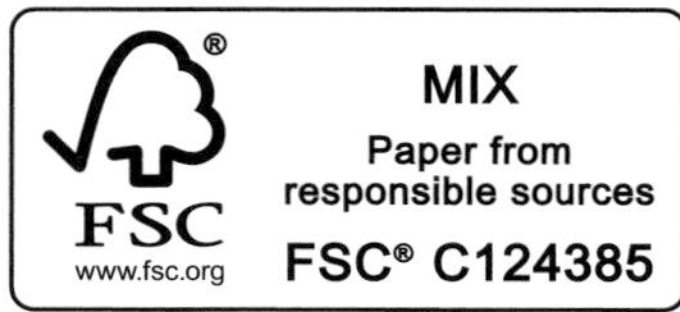

Contents

Foreword to the Second Edition

More than three decades ago, I was fortunate to have a wonderful post-residency clinical experience at the *Universitätsklinik für Orthopädie* in Innsbruck, Austria. In addition to an opportunity to perform complex operative procedures with extraordinary surgeons such as Rudolf Bauer and Fridun Kerschbaumer, I became enamored with their institution's scientific environment of excellence and intellectual curiosity that inspires my surgical acumen even to this day. However, the greatest gift that my Tyrolean colleagues bestowed upon me was actually an English version of *Operative Approaches in Orthopedic Surgery and Traumatology.*

The impetus for this textbook was an extremely successful medical school musculoskeletal anatomy lecture series that evolved into a mission to provide surgeons, regardless of their level of experience, with a unique, visually appealing atlas of orthopedic surgical approaches. Drs. Bauer and Kerschbaumer, in collaboration with anatomist Sepp Poisel, painstakingly amassed 593 high-quality illustrations supported by succinct text which covered all of the salient aspects of any surgical procedure—its indications, positioning, incisions, hazards, wound closure, and complications.

The first English edition of this exemplary atlas has not only garnered worldwide acclaim, it redefined the standard by which surgical exposures should be taught. Throughout my academic career, this monograph has always been in proximity to the operating room, and considered an invaluable reference I shared with all members of the surgical team. In fact, my surgery colleagues commonly referred to it as simply "The Book".

Since the first edition, Dr. Poisel has passed away, and Dr. Bauer has retired. I applaud Dr. Kerschbaumer for his vision to update the original textbook for the new millennium. In the second English edition, the indications have been updated, and the operative approaches expanded to include the soft-tissue sparing and minimally-invasive endoscopic and arthroscopic techniques as new standards of modern practice. In this latest edition, the clarity and organization of more than 700 topographic anatomical illustrations comprehensively depict the surgeon's perspective of any orthopedic operative procedure.

The second edition has also benefitted from its transition from an "authored" to an "edited" textbook. A highly accomplished group of international contributors with extensive surgical experience in their respective fields have created this comprehensive, state-of-the-art resource. The four renowned editors (Kerschbaumer, Weise, Wirth, and Vaccaro) have truly succeeded in enhancing the quality of this latest edition while retaining the spirit of the original text.

This textbook has already established itself as a remarkable asset for present-day musculoskeletal surgeons and trainees worldwide. I am confident that future generations will also come to appreciate the educational merits of "The Book".

Ronald W. Lindsey, MD

Foreword to the First Edition

Textbooks on surgical approaches for orthopedic surgeons are not uncommon. In fact, each year an ever increasing number of textbooks on surgical approaches in anatomy are distributed to the medical audience. Why, one might ask, is another book really necessary? Are not all these texts pretty much the same? Can one just not go back to a rather standardized anatomical text and glean from that the relevant information necessary for a particular surgical anatomical exposure?

For this Professor Bauer and his colleagues have an answer, and it is a resounding no. They have, in effect, provided us with one of the most useful and exciting textbooks on anatomical approaches in surgery that I have ever had the pleasure of reading. We are indeed fortunate that such a superb textbook has been translated for the English speaking world.

As Professor Bauer and his colleagues have stated, the atlas has been organized to show and demonstrate standardized approaches from the skin incision to the particular target organ supplemented with detailed illustrations outlining the relevant anatomy. The exposure is well described in a concise fashion making it easy for the reader to follow the illustrations sequentially. I particularly liked the illustrations which were drawn in a manner in which the surgeon visualizes the anatomy, rather than in the usual upright profile of most published textbooks. Illustrations from both the right and left side, particularly in the cervical spine, are tremendously helpful. The organization structure describing exposures, discussing complications and outlining the dangers of particular approaches is most useful.

It is apparent that Professor Bauer and his colleagues have drawn on extensive experience in producing this atlas. Professor Bauer is well-known in orthopedic circles in the English speaking world. Born in Vienna, December 25, 1937, he studied medicine at the University of Vienna and obtained his medical doctorate in 1962. He was appointed as Associate Professor at the University of Innsbruck in 1974, being made Professor at the University Hospital in 1976. He is the author of over 200 scientific papers and has written textbooks and monographs in a variety of fields. He is a corresponding member of numerous orthopedic societies, both in Europe and North America. He is well respected for his work in trauma, spine, and pediatric and adult reconstructive surgery.

We are indeed fortunate that this textbook has been translated into English. It is a unique, outstanding contribution and I feel should be an important and useful addition to the libraries of all orthopedic surgeons and medical centers.

Autumn 1987 *David S. Bradford, MD*

Preface

Knowledge of the operative approaches in orthopedic and trauma surgery is an essential prerequisite for the success of any surgical procedure. Twenty-seven years ago the authors Rudolf Bauer, Fridun Kerschbaumer, and Sepp Poisel published an illustrated textbook for the English-speaking world. The quality of the surgical topographic illustrations drawn by the late Professor Gerhard Spitzer is still unique.

Recent advances in less invasive techniques and in endoscopic and arthroscopic procedures are the main reason for publishing a new edition including these approaches. Furthermore, soft-tissue-sparing techniques used in trauma surgery have been added. This new edition was written by seventeen authors reflecting their special topographic experience and illustrated by Professor Spitzer, Holger Vanselow, and Reinhold Henkel.

As was done with the original edition, all new surgical approaches were either documented step by step in the operating theater or the authors demonstrated them on cadavers in the presence of the illustrator.

The anatomical labels of the new illustrations were written by anatomists in the Department of Surgical Anatomy at the University of Tübingen, Germany. The indications for the surgical approaches and the references have been adapted and updated.

This new edition would not have been possible without the support of Dr. Albrecht Hauff, Dr. Udo Schiller, Antje-Karen Richter, and Silvia Haller at Georg Thieme Verlag, Angelika-Marie Findgott and Dr. Martina Habeck at Thieme Publishers, and Geraldine O'Sullivan, who translated these new chapters.

We are very grateful to Professor Bernhard Hirt, Head of the Department for Surgical Anatomy at the University of Tübingen, for allowing us to use his laboratory for the anatomical dissections and the audiovisual documentation. We thank Mr. Vanselow, our illustrator, for his drawings of the new operative approaches and for staying so close to the style of the original illustrations drawn by Professor Spitzer.

Fridun Kerschbaumer, MD
Kuno Weise, MD
Carl Joachim Wirth, MD
Alexander R. Vaccaro, MD, PhD

Contributors

Rudolf Bauer, MD
Professor
Formerly Department of Orthopaedic Surgery
Medical University of Innsbruck
Innsbruck, Austria

Michael Dienst, MD
Associate Professor
OCM Orthopaedic Surgery Munich
Munich, Germany

Oliver Eberhardt, MD
Department of Orthopaedic Surgery
Olgahospital
Stuttgart, Germany

Karin Häringer, MD
Center for Orthopaedic Surgery and Traumatology
Städtisches Klinikum München Bogenhausen
Munich, Germany

Bernhard Hirt, MD
Professor
Head of the Department of Clinical Anatomy
Institute of Anatomy
University of Tübingen
Tübingen, Germany

Dankward Höntzsch, MD
Professor
Department of Medical Technology Development
BG Trauma Hospital Tübingen
University of Tübingen
Tübingen, Germany

Frank Kandziora, MD
Professor
Head of the Center for Spinal Surgery
BG Trauma Hospital Frankfurt
Frankfurt, Germany

Fridun Kerschbaumer, MD
Professor
Head of the Orthopaedic Surgery and Rheumatology Department
Red Cross Hospital
Frankfurt, Germany

Dieter Kohn, MD
Professor
Head of the Department of Orthopaedic Surgery
Saarland University
Homburg, Germany

Philipp Lobenhoffer, MD
Professor
Sportsclinic Germany
Hannover, Germany

Markus Michel, MD
Orthopaedic Center Münsingen
Münsingen, Switzerland

Sepp Poisel, MD†
Professor
Formerly Institute of Anatomy
University of Innsbruck
Innsbruck, Austria

Andreas Roth, MD
Professor
Head of the Division for Total Joint Replacement
University Hospital Leipzig
Leipzig, Germany

Fabian Stuby, MD
Senior Surgeon at the Department for Trauma and Reconstructive Surgery
BG Trauma Hospital Tübingen
University of Tübingen
Tübingen, Germany

Alexander R. Vaccaro, MD, PhD
Richard H. Rothman Professor and Chairman of Orthopaedic Surgery
Professor of Neurosurgery
Co-Director of the Delaware Valley Spinal Cord Injury Center
Co-Chief of Spine Surgery
Co-Director of the Spine Fellowship Program
President of the Rothman Institute
Thomas Jefferson University
Philadelphia, Pennsylvania, USA

Kuno Weise, MD
Professor
Formerly Head of the BG Trauma Hospital Tübingen
University of Tübingen
Tübingen, Germany

Carl Joachim Wirth, MD
Professor
Formerly Head of the Department of Orthopaedic Surgery
Hannover Medical School
Hannover, Germany

Thomas Wirth, MD
Professor
Head of the Department of Orthopaedic Surgery
Olgahospital
Stuttgart, Germany

Oleg Yastrebov, MD
Department for Trauma and Reconstructive Surgery
Diakoniekrankenhaus Henriettenstiftung
Hannover, Germany

Spine, Anterior Approaches

1 Cervical Spine and Cervicothoracic Junction

1.1 Transoropharyngeal Approach C1–C2 (C3)

R. Bauer, F. Kerschbaumer, S. Poisel

1.1.1 Principal Indications

- Posttraumatic states, dens fractures, or pseudarthroses
- Tumors
- Osteomyelitis
- Os odontoideum

1.1.2 Preparation of Patient, Positioning, Anesthesia, Incision

This approach continues to present the problem of opening spongy bone cavities in an area colonized by pathogens. Thorough oral disinfection is therefore required before the start of the operation. The procedure is performed under antibiotic protection, and antibiotics are applied locally before closure of the wound. The patient is placed in a supine position with the head lowered and the cervical spine slightly overextended. The anesthesiology team stands on one side of the patient, and the operator at the head, with the assistants standing on both sides of the head.

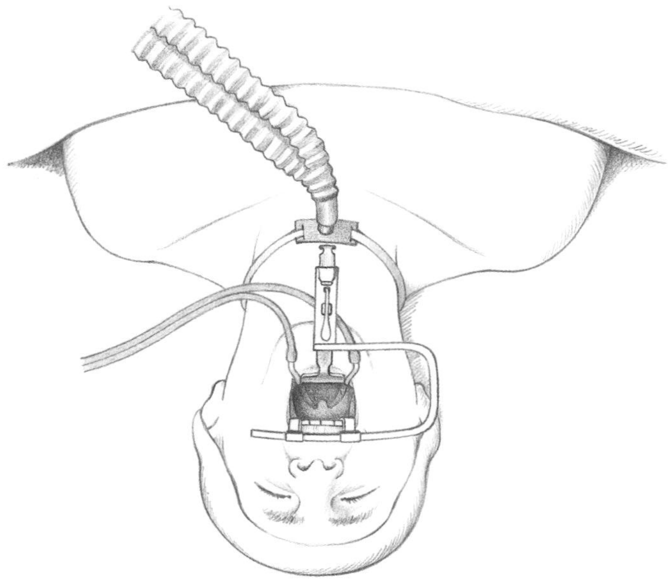

Fig. 1.1 The transoropharyngeal approach. Appearance after tracheotomy, with gag and tongue plate inserted.

The transoral approach is facilitated by prior creation of a tracheotomy for anesthetic purposes. Tracheotomy is not absolutely necessary: the operation can also be performed without special problems with a transnasal or transoral tube that is laterally retracted by means of a long spatula. A gag is then inserted with a special plate that holds down the tongue (**Fig. 1.1**). A hook is used to pull the soft palate up.

1.1.3 Exposure of the Vertebrae

An incision of the posterior pharyngeal wall is made with a scalpel in the midline, beginning at the readily palpable anterior tubercle of the atlas and extending to the level of C2 or C3. The length of the cut is approximately 5–6 cm (**Fig. 1.2**). The longus colli muscle now becomes visible (**Fig. 1.3**); it is split in the midline. Using a rasp, the soft tissue on the anterior side of C1 and C2 (possibly also C3) is now retracted laterally, beginning at the midline. This brings the anterior tubercle as well as the lateral mass of the atlas and the body of the axis into view. The operative area is kept open with flexible spatulas, and hemostasis is effected by diathermy (**Fig. 1.4**). The atlas can be exposed to at most 2 cm laterally from the midline, but vertebrae C2 and C3 to no more than 1 cm. At the inferior border of C2 in particular, there is a danger of injury to the vertebral artery (**Fig. 1.5**). On the side of the lateral mass of the atlas, the rasp may penetrate the retromandibular fossa, and this may lead to injuries of the ninth and 12th cranial nerves.

1.1.4 Wound Closure

Wound closure is performed in two layers with absorbable interrupted sutures.

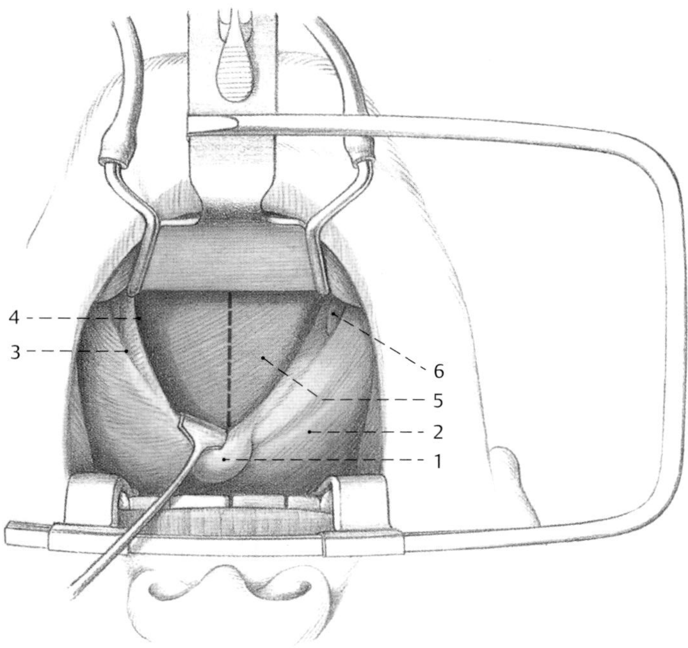

Fig. 1.2 Retraction of the soft palate; longitudinal incision of the posterior pharyngeal wall.

1 Uvula
2 Soft palate
3 Palatoglossal arch
4 Palatopharyngeal arch
5 Posterior pharyngeal wall with mucosa
6 Palatine tonsil

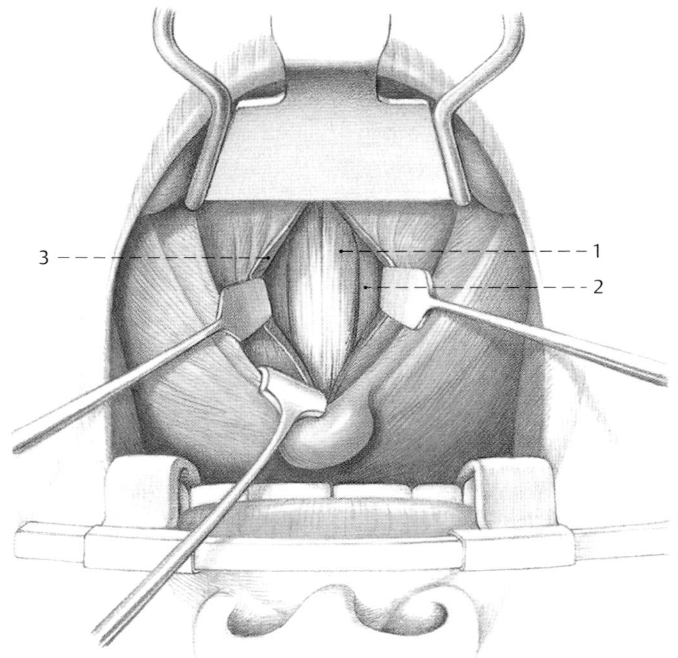

Fig. 1.3 Appearance after splitting of the posterior pharyngeal wall.

1 Longus colli
2 Longus capitis
3 Superior constrictor muscle of the pharynx

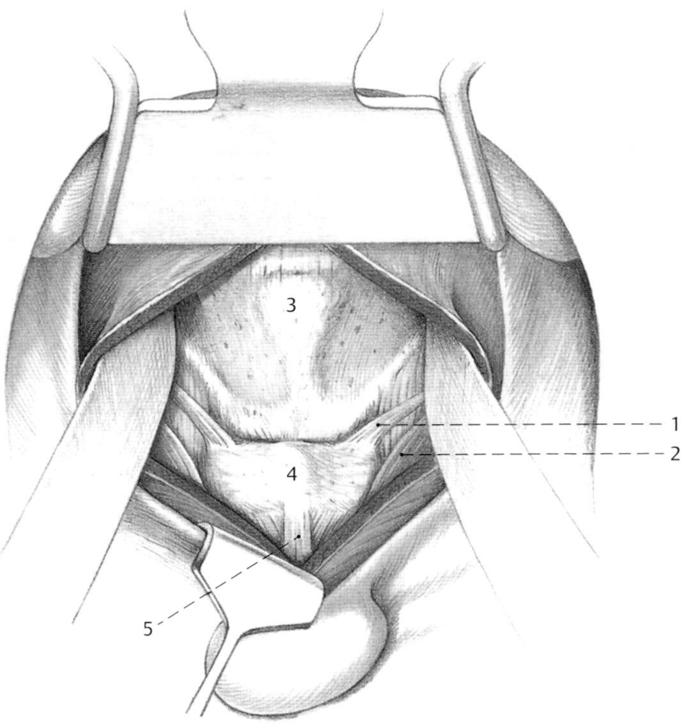

Fig. 1.4 Exposure of the atlas and axis.

1 Longus colli
2 Longus capitis
3 Body of the axis
4 Anterior tubercle of the atlas
5 Anterior atlantooccipital membrane

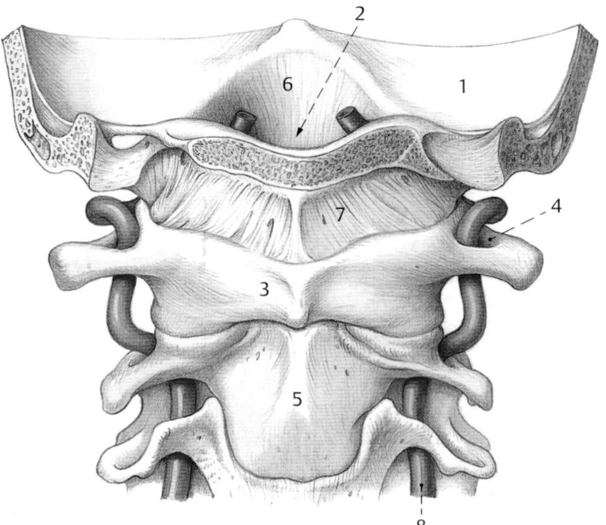

Fig. 1.5 Anatomical site of C1 and C2 with the vertebral artery, as seen from the front.

1 Squamous part of the occipital bone
2 Foramen magnum
3 Anterior tubercle of the atlas
4 Foramen transversarium
5 Body of the axis
6 Tectorial membrane
7 Anterior atlantooccipital membrane
8 Vertebral artery

1.2 Anterior Approach to the Cervical Spine C3–T2

R. Bauer, F. Kerschbaumer, S. Poisel

1.2.1 Principal Indications

- Trauma
- Degenerative changes
- Tumors
- Spondylitis

1.2.2 Choice of Side of Approach

For the upper and middle portions of the cervical spine, an approach is possible from either side. This also depends, however, on the side of the lesion. Right-handed persons generally prefer a right-sided approach, although for exposure of the cervical spine from C6 and below, the left-sided approach is preferable so that injury to the recurrent laryngeal nerve, which runs irregularly and at a higher level on the right side, may be avoided.

1.2.3 Positioning and Incision

The patient is placed in a supine position, generally without skeletal extension except in the presence of fresh trauma. A cushion is placed between the shoulder blades; if hyperextension is desired, a rolled-up pad is put beneath the cervical spine. The head is turned slightly toward the contralateral side, and both shoulders are pulled down with strips

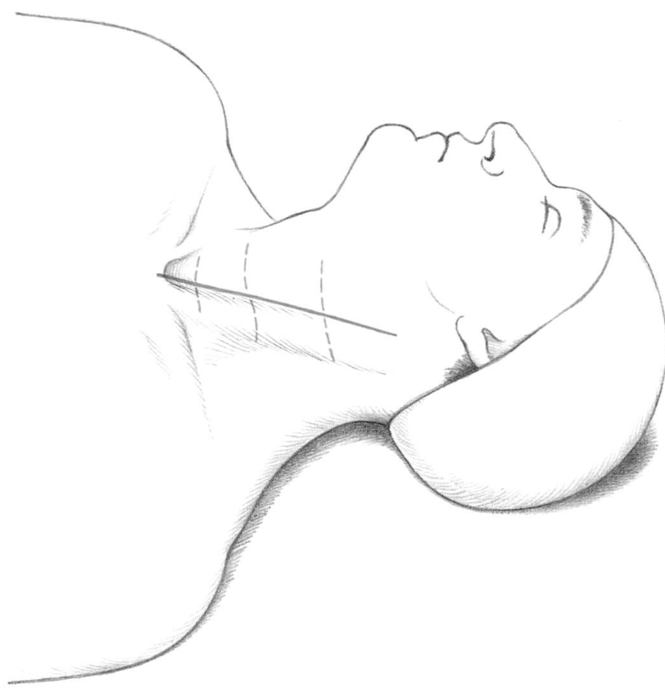

Fig. 1.6 Anterior approach to the cervical spine. Longitudinal incision and alternative transverse incisions. Supine position with the head turned to the side and slight overextension of the cervical spine.

Fig. 1.7 After longitudinal transection of the subcutaneous tissue and platysma, the anterior border of sternocleidomastoid is identified, and the superficial cervical fascia is transected parallel to it. Ligation of the transverse veins and branches of the superficial ansa cervicalis.

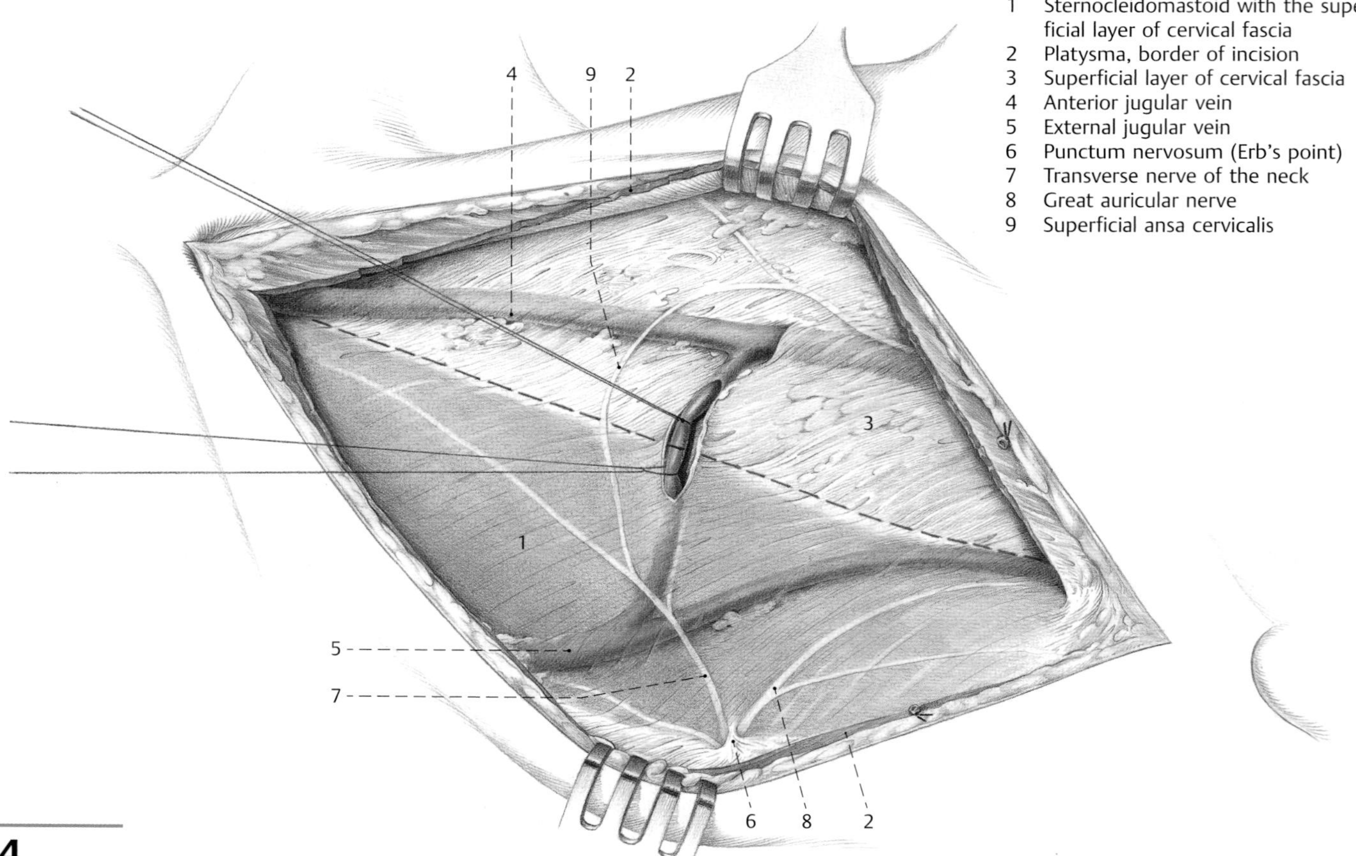

1 Sternocleidomastoid with the superficial layer of cervical fascia
2 Platysma, border of incision
3 Superficial layer of cervical fascia
4 Anterior jugular vein
5 External jugular vein
6 Punctum nervosum (Erb's point)
7 Transverse nerve of the neck
8 Great auricular nerve
9 Superficial ansa cervicalis

of adhesive tape. The operation is performed under endotracheal anesthesia.

The type of incision used depends on the desired extent of the vertebral exposure. If an exposure of only one or two segments suffices, a transverse skin incision parallel to the skin creases of the neck is recommended. The level of the transverse incision may be chosen according to the following guide:

- C3 and C4: incision two fingerbreadths caudal to the mandible at the level of the hyoid bone
- C4 and C5: incision at the level of the thyroid cartilage
- C5 and C6: incision at the level of the cricoid cartilage
- C6 and T1: incision two fingerbreadths cranial to the clavicle

For a long exposure of the cervical spine involving several segments, a longitudinal incision in front of the sternocleidomastoid is preferred. The skin incision begins at the level of the mandibular angle and extends distally as far as the manubrium of the sternum (**Fig. 1.6**). The platysma is split in the same direction and moved to the two sides to expose the superficial cervical fascia. This is now transected longitudinally at the anterior border of the sternocleidomastoid. This usually also requires sectioning of transversely coursing cervical veins and branches of the transverse cervical nerve (**Fig. 1.7**). The sternocleidomastoid is then retracted laterally and the subhyoid medially. The upper belly of omohyoid now extends transversely across the operative site (**Fig. 1.8**). Undermining this belly, it is transected between two ligatures and retracted on both sides. Then the pretracheal layer of the cervical fascia is opened by blunt scissor dissection. The cervical vertebrae can now be palpated with the finger. Veins running transversely deep to the fascia (middle thyroid veins) often need to be transected between ligatures (**Fig. 1.9**). The pretracheal fascia should then be bluntly dissected cranially and caudally, sacrificing transverse branches of the deep ansa cervicalis. The pulse of the common carotid artery can be palpated laterally with the finger. The neurovascular bundle (common carotid artery, internal jugular vein, vagus nerve) is cautiously retracted laterally, while the visceral structures (trachea, larynx, thyroid, and sternohyoid and sternothyroid muscles) are retracted medially (**Figs. 1.9** and **1.10**).

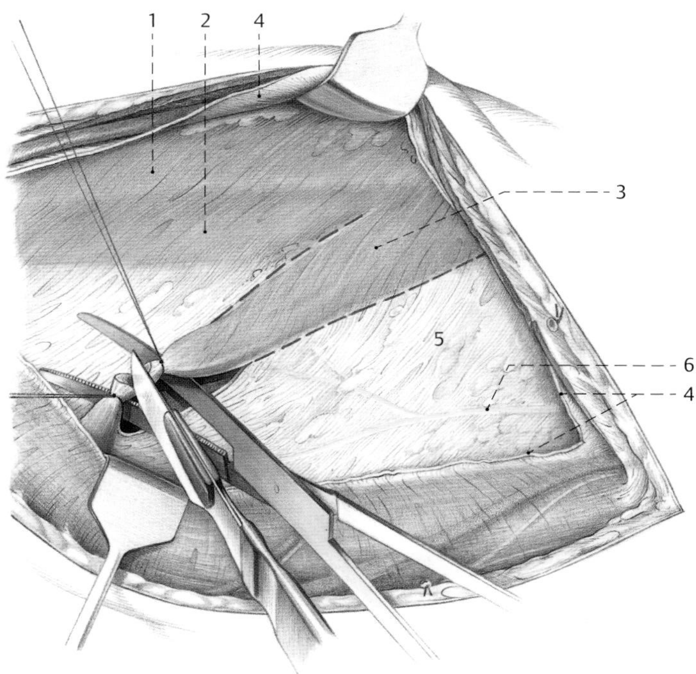

Fig. 1.8 Undermining and transection of the upper belly of omohyoid between two ligatures.

1 Sternohyoid
2 Sternothyroid
3 Omohyoid
4 Cervical fascia, superficial layer
5 Cervical fascia, pretracheal layer
6 Deep ansa cervicalis

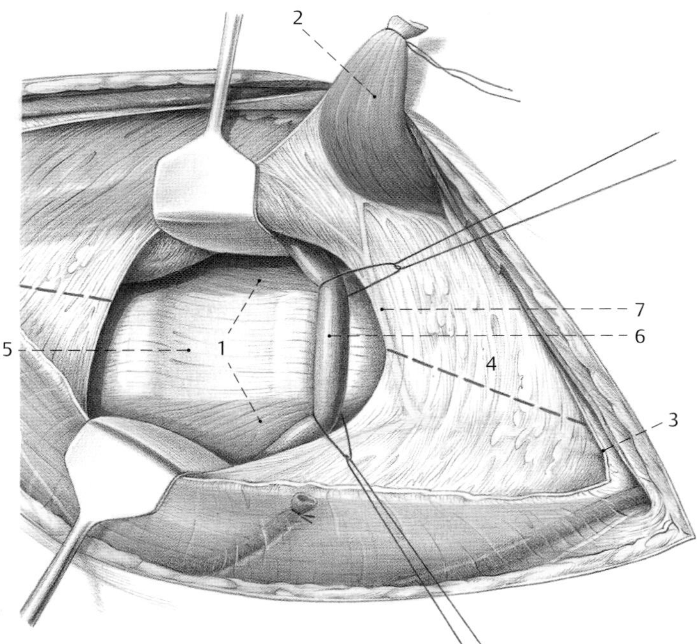

Fig. 1.9 Blunt division of the pretracheal cervical fascia; ligation and transection of the transverse veins and branches of the deep ansa cervicalis. Insertion of blunt hooks, and further dissection between the lateral neurovascular bundle and medial visceral structures.

1 Longus colli
2 Omohyoid
3 Cervical fascia, superficial layer
4 Cervical fascia, pretracheal layer
5 Sixth cervical vertebra with prevertebral cervical fascia
6 Middle thyroid vein
7 Deep ansa cervicalis

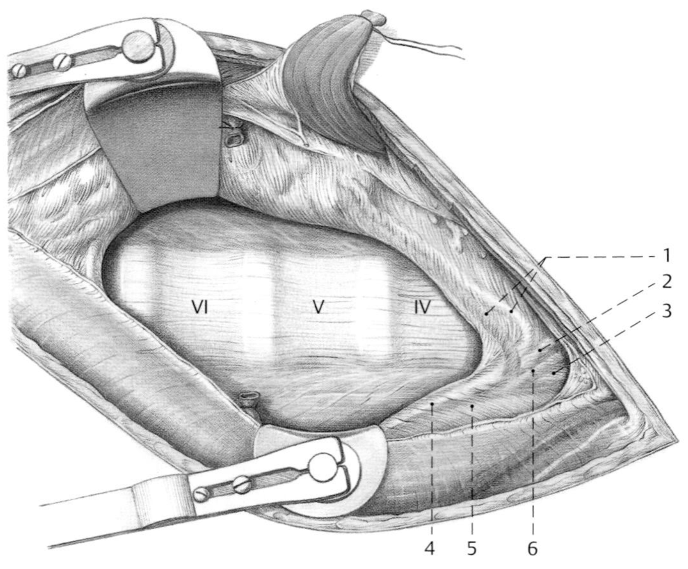

Fig. 1.10 Exposure of the prevertebral cervical fascia and the anterior aspects of the fourth, fifth and sixth cervical vertebrae by retraction with Cloward spreaders.

1 Superior thyroid artery and vein
2 Lingual artery
3 External carotid artery
4 Common carotid artery
5 Internal jugular vein
6 Facial vein
IV–VI Cervical vertebrae

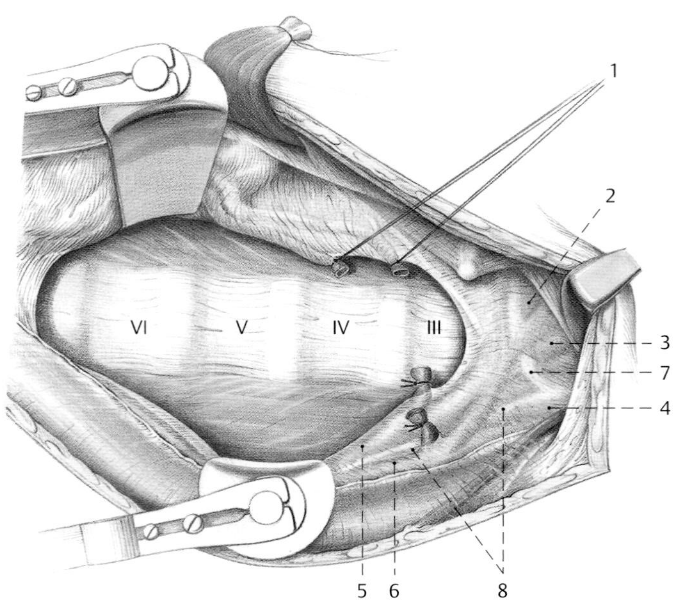

Fig. 1.11 Exposure of the cervical vertebrae above C4 requires ligation and transection of the superior thyroid artery.

1 Superior thyroid artery and vein
2 Lingual artery
3 Facial artery
4 External carotid artery
5 Common carotid artery
6 Internal jugular vein
7 Hypoglossal nerve
8 Deep ansa cervicalis
III–VI Cervical vertebrae

1.2.4 Exposure of Cervical Vertebrae C2–C6

Further dissection, in the medial and cranial directions, between the prevertebral layer of the cervical fascia on the one hand, and the esophagus and larynx on the other hand, is best done with the finger. If further dissection in a cranial direction for exposure of the third or second cervical vertebra is required, the superior thyroid artery must be found, ligated, and transected (**Fig. 1.11**).

1.2.5 Anatomical Site

(**Figs. 1.12** and **1.13**)

The following anatomical structures need to be considered when exposing the proximal segments of the cervical spine: superior thyroid artery, lingual artery, and facial artery, all of which branch off from the external carotid artery and may be ligated if necessary. The hypoglossal nerve, which runs from its cranial origin caudally and then takes a medial turn in front of the external carotid artery to enter the lingual muscles, should be spared.

The superior laryngeal nerve with its external and internal branches originates from the vagus nerve and courses deep to the lingual and facial arteries before entering the larynx. Further cranially, coursing in a medial direction from the base of the skull, the glossopharyngeal nerve runs into the superior constrictor muscle of the pharynx.

The irregularly coursing veins may be ligated if necessary (**Fig. 1.14**).

The approaches are represented schematically in **Figs. 1.15** and **1.16** (red arrows).

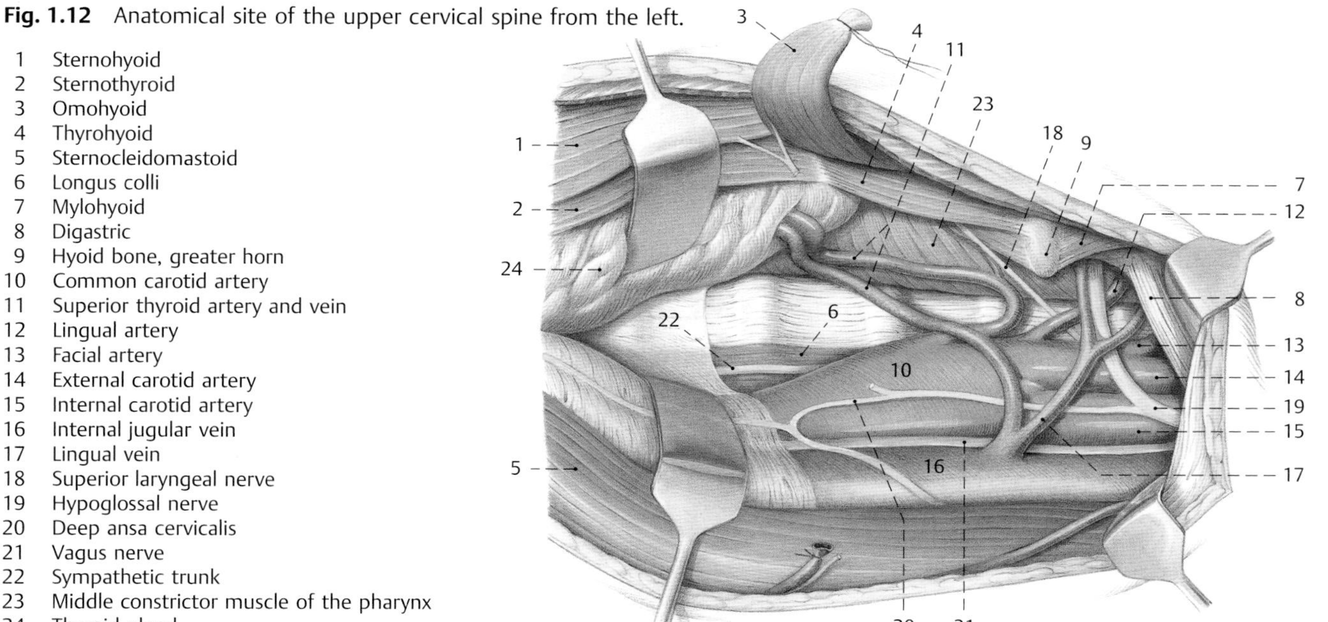

Fig. 1.12 Anatomical site of the upper cervical spine from the left.

1 Sternohyoid
2 Sternothyroid
3 Omohyoid
4 Thyrohyoid
5 Sternocleidomastoid
6 Longus colli
7 Mylohyoid
8 Digastric
9 Hyoid bone, greater horn
10 Common carotid artery
11 Superior thyroid artery and vein
12 Lingual artery
13 Facial artery
14 External carotid artery
15 Internal carotid artery
16 Internal jugular vein
17 Lingual vein
18 Superior laryngeal nerve
19 Hypoglossal nerve
20 Deep ansa cervicalis
21 Vagus nerve
22 Sympathetic trunk
23 Middle constrictor muscle of the pharynx
24 Thyroid gland

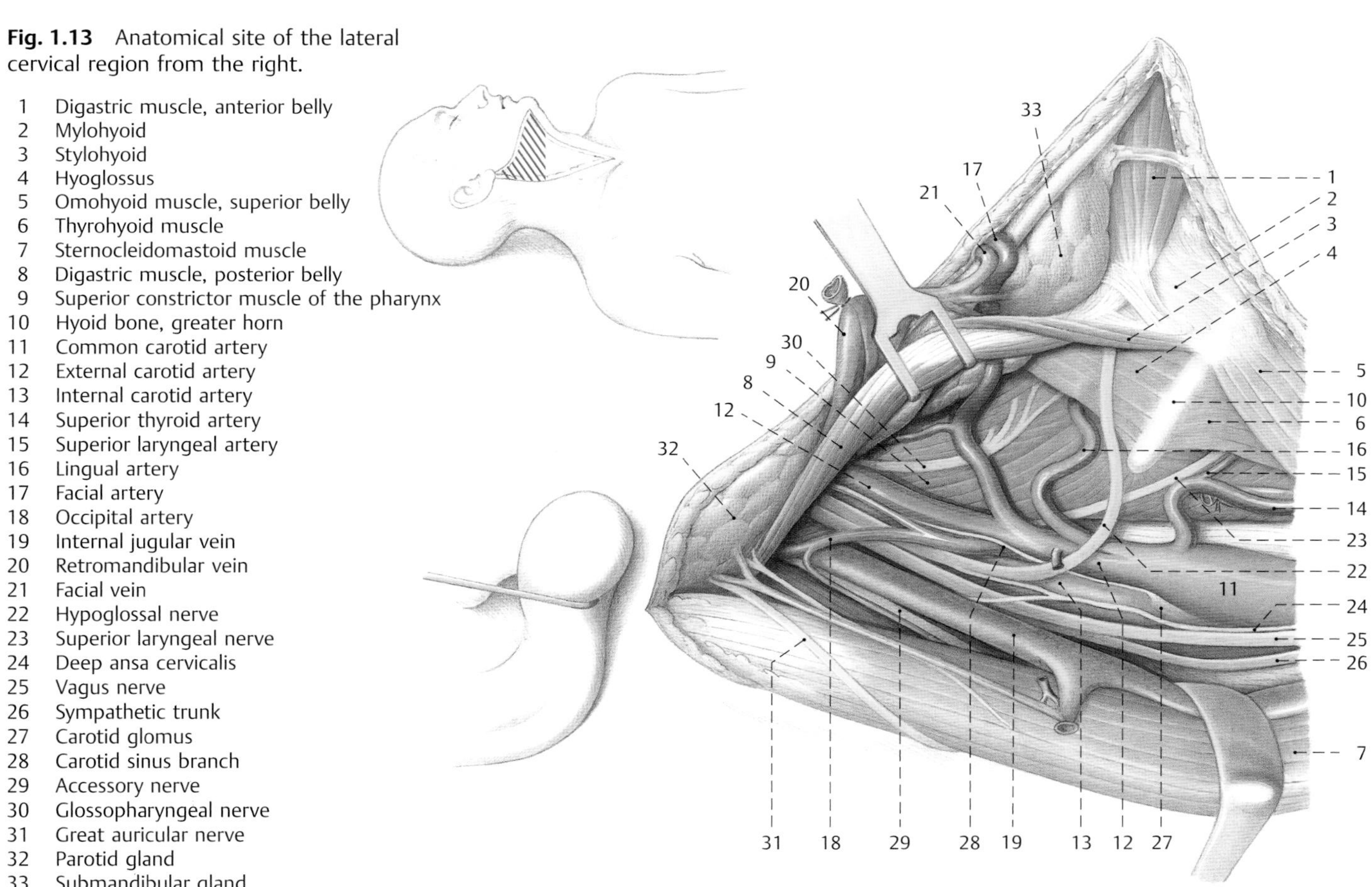

Fig. 1.13 Anatomical site of the lateral cervical region from the right.

1 Digastric muscle, anterior belly
2 Mylohyoid
3 Stylohyoid
4 Hyoglossus
5 Omohyoid muscle, superior belly
6 Thyrohyoid muscle
7 Sternocleidomastoid muscle
8 Digastric muscle, posterior belly
9 Superior constrictor muscle of the pharynx
10 Hyoid bone, greater horn
11 Common carotid artery
12 External carotid artery
13 Internal carotid artery
14 Superior thyroid artery
15 Superior laryngeal artery
16 Lingual artery
17 Facial artery
18 Occipital artery
19 Internal jugular vein
20 Retromandibular vein
21 Facial vein
22 Hypoglossal nerve
23 Superior laryngeal nerve
24 Deep ansa cervicalis
25 Vagus nerve
26 Sympathetic trunk
27 Carotid glomus
28 Carotid sinus branch
29 Accessory nerve
30 Glossopharyngeal nerve
31 Great auricular nerve
32 Parotid gland
33 Submandibular gland

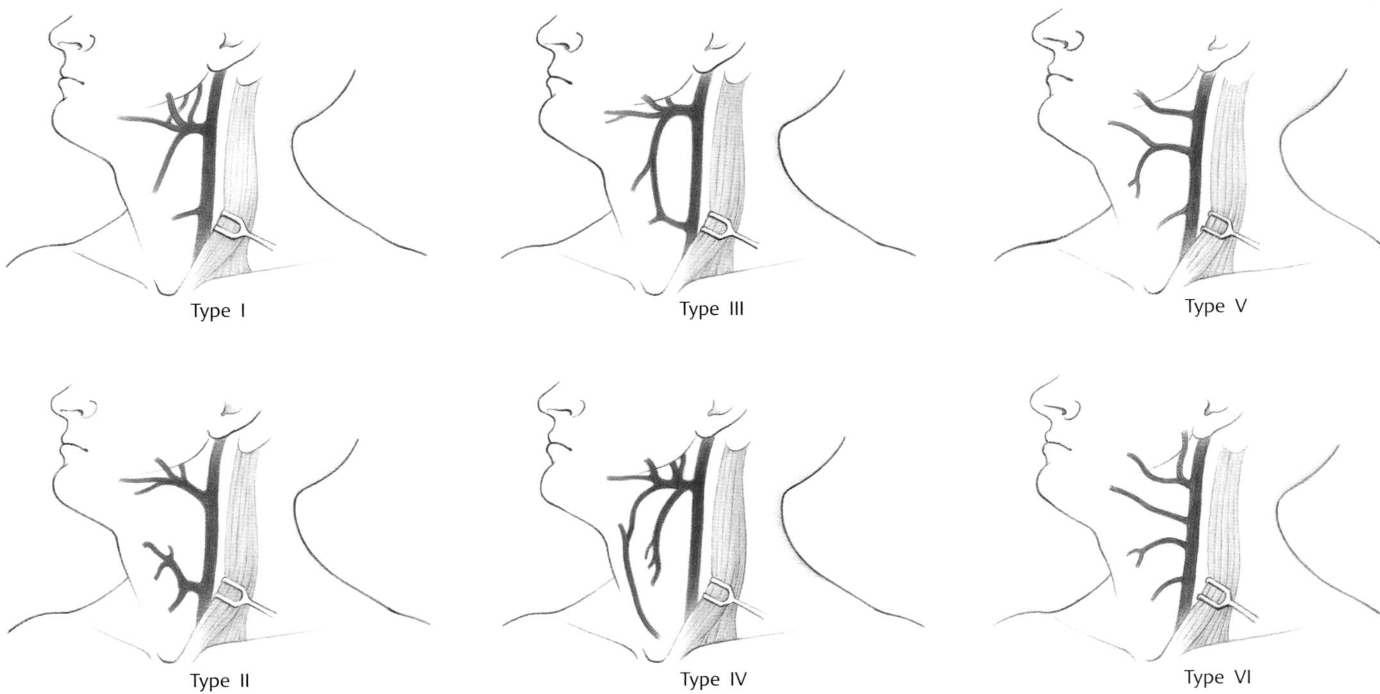

Fig. 1.14 Variations in venous drainage to the internal jugular vein.

Type I Thyrolinguofacial trunk (45%)
Type II Linguofacial trunk (9%)
Type III Linguofacial trunk with arcade (12%)
Type IV Thyrolinguofacial trunk with connection to the anterior jugular vein (15%)
Type V Thyrolingual trunk (7%)
Type VI Independent afferent course of all three veins (12%)

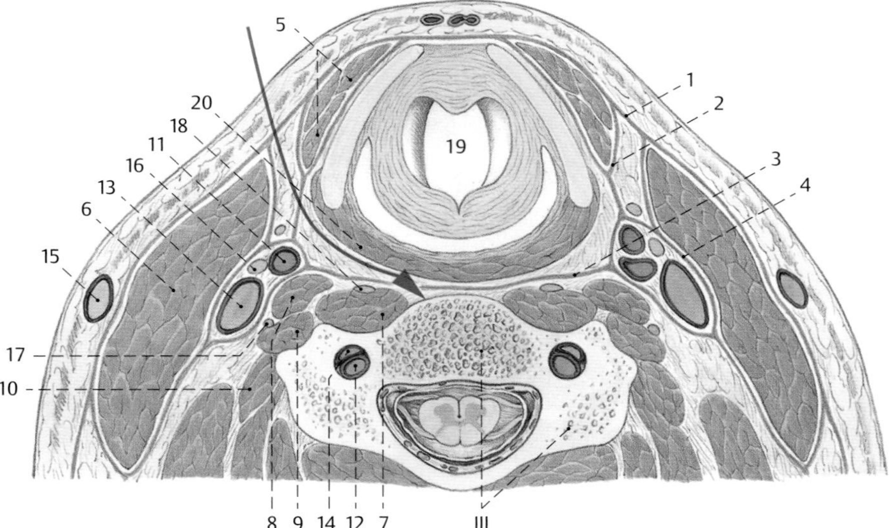

Fig. 1.15 Anatomical cross-section at the level of the third cervical vertebra.

1 Cervical fascia, superficial layer
2 Cervical fascia, pretracheal layer
3 Cervical fascia, prevertebral layer
4 Cervical fascia, carotid sheath
5 Infrahyoid muscles
6 Sternocleidomastoid
7 Longus colli
8 Longus capitis
9 Anterior scalene muscle
10 Middle scalene muscle
11 Common carotid artery
12 Vertebral artery
13 Internal jugular vein
14 Vertebral vein
15 External jugular vein
16 Vagus nerve
17 Phrenic nerve
18 Sympathetic trunk
19 Larynx
20 Pharynx
III Cervical vertebra

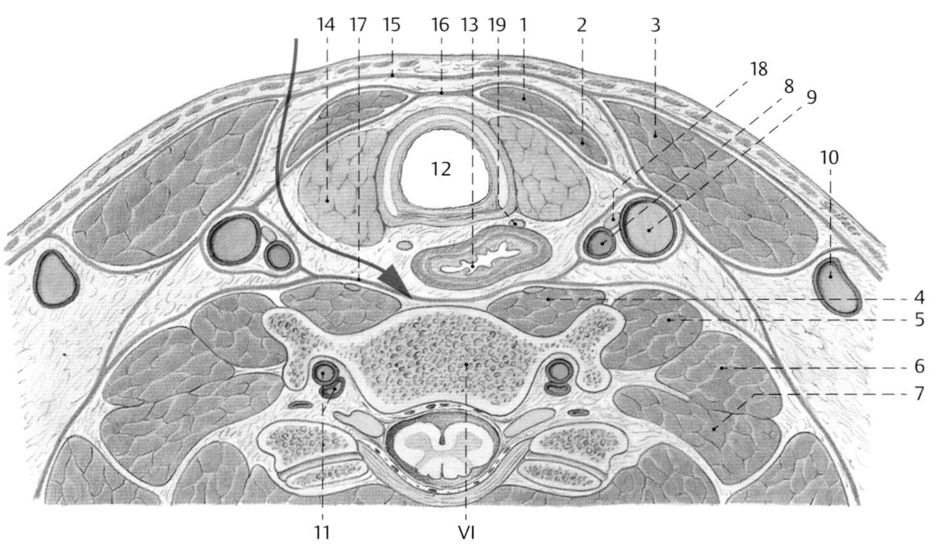

Fig. 1.16 Anatomical cross-section at the level of the sixth cervical vertebra.

1 Sternohyoid
2 Sternothyroid
3 Sternocleidomastoid
4 Longus colli
5 Anterior scalene muscle
6 Middle scalene muscle
7 Posterior scalene muscle
8 Common carotid artery
9 Internal jugular vein
10 External jugular vein
11 Vertebral vessels
12 Trachea
13 Esophagus
14 Thyroid gland
15 Cervical fascia, superficial layer
16 Cervical fascia, pretracheal layer
17 Cervical fascia, prevertebral layer
18 Vagus nerve
19 Recurrent laryngeal nerve
VI Cervical vertebra

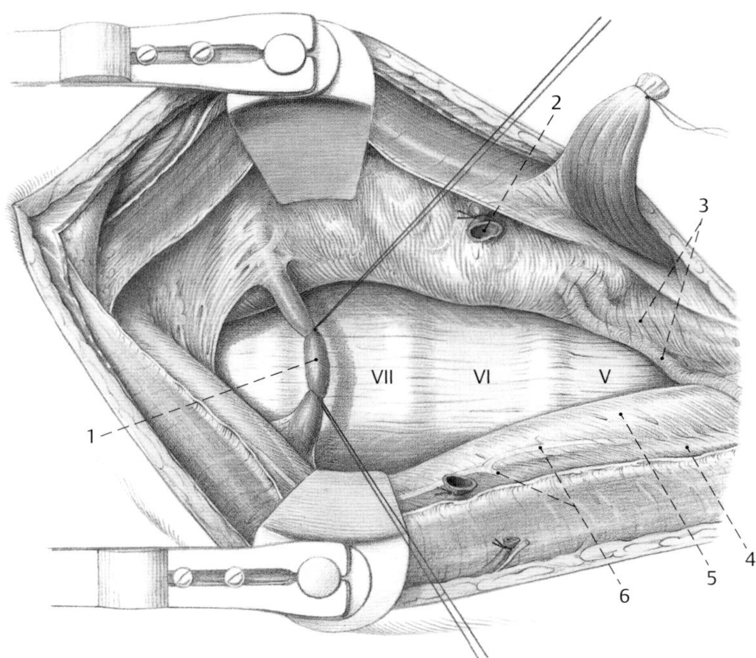

Fig. 1.17 Exposure of the lower cervical spine and cervicothoracic junction (C6–T2); ligation and transection of the inferior thyroid artery.

1 Inferior thyroid artery
2 Middle thyroid vein
3 Superior thyroid artery and vein
4 Internal jugular vein
5 Common carotid artery
6 Deep ansa cervicalis
V–VII Cervical vertebrae

1.2.6 Exposure of Vertebrae C7–T2

If exposure of the caudally situated cervical vertebrae and the two superior thoracic vertebrae is required, the inferior thyroid artery has to be located and ligated. Further exposure of the pretracheal cervical fascia in a caudal direction is performed bluntly with scissors, cotton balls, and, partly, with the finger (**Fig. 1.17**).

1.2.7 Anatomical Site

The anterior aspect of the lower cervical and upper thoracic vertebrae is covered by the following structures, in descending order from cranial:

On the left side (**Figs. 1.18** and **1.19**): The inferior thyroid artery, which arises from the thyrocervical trunk or the subclavian artery and runs transversely across the anterior surface of the vertebrae, enters the inferior pole of the thyroid. The sympathetic trunk with the stellate ganglion is located at approximately the same level on the anterior aspect of longus colli, and the vertebral artery is situated lateral to it. More

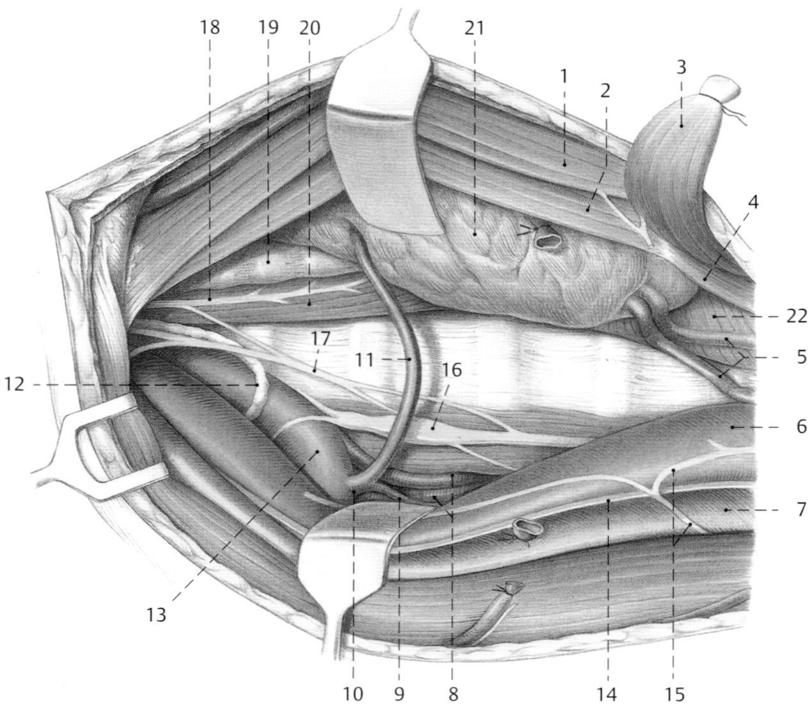

Fig. 1.18 Anatomical site of the lower cervical spine as seen from the left. Note the course of the recurrent nerve and thoracic duct. The cervical fascia is not shown.

1 Sternohyoid
2 Sternothyroid
3 Omohyoid
4 Thyrohyoid
5 Superior thyroid artery and vein
6 Common carotid artery
7 Internal jugular vein
8 Vertebral artery and vein
9 Ascending cervical artery
10 Thyrocervical trunk
11 Inferior thyroid artery
12 Thoracic duct
13 Subclavian artery
14 Vagus nerve
15 Deep ansa cervicalis
16 Stellate ganglion
17 Sympathetic trunk
18 Recurrent laryngeal nerve
19 Trachea
20 Esophagus
21 Thyroid gland
22 Pharynx

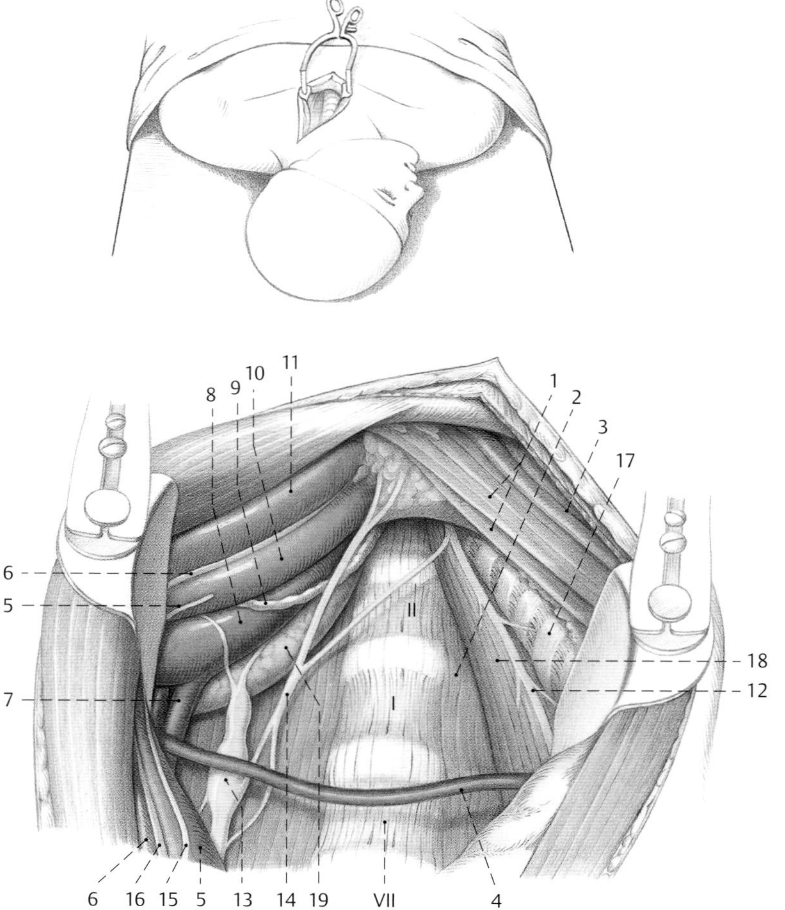

Fig. 1.19 Anatomical site of the cervicothoracic junction seen from above left. Note the relation of the cupula of the pleura to the vertebrae. The cervical fascia is not shown.

1 Sternohyoid and sternothyroid muscles
2 Longus colli
3 External jugular vein
4 Left inferior thyroid artery
5 Common carotid artery
6 Internal jugular vein
7 Vertebral artery
8 Subclavian artery
9 Thoracic duct
10 Common carotid artery
11 Internal jugular vein
12 Recurrent laryngeal nerve
13 Stellate ganglion
14 Sympathetic trunk
15 Deep ansa cervicalis
16 Vagus nerve
17 Trachea
18 Esophagus
19 Cupula of the pleura
I, II Thoracic vertebrae
VII Cervical vertebra

caudally situated is the thoracic duct, which, coming from the thorax, courses anteriorly across the subclavian artery and subsequently opens into the venous angle. The cupula of the pleura lies approximately at the level of the first thoracic vertebra between the longus colli and the subclavian artery. The recurrent laryngeal nerve, arising from the vagus nerve, curves around the aortic arch on the left side and then ascends to the larynx between the trachea and the esophagus. Among the anatomical structures enumerated above, only the inferior thyroid artery may be ligated. All the nerves with the exception of anastomoses between the sympathetic trunk and the recurrent laryngeal nerve have to be spared, as does the thoracic duct.

The prevertebral cervical fascia should now be split in the midline and dissected on both sides as far as the longus colli. With the aid of a broad raspatory, the longus colli is then retracted on both sides of the anterior longitudinal ligament as far as the base of the transverse processes (**Figs. 1.20** and **1.21**). The anterior surface of the cervical vertebrae may also be exposed subperiosteally by first transecting the anterior longitudinal ligament in a longitudinal direction with the diathermy scalpel and then retracting it with the raspatory. This method of dissection causes bleeding from the nutrient foramina of the anterior aspect of the cervical vertebrae, which can be stopped by means of bone wax. The level can be most reliably located at operation with the aid of an image converter or a lateral radiograph after insertion of a needle into the intervertebral disk. The prominent transverse process of the sixth cervical vertebra (carotid tubercle, Chassaignac's tubercle) can, as a rule, be readily palpated laterally below

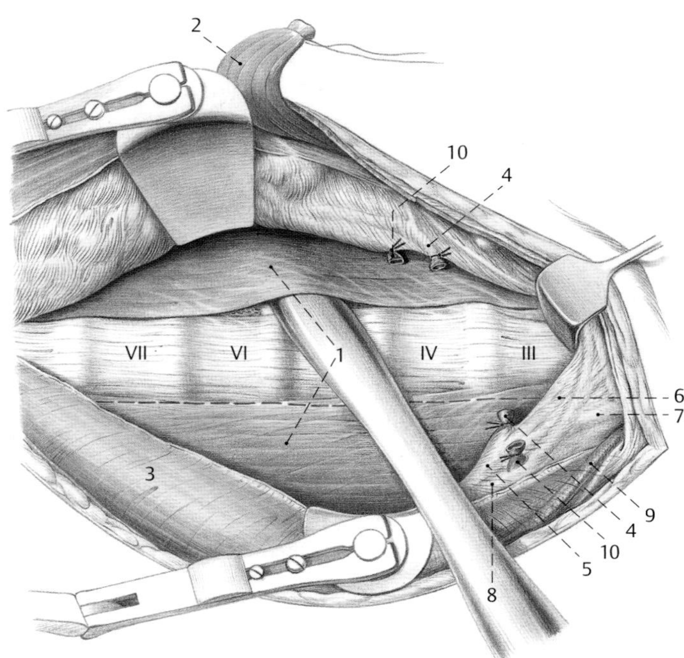

Fig. 1.20 Appearance after division of the prevertebral cervical fascia; exposure of the vertebrae as far as the base of the transverse processes by bilateral detachment of longus colli. Alternative method: subperiosteal exposure of the vertebrae by detachment of the anterior longitudinal ligament. View from the left.

1 Longus colli
2 Omohyoid
3 Sternocleidomastoid
4 Superior thyroid artery
5 Common carotid artery
6 Lingual artery
7 External carotid artery
8 Internal jugular vein
9 External jugular vein
10 Superior thyroid vein
III–VII Cervical vertebrae

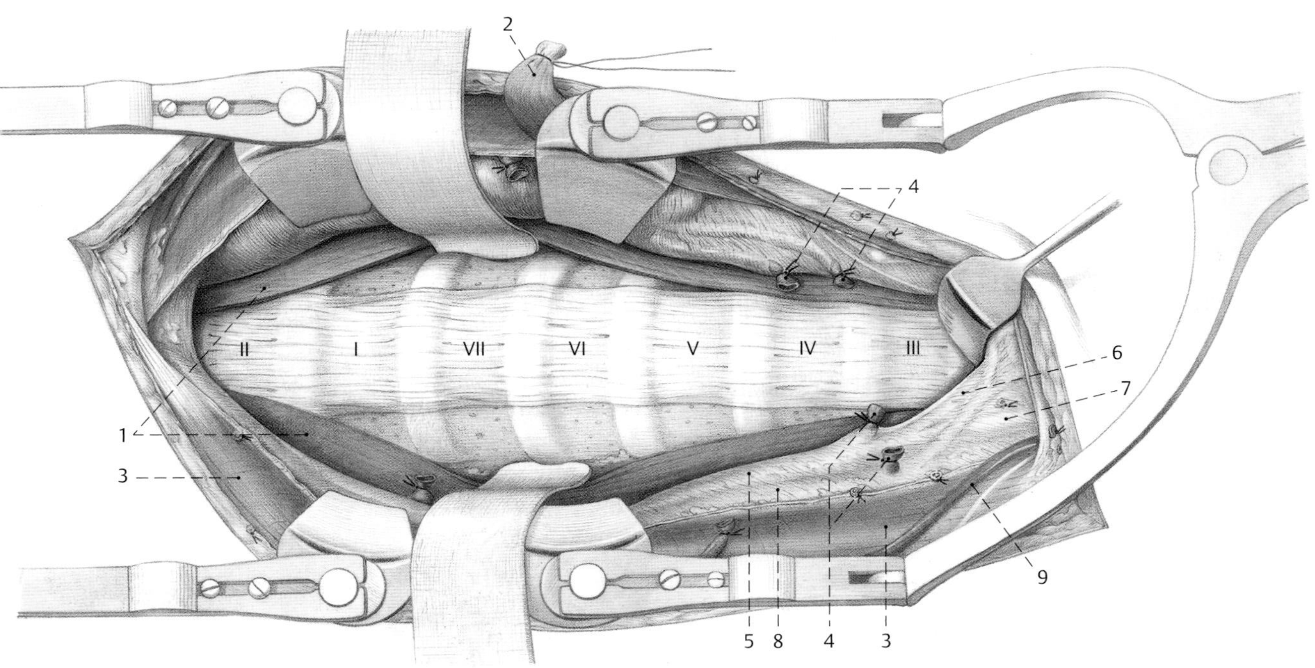

Fig. 1.21 Exposure of the cervical spine from C3 to T2 by a left anterior approach after bilateral mobilization of the longus colli.

1 Longus colli
2 Omohyoid
3 Sternocleidomastoid
4 Superior thyroid vessels
5 Common carotid artery
6 Lingual artery
7 External carotid artery
8 Internal jugular vein
9 External jugular vein
III–VII Cervical vertebrae
I, II Thoracic vertebrae

the longus colli. However, in fewer than 10% of cases, the seventh cervical vertebra may also have a prominent transverse process if the vertebral artery runs in the cervical vertebral foramen from C7. **Fig. 1.21** shows the operative site of the cervical spine from the left anterior approach over an area from C3 to T2. Besides Cloward's retractors, flexible spatulas with a wide contact surface, which can be laterally applied to the base of the transverse processes, have been found useful for broad exposure of the spine.

On the right side: The principal difference between the right and the left approach lies in the different course of the recurrent laryngeal nerve (**Fig. 1.22**). On the right side, it may leave the vagus nerve at varying levels. It runs deep to the subclavian artery and then courses obliquely over the anterior surface of the vertebral body toward the groove between the trachea and esophagus. Normally, the nerve passes beneath the inferior thyroid artery, but in exceptional cases it may pass in front of the artery, where it may be damaged or transected by pressure from a surgical hook.

1.2.8 Wound Closure

During closure of the wound, the transected omohyoid muscle has to be rejoined by suture. Use of a Redon drain is recommended.

1.2.9 Dangers

Excessive traction on the visceral structures may cause injuries to the thin-walled esophagus or pharyngeal edema. Retractor pressure (beware of unduly short retractors) may also lead to damage of the recurrent laryngeal nerve resulting in paresis of the vocal cords. In exposure of the cranial cervical vertebrae, the hypoglossal nerve may be injured, which would cause unilateral paralysis of the lingual muscles. A lesion of the superior laryngeal nerve, particularly its external branch, may lead to disorders of sensation in the laryngeal mucosa and to paralysis of the cricothyroid muscle. This may entail postoperative hoarseness and voice disorders. Horner's syndrome develops as a result of injuries to the sympathetic trunk, especially in the area of the stellate ganglion, if dissection has gone too far laterally. The vertebral artery may be damaged if the rasps used for dissection are too narrow and slip between the transverse processes. In exposure of the cervicothoracic junction using the anterior approach, the thoracic duct or the cupula of the pleura may be injured, with the possible consequence of chylothorax or pneumothorax.

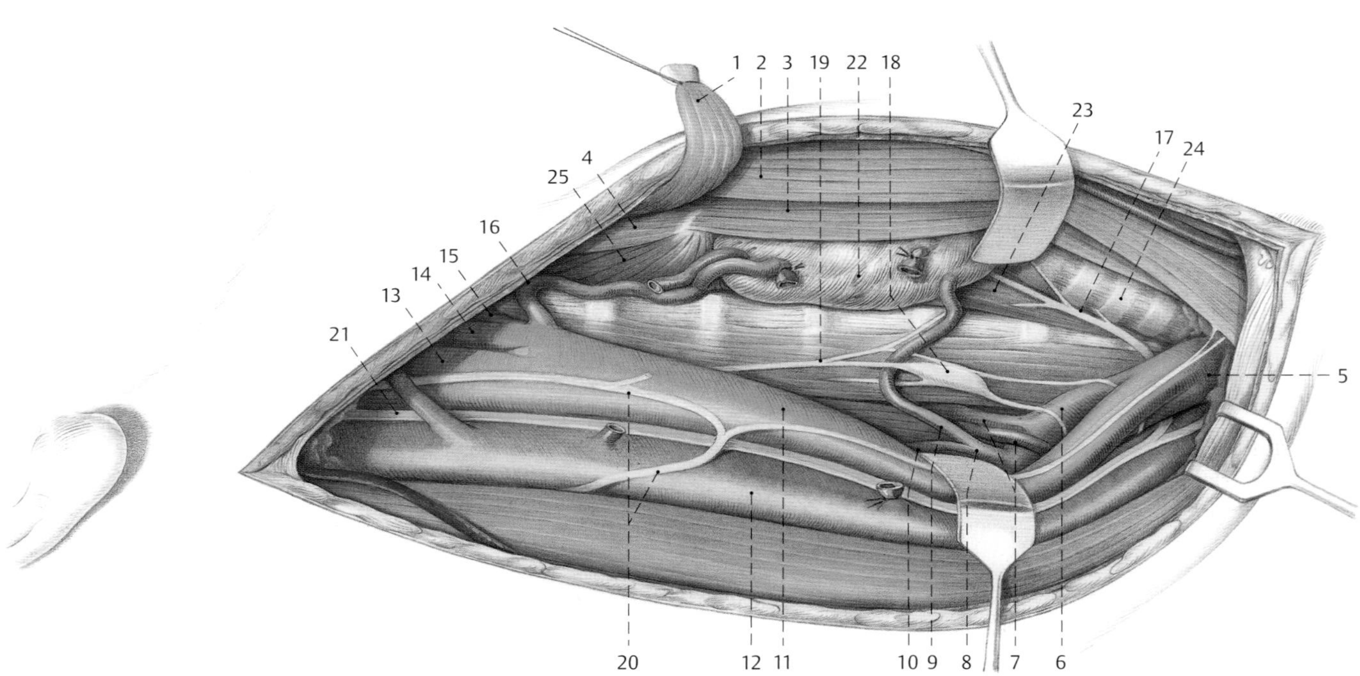

Fig. 1.22 Anatomical site of the cervical spine as seen from the right side. Note the course of the recurrent laryngeal nerve.

1 Omohyoid
2 Sternohyoid
3 Sternothyroid
4 Thyrohyoid
5 Brachiocephalic trunk
6 Subclavian artery
7 Vertebral artery and vein
8 Thyrocervical trunk
9 Inferior thyroid artery
10 Ascending cervical artery
11 Common carotid artery
12 Internal jugular vein
13 Internal carotid artery
14 External carotid artery
15 Lingual artery
16 Superior thyroid artery
17 Recurrent laryngeal nerve
18 Stellate ganglion
19 Sympathetic trunk
20 Deep ansa cervicalis
21 Vagus nerve
22 Thyroid gland
23 Esophagus
24 Trachea
25 Pharynx

1.2.10 Note

With adequate knowledge of the anatomy, the approach described is easy and is associated with a low rate of complications. It is therefore the standard approach for anterior exposure of the cervical spine. Other anterior and lateral approaches have been described by Henry, Whitesides and Kelly, Verbiest, Nanson, Hodgson, and others. These approaches are suitable particularly for exposure of the spinal nerves, the vertebral artery, and the scalene muscle lacunae, and less suitable for clear exposure of the cervical spine from the front. For exposure of the upper cervical spine, and the craniocervical junction in particular, Riley has described an approach that, in addition to extensive skeletization of the submandibular space, involves dislocation of the temporomandibular joint and removal of the submandibular gland.

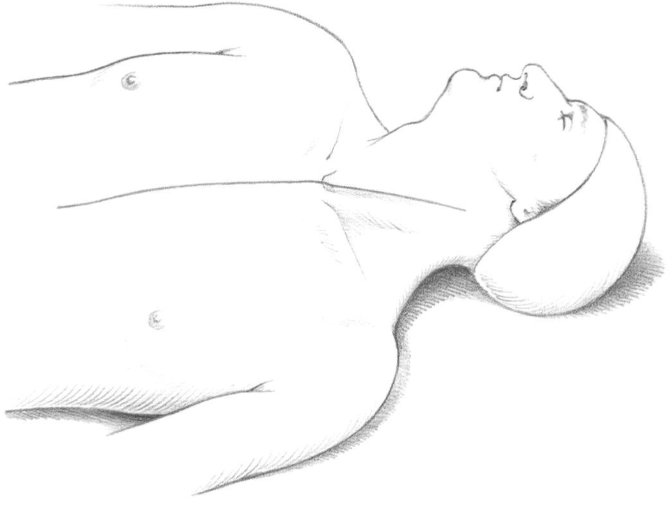

Fig. 1.23 Cervicosternotomy. A skin incision is made in the midline over the sternum and on the anterior border of the left sternocleidomastoid.

1.3 Anterior Approach to the Lower Cervical and Upper Thoracic Spine C4–T3 According to Cauchoix, Binet, and Evrard

R. Bauer, F. Kerschbaumer, S. Poisel

1.3.1 Principal Indications

- Internal fixation of fracture dislocations
- Tumors
- Spondylitis

1.3.2 Choice of Side of Approach

The cervical portion of the approach is from the left side.

1.3.3 Positioning and Incision

(**Fig. 1.23**)

Positioning is the same as that for the anterior approach to the cervical spine: the patient is placed in a supine position, head turned to the right, and the cervical spine is extended by placing a cushion between the shoulder blades and under the neck.

The skin incision is made medially over the sternum from the tip of the xiphoid process to the manubrium and is continued upward to the left along the anterior border of the sternocleidomastoid, extending as far as for the anterior approach to the cervical spine (see **Figs. 1.7**, **1.8**, **1.9**, **1.10**). After division of the subcutaneous tissue and the platysma, the superficial cervical fascia is opened at the anterior border of the sternocleidomastoid.

The anterior side of the inferior cervical spine is then exposed by blunt dissection between the laterally situated neurovascular bundle on one hand, and the medial visceral structures on the other. Using cotton applicators, the retrosternal fat and thymus remnants are retracted from the manubrium of the sternum from cranial to caudal. The tip of the xiphoid process is detached from the caudal muscular aponeuroses, and the retrosternal fat is bluntly dissected from caudal to cranial. Median sternotomy may now be performed with a sternotome or sternotomy saw. After hemostasis of the sternal periosteum, a thoracic retractor is inserted and opened slowly. Injury to the pleura must be avoided. Subsequently, the sternohyoid, sternothyroid, and omohyoid are exposed, undermined, and transected between two ligatures (**Figs. 1.24** and **1.25**). The previously opened pretracheal cervical fascia is now bluntly dissected further caudally until the left brachiocephalic vein (left innominate vein) is exposed. This may be exposed, doubly ligated bilaterally, and transected as needed. If an accessory hemiazygos vein is present (**Fig. 1.26**), an adequate venous return is possible.

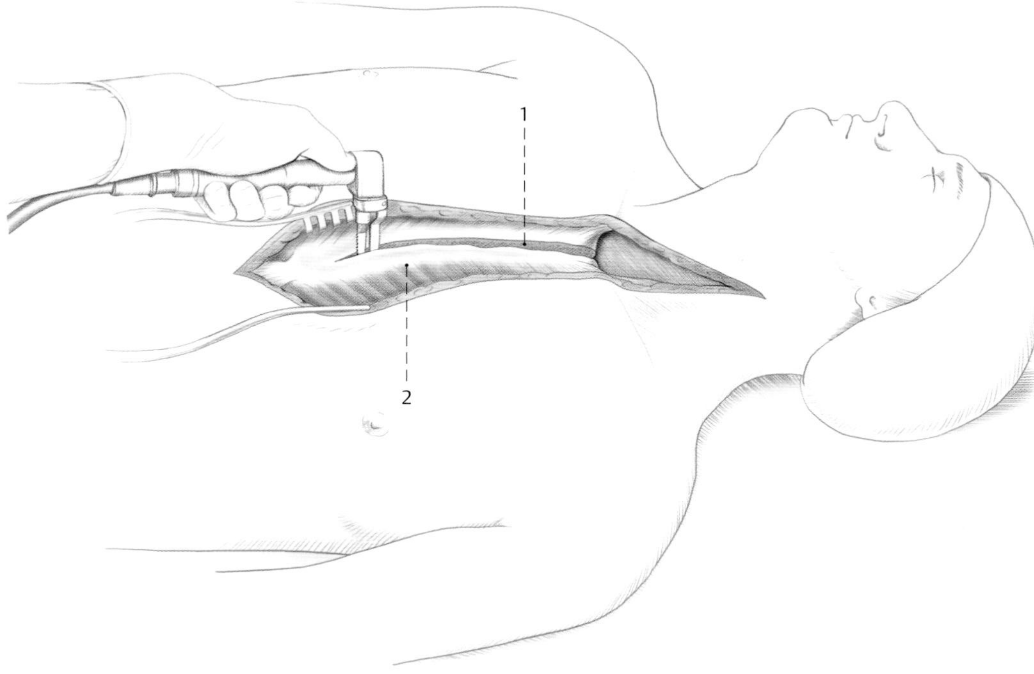

Fig. 1.24 After incision of platysma and the superficial and pretracheal cervical fascia, the sternum is bluntly undermined first below the manubrium and then below the xiphoid process, and is subsequently transected in the midline with a sternotomy saw.

1 Sternum
2 Pectoralis major

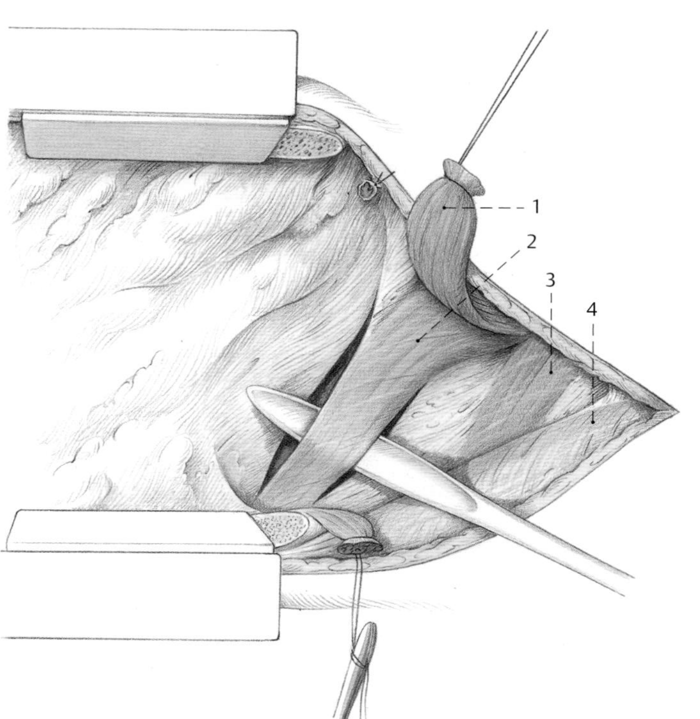

Fig. 1.25 Transection of the lower portion of the sternohyoid and sternothyroid as well as the omohyoid. The sternum is slowly spread with a thoracic retractor, and the pleura, anterior portion of pericardium, and remnants of the thymus are bluntly retracted.

1 Sternohyoid
2 Sternothyroid
3 Omohyoid
4 Sternocleidomastoid

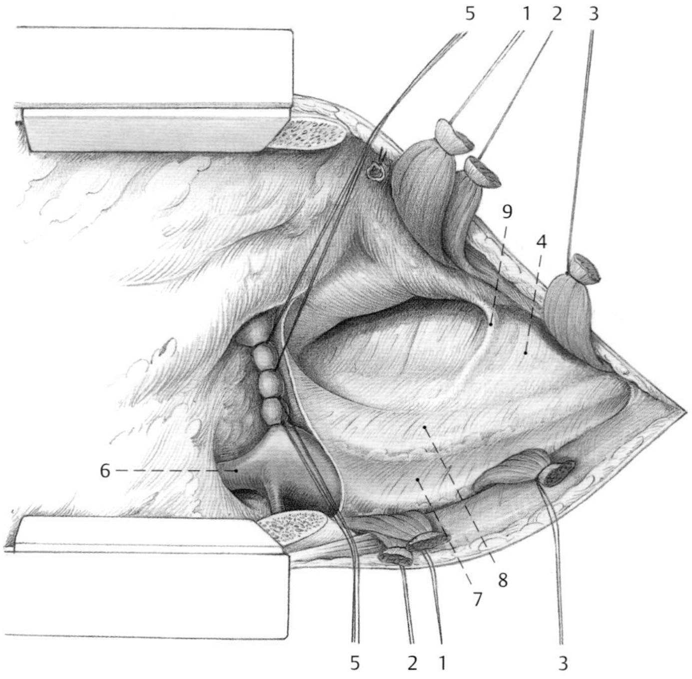

Fig. 1.26 Exposure and double ligation of the left brachiocephalic vein. Caudad dissection of the pretracheal cervical fascia and exposure of the prevertebral cervical fascia.

1 Sternothyroid
2 Sternohyoid
3 Omohyoid
4 Cervical fascia, prevertebral layer
5 Left brachiocephalic vein
6 Accessory hemiazygos vein
7 Internal jugular vein
8 Common carotid artery
9 Inferior thyroid artery

1.3.4 Anatomical Site

In cranial to caudal order, the following structures lie in front of the C6–T3 vertebrae that are to be exposed (**Fig. 1.27**):

- The inferior thyroid and vertebral arteries.
- The sympathetic trunk with the stellate ganglion.
- The cupula of the pleura at the level of Tl.
- The thoracic duct, which passes into the left venous angle between the subclavian artery and the common carotid artery.
- The brachiocephalic vein.
- The aortic arch with the brachiocephalic trunk as well as the origins of the left common carotid artery and left subclavian artery.
- The vagus nerve, which runs in a caudal direction in the perivascular sheath of the common carotid artery and the internal jugular vein and, under the aortic arch, gives off the left recurrent laryngeal nerve, which then ascends cranially toward the larynx between the trachea and esophagus.

1.3.5 Exposure of the Vertebrae

(**Fig. 1.28**)

For clear exposure of the vertebrae, the inferior thyroid artery is identified, ligated, and transected. Using cotton applicators, the prevertebral cervical fascia is now exposed, proceeding from the cranial toward the caudal portion. The esophagus and the trachea as well as the cervical pleura are cautiously diverted medially, while the thoracic duct and the vessels are retracted laterally. The pretracheal fascia is now split in the middle and retracted. Subsequently, the longus colli is retracted with a rasp toward both sides as far as the base of the transverse processes or the costovertebral joints. Flexible spatulas are used to retract the vessels laterally and the visceral structures medially without application of pressure.

1.3.6 Wound Closure

(**Fig. 1.29**)

The sternotomy is closed with transosseous wire sutures; the omohyoid, sternohyoid, and sternothyroid muscles are rejoined using retention sutures; and the platysma is closed by interrupted sutures. The use of two Redon drains is recommended.

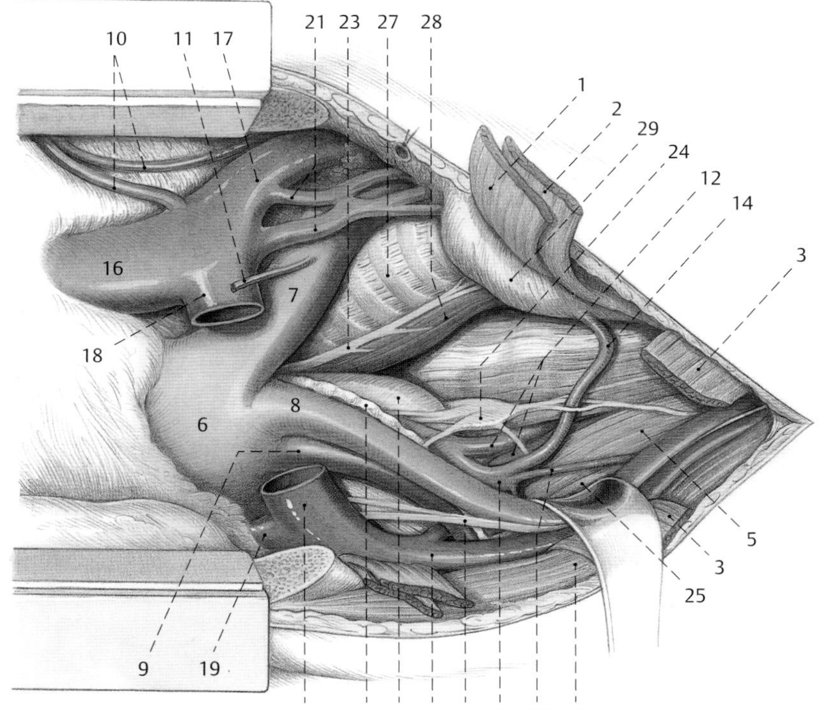

Fig. 1.27 Anatomical site of the cervicothoracic junction. View from the left.

1 Sternothyroid
2 Sternohyoid
3 Omohyoid
4 Sternocleidomastoid
5 Anterior scalene muscle
6 Aortic arch
7 Brachiocephalic trunk
8 Left common carotid artery
9 Left subclavian artery
10 Internal thoracic vessels
11 Thymic branch
12 Vertebral artery and vein
13 Thyrocervical trunk
14 Inferior thyroid artery
15 Ascending cervical artery
16 Superior vena cava
17 Right brachiocephalic vein
18 Left brachiocephalic vein
19 Accessory hemiazygos vein
20 Internal jugular vein
21 Unpaired thyroid plexus
22 Thoracic duct
23 Recurrent laryngeal nerve
24 Stellate ganglion
25 Phrenic nerve
26 Vagus nerve
27 Trachea
28 Esophagus
29 Thyroid gland
30 Cupula of the pleura

1.3.7 Dangers

There is a danger of injury to the pleura, to the recurrent laryngeal nerve due to excessive retractor pressure, and to the thoracic duct.

1.3.8 Note

Disadvantages of this approach are the amount of work involved in the median sternotomy, and the transection of the brachiocephalic vein, which may lead postoperatively to disturbances of venous reflux in the region of the left arm. Exposure of the third thoracic vertebra is possible without transection of the brachiocephalic vein. However, this becomes necessary in resection of vertebral bodies or internal fixation.

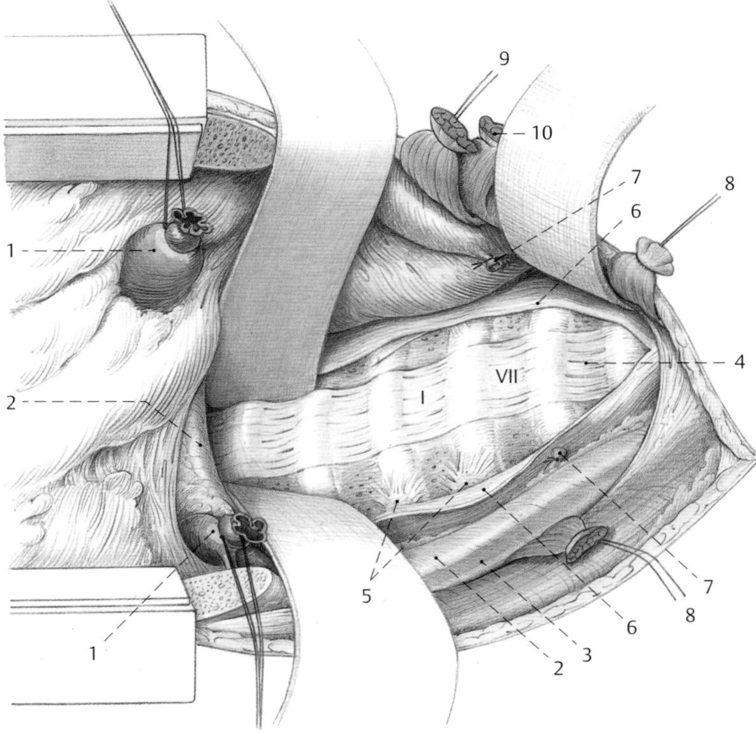

Fig. 1.28 Exposure of the cervicothoracic junction C6–T3. Vessels and visceral structures are loosely retracted laterally with flexible spatulas.

1 Left brachiocephalic vein
2 Left common carotid artery
3 Left internal jugular vein
4 Anterior longitudinal ligament
5 Radiate ligament of the head of the rib
6 Longus colli
7 Inferior thyroid artery
8 Omohyoid
9 Sternothyroid
10 Sternohyoid
VII Cervical vertebra
I Thoracic vertebra

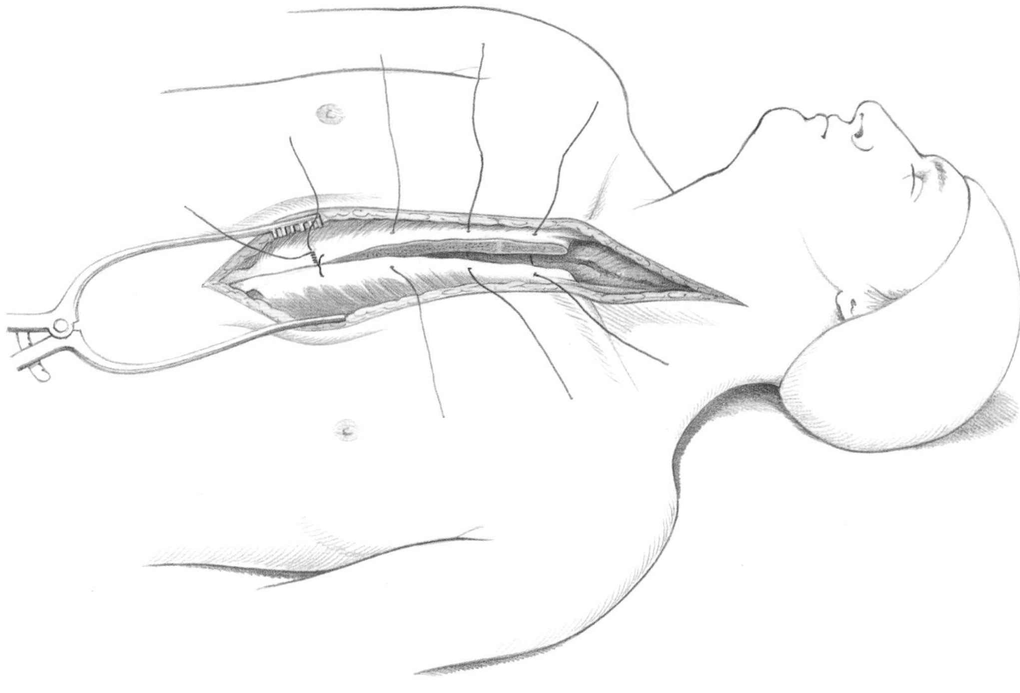

Fig. 1.29 Closure of a sternotomy with wire sutures.

2 Thoracic Spine

2.1 Transthoracic Approach to the Thoracic Spine T4–T11

R. Bauer, F. Kerschbaumer, S. Poisel

2.1.1 Indications

- Kyphosis
- Scoliosis
- Vertebral body fractures
- Tumors
- Spondylitis

2.1.2 Choice of Side of Approach

Generally speaking, the thoracic spine can be approached using either right-sided or left-sided thoracotomy. Unless the indication prescribes the side to be used, right-sided thoracotomy is preferable because of the vascular anatomy (the left-sided course of the aorta). However, in the case of scoliosis, thoracotomy is always performed on the side of the convexity.

2.1.3 Dorsolateral Thoracotomy with Rib Resection

With orthopedic indications, the thoracotomy is generally performed with rib resection. This creates better exposure in adult patients and in the case of thoracic deformities associated with spinal deformities. In addition, the resected rib may serve as graft material for vertebral fusion.

2.1.4 Choice of Rib to be Resected

Entry is generally made two ribs above the level of the center of the lesion. Owing to the descending course of the ribs, it is easier to cut along the lower rib in a caudal direction rather than toward the proximal end. If a rib is chosen whose location is too distal, it is difficult to reach the upper end of the deformity. In younger individuals and those in whom the ribs are mobile, it may be possible to reach the vertebra corresponding to the resected rib. If this proves difficult, the segment close to the spine of the next higher rib may be resected through the same approach. The following vertebrae can be reached in favorable circumstances:

- Resection of the fifth rib: a T5–T11 approach
- Resection of the sixth rib: a T6–T12 approach
- Resection of the seventh rib: a T7–L1 approach

However, there are exceptions to this rule. In patients with horizontally coursing ribs, resection of the sixth rib may allow vertebrae T5–T11 to be reached. On the other hand, if the ribs describe a sharply descending course, resection of the fifth rib only permits exposure of T6–T11. Finally, in patients with severe spinal curvatures and commensurate thoracic deformities, rib resection thoracotomy may provide access to only two or three vertebrae.

2.1.5 Positioning and Incision

The patient is placed on his or her side. Elevation of the kidney rest or slight tilting of the operating table allows for good extension in the operative field. The skin incision made over the selected rib is slightly S-shaped, curving caudally around the scapula. It is started about four fingerbreadths lateral to the spinous processes and continues forward as far as the chondrocostal border (**Fig. 2.1**). Next, latissimus dorsi is completely divided transversely to its course (**Fig. 2.2**). Because of the nerve supply (thoracodorsal nerve) this should be done as far caudally as possible (see **Figs. 2.32** and **2.33**).

Serratus anterior is exposed in the anterior area of the wound. It is now possible to reach behind this muscle under the scapula with the hand and to count off the ribs from cranial to caudal. The first rib usually cannot be palpated, and the first palpable one is therefore, as a rule, the second rib. Serratus anterior is likewise transected, as far caudally as possible to spare, if possible, the long thoracic nerve (**Fig. 2.3**). The periosteum of the selected rib is divided from posterior to anterior as far as the chondrocostal border, using cutting diathermy

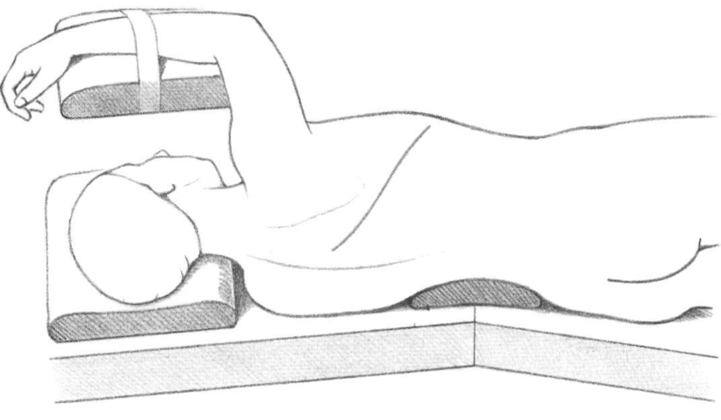

Fig. 2.1 Positioning and incision.

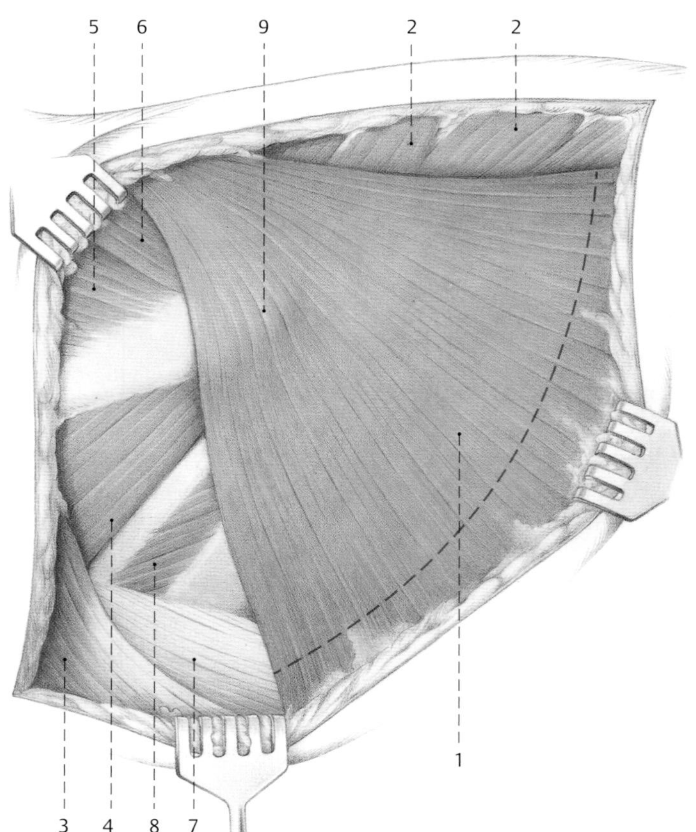

Fig. 2.2 Anatomical exposure of the operative field after transection of the skin and subcutaneous tissue. The muscle fasciae have been removed.

1 Latissimus dorsi
2 Serratus anterior
3 Trapezius
4 Rhomboid major
5 Infraspinatus
6 Teres major
7 Iliocostalis thoracis
8 External intercostal muscle
9 Inferior angle of the scapula

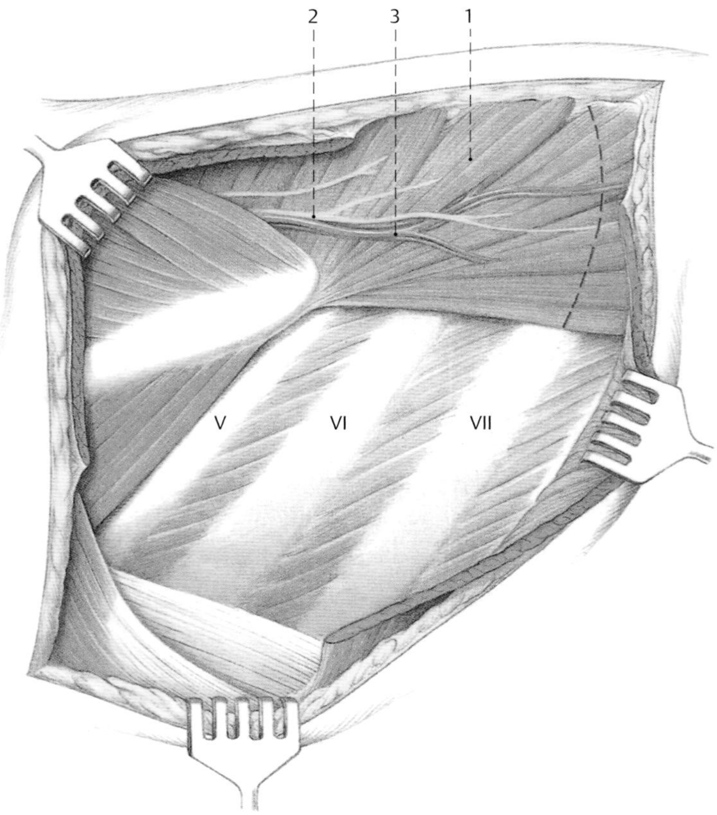

Fig. 2.3 Anatomical exposure of the operative field after transection of latissimus dorsi and before incision of serratus anterior. The appropriate site of incision is identified by the dashed line.

1 Serratus anterior
2 Long thoracic nerve
3 Lateral thoracic vessels.
V–VII Ribs

(**Fig. 2.4**), and is initially retracted with a straight raspatory. At the superior margin of the rib, the direction of the cut, in accordance with the course of the intercostal muscles, is from posterior to anterior; at the lower border, it is from anterior to posterior. Hereafter, the rib is completely exposed with a rib raspatory (**Fig. 2.5**).

Following this preparation, the rib is transected anteriorly at the osseocartilaginous boundary and elevated; posteriorly, it is resected with rib shears about two fingerbreadths laterally from the costotransverse joint. The thoracic cavity can now be opened within the bed of the resected rib (**Fig. 2.6**).

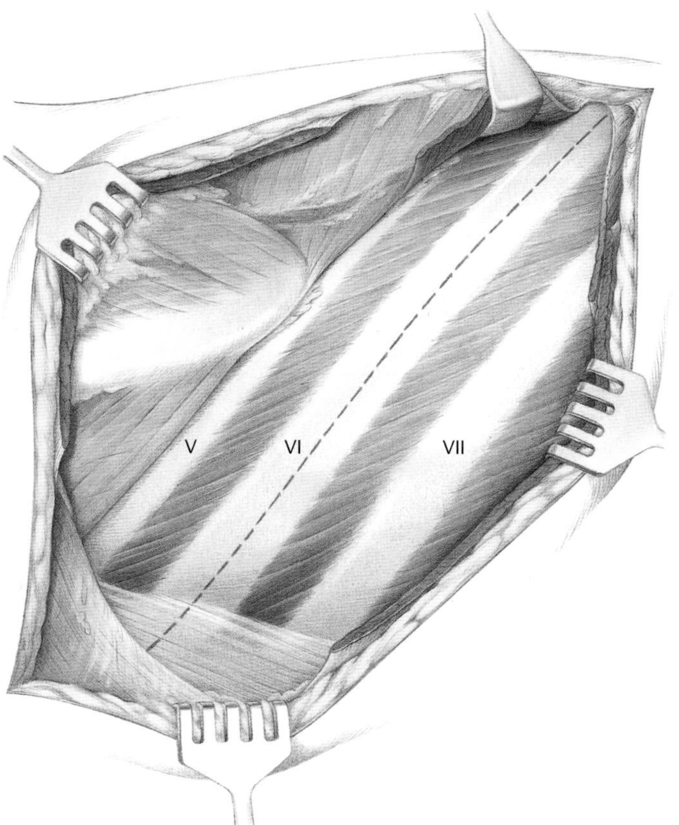

Fig. 2.4 Operative site following transection of serratus anterior. The periosteum is split over the sixth rib along the red dashed line.

V–VII Ribs

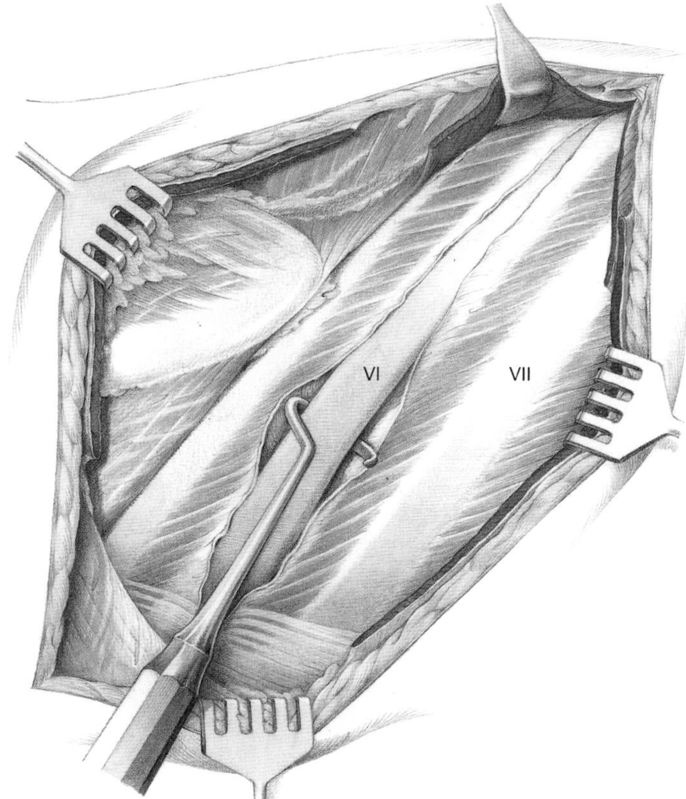

Fig. 2.5 Operative site following division of the periosteum and enucleation of the sixth rib with a rib raspatory.

VI, VII Ribs

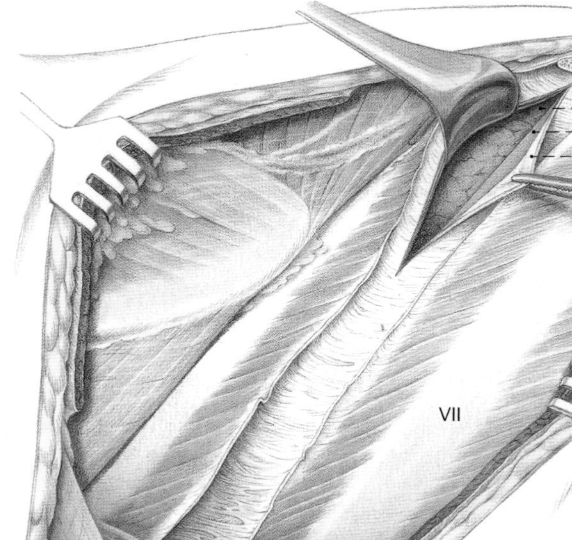

Fig. 2.6 Operative site following rib resection and partial division of the periosteum and costal pleura.

1 Resection stump of the sixth rib
2 Costal pleura
3 Periosteum
4 Lung
VII Rib

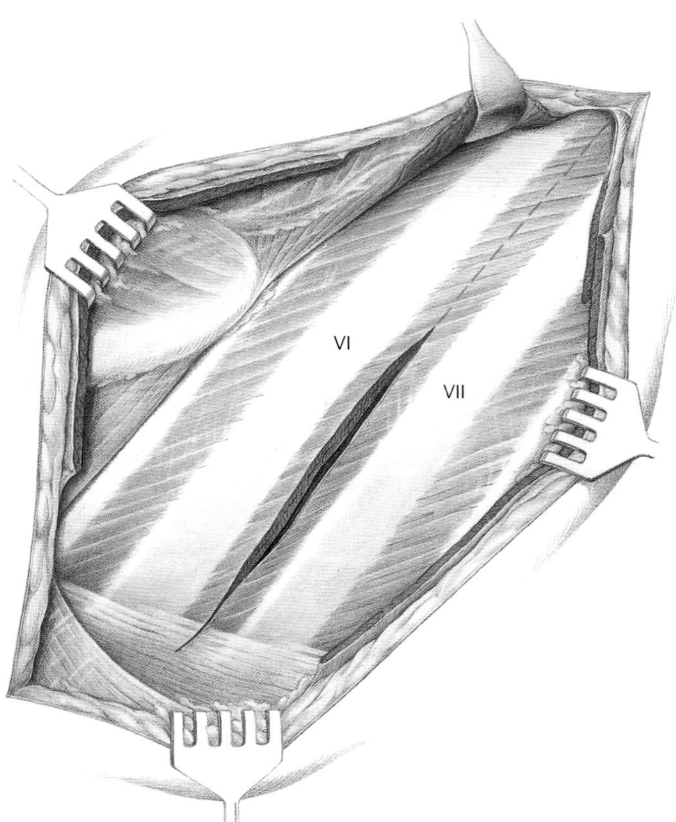

Fig. 2.7 Intercostal approach to the pleural cavity. The intercostal muscles are transected between the sixth and seventh ribs. Care should be taken to make the incision at the upper border of the lower rib to avoid injury to the intercostal vessels and intercostal nerve.

VI, VII Ribs

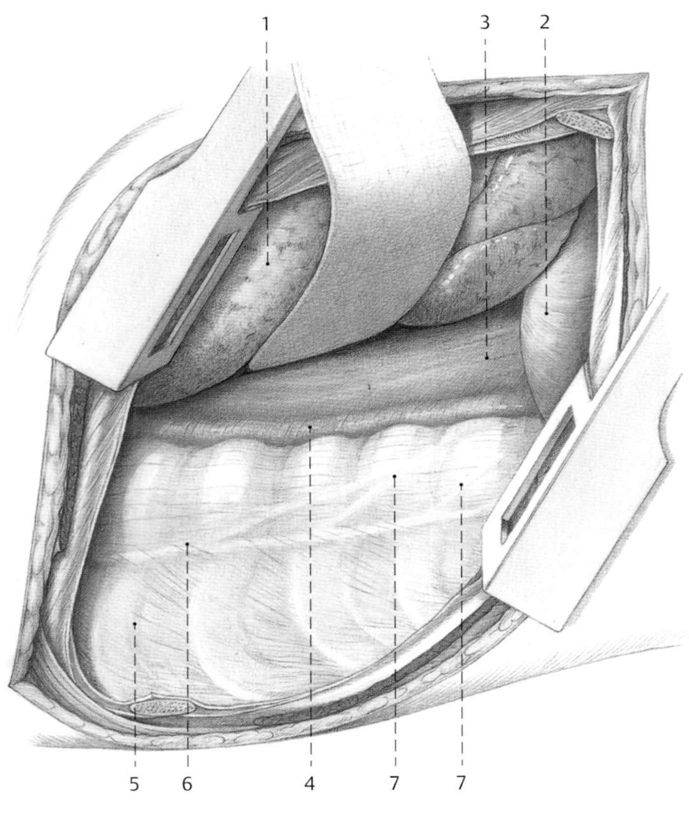

Fig. 2.8 Operative site after opening the pleural cavity. The parietal pleura (costal and mediastinal pleura) is preserved.

1 Right lung
2 Diaphragm
3 Esophagus
4 Azygos vein
5 Intercostal vessels
6 Sympathetic trunk
7 Greater splanchnic nerve

(3–7: visible through the parietal pleura)

2.1.6 Intercostal Thoracotomy

In children and adolescents with a mobile thorax, the thoracotomy may also be performed intercostally. This is indicated especially if only a few vertebrae need to be exposed and the rib is not needed as graft material. Positioning of the patient and the type of incision conform to those used in dorsolateral thoracotomy with rib resection. Following transection of the latissimus dorsi and serratus anterior, the selected intercostal space is entered. As a rule, a plastic probe is inserted between the intercostal muscles and the parietal pleura, above which the intercostal muscles can then be divided with cutting diathermy (**Fig. 2.7**). The procedure after transection of the parietal pleura again conforms to that for thoracotomy with rib resection.

After complete transection of the pleura, a thoracotomy spreader is inserted, and the thorax is then slowly and cautiously spread. The lung is retracted anteriorly, and a good view is obtained of the vertebrae covered by the parietal pleura (**Fig. 2.8**).

2.1.7 Anatomical Site

The anatomy of the posterior mediastinum and retropleural cavity is shown in **Figs. 2.9**, **2.10**, **2.11**.

A brief discussion of the most important anatomical variations of the structures in the posterior mediastinum now follows (**Figs. 2.12** and **2.13**). Injury to the thoracic duct during exposure of the vertebral bodies should be avoided if at all possible. Chylothorax may otherwise develop as a complication. **Fig. 2.12** shows variations in the course of the thoracic duct. This makes it clear that the thoracic duct essentially follows the course of the aorta on the right side. Variations of the azygos and hemiazygos veins are shown in **Fig. 2.13**. As a rule, the vertebrae can be accessed through a median transection of the intercostal veins without touching the longitudinal venous systems.

Fig. 2.9 Anatomical site of the posterior mediastinum and retropleural cavity as seen from the anterior.

1 Ascending aorta
2 Arch of the aorta
3 Brachiocephalic trunk
4 Left internal carotid artery
5 Thoracic aorta
6 Intercostal arteries
7 Abdominal aorta
8 Celiac trunk
9 Superior vena cava
10 Opening of the azygos vein
11 Right brachiocephalic vein
12 Left brachiocephalic vein
13 Accessory hemiazygos vein
14 Azygos vein
15 Hemiazygos vein
16 Intercostal veins
17 Thoracic duct
18 Right vagus nerve
19 Left vagus nerve
20 Esophageal plexus
21 Vagal trunks
22 Sympathetic trunk with ganglia
23 Greater splanchnic nerve
24 Lesser splanchnic nerve
25 Intercostal nerves
26 Subcostal nerve
27 Trachea
28 Esophagus
29 Diaphragm
V–XII Ribs

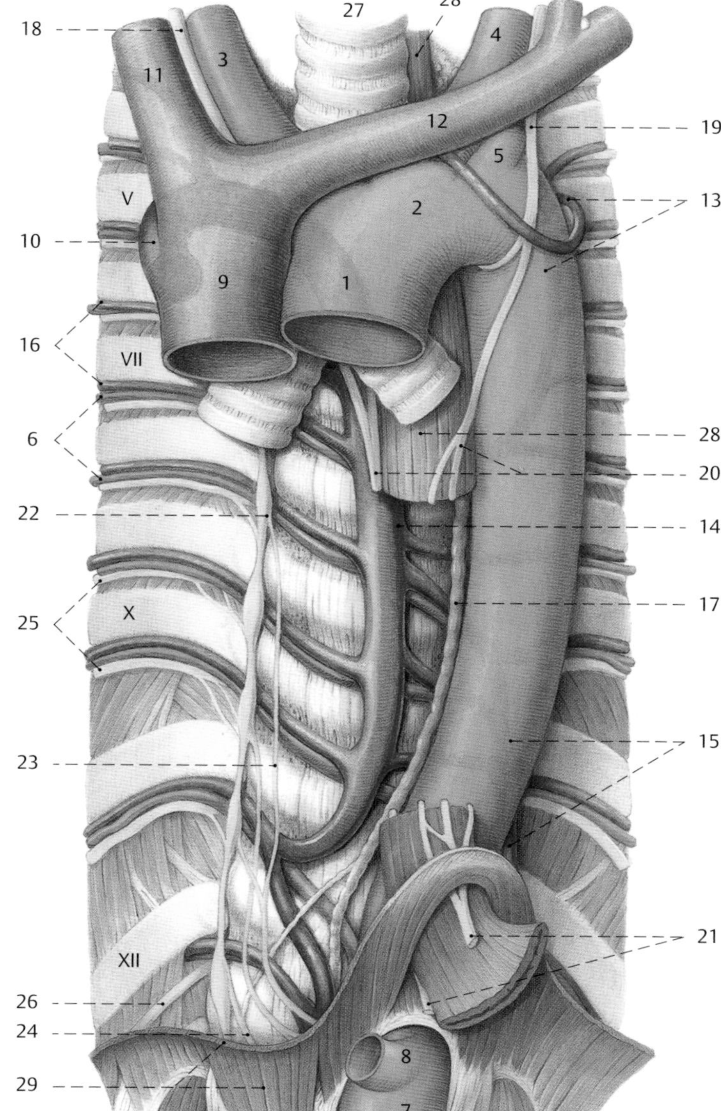

Fig. 2.10 Anatomical site of the right half of the posterior mediastinum and right retropleural space.

1 Right lung
2 Esophagus
3 Cut edge of the parietal pleura
4 Esophageal plexus of the vagus nerves
5 Thoracic diaphragm
6 Azygos vein
7 Intercostal vessels
8 Sympathetic trunk
9 Greater splanchnic nerve
10 Communicating branches
11 Intercostal nerve
I–X Ribs

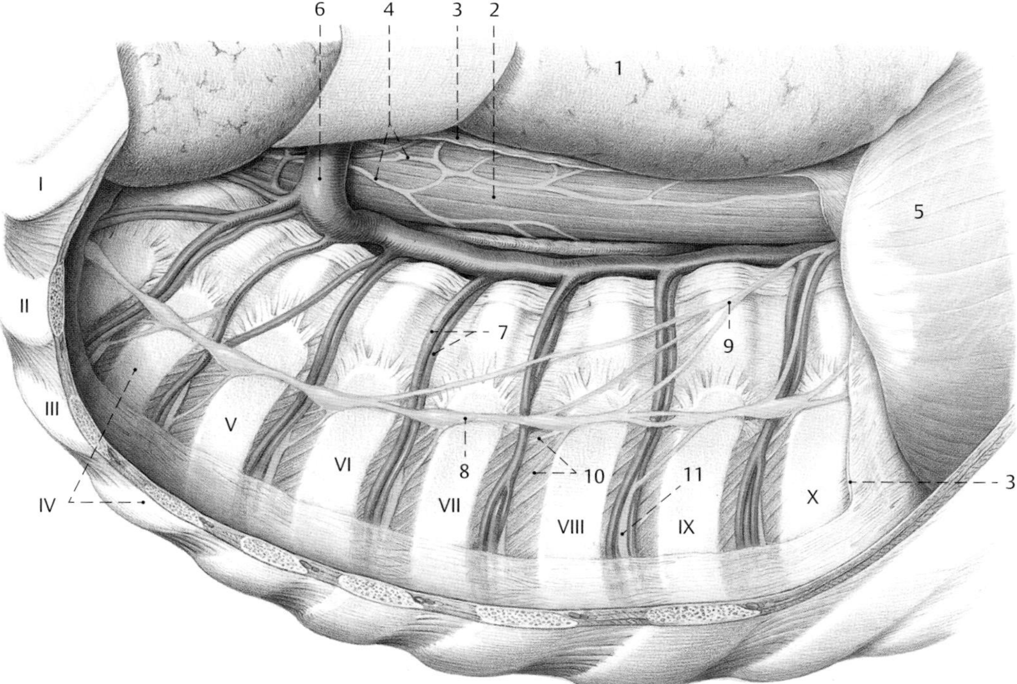

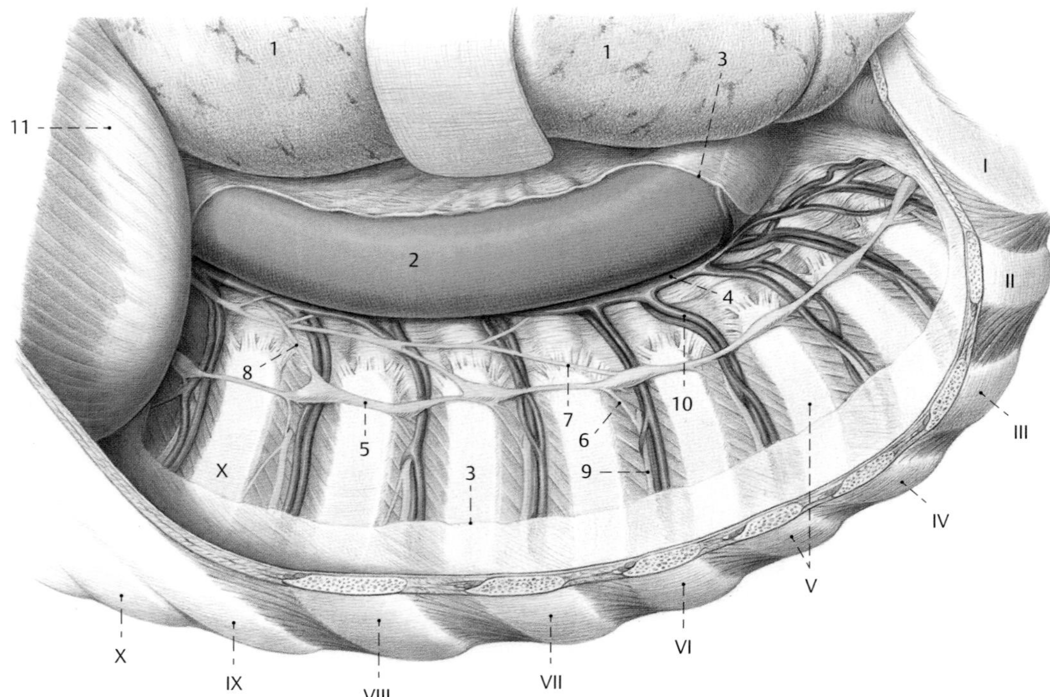

Fig. 2.11 Anatomical site of the left half of the posterior mediastinum and left retropleural space.

1 Left lung
2 Thoracic aorta
3 Cut edge of the parietal pleura
4 Accessory hemiazygos vein
5 Sympathetic trunk
6 Communicating branches
7 Greater splanchnic nerve
8 Lesser splanchnic nerve
9 Intercostal nerve
10 Intercostal vessels
11 Thoracic diaphragm
I–X Ribs

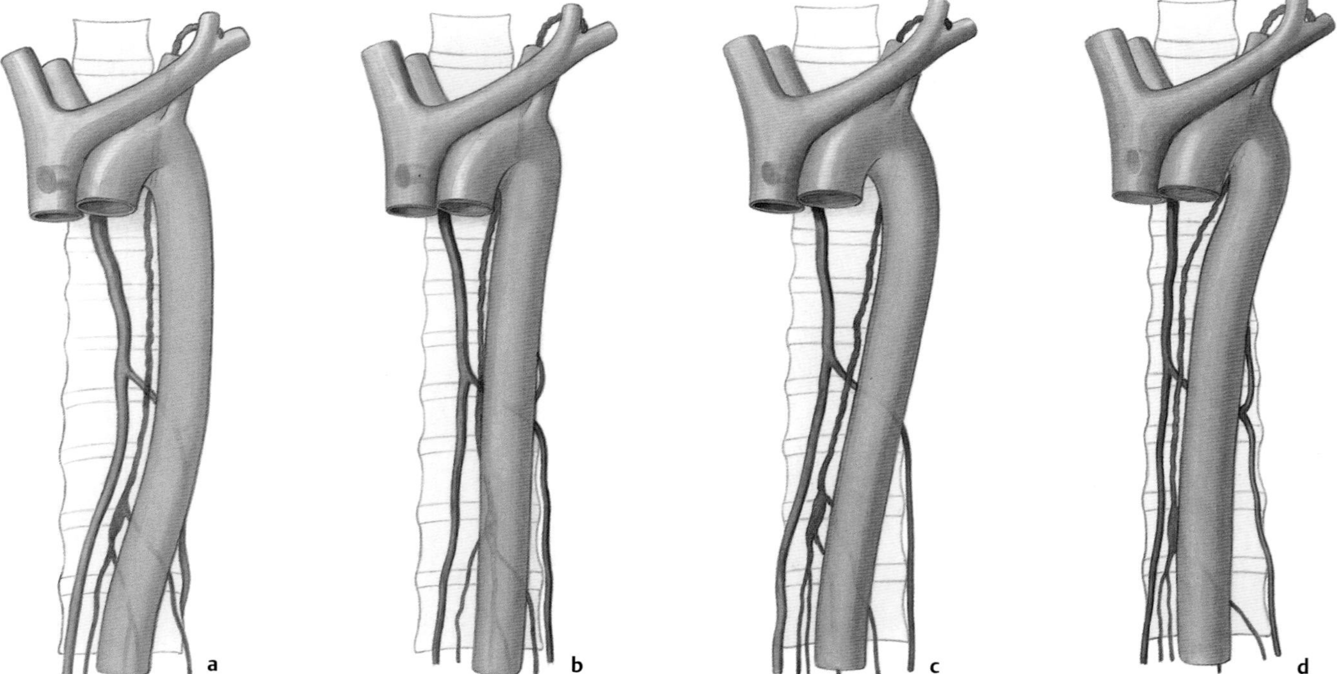

Fig. 2.12 a–d Positional variants of the thoracic aorta, azygos vein, and thoracic duct in relation to the thoracic spine (according to Kubik, 1975). The left-sided position of the topographic unit of thoracic duct–aorta–azygos vein may be regarded as an age-related displacement (83 % of individuals with a left-sided position were over 70 years old).

a Left-sided position (36 %).
b Middle position (20 %).
c Oblique position (17 %).
d Right-sided position (6 %).

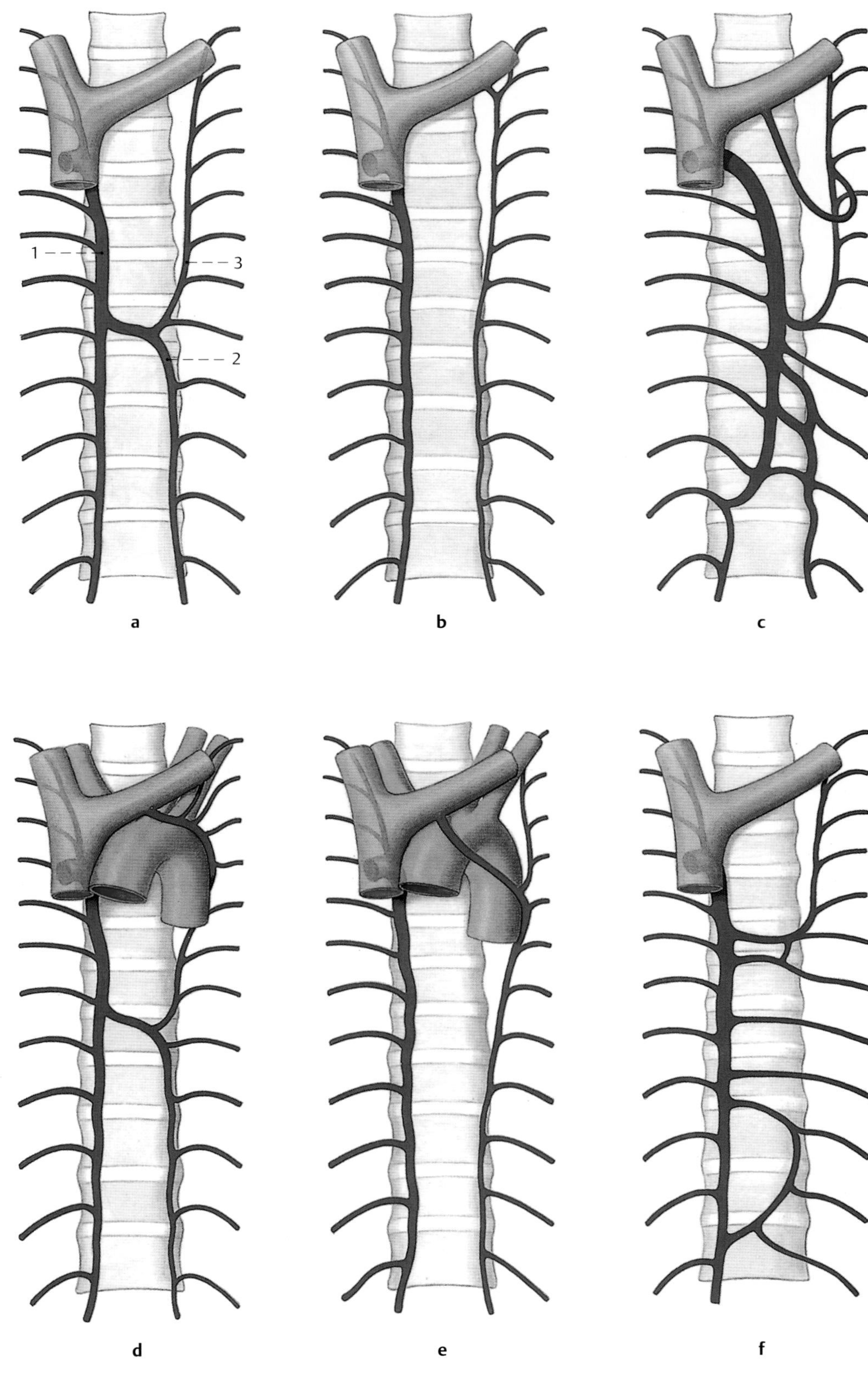

Fig. 2.13 a–f Morphologic and positional variants of the azygos and hemiazygos vein system (according to Adachi, 1933; Cordier et al., 1938; and our own observations).

a "Classic type."
  1 Azygos vein
  2 Hemiazygos vein
  3 Accessory hemiazygos vein

b Absence of anastomosis between the azygos and hemiazygos veins.
c Multiple arcade formations and age-related arcuate leftward displacement of the azygos vein.
d Cranioaortic arc of the hemiazygos vein.
e Lateroaortic arc of the azygos vein and absence of communication between the azygos and hemiazygos veins.
f Multiple prevertebral anastomoses; absence of the hemiazygos vein.

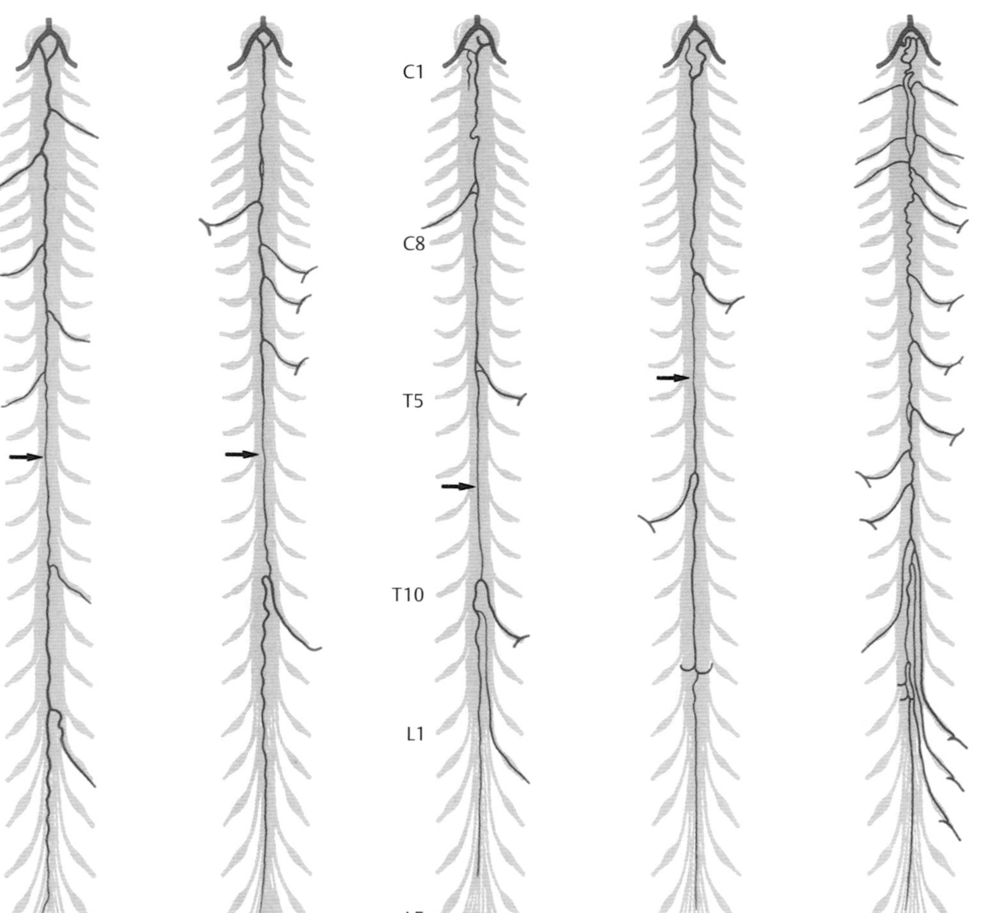

Fig. 2.14 Schematic representation of the segmental blood supply of the spinal cord. The "critical supply zone" is indicated by an arrow (according to Dommisse, 1974 and Kahle et al., 1976).

C1, C8, T5, T10, L1, L5 Spinal nerves

2.1.8 Blood Supply of the Spinal Cord

The vascular supply of the spinal cord is of special significance for spinal surgery. The major supply systems will therefore be briefly discussed below (**Figs. 2.14** and **2.15**).

The spinal cord is supplied by two different arterial systems; on the one hand, by the vertebral arteries, which give off in a caudal direction two posterior spinal arteries and one anterior spinal artery, and on the other hand, by branches of the posterior intercostal arteries.

With respect to the transthoracic approach to the spine, only the latter arteries will be considered—these are the spinal branches of the posterior branches of the posterior intercostal arteries (cf. **Fig. 2.15**). The segmental arteries, which reach the spinal cord via the interspinal foramina and anastomose with the anterior spinal artery, are exceedingly variable in number and caliber so that a division into types does not appear possible. At least two and at most 16 spinal branches have been observed (Domisse, 1974) that advance toward the spinal cord at various levels and contribute to its blood supply. The vessel with the largest caliber is the great radicular artery (Adamkiewicz's artery), which in 80% of cases arises from a left posterior intercostal artery between the seventh thoracic and the fourth lumbar vertebra (most often between the ninth and 11th thoracic vertebrae).

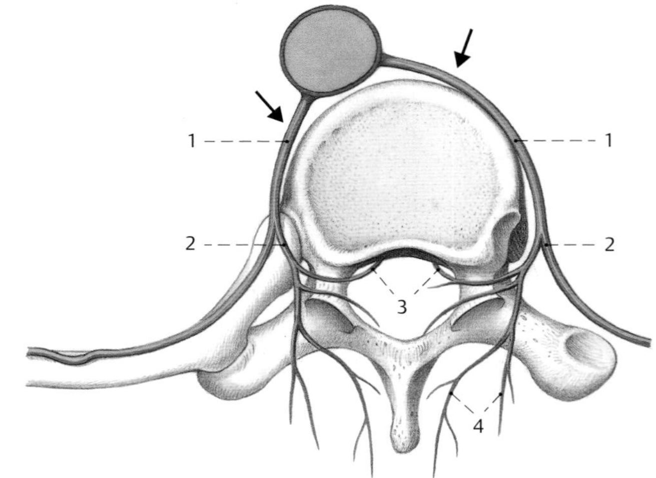

Fig. 2.15 Schematic representation of the blood supply of the vertebral canal and spinal cord on a transverse section (according to Crock et al., 1977). The arrows point to the appropriate ligation sites.

1 Posterior intercostal artery
2 Posterior branch
3 Spinal branches
4 Muscular and cutaneous branches

It should be noted, without minimizing the importance of Adamkiewicz's artery, that it alone is hardly sufficient to supply the caudal segments of the spinal cord. There are in fact several medullary nutrient arteries at different levels that play a vital role in maintaining the supply of the spinal cord. This is consistent with the experience of spinal surgeons who, particularly in the treatment of scoliosis, have ligated between four and 16 segmental arteries without causing any neurologic dysfunction. At any rate, it seems prudent to protect the segmental spinal arteries insofar as the surgical procedure allows.

In the spinal cord, there is a zone of cervical enlargement, a thoracic zone, and a zone of lumbar enlargement. The number and size of the branches supplying the cervical and lumbar cord are greater than those in the thoracic cord. Thus, the thoracic cord is described as a watershed. The "critical supply zone" of the spinal cord generally lies between the fourth and ninth thoracic vertebrae. It is in this zone that the greatest caution should be exercised during surgery.

In exposing vertebrae by the anterior approach, it is important to transect the segmental arteries as far forward as possible; also, the vessels should be dissected free only over a short distance in a posterior direction (**Fig. 2.15**). The arterial arcades that join the segmental arteries outside and inside the vertebral canal are thus preserved. To avoid damage to the spinal branches, the vessels should not be electrocoagulated near the intervertebral foramen.

2.1.9 Site of Thoracotomy in Scoliosis

(**Figs. 2.16** and **2.17**)

In scoliosis, thoracotomy is always performed on the side of the convexity. Owing to the severe torsion of the vertebral bodies and the posterior rib-hump on the convex side, contact is often made immediately after thoracotomy with the spine, which is situated only a few centimeters under the resected rib. The large thoracic vessels generally do not, or do not completely, follow the line of the curvature, and are therefore usually found on the concave side. This means that in left-sided thoracotomy for thoracic scoliosis with a left-sided convexity, the aorta is generally located on the right of the spine.

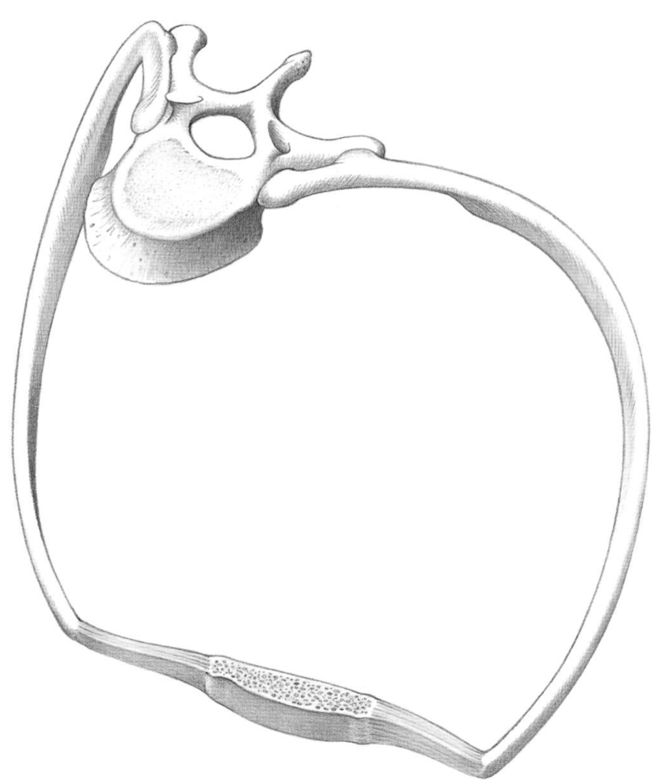

Fig. 2.16 Schematic representation of a costovertebral segment in severe right-sided scoliosis of the thoracic spine. The body of the right rib nearly abuts the thoracic vertebra.

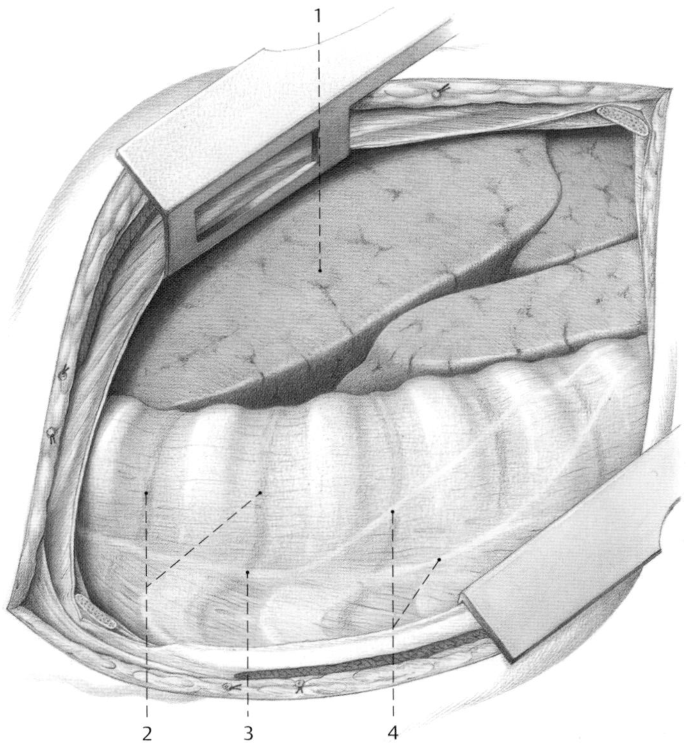

Fig. 2.17 Operative site in scoliosis with right convexity after opening of the pleural cavity. The vertebral pleura is not split; the spine protrudes into the right pleural cavity, and the right lung is displaced toward the left.

1 Right lung
2 Intercostal vessels
3 Sympathetic trunk
4 Greater splanchnic nerve

2.1.10 Exposure of Individual Vertebrae

After the thoracotomy, the parietal pleura should, if possible, be split over the midline of the vertebral bodies; in scoliosis in particular, vertebral torsion should be taken into consideration (see **Fig. 2.16**). The segmental vessels are exposed, ligated and transected in the midline. The vertebral bodies and intervertebral disks are then accessible over the entire anterior circumference (**Fig. 2.18**).

2.1.11 Closure of Thoracotomy with Rib Resection

(**Fig. 2.19**)

A chest drain is inserted and a rib approximator applied. The pleura, periosteum, and intercostal muscles are then as a rule sutured continuously (**Fig. 2.19**), followed by continuous suture of the lateral serratus and the latissimus dorsi (**Fig. 2.20**).

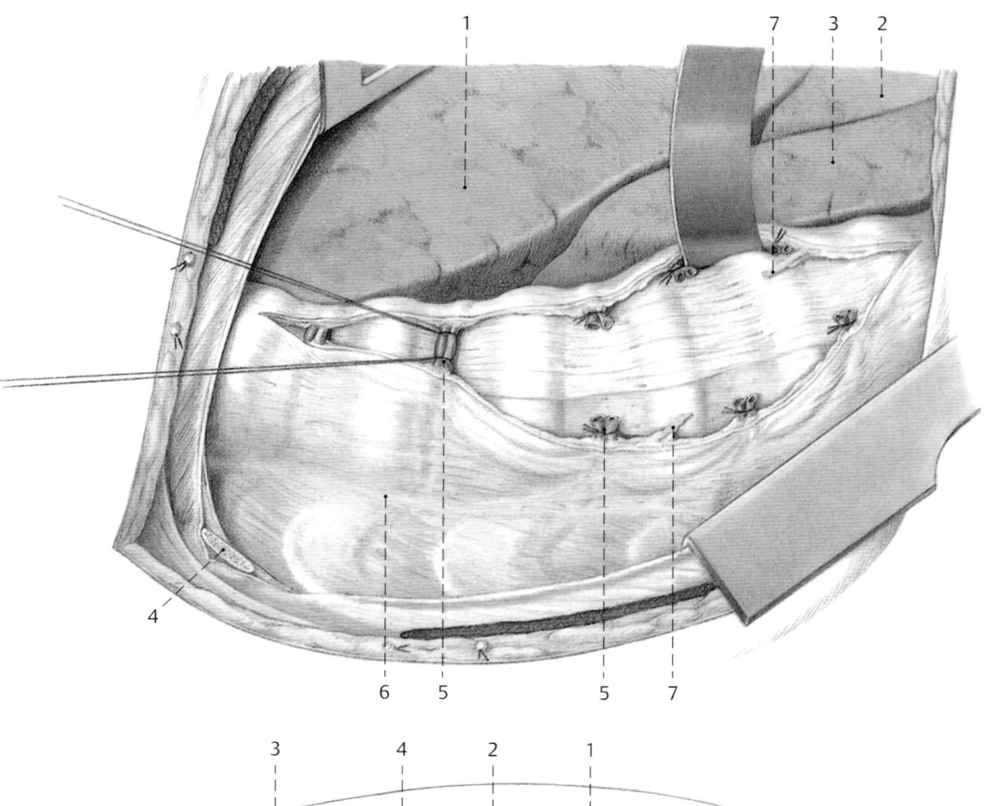

Fig. 2.18 Operative site: the vertebral pleura is split, and the intercostal vessels are partly tied off or transected.

1 Superior lobe } of the right lung
2 Middle lobe } of the right lung
3 Inferior lobe } of the right lung
4 Resection stump of the sixth rib
5 Intercostal vessels
6 Sympathetic trunk visible through the parietal pleura
7 Greater splanchnic nerve

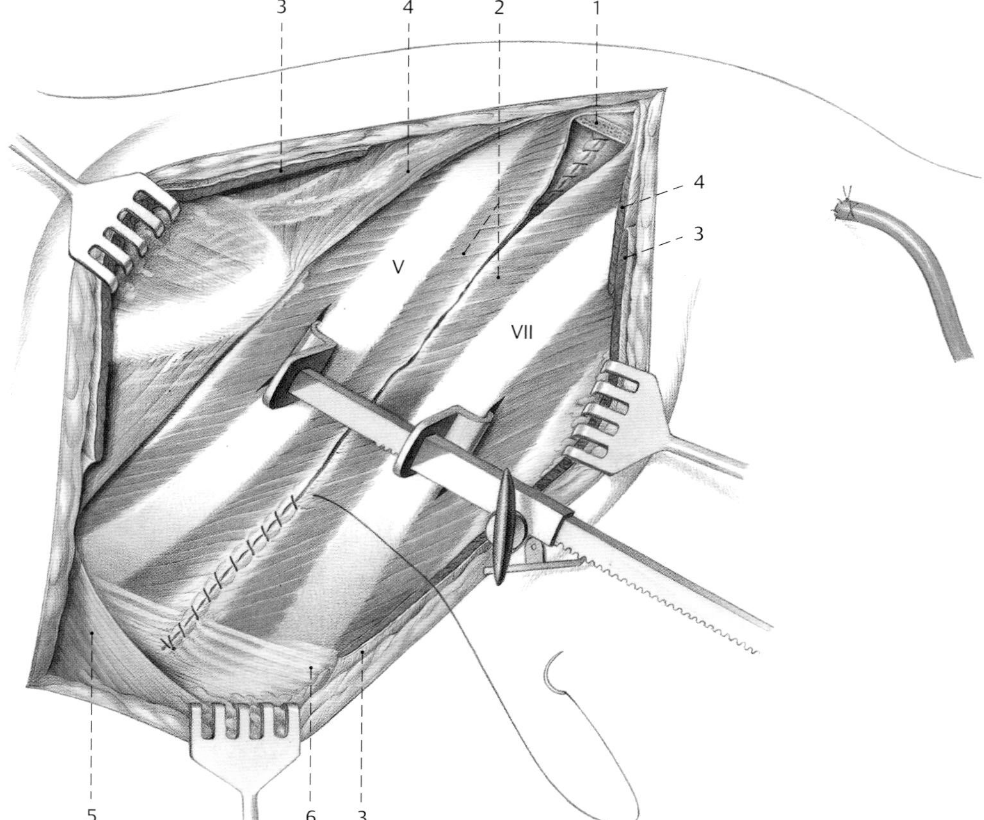

Fig. 2.19 Closure of the thorax using a rib approximator.

1 Resection stump of the sixth rib
2 External intercostal muscle
3 Latissimus dorsi
4 Serratus anterior
5 Trapezius
6 Iliocostalis thoracis
V, VII Ribs

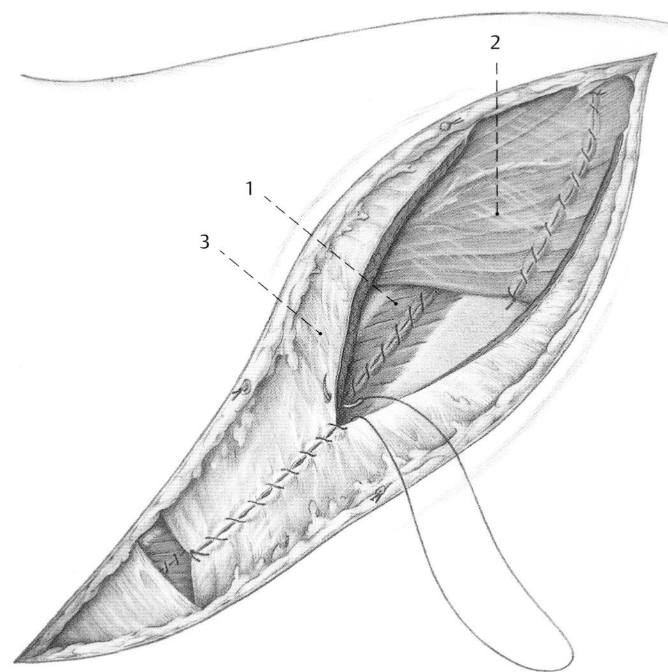

Fig. 2.20 Suture of the extremity muscles of the thorax.

1 External intercostal muscle
2 Serratus anterior
3 Latissimus dorsi

2.1.12 Closure of Intercostal Thoracotomy

(**Fig. 2.21**)

Pericostal absorbable sutures are introduced but not tied. To avoid injury to the intercostal artery and postoperative bleeding, the suture should not be placed directly underneath the caudal rib. With the use of the rib approximator, the pleura and intercostal muscle are sutured, and the pericostal sutures are subsequently tied. Further closure is performed as for thoracotomy with rib resection.

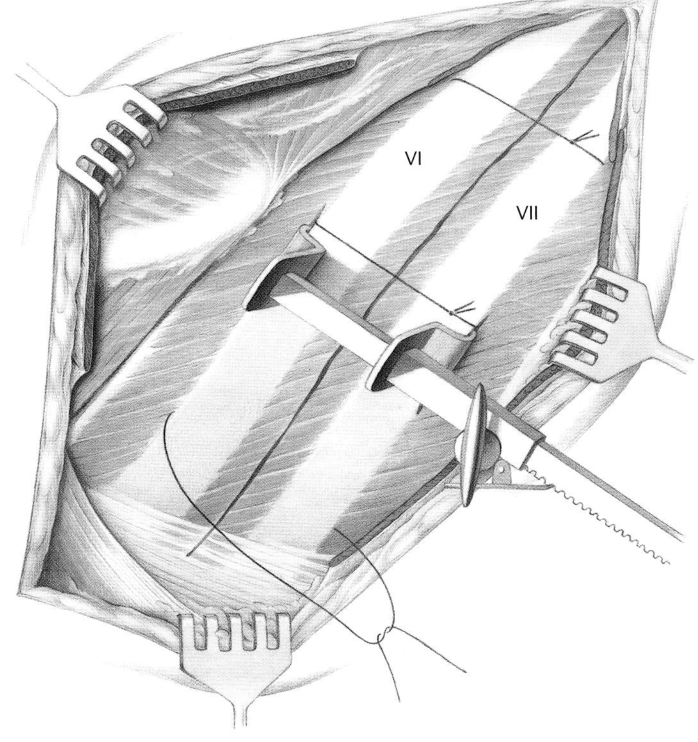

Fig. 2.21 Closure of the thorax after an intercostal thoracotomy.

VI, VII Ribs

2.2 Anterior Transpleural Approach to the Spine T3–T11 According to Louis

R. Bauer, F. Kerschbaumer, S. Poisel

2.2.1 Principal Indications

- Vertebral fractures
- Tumors
- Spondylitis

2.2.2 Choice of Side of Approach

As a general rule, this operation is performed from the right side.

2.2.3 Positioning, Choice of Rib Osteotomy, and Incision

(**Fig. 2.22**)

With the patient in the supine position, the right arm is angulated and moved proximally until the forearm is approximately at the level of the mandible. The forearm is secured by a metal stirrup.

A caudally convex skin incision curving around the right breast is made. The incision begins laterally at the midaxillary line and ends at the right lateral border of the sternum. From here, it may, if necessary, be extended by one or two rib segments cranially parallel to the sternum. The skin incision generally follows the anterior portion of the fourth rib but varies according to the vertebral area to be reached. In women, the skin incision is made in the inframammary crease independently of the level of the rib transection, the breast being displaced upward. Depending on the target area, the following costal cartilages are transected:

- Transection of the second and third ribs: a T3–T9 approach
- Transection of the third and fourth ribs: a T4–T10 approach
- Transection of the fourth and fifth ribs: a T6–T11 approach

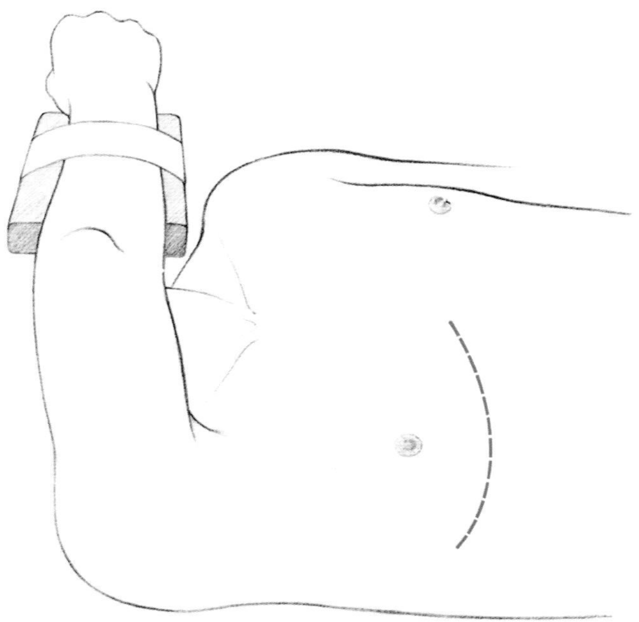

Fig. 2.22 Anterior thoracotomy according to Louis. Positioning and incision.

Incision of the skin and subcutaneous tissue is followed by a parallel incision dividing the superficial muscle layers with the diathermy scalpel (pectoralis major and serratus anterior, **Fig. 2.23**). The periosteum over the fifth rib is now split with the same instrument along the rib axis. The upper half of the costal periosteum is separated with a raspatory, the fibromuscular structures of the intercostal space being stripped off the upper border of the selected rib, moving from lateral to medial. The raspatory should not be moved closer than 1.5 cm from the lateral margin of the sternum as this produces a risk of injuring the internal thoracic artery.

Subsequently, the fourth rib is exposed subperiosteally. The structures of the intercostal space are transected between two ligatures at least 13 mm lateral to the sternal border.

A grooved director is now passed below the fourth or fifth costal cartilage, which is then transected with a scalpel at a point 1.5 cm to the side of the sternal border. Subsequently, a thoracic retractor is inserted (**Fig. 2.24**). Transection of only two cartilage segments permits good distraction of the thoracic retractor between the fourth and fifth ribs. For exposure of a wider area, an additional costal cartilage, placed more cranially or more caudally, may be exposed.

2.2.4 Exposure of the Vertebrae

The right lung is displaced medially and held with flexible spatulas (**Fig. 2.24**). The dome of the diaphragm has to be retracted caudally, using a curved retractor; the azygos vein, which can be seen through the parietal pleura, is now identified. The pleura is split longitudinally to the left of the azygos vein, as described by Louis. In the region of the upper thoracic spine, this approach has the advantage of not requiring ligation of the segmental veins (**Fig. 2.25**). The segmental arteries in the desired area are transected after ligation (**Fig. 2.26**), and the vertebral bodies are then exposed in the usual manner over the entire circumference.

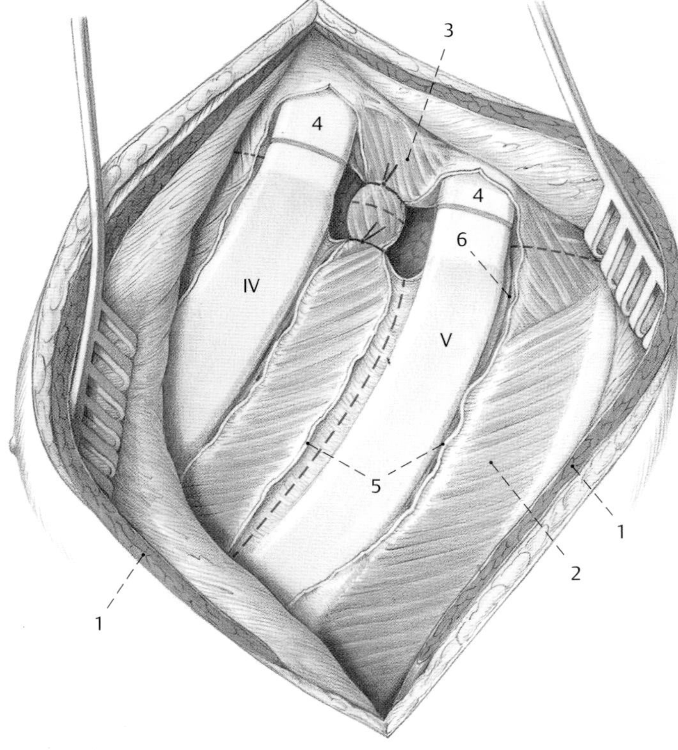

Fig. 2.23 Operative site after transection of pectoralis major. The periosteum over the fourth and fifth ribs is split. The ribs are transected at the level of the costal cartilage. Transection of the intercostal tissue is shown by a dashed line.

1 Pectoralis major
2 External intercostal muscle
3 Internal intercostal muscle
4 Costal cartilage
5 Periosteum
6 Intercostal vein
IV, V Ribs

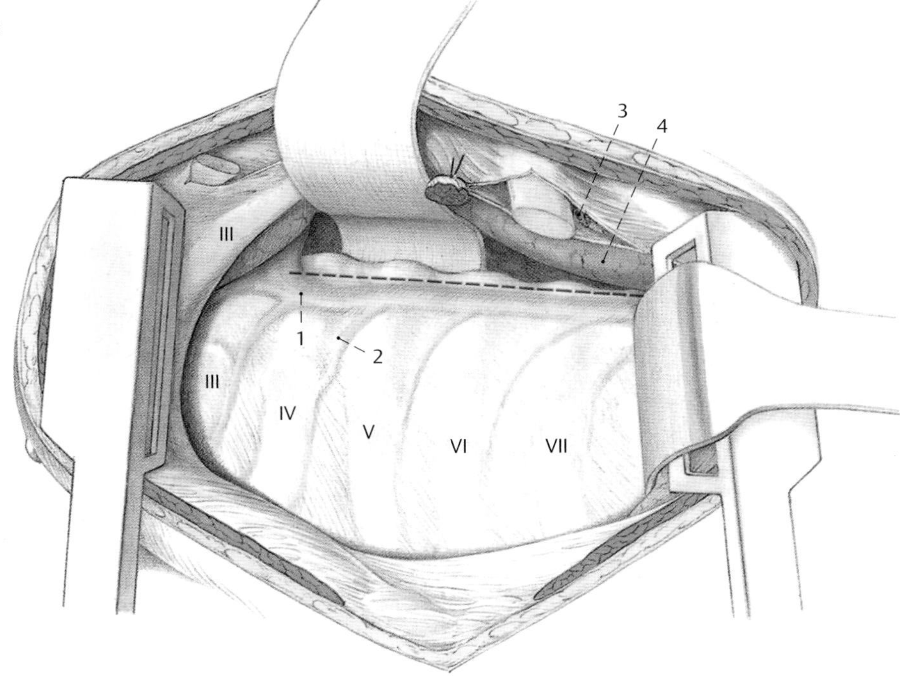

Fig. 2.24 Operative site after opening of the pleural cavity and insertion of a rib spreader. The parietal pleura is split over the spine on the left side of the azygos vein (dashed line).

1 Azygos vein
2 Intercostal vein
3 Intercostal vessels
4 Lung
III–VII Ribs

If vertebrae T3 and T4 have to be reached, their exposure is hampered by the fact that both the segmental veins and the arteries course obliquely to vertically above these vertebrae, so that several vessels overlie a single vertebra (see **Fig. 2.10**). To avoid the dissection of several segmental arteries, the parietal pleura may be incised slightly diagonally between two segmental arteries at the level of the arch of the azygos vein (**Fig. 2.27**). The vertebral body is essentially accessible between the segmental arteries; the arch of the azygos vein may be ligated and transected.

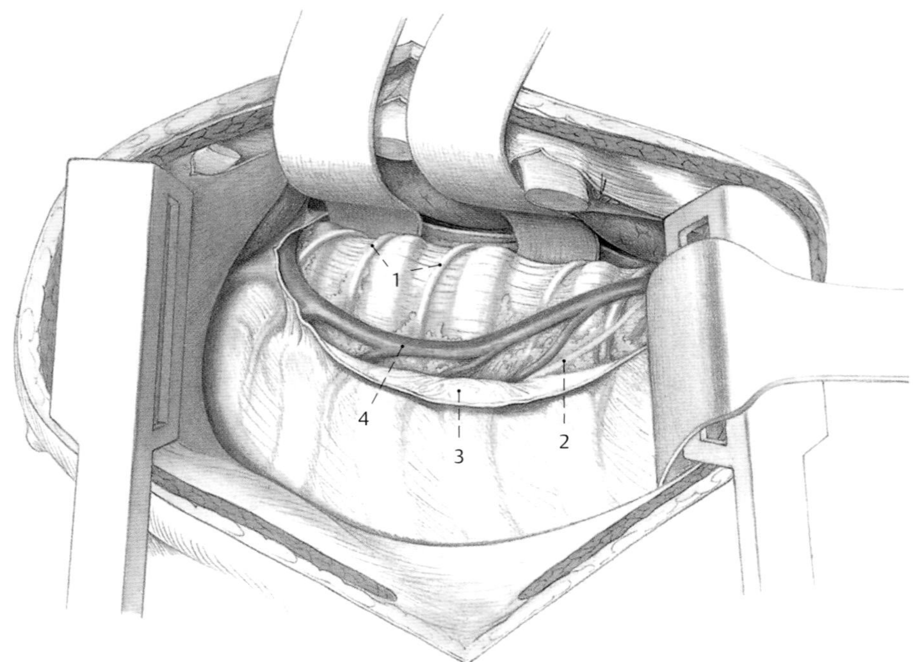

Fig. 2.25 Operative site after splitting of the parietal pleura. The segmental arteries are visible.

1 Intercostal arteries
2 Greater splanchnic nerve
3 Parietal pleura
4 Azygos vein

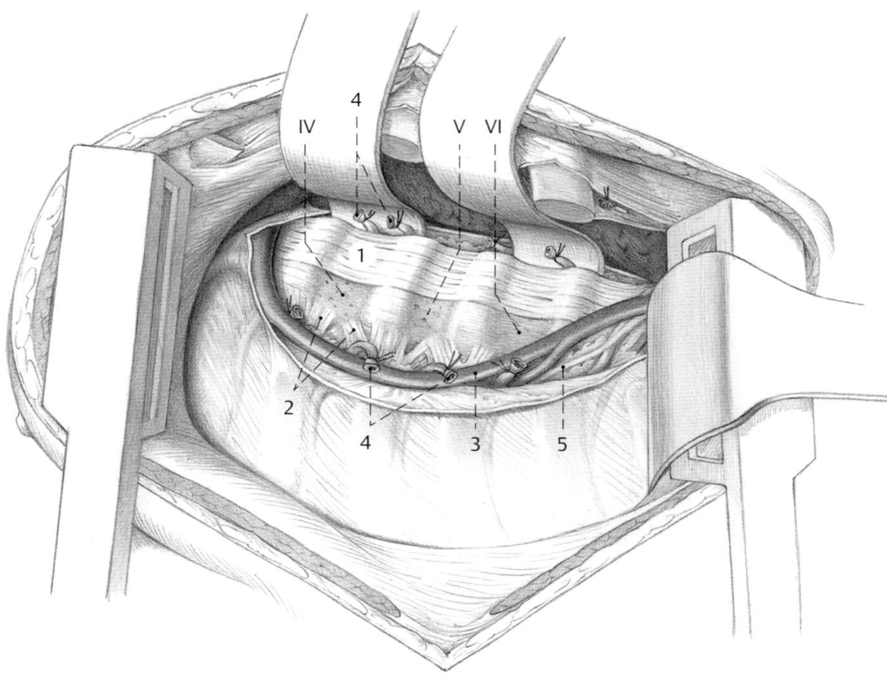

Fig. 2.26 Operative site after transection of the segmental arteries. Vertebrae T4–T6 are exposed.

1 Anterior longitudinal ligament
2 Radiate ligament of the head of the rib
3 Azygos vein
4 Posterior intercostal arteries
5 Greater splanchnic nerve
IV–VI Vertebral bodies

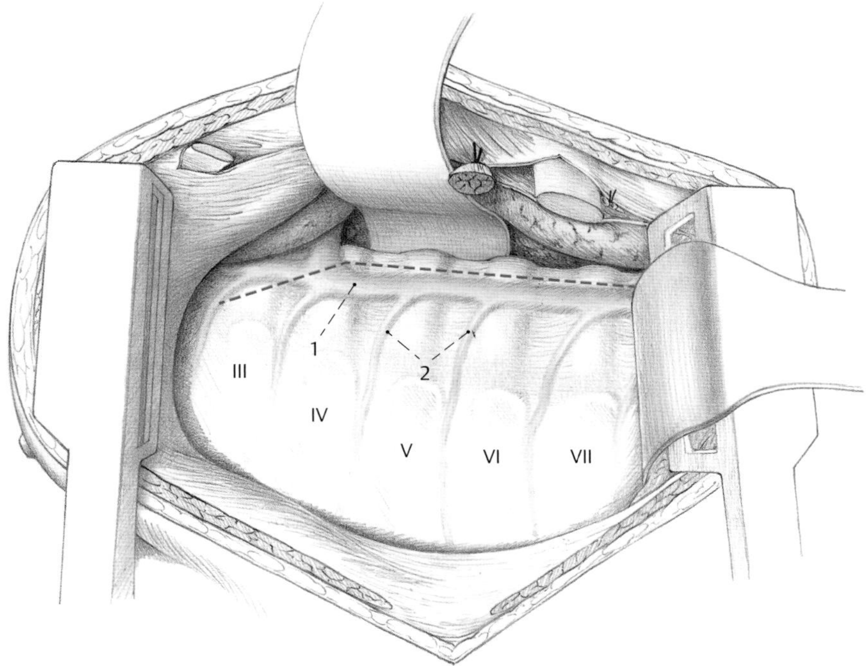

Fig. 2.27 The arch of the azygos vein may be transected for exposure of vertebrae T3 and T4. This makes it possible to reach the vertebrae between the obliquely running arteries.

1 Azygos vein
2 Posterior intercostal veins
III–VII Ribs

2.3 High Thoracotomy T1–T4

R. Bauer, F. Kerschbaumer, S. Poisel

2.3.1 Principal Indications

- Tuberculous spondylitis
- Tumors

Access to this area is difficult. If several vertebrae at the cervicothoracic junction have to be exposed, including the inferior cervical spine, an available alternative is the trans-sternal approach according to Cauchoix and Binet (see Section 1.3, **Figs. 1.23–1.29**).

For anatomical reasons, however, the combination of an anterior approach to the cervical spine with a Louis thoracotomy (**Fig. 2.28**) or high thoracotomy (**Fig. 2.29**), which is described below, seems more advantageous to us in this case.

2.3.2 Choice of Side of Approach

Generally speaking, the upper thoracic spine can be reached from the right as well as from the left side.

2.3.3 Positioning and Incision

The operation is performed from the right, with the patient lying on the left side (the analogous approach may of course be made from the left with the patient lying on the right side). The right arm is placed as far proximally as possible. The skin incision is begun in the area of the upper thoracic spine near the spinous processes, and then curves in an arc around the inferior angle of the scapula (**Fig. 2.30**). After this, as shown in **Fig. 2.31**, the trapezius is dissected along a curved line that, because of the innervation, is as close to the spine as possible. The latissimus dorsi is also dissected, as far caudally as possible (**Figs. 2.32** and **2.33**). On the next level, rhomboid major is divided near the scapula, while serratus anterior is divided as far caudally as possible, to avoid the long thoracic nerve (**Fig. 2.34**; see also **Fig. 2.3**). The scapula can now be elevated with a hook (**Fig. 2.35**); the topmost ribs are exposed and can be counted off in typical fashion from the cranial toward the caudal end. Depending on the level of the vertebra to be exposed, the third or, as shown in **Fig. 2.35**, the fourth rib may now be resected subperiosteally in the customary manner. If T1 and perhaps C7 have to be reached, the third rib is resected and, in addition, the insertion of the middle scalene muscle may be detached and the second rib excised to improve the approach. After this, a thoracic retractor is inserted (**Fig. 2.36**).

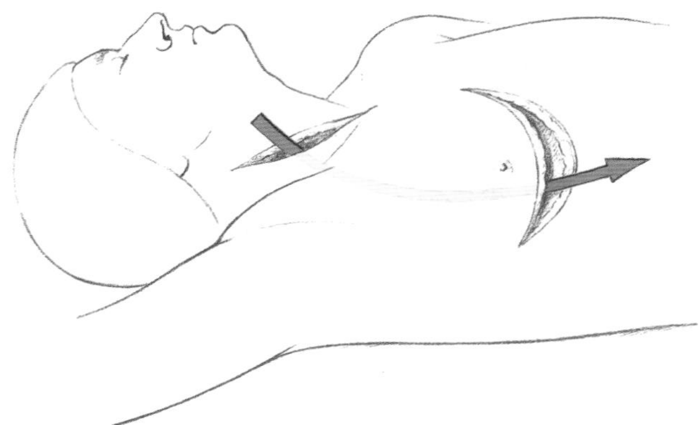

Fig. 2.28 Schematic representation of the approach to the cervicothoracic junction by an anterolateral approach to the cervical spine combined with a thoracotomy according to Louis.

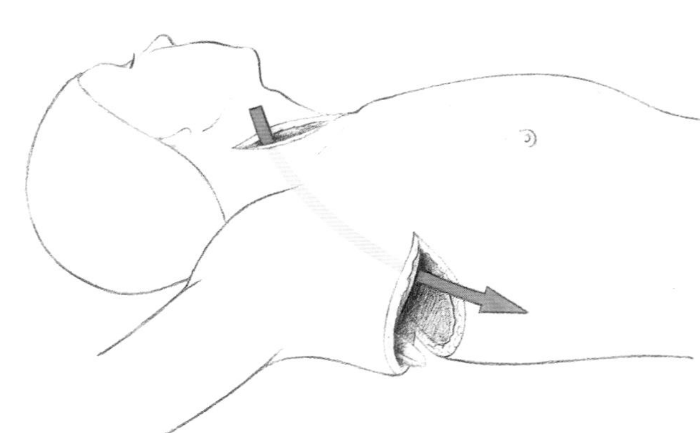

Fig. 2.29 Schematic representation of the approach to the cervicothoracic junction by an anterolateral approach to the cervical spine combined with a high thoracotomy.

2.3.4 Exposure of the Vertebrae

The parietal pleura over the upper thoracic spine is split longitudinally, and the segmental vessels are transected after ligation. It should be borne in mind that, in the upper thoracic spine, the intercostal vessels pass over the vertebrae at a slant so that several segmental vessels are found over a single vertebral body. This situation has been discussed in connection with the Louis approach (see Section 2.2.4) and is depicted in **Fig. 2.10**.

2.3.5 Wound Closure

A chest drain is inserted and a typical wound closure performed (see Sections 2.1.11 and 2.1.12, **Figs. 2.19**, **2.20**, and **2.21**).

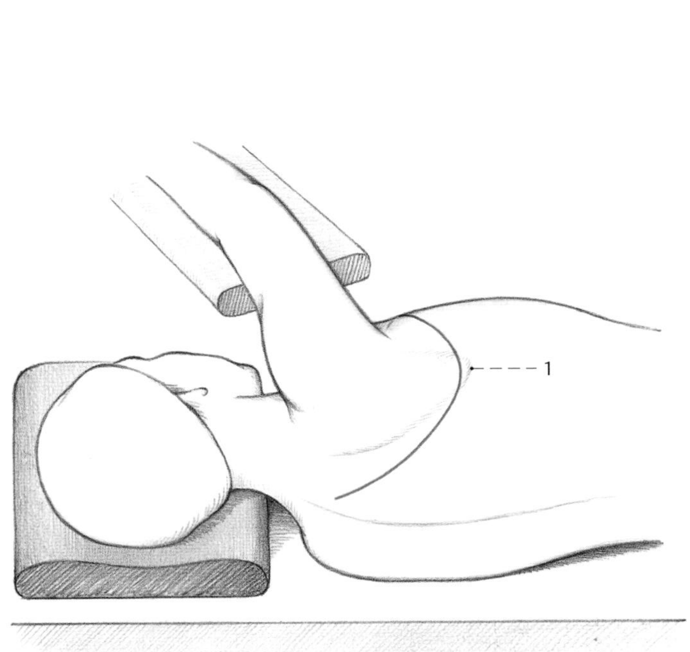

Fig. 2.30 High thoracotomy. Positioning and incision.

1 Inferior angle of scapula

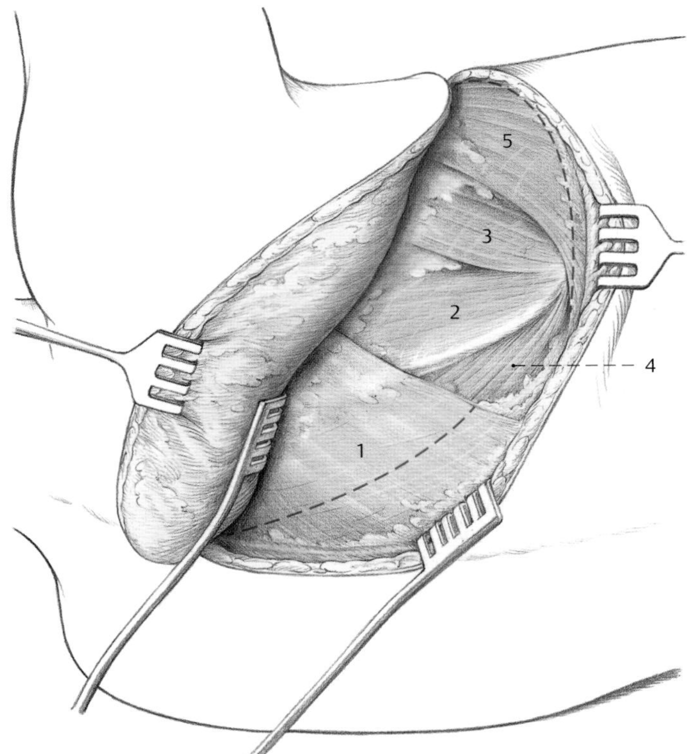

Fig. 2.31 Exposure of the operative field after transection of the skin and subcutaneous tissue. Division of trapezius and latissimus dorsi occurs along the dashed line.

1 Trapezius
2 Infraspinatus
3 Teres major
4 Rhomboid major
5 Latissimus dorsi

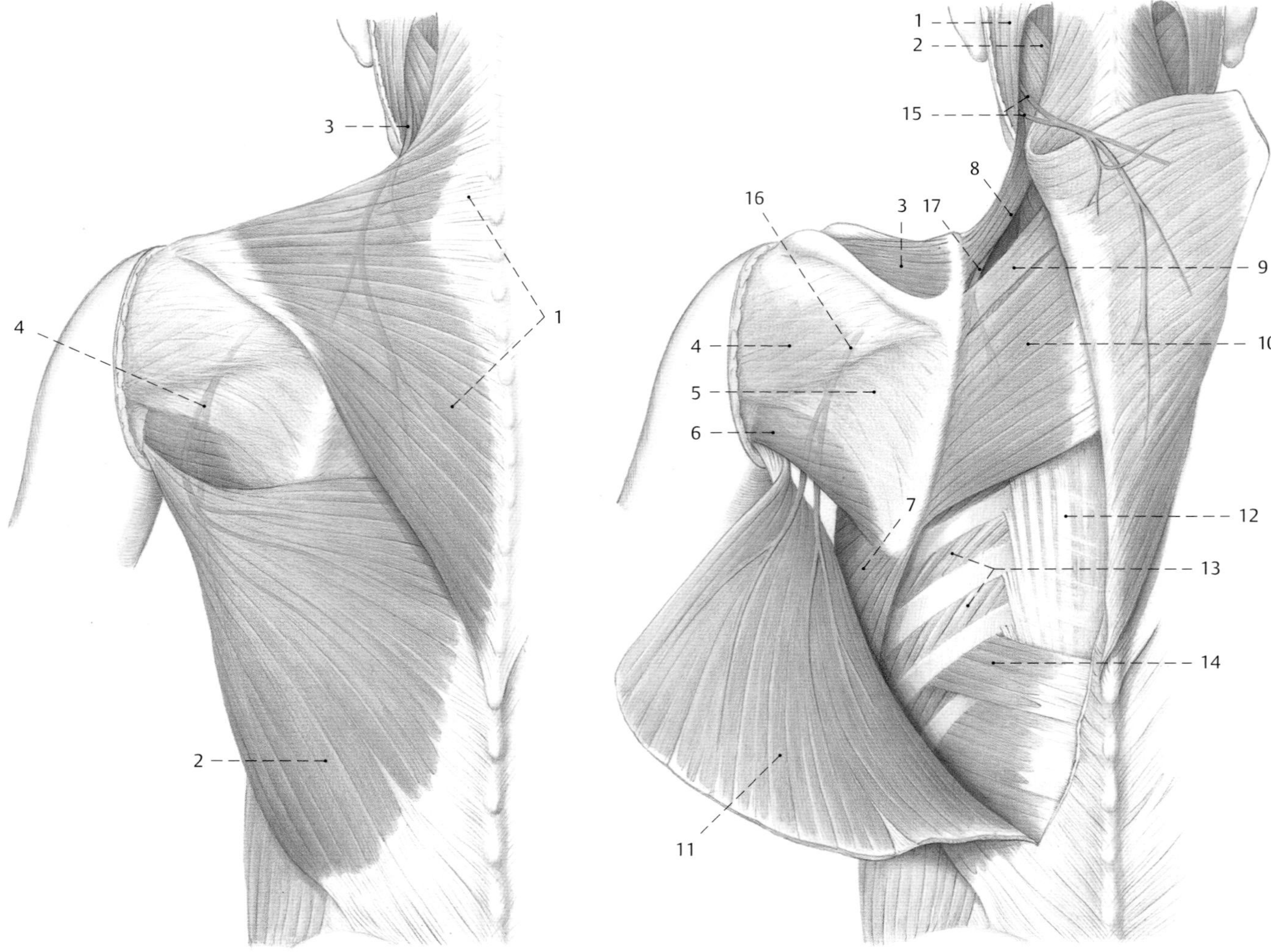

Fig. 2.32 Schematic representation of the nerve supply of trapezius and latissimus dorsi.

1 Trapezius
2 Latissimus dorsi
3 Accessory nerve
4 Thoracodorsal nerve

Fig. 2.33 For better exposure of the nerve supply, some muscle origins have been detached and opened up.

1 Sternocleidomastoid
2 Splenius capitis
3 Supraspinatus
4 Deltoid
5 Infraspinatus
6 Teres major
7 Serratus anterior
8 Levator scapulae
9 Rhomboid minor
10 Rhomboid major
11 Latissimus dorsi
12 Iliocostalis
13 External intercostal muscles
14 Serratus posterior superior
15 Accessory nerve and trapezius branch
16 Thoracodorsal nerve
17 Posterior nerve of the scapula

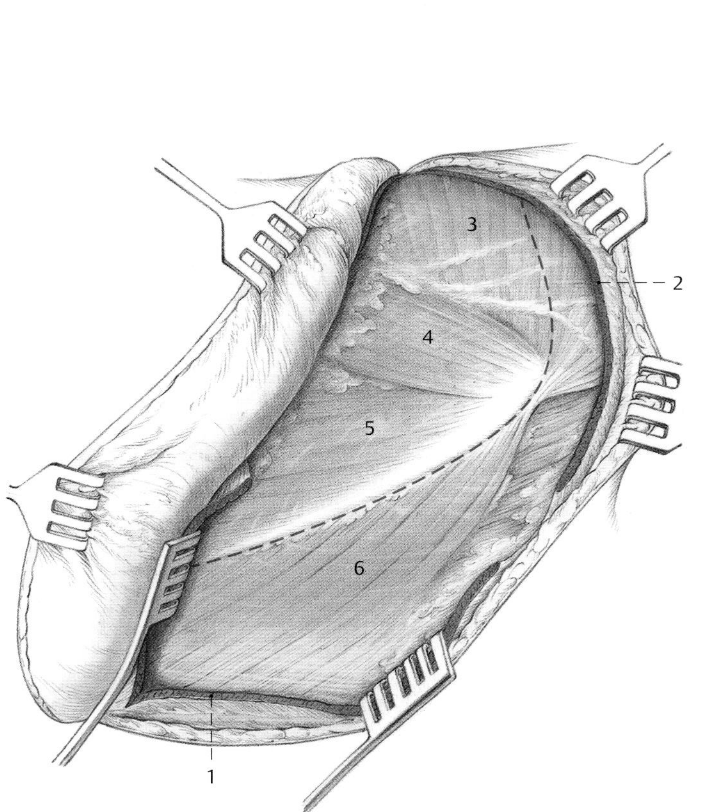

Fig. 2.34 Operative site after transection of the superficial muscle layer, an incision around the scapula along the dashed line, and transection of rhomboid major and serratus anterior.

1 Trapezius
2 Latissimus dorsi
3 Serratus anterior
4 Teres major
5 Infraspinatus
6 Rhomboid major

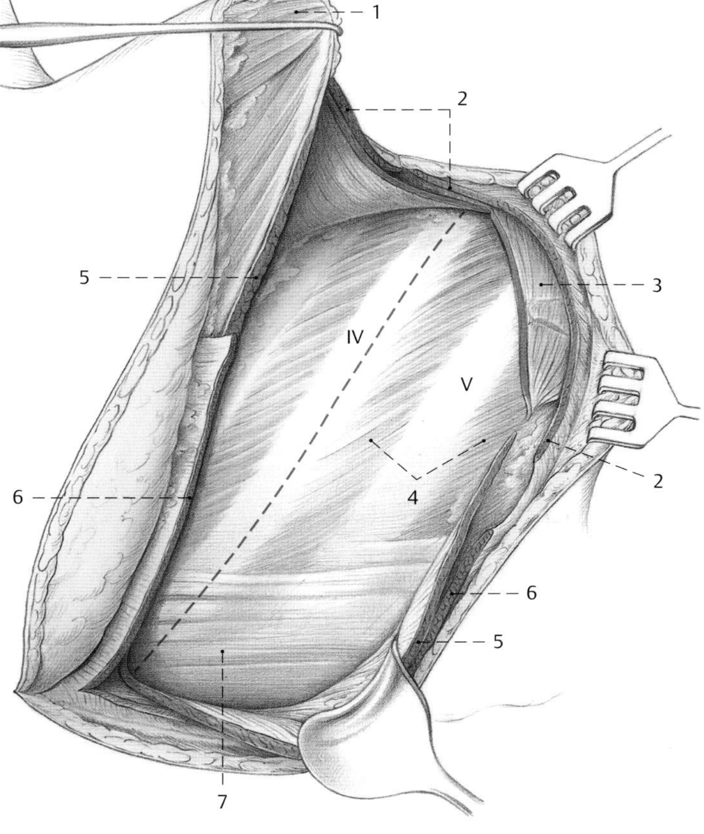

Fig. 2.35 Operative site with exposure of the fourth rib, which is exposed subperiosteally along the dashed line.

1 Teres major
2 Latissimus dorsi
3 Serratus anterior
4 External intercostal muscles
5 Rhomboid major
6 Trapezius
7 Iliocostalis
IV, V Ribs

Fig. 2.36 Operative site after opening of the pleural cavity. The uppermost thoracic vertebrae are exposed after splitting of the parietal pleura and transection of the segmental vessels.

1 Trapezius
2 Rhomboid major
3 Longus colli
4 Intrinsic muscles of the back
5 Anterior longitudinal ligament overlying the second and third thoracic vertebrae
6 Intercostal vessels
7 Sympathetic trunk
IV Rib

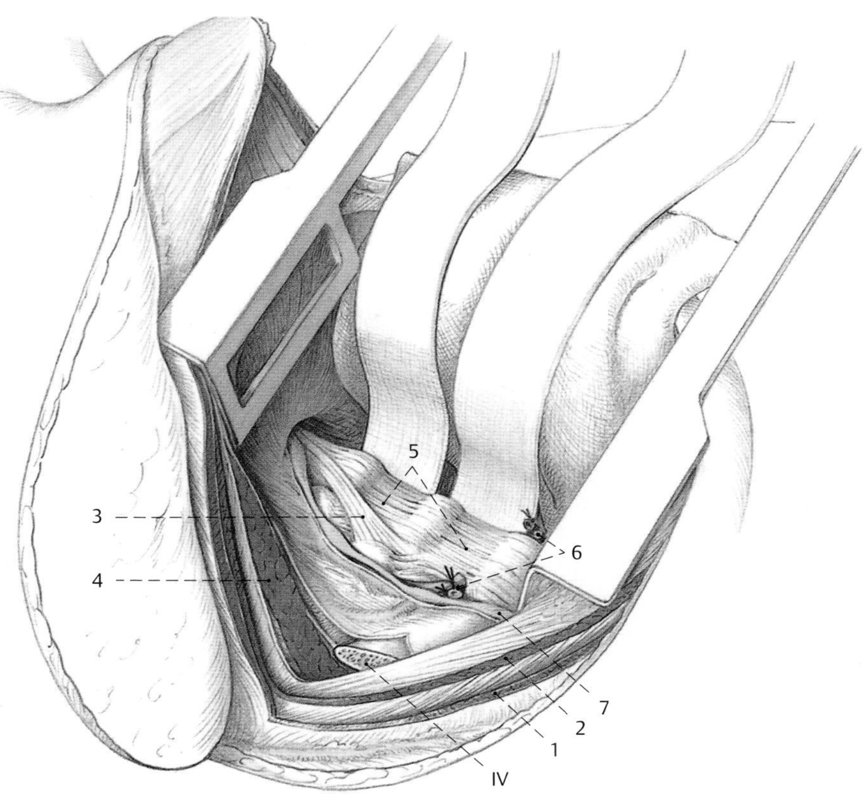

2.4 Thoracoscopic and Minimally Invasive, Thoracoscopy-Assisted Access to the Thoracic Spine

F. Kandziora

2.4.1 Principal Indications

- Kyphosis
- Scoliosis
- Vertebral fractures
- Tumors
- Spondylitis and spondylodiskitis
- Disk prolapse
- Segmental degeneration

2.4.2 Preoperative Preparation

In addition to correct positioning, single-lung ventilation is required, especially when the procedure is entirely thoracoscopic. Correct placement of the double-lumen tube must be checked by bronchoscopy preoperatively and after the patient has been positioned. In exceptional cases of a far caudal left-sided approach (T12, L1, L2), single-lung ventilation may be omitted, particularly when minimally invasive, thoracoscopy-assisted access is planned. However, it must then be ensured that the positive end-expiratory pressure is kept as low as possible to allow better retraction of the lung.

2.4.3 Choice of Side of Approach

Because of the course of the thoracic aorta, the purely thoracoscopic and the minimally invasive thoracoscopy-assisted approach to the thoracic spine is between T1 and T10 on the right and between T11 and L2 on the left. Exceptions to this approach may be chosen in the case of scoliosis, where the approach is normally from the side of the convexity; deviation from this rule may also be considered in special cases such as unilateral tumor or disk prolapse.

2.4.4 Positioning

For thoracoscopic spinal surgery and the minimally invasive, thoracoscopy-assisted approach to the thoracic spine on the right, the patient is placed in stable left lateral position. A stable right lateral position is required for the left-sided approach.

In the description of the operation that follows, we shall concentrate on the left-sided approach (**Figs. 2.37** and **2.38**); the right-sided approach is analogous.

For the left-sided procedure, the left arm must be abducted and elevated. Abduction must not exceed 90°, to avoid brachial plexus damage. The operating table should be hinged so that it can be angled below the instrumented regions to allow widening of the intercostal spaces if necessary. However, angling of the table must not cause scoliotic flexion of the spine, especially when instrumentation is planned to avoid the risk of spinal fixation in an incorrect position. The C-arm must be freely mobile around the patient. In thoracoscopic procedures, the video monitor is at the patient's feet, the surgeon is at the patient's back, and the assistant is in front of the patient.

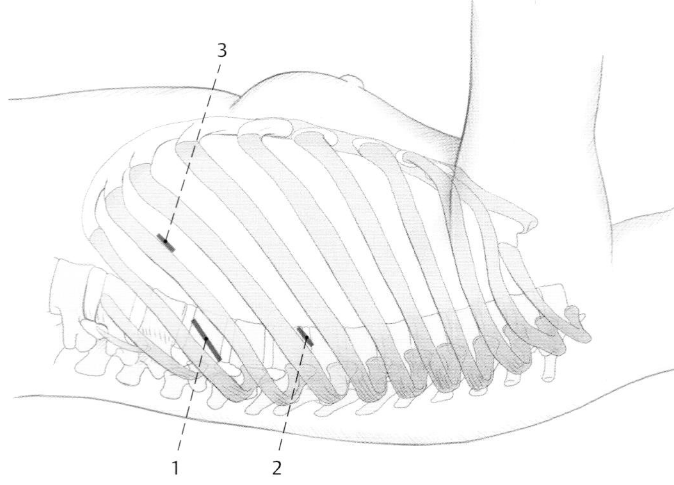

Fig. 2.37 Incision for a minimally invasive, thoracoscopy-assisted operation.

1 Minithoracotomy
2 Optic portal
3 Retractor portal

2.4.5 Localization

The C-arm is used to locate the radiographic landmarks of the region being operated on; these are projected and drawn on the skin. For example, when corpectomy is planned, the cranial and caudal boundaries and the anterior and posterior walls of the affected vertebral body and the two adjacent ones are drawn on the skin.

In the **minimally invasive, thoracoscopy-assisted operation** (**Fig. 2.37**) the minithoracotomy is drawn centered over the area in question and in the line of the overlying rib (**Fig. 2.37**, number 1). The thoracoscopy (optic) portal is also drawn (**Fig. 2.37**, number 2). In a left-sided thoracotomy, this portal is two or three intercostal spaces cranial to the marked skin incision, and is located two or three intercostal spaces caudal to the marked incision in the case of a right-sided thoracotomy. The optic portal is normally placed at the center of the skin incision in an anteroposterior direction. However, if necessary, the 30° optic may be placed somewhat further anteriorly to allow better visualization of the posterior wall of the vertebral body. A portal for the endoscopic fan retractor is optional (retractor portal; **Fig. 2.37**, number 3). In a left-sided thoracoscopy-assisted procedure, this portal is sited approximately 10–15 cm anterior to the working portal. The diaphragm and/or lung can be held away with the fan retractor in addition to the retractor system.

In the **purely thoracoscopic operation** (**Fig. 2.38**), the first thoracoscopy portal (working portal; **Fig. 2.38**, number 1) is marked directly over the site of the pathology at the upper border of the corresponding rib. The second access for the optic (optic portal; **Fig. 2.38**, number 2) is two or three spaces cranial to the working portal in a left-sided thoracoscopic procedure. The optic portal can be moved in an anteroposterior direction depending on the pathology. Access 2–3 cm further anteriorly facilitates visualization of the posterior border of the vertebral body, while access further posteriorly can improve visualization of the spinal canal if there is disk prolapse. A further portal for the endoscopic fan retractor is required (retractor portal; **Fig. 2.38**, number 3). In a left-sided thoracoscopic procedure, this portal is sited approximately 10–15 cm anterior to the working portal, usually one or two intercostal spaces cranially. The fan retractor is used to hold the diaphragm and lung. Finally, a fourth portal is opened for suction and irrigation (suction portal; **Fig. 2.38**, number 4), usually half way along a line between the optic portal and the retractor portal. Different portal planning is possible in individual cases.

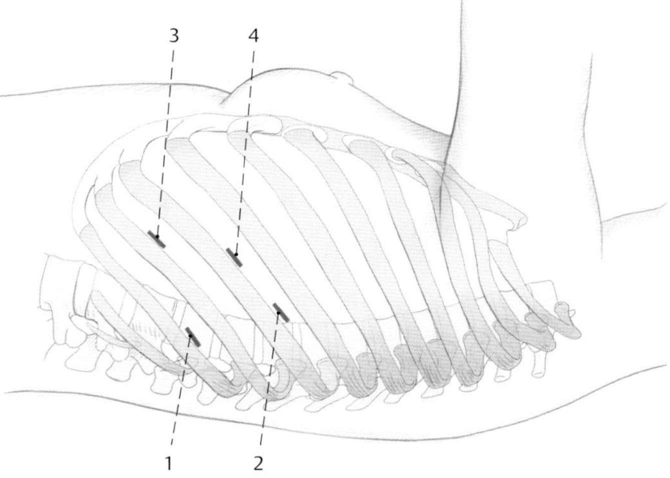

Fig. 2.38 Incisions for a purely thoracoscopic operation.

1 Working portal
2 Optic portal
3 Retractor portal
4 Suction portal

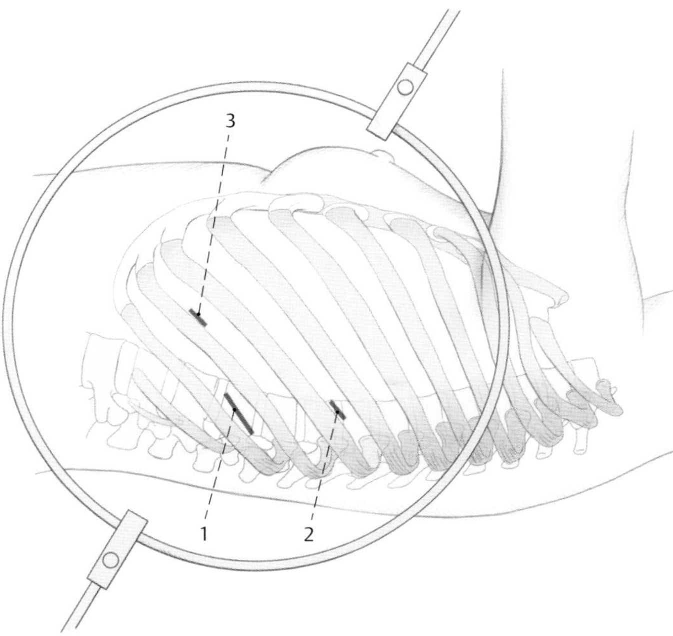

Fig. 2.39 Placement of a retractor system over the operation site.

1 Working portal
2 Optic portal
3 Retractor portal

2.4.6 Incision

In the **minimally invasive, thoracoscopy-assisted operation**, use of a retractor system is obligatory (**Fig. 2.39**). The skin incision is made slightly obliquely from anterocaudal to posterocranial, directly over the corresponding rib and centered over the pathology. A roughly 4–8 cm skin incision suffices. The minithoracotomy is performed as an intercostal thoracotomy. Rib resection is not necessary. After dividing the latissimus dorsi and serratus anterior (**Fig. 2.40**), the intercostal muscles (**Fig. 2.41**) are divided at the upper border of the rib, followed by division of the parietal pleura (**Fig. 2.42**), protecting the lung.

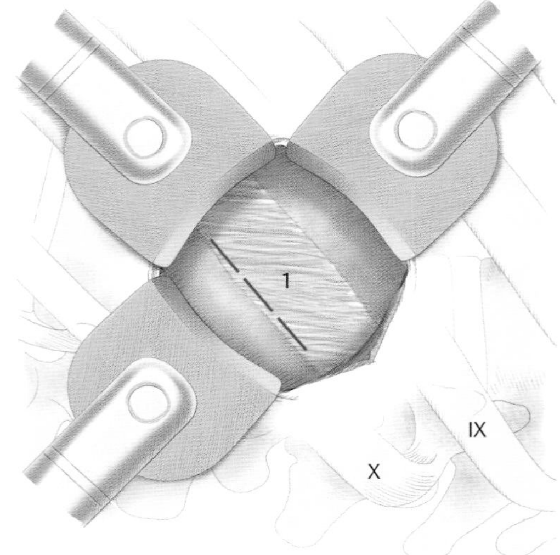

Fig. 2.41 Division of the intercostal muscles at the upper border of the rib.

1 External intercostal muscle
IX, X Ribs

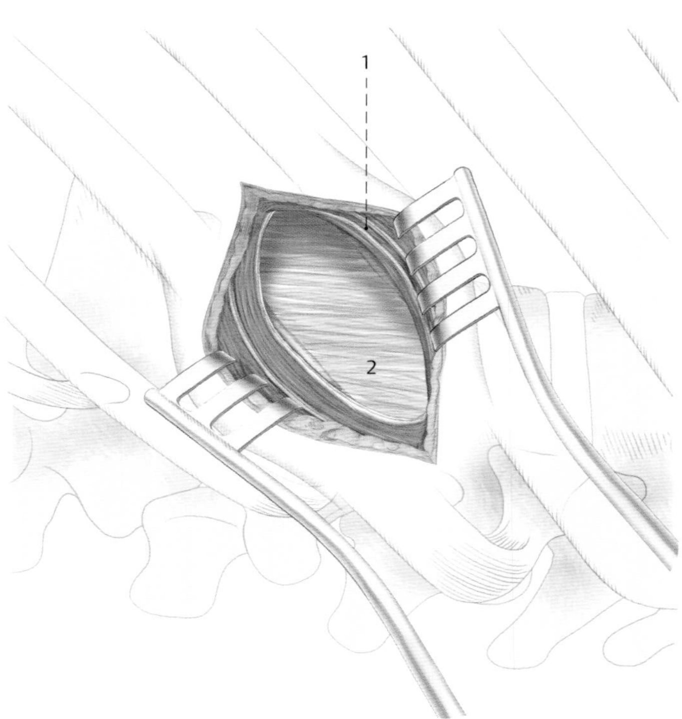

Fig. 2.40 Intercostal minithoracotomy: division of latissimus dorsi and serratus anterior.

1 Serratus anterior
2 External intercostal muscle

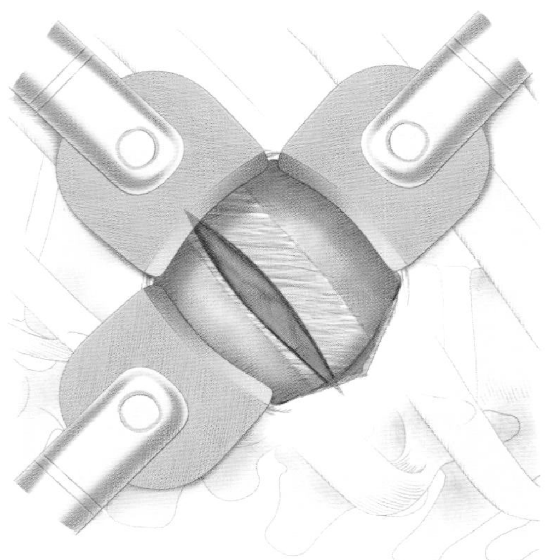

Fig. 2.42 Division of the parietal pleura, protecting the lung.

2.4.7 Operative Procedure

Before dividing the parietal pleura, single-lung ventilation is started to avoid accidental injury of the lung when dividing the parietal pleura.

In the **minimally invasive, thoracoscopy-assisted operation**, the thoracoscope is first introduced through the minithoracotomy, and the entire thoracic space is evaluated (**Fig. 2.43**). Single-lung ventilation with adequate lung collapse must be ensured and, if necessary, the lung may be further evacuated by bronchoscopic aspiration. The optic portal is then placed under thoracoscopic visualization. The location of the previously marked incision site can be checked by palpation of the intercostal space under thoracoscopic vision (**Fig. 2.43**), when it appears as a depression in the intercostal space. After establishing the incision site, a stab incision approximately 2 cm long is made. The precostal muscles on the corresponding rib are then spread bluntly, and the thoracic space is entered bluntly at the upper border of the rib under thoracoscopic vision. The parietal pleura is opened bluntly under thoracoscopic vision by opening the scissors (**Fig. 2.44**), and finally a trocar is advanced into the thorax. The thoracoscope is then removed from the minithoracotomy and switched to the introduced trocar (optic portal) (**Fig. 2.45**).

To facilitate exposure, a self-retaining retractor system can now be placed in the minithoracotomy. Alternatively, an additional portal may be placed approximately 10–15 cm anteriorly through which a fan retractor is introduced (retractor portal; **Fig. 2.45**). This can be used to hold down the lung and also the diaphragm, if necessary.

Should the minithoracotomy prove insufficient in size to fully expose the pathology, rib osteotomy may be performed in addition to stretching the intercostal space with retractors and extending the skin incision. The site of the osteotomy can be both anterior and posterior to the border of the access region, depending on the required space. The intercostal neurovascular bundles should be spared during rib osteotomy. Partial rib resection is not normally necessary.

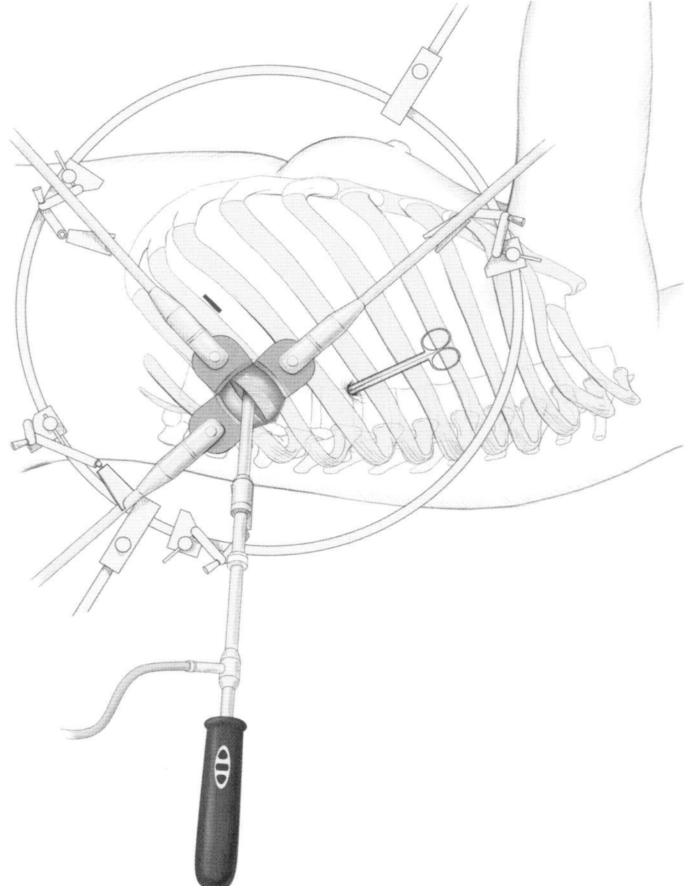

Fig. 2.43 Introduction of the thoracoscope through the minithoracotomy and thoracoscopic evaluation of the thorax.

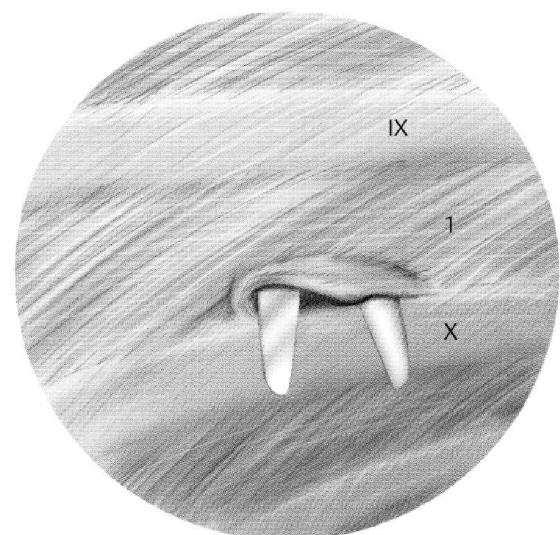

Fig. 2.44 Entering the thorax with scissors under thoracoscopic vision.

1 Internal intercostal muscle
IX, X Ribs

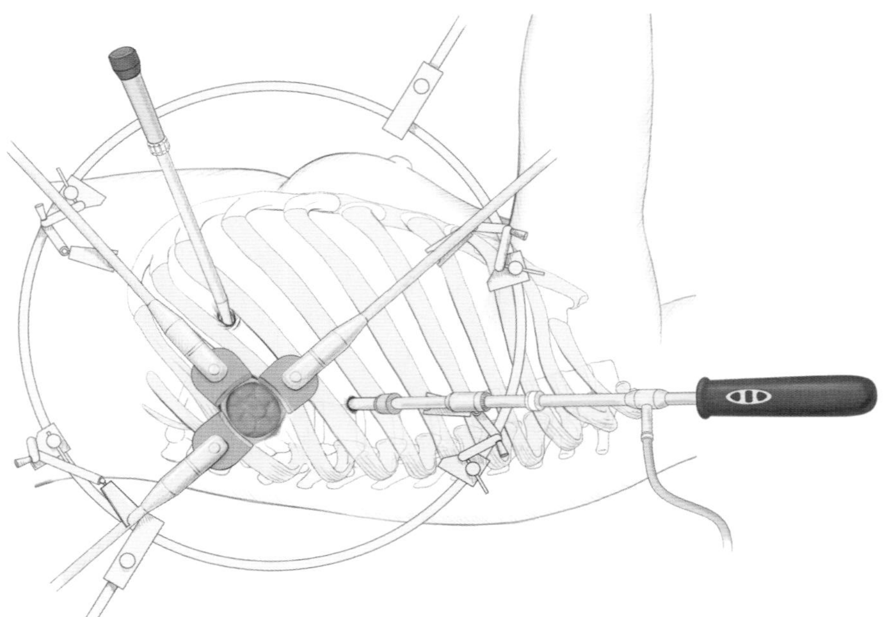

Fig. 2.45 Switching the thoracoscope to the optic portal. The retractor system is placed more deeply. If necessary, a retractor portal can also be placed.

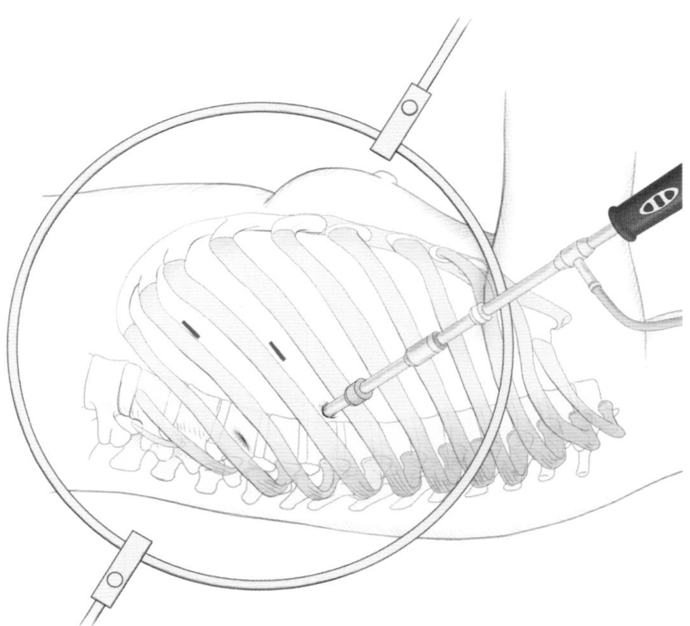

Fig. 2.46 Switching the thoracoscope from the working portal to the optic portal.

In the **purely thoracoscopic operation**, the working portal is first placed (see **Fig. 2.38**, number 1). The length of the skin incision for the working portal depends on the nature and extent of the planned instrumentation. For example, if it is necessary to introduce an expandable vertebral body replacement, the working portal can be extended to a length of approximately 4 cm. Alternatively, extension of the working portal for introduction of the implant can take place at the end of the purely thoracoscopic procedure. The working portal is placed by dividing the parietal pleura under vision after making a 2–3 cm stab incision and introducing two Langenbeck retractors. Single-lung ventilation must be ensured prior to this. After the first portal has been placed under vision, the optic is introduced through this portal. All other portals are then placed under thoracoscopic vision, as described above (see **Fig. 2.44**). The thoracoscope is then switched from the working portal to the optic portal (**Fig. 2.46**). Finally, the fan retractor, suction catheter, and instruments are introduced through the other portals (**Fig. 2.47**).

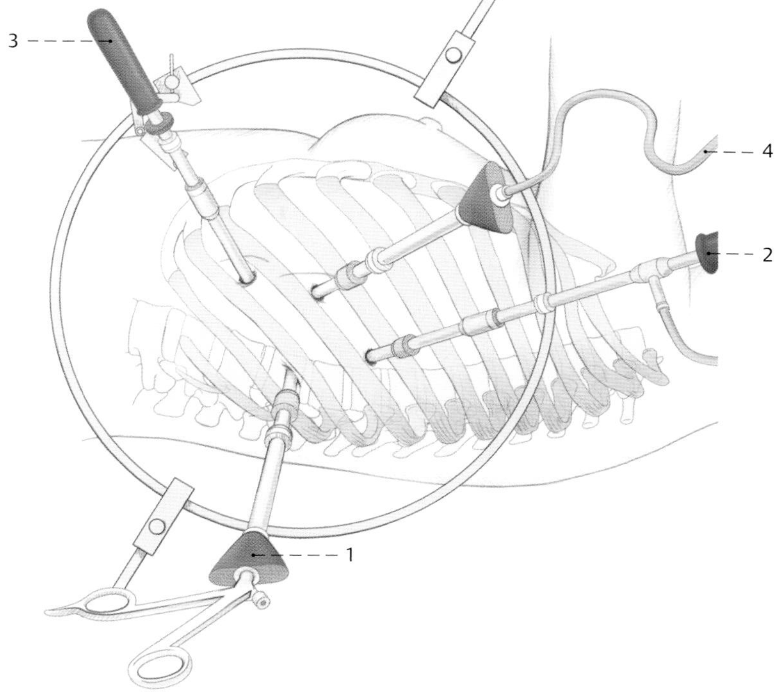

Fig. 2.47 Placement of portals and introduction of instruments.

1 Working portal with grasping forceps
2 Optic portal with thoracoscope
3 Retractor portal with fan retractor
4 Suction portal with suction catheter

2.4.8 Prevertebral Dissection

Prevertebral dissection is identical in both approaches. The correct location of the pathology must first be identified. Orientation points that can be visualized thoracoscopically (e.g., spondylophytes) or a prevertebral hematoma following trauma can be helpful. Otherwise, a Kirschner wire is placed in the intervertebral disk over the suspected location, and its correct position is evaluated with an image converter. Insertion of the Kirschner wire in the anterior part of the vertebral body is not recommended as the segmental vessels could be injured there.

After the height has been correctly located by means of the Kirschner wire, the optic is adjusted so that the structures shown in **Fig. 2.48** can be identified. It must be ensured that the monitor shows the operation site as visualized by the operator: in a left-sided minithoracotomy, the aorta appears cranially on the monitor, with the diaphragm on the left and the costotransverse joints posteriorly. A longitudinal incision is then made in the parietal pleura over the area of pathology. A central incision is ensured by palpation of the anterior border of the vertebral body and of the costotransverse joints. If incision of the diaphragm is necessary (dissection at the level of L1 and L2), the incision line is first marked by bipolar cautery, and a curved incision is then made in the diaphragm. A margin of at least 1 cm should be left on the lateral thoracic wall to allow reapproximation. The intersegmental vessels (**Fig. 2.49**) are then exposed by blunt dissection with a swab and coagulated; the arteries are clipped and divided (**Fig. 2.50**). Using the swab, the prevertebral tissue is pushed bluntly off the intervertebral disk compartments, and then in the plane between the segmental vessels and the vertebral body. Finally, the complete vertebral body is exposed.

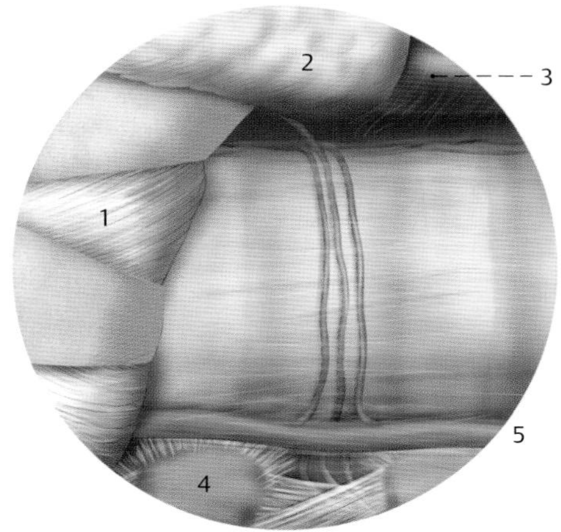

Fig. 2.48 Thoracoscopic visualization of the site: the lung and aorta are cranial, the diaphragm is on the left, and the costotransverse joints are posterior.

1 Diaphragm
2 Lung
3 Thoracic aorta
4 Costotransverse joints
5 Hemiazygos vein

In the minimally invasive, thoracoscopy-assisted operation using a retractor system, the retractors can now be moved to keep the operation site free. Instruments and optics introduced thoracoscopically can also be fixed to many retractor systems. This often facilitates and stabilizes the optic, which is otherwise done regularly by the assistant.

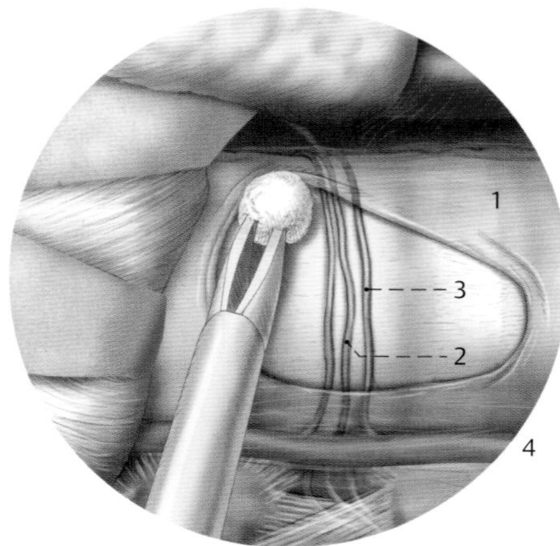

Fig. 2.49 Longitudinal incision of the parietal pleura and blunt exposure of the segmental vessels.

1 Parietal pleura
2 Posterior intercostal artery
3 Anterior external vertebral venous plexus
4 Hemiazygos vein

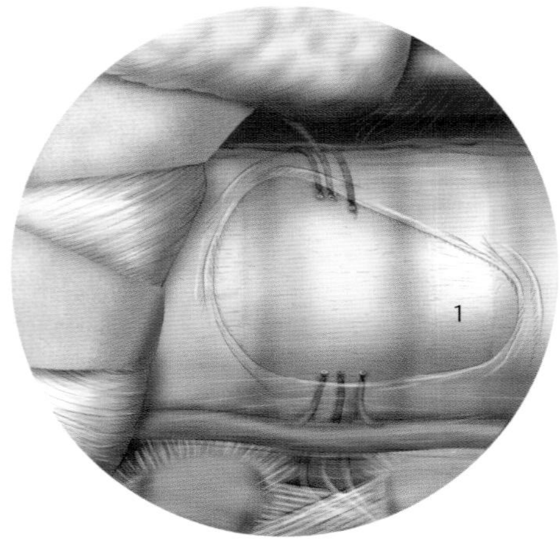

Fig. 2.50 Division of the segmental vessels and exposure of the vertebral body.

1 Intervertebral disk

2.4.9 Wound Closure

The minithoracotomy in the minimally invasive, thoracoscopy-assisted operation is closed similarly to a standard thoracotomy.

The trocar portals are closed in two layers, first a muscle suture and then a deeply placed skin back-and-forth suture. If a drain is placed through the trocar portal, a purse-string suture is recommended; this is tightened after removal of the drain.

3 Thoracolumbar Junction

3.1 Retroperitoneal Extrapleural Approach to the Thoracolumbar Spine T9–L5 According to Hodgson

R. Bauer, F. Kerschbaumer, S. Poisel

3.1.1 Principal Indications

- Scoliosis
- Kyphosis
- Vertebral body fractures
- Tumors
- Spondylitis

3.1.2 Choice of Side of Approach

Generally speaking, exposure of the thoracolumbar junction is possible using a right-sided as well as a left-sided approach. If the given indication does not prescribe the side to be used, the left-sided approach is preferable for anatomical reasons: the left dome of the diaphragm lies lower, and a right-sided exposure of the vertebrae is hampered by the liver and by the easily torn inferior vena cava. In cases of scoliosis, entry is made, as a general rule, from the side of the convexity.

3.1.3 Choice of Rib to be Resected

The standard approach in this technique, which is employed mainly in the surgical treatment of scoliosis, is at the level of the ninth or 10th rib. By resecting the 10th rib, T11 and possibly T10 can be reached; if the ninth rib is chosen for the approach, one naturally reaches a more cranial segment. In younger individuals with mobile ribs, it may be possible to gain access to the vertebra corresponding to the resected rib. If this should prove difficult, the segment close to the spine of the next higher rib is removed by the same approach. In favorable circumstances the following vertebrae can be reached:

- Resection of the ninth rib: access to T9–L5
- Resection of the 10th rib: access to T10–L5

3.1.4 Positioning and Incision

(**Fig. 3.1**)

The patient is placed on the right side. The skin incision begins posteriorly near the midline and follows the course of the 10th rib as far as the costal cartilage, continuing obliquely and distally in the epigastric and mesogastric regions in the direction of the segmental nerves (**Fig. 3.2**). It usually ends at a level between the umbilicus and the pubic symphysis. If only the thoracolumbar junction of the spine is to be exposed, the incision may be commensurately shorter. After transection of the skin, the incision is continued with a diathermy scalpel; visible vessels are immediately grasped by forceps and coagulated. Thorough hemostasis has to be assured during the operation. The latissimus dorsi is then transected along the

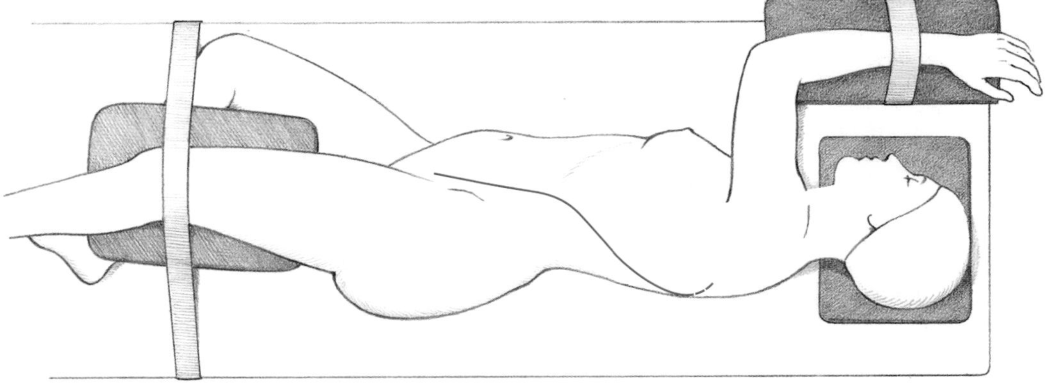

Fig. 3.1 Hodgson's approach to the thoracolumbar spine. Positioning and incision.

course of the 10th rib (**Fig. 3.3**, see also **Figs. 2.32** and **2.33**). More distally, the external oblique muscle of the abdomen is split in the direction of the fibers, exposing the 10th rib (**Fig. 3.4**).

During the ensuing operation, it proves advantageous first to expose the peritoneum from the side of the abdomen. The deep abdominal muscle layers (internal oblique and transversus abdominis) are generally forced apart by opening of the scissors, and two blunt hooks are inserted (**Fig. 3.4**). The peritoneum, now visible in the depths, is retracted medially from the lateral abdominal wall with a cotton applicator. Further exposure of the deep abdominal muscle layers is carried out in the direction of the costal arch parallel to the course of the vessels and nerves with the aid of a director. In this fashion, the upper lumbar spine is exposed retroperitoneally (**Fig. 3.5**). After this, the peritoneum is also detached from the inferior surface of the diaphragm.

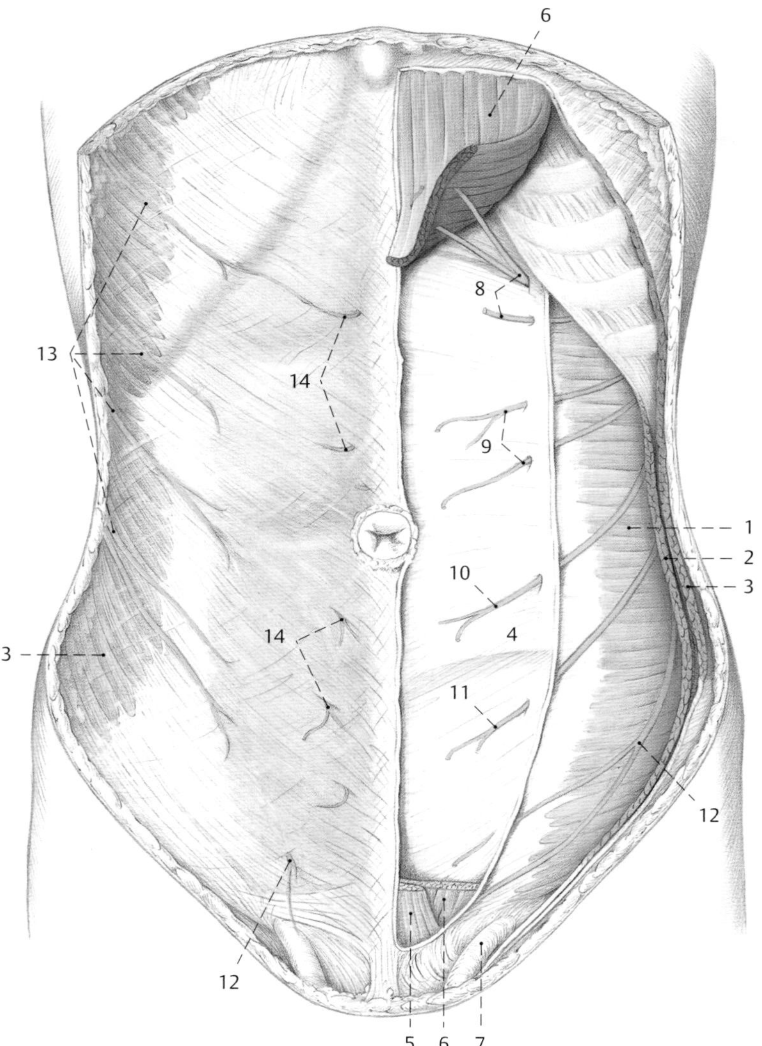

Fig. 3.2 Exposure of the nerve supply of the anterior abdominal wall.

1 Transversus abdominis
2 Internal oblique
3 External oblique
4 Rectus sheath, posterior layer
5 Pyramidalis
6 Rectus abdominis
7 Spermatic cord
8 Ninth intercostal nerve
9 Tenth intercostal nerve
10 Eleventh intercostal nerve
11 Subcostal nerve
12 Iliohypogastric nerve
13 Lateral cutaneous branches
14 Anterior cutaneous branches

Fig. 3.3 Anatomical exposure of the operative area after transection of the skin and subcutaneous tissue. ►

1 Serratus anterior
2 Latissimus dorsi
3 External oblique
X, XI Rib locations

Fig. 3.4 Operative site after transection of the latissimus dorsi, serratus anterior, external oblique, and deep abdominal muscle layers. ►

1 Serratus anterior
2 External oblique
3 Latissimus dorsi
4 Internal oblique and transversus abdominis
5 Peritoneum with preperitoneal fat
6 External intercostal muscle
X Rib

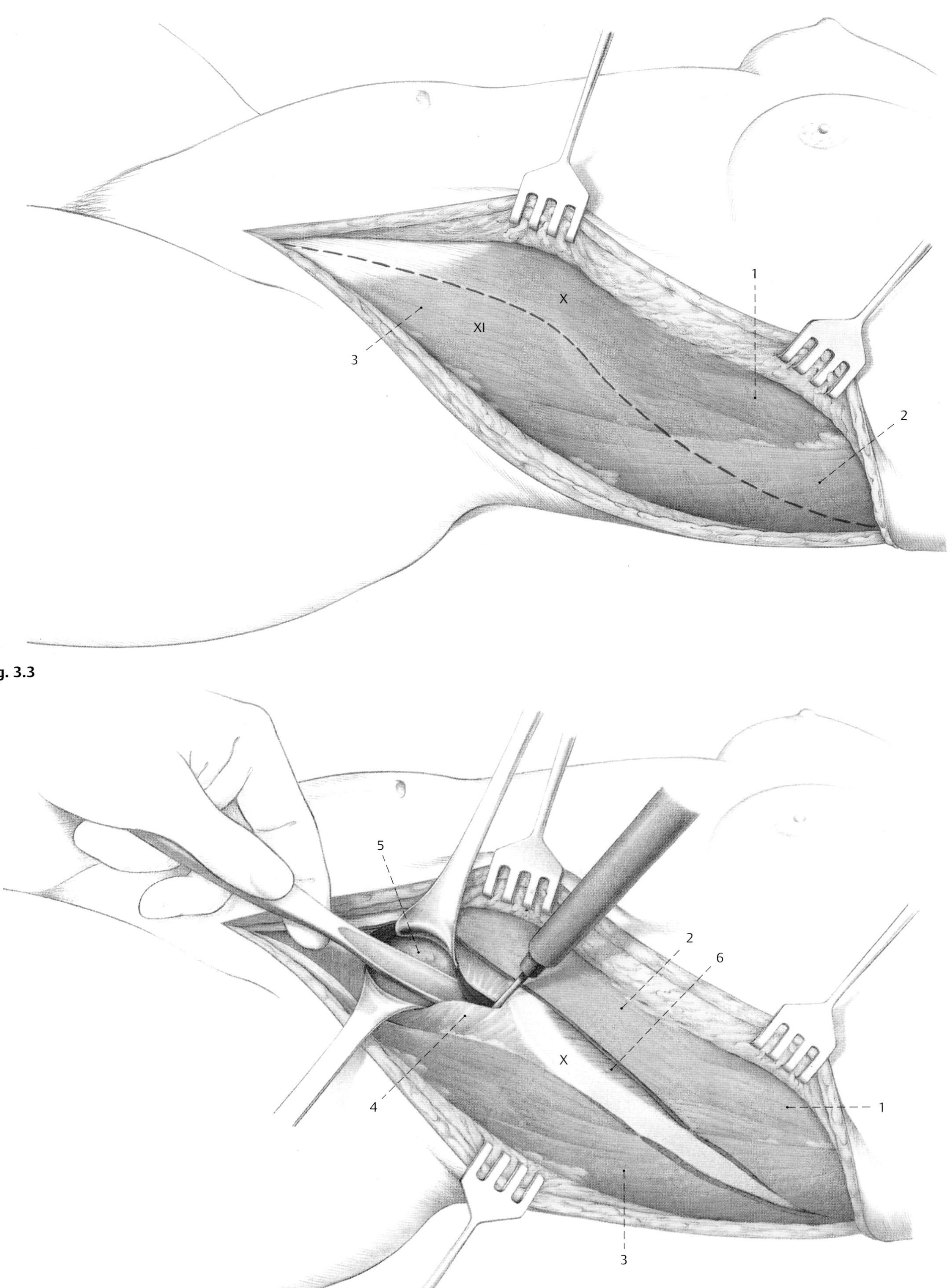

Fig. 3.3

Fig. 3.4

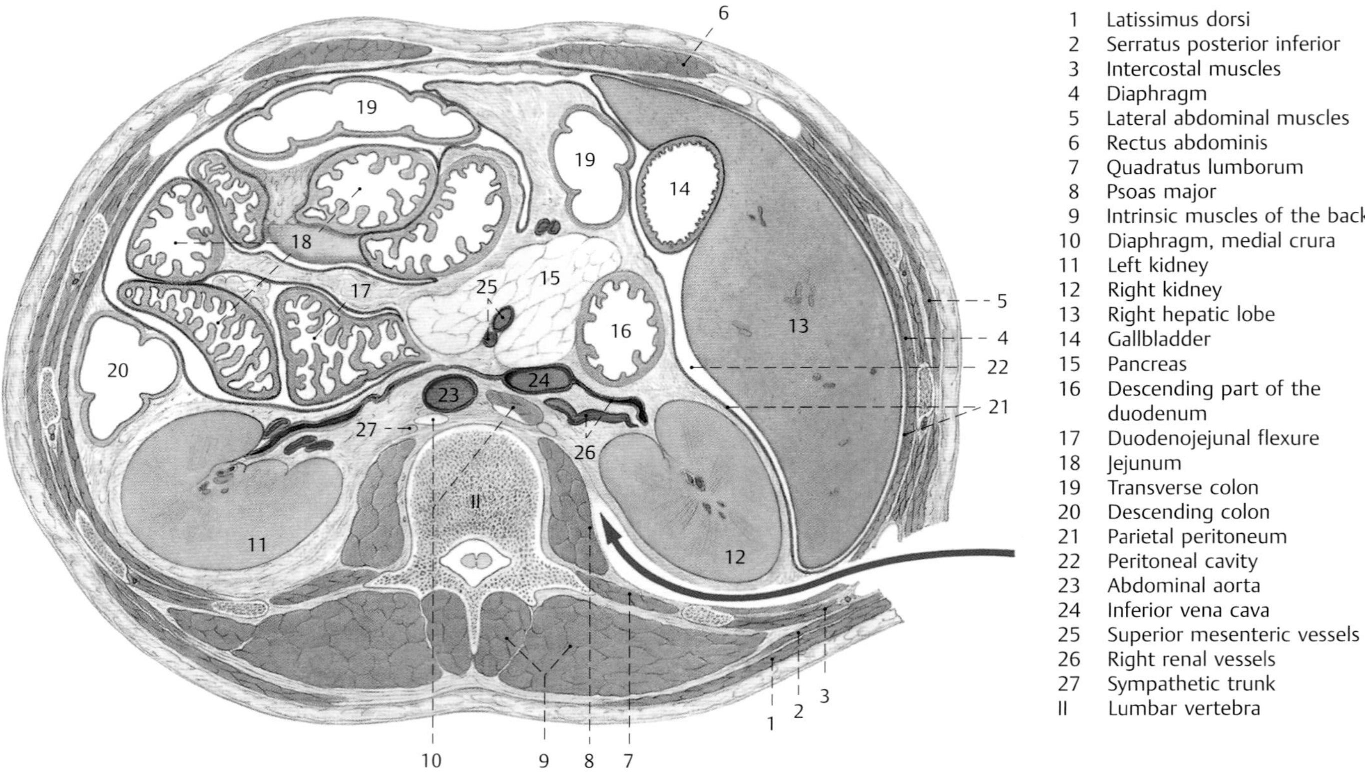

1 Latissimus dorsi
2 Serratus posterior inferior
3 Intercostal muscles
4 Diaphragm
5 Lateral abdominal muscles
6 Rectus abdominis
7 Quadratus lumborum
8 Psoas major
9 Intrinsic muscles of the back
10 Diaphragm, medial crura
11 Left kidney
12 Right kidney
13 Right hepatic lobe
14 Gallbladder
15 Pancreas
16 Descending part of the duodenum
17 Duodenojejunal flexure
18 Jejunum
19 Transverse colon
20 Descending colon
21 Parietal peritoneum
22 Peritoneal cavity
23 Abdominal aorta
24 Inferior vena cava
25 Superior mesenteric vessels
26 Right renal vessels
27 Sympathetic trunk
II Lumbar vertebra

Fig. 3.5 Transverse section at the level of the second lumbar vertebra. The approach for retroperitoneal dissection is identified by an arrow (right-sided approach).

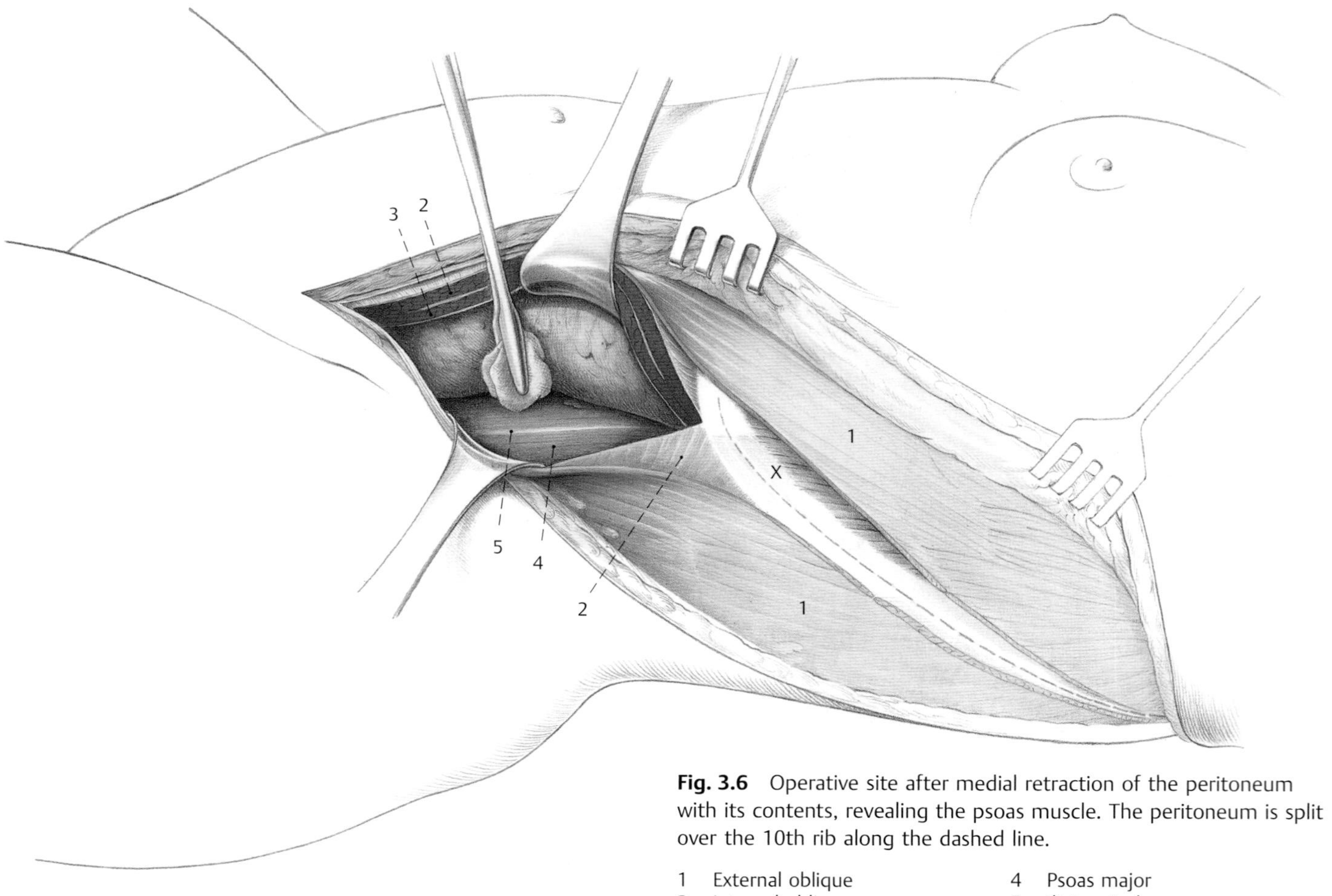

Fig. 3.6 Operative site after medial retraction of the peritoneum with its contents, revealing the psoas muscle. The peritoneum is split over the 10th rib along the dashed line.

1 External oblique
2 Internal oblique
3 Transversus abdominis
4 Psoas major
5 Ilioinguinal nerve
X Rib

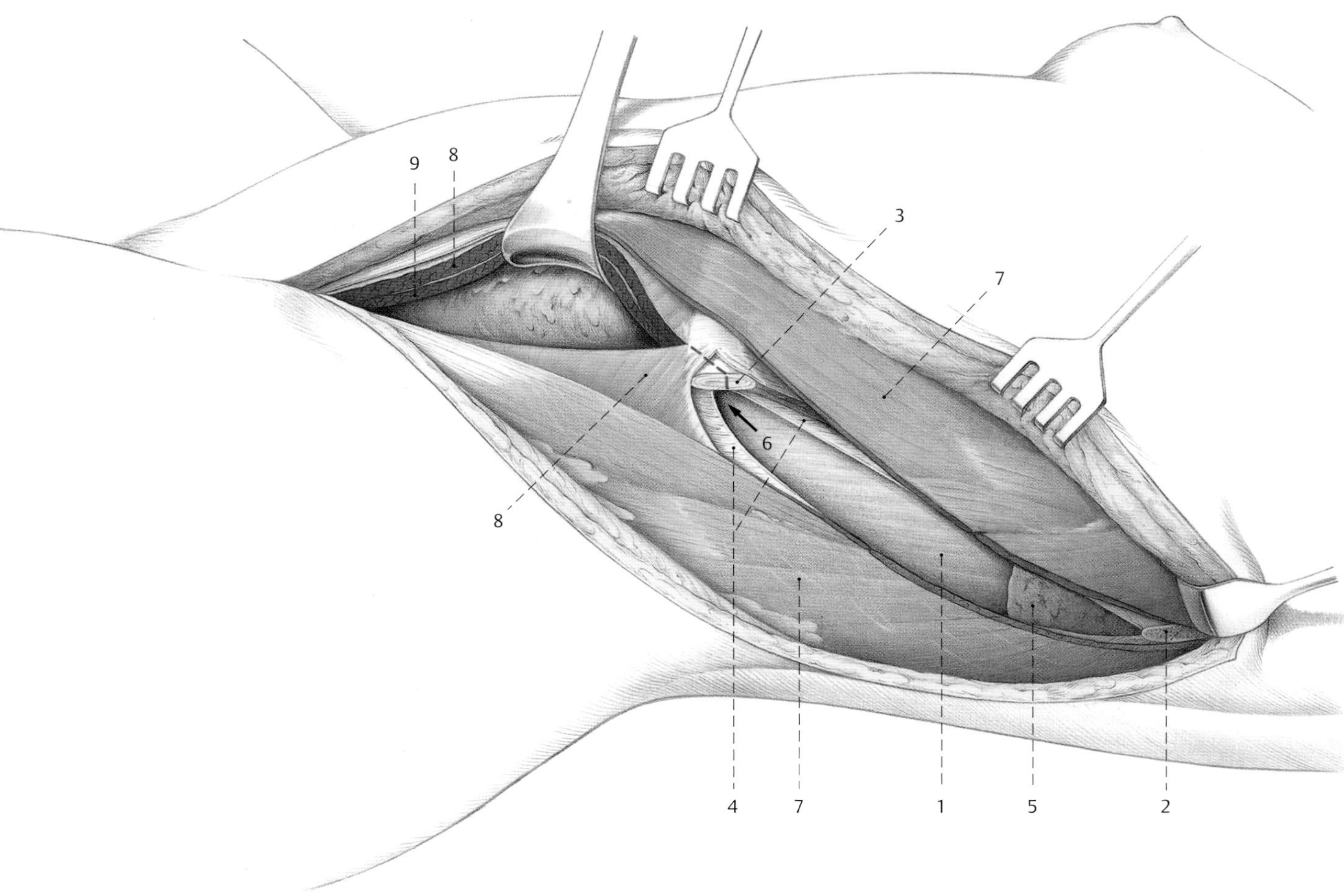

Fig. 3.7 Operative site after resection of the 10th rib and opening of the thorax in its bed. The costal cartilage is transected along the dashed line.

1 Diaphragm with diaphragmatic pleura
2 Stump of the 10th rib
3 Cartilage of the 10th rib
4 Periosteum of the rib and costal pleura
5 Left lung, inferior lobe
6 Costodiaphragmatic recess
7 External oblique
8 Internal oblique
9 Transversus abdominis

Subsequently, the periosteum of the 10th rib is transected using cutting diathermy along its entire length (**Fig. 3.6**), and the rib is then exposed with a raspatory in customary fashion. This is done in the direction of the fibers at the muscle insertion; that is, the rib is exposed cranially from posterior to anterior, and caudally from anterior to posterior. Finally, the 10th rib is divided transversely with a scalpel at the costochondral border, elevated, posteriorly transected with rib shears, and removed. The thorax is now opened by longitudinal division of the parietal pleura in the bed of the 10th rib (see Section 2.1.4, **Figs. 2.4**, **2.5**, **2.6**). By extending the thoracotomy incision, the remaining posterior part of the rib may be further exposed and resected if necessary near the costotransverse joint with a rib cutter. Enucleation of the head of the rib should be omitted since this can lead to severe bleeding. The costal cartilage is then divided with a scalpel; it will serve later as a landmark for wound closure (**Fig. 3.7**).

The peritoneum having previously been stripped off the inferior surface of the diaphragm, the diaphragm can now be transected under vision in a curved line beginning at a point approximately 2 cm away from the rib attachment and extending posterior to the spine (**Fig. 3.8**). Damage to the phrenic vessels and the branches of the phrenic nerve can thus be avoided (**Fig. 3.9**).

It is advantageous to place occasional marking sutures, which facilitate perfect approximation during wound closure (**Fig. 3.10**). A rib spreader is then inserted. The peritoneal contents and the lung are retracted manually by an assistant or with the aid of a suitable spatula.

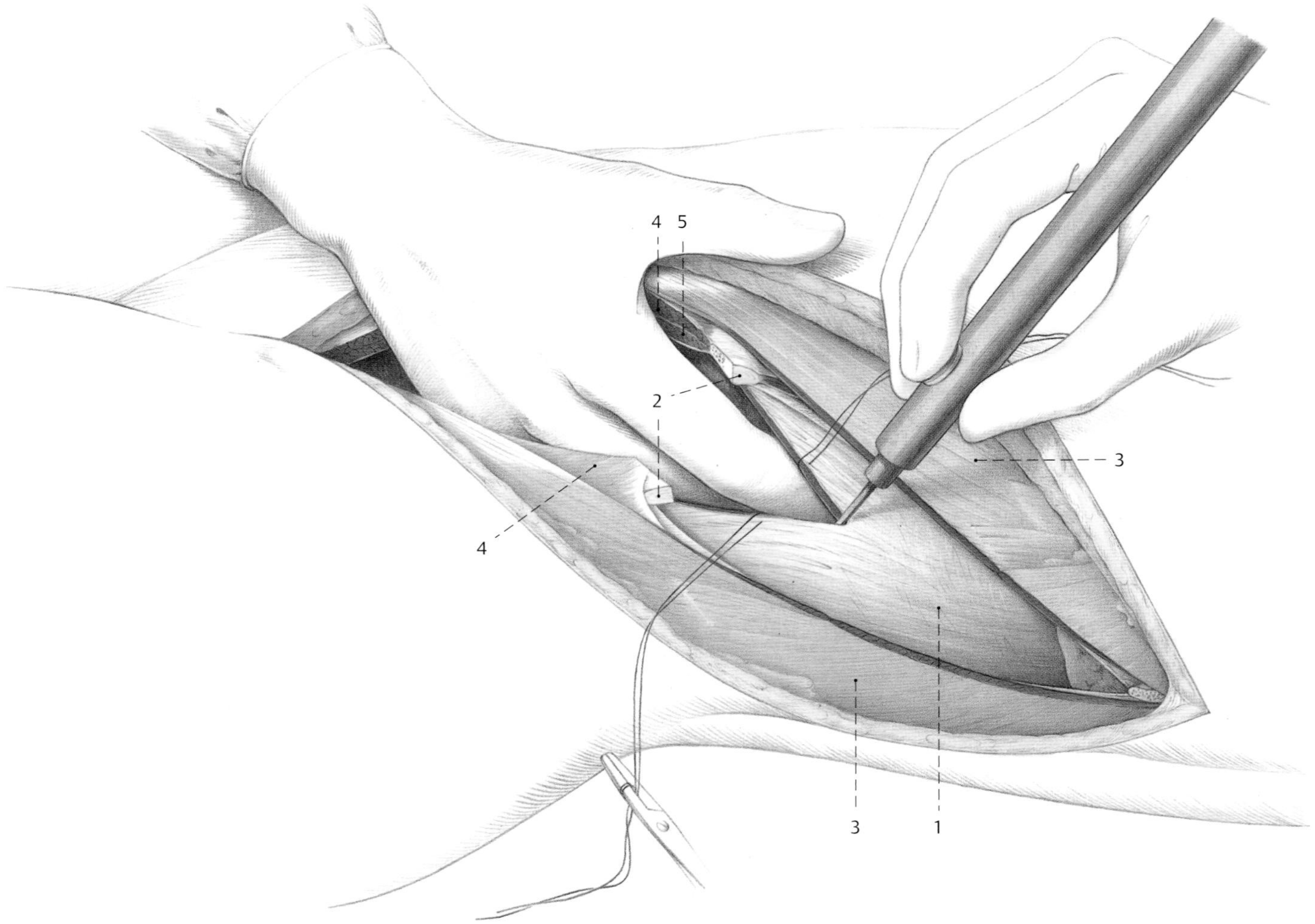

Fig. 3.8 Operative site after thoracotomy. The diaphragm is transected with the diathermy scalpel in a curved incision.

1 Diaphragm
2 Split cartilage of the 10th rib
3 External oblique
4 Internal oblique
5 Transversus abdominis

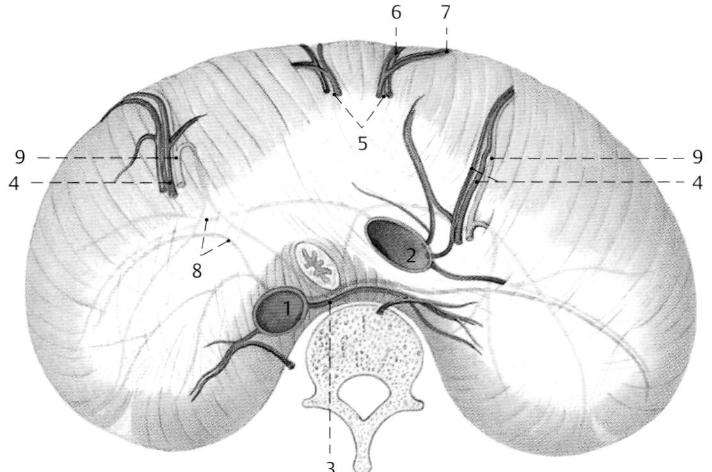

Fig. 3.9 Schematic representation of the diaphragm with the vascular and nerve supply viewed from the cranial direction.

1 Aorta
2 Inferior vena cava
3 Superior phrenic artery
4 Pericardiacophrenic vessels
5 Internal thoracic vessels
6 Superior epigastric vessels
7 Musculophrenic vessels
8 Inferior phrenic vessels
9 Phrenic nerve

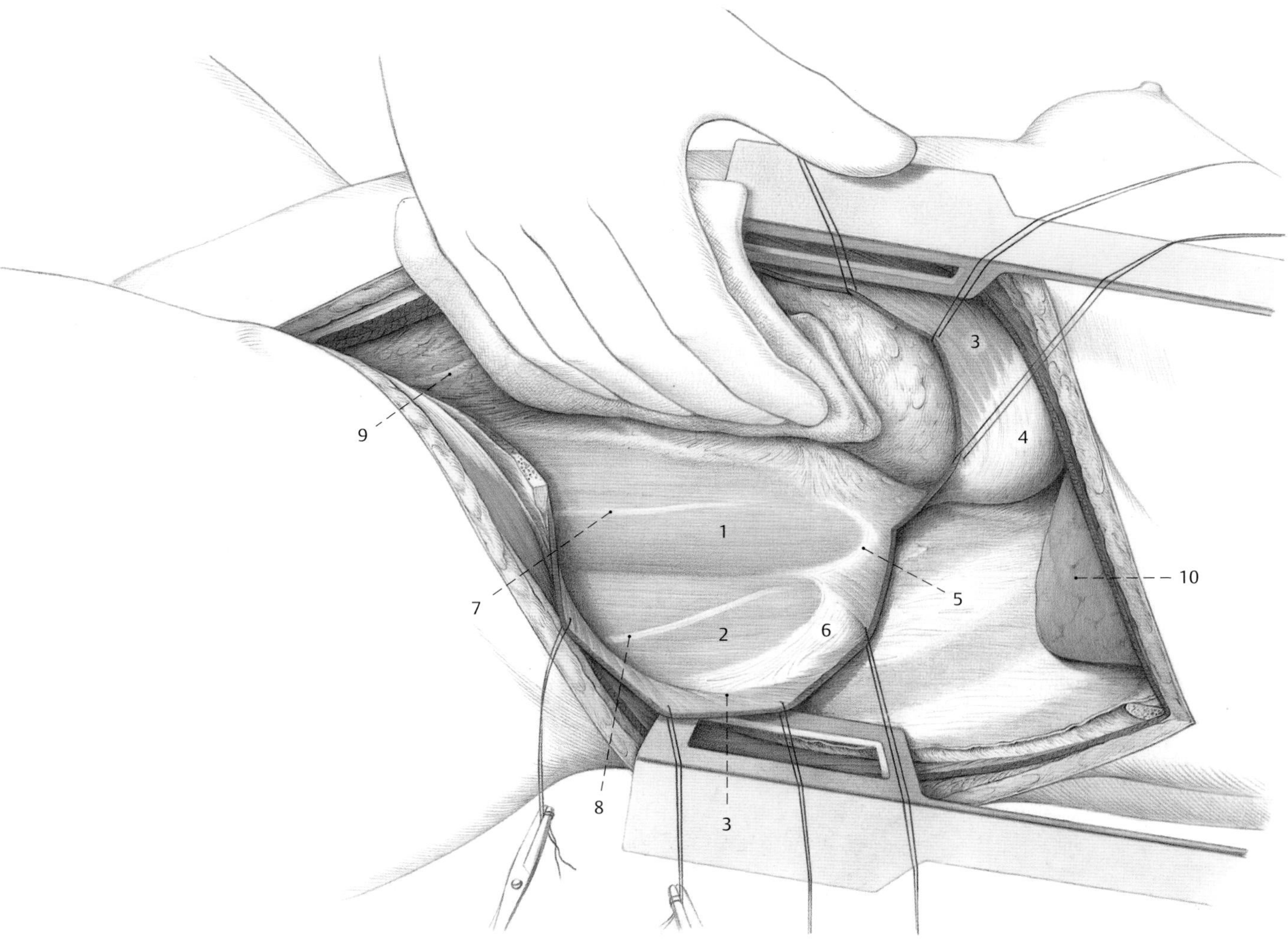

Fig. 3.10 Operative site after thoracotomy and exposure of the left retroperitoneal space.

1 Psoas major
2 Quadratus lumborum
3 Diaphragm
4 Diaphragm, central tendon
5 Medial arcuate ligament
6 Lateral arcuate ligament
7 Ilioinguinal nerve
8 Iliohypogastric nerve
9 Ureter
10 Lung

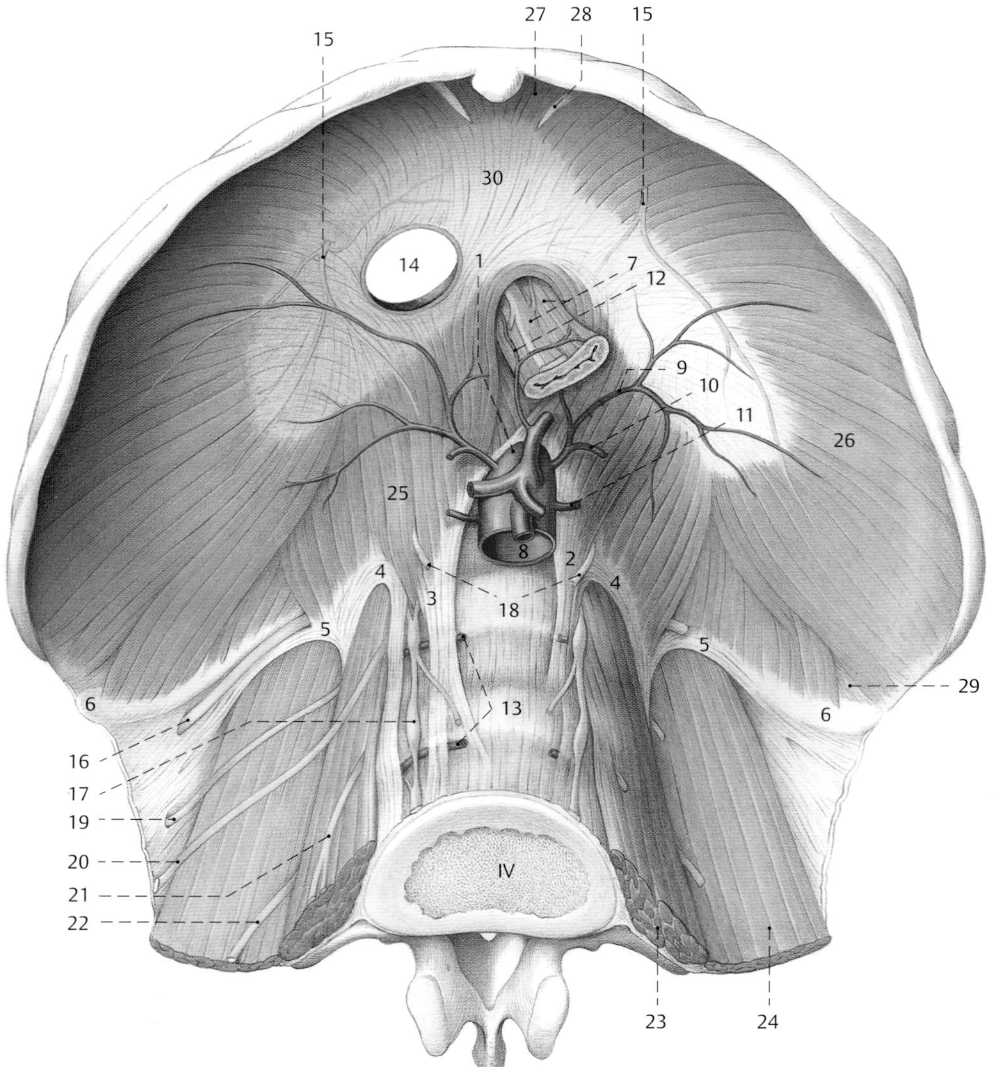

Fig. 3.11 Anatomical exposure of the diaphragm and the structures that traverse it.

1 Median arcuate ligament
2 Left crus
3 Right crus
4 Medial arcuate ligament
5 Lateral arcuate ligament
6 Twelfth rib
7 Esophagus and anterior vagal trunk
8 Aorta with celiac trunk and superior mesenteric artery
9 Inferior phrenic artery
10 Superior suprarenal artery
11 Middle suprarenal artery
12 Left gastric artery, esophageal branch
13 Lumbar arteries
14 Inferior vena cava
15 Phrenic nerve
16 Subcostal nerve
17 Sympathetic trunk
18 Greater splanchnic nerve
19 Iliohypogastric nerve
20 Ilioinguinal nerve
21 Genitofemoral nerve
22 Lateral cutaneous nerve of the thigh
23 Psoas major
24 Quadratus lumborum
25 Diaphragm, lumbar part
26 Diaphragm, costal part
27 Diaphragm, sternal part
28 Sternocostal triangle
29 Lumbocostal triangle
30 Tendinous center
IV Lumbar vertebra

In the next step, the lumbar part of the diaphragm with the left crus is transected. To subsequently undertake the appropriate procedure, the following structures first need to be identified (**Fig. 3.11**). The greater splanchnic nerve passes through the diaphragm with the ascending lumbar vein (or the azygos vein) between the medial and intermediate crus, and runs distally and medially to the celiac plexus. Somewhat more laterally, the sympathetic trunk passes through the diaphragm between the intermediate crus and the lateral crus. The left diaphragmatic crus is dissected approximately 1.5 cm above the lateral or medial arcuate ligament. Preferably, a grooved director or a curved clamp is inserted into the aortic hiatus directly underneath the diaphragmatic crus. The diaphragm is transected in the direction of the grooved director in such a way that the greater splanchnic nerve cranially and the sympathetic trunk caudally remain undamaged (**Fig. 3.12**). Occasionally, segmental vessels or branches of the ascending lumbar vein have to be ligated and transected.

The retroperitoneal tissue and/or the parietal pleura on the spine is now elevated with forceps, and a scissor incision is made along the axis of the vertebral column. The parietal pleura is then slightly retracted bilaterally; a curved clamp is passed beneath the segmental vessels that run transversely over the vertebral bodies, and these are then transected between the ligatures (**Fig. 3.13**).

Fig. 3.12 Operative site after complete transection of the left half of the diaphragm and of the left diaphragmatic crus. Exposure of the vertebrae by splitting of the retroperitoneal tissue or of the parietal pleura along the dashed line. ►

1 Diaphragm
2 Right crus
3 Left crus
4 Abdominal aorta
5 Lumbar vessels
6 Ascending lumbar vein
7 Sympathetic trunk
8 Greater splanchnic nerve

Fig. 3.13 Operative site after transection of the segmental vessels. Exposure of the vertebral bodies. ►

1 Psoas major laterally retracted from the spine
2 Anterior longitudinal ligament
3 Lumbar vessels
4 Greater splanchnic nerve
5 Sympathetic trunk
II–IV Lumbar vertebrae

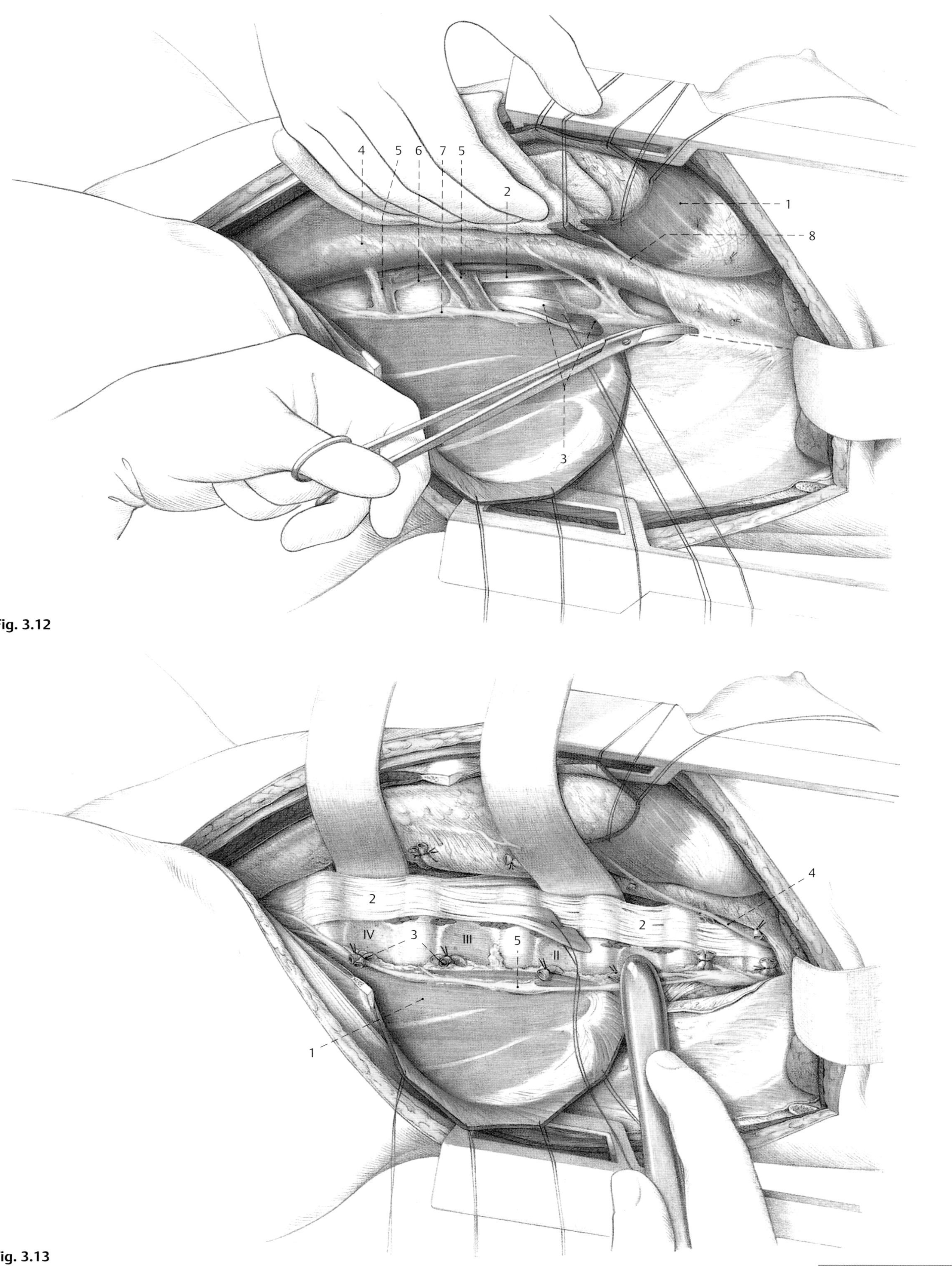

Fig. 3.12

Fig. 3.13

3.1.5 Exposure of Individual Vertebrae

The vertebrae may now be exposed. The process always begins over the intervertebral disks, which are the prominent areas, since no vessels are found here. A cotton applicator is inserted above the intervertebral disks or above the vertebral bodies, and the tissue is retracted until the base of the transverse processes is reached on both sides. The sympathetic trunk is laterally retracted (see **Fig. 3.13**). The origins of psoas are detached from the intervertebral disks in the region of the lumbar spine so that these can be exposed as far as the intervertebral foramina. **Fig. 3.14** presents the anatomical situation in this approach.

With a sufficiently long incision, this approach also gives access to the promontory and cranial portions of the sacrum (**Fig. 3.15**). Particular importance should be attached to exposure and ligation of the iliolumbar vessels.

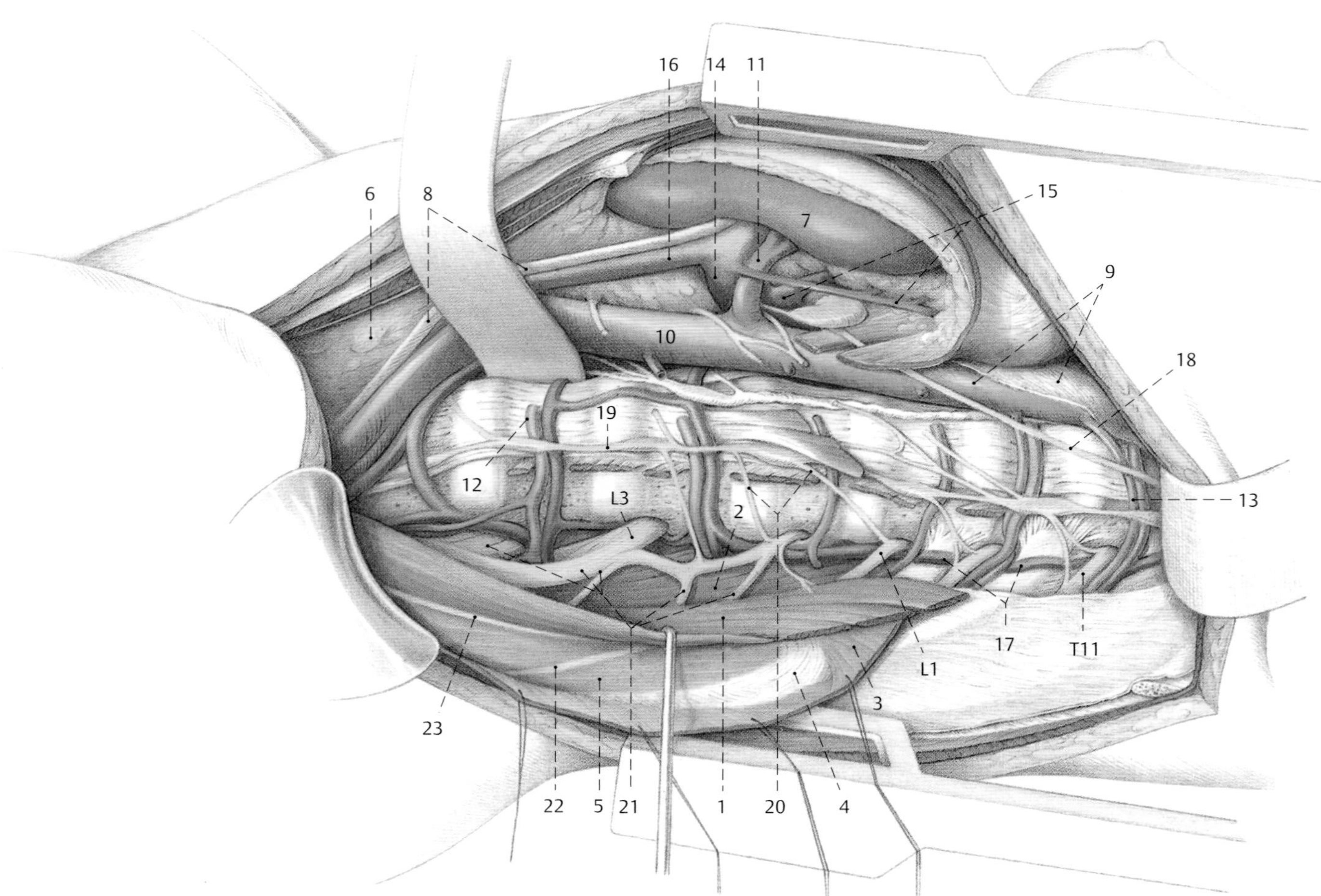

Fig. 3.14 Anatomical site of the left retroperitoneal space and left retropleural space.

1 Psoas major, superficial origin
2 Psoas major, deep origin
3 Diaphragm
4 Lateral arcuate ligament
5 Quadratus lumborum
6 Peritoneum
7 Left kidney
8 Ureter
9 Thoracic aorta
10 Abdominal aorta
11 Renal artery
12 Lumbar artery
13 Intercostal artery
14 Renal vein
15 Suprarenal veins
16 Ovarian vein
17 Ascending lumbar vein
18 Greater splanchnic nerve
19 Sympathetic trunk
20 Communicating branches
21 Lumbar plexus
22 Iliohypogastric nerve
23 Ilioinguinal nerve
T11, L1, L3 Spinal nerves, anterior branches

3.1.6 Wound Closure

The psoas is reinserted into the area of origin. Anatomical restoration of the left diaphragmatic crus is important (**Fig. 3.16**). In the thoracic region, the parietal pleura is then closed over the spine by a continuous suture. Using interrupted sutures tied extrathoracically, the diaphragm is closed from medial posterior to lateral anterior. Finally, the cartilage of the 10th rib, which served as a landmark, is sutured (**Fig. 3.17**). A chest drain is then inserted, a rib approximator is applied, the parietal pleura is sutured within the bed of the resected rib, and the thoracic wall (intercostal muscles, latissimus dorsi, serratus anterior) as well as the abdominal muscles are sutured in layers.

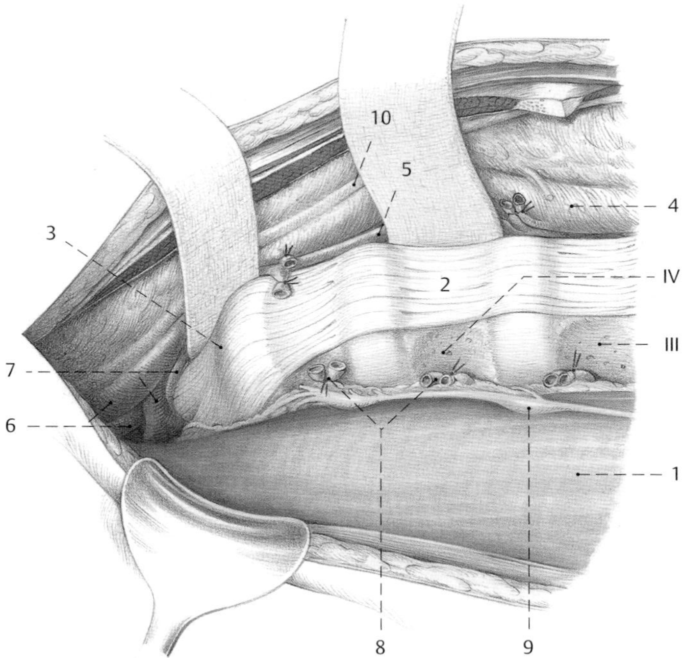

Fig. 3.15 Operative site in exposure of the lumbosacral junction.

1 Psoas major
2 Anterior longitudinal ligament
3 Promontory
4 Abdominal aorta
5 Inferior vena cava
6 External iliac artery and vein
7 Internal iliac artery and vein
8 Lumbar artery and vein
9 Sympathetic trunk
10 Ureter
III, IV Lumbar vertebrae

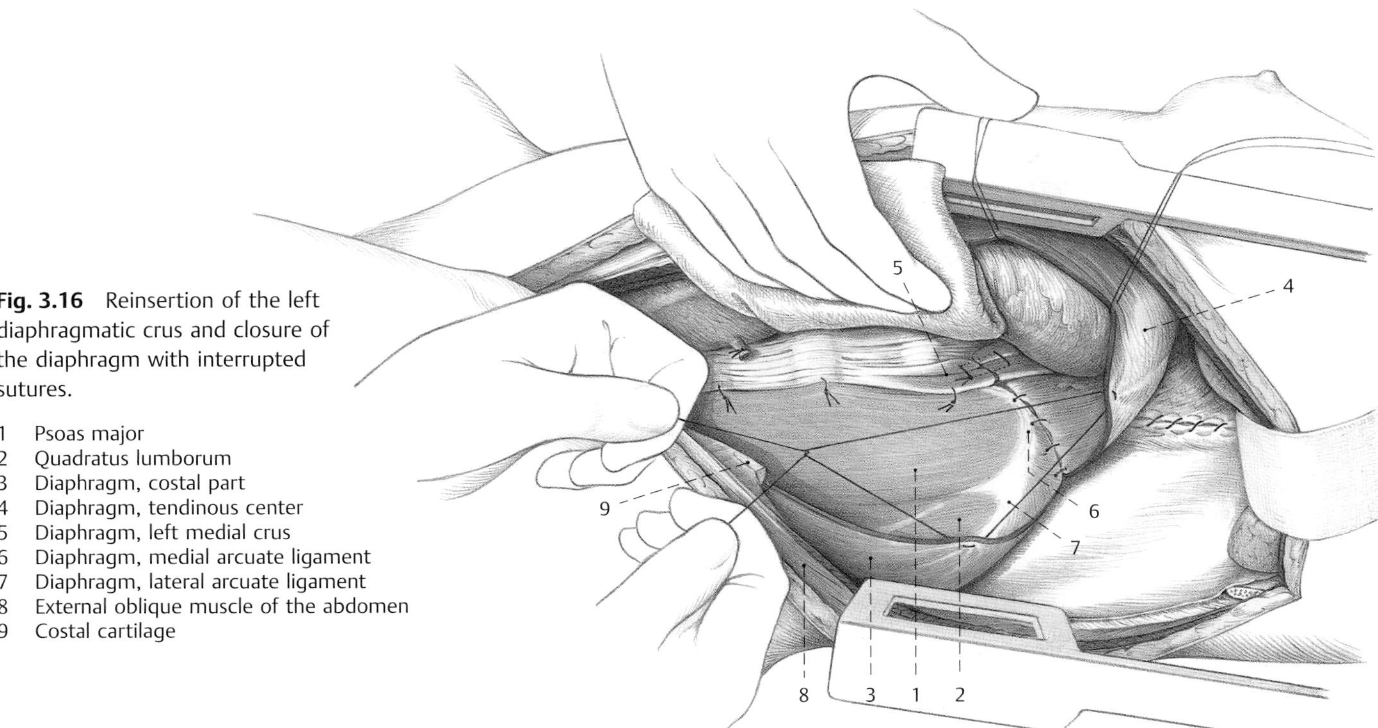

Fig. 3.16 Reinsertion of the left diaphragmatic crus and closure of the diaphragm with interrupted sutures.

1 Psoas major
2 Quadratus lumborum
3 Diaphragm, costal part
4 Diaphragm, tendinous center
5 Diaphragm, left medial crus
6 Diaphragm, medial arcuate ligament
7 Diaphragm, lateral arcuate ligament
8 External oblique muscle of the abdomen
9 Costal cartilage

3.1.7 Approach to the Thoracolumbar Spine According to Hodgson from the Right

The operation is performed similarly to the left-sided approach but with the sides reversed (see **Fig. 3.5**). The main differences arise in the exposure of the diaphragm from the abdomen. The diaphragmatic aspect of the right hepatic lobe is fused with the right diaphragm over an approximately palm-sized area. Therefore, only a relatively narrow portion of the diaphragm near the rib can be exposed. In this area, the diaphragm is incised, and the liver is mobilized with the diaphragm step by step and retracted toward the left. The inferior vena cava may cause difficulties: not until transection of the right lumbar veins is it possible to retract the vena cava toward the left (see Section 3.2.4, **Figs. 3.20** and **3.21**).

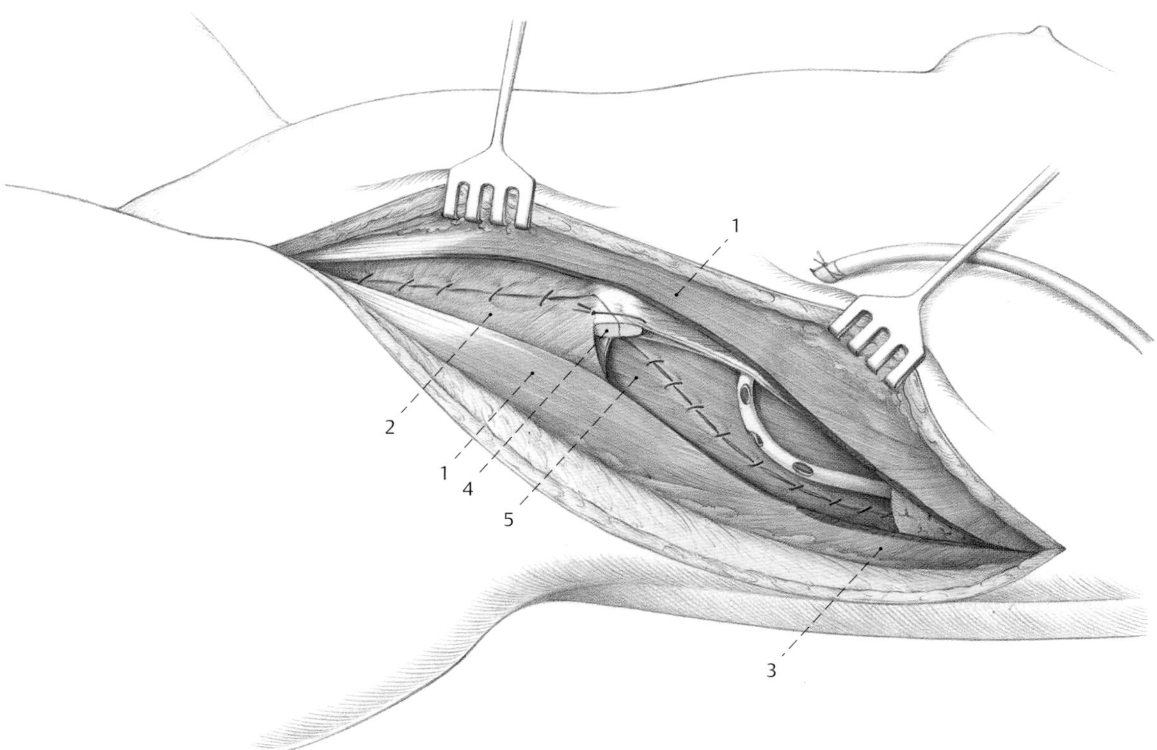

Fig. 3.17 Suture of the diaphragm and abdominal muscles.

1 External oblique
2 Internal oblique
3 Latissimus dorsi
4 Cartilage of the 10th rib
5 Diaphragm

3.2 Approach to Thoracolumbar Spine with Two-fold Thoracotomy T4–L5 According to Bauer

R. Bauer, F. Kerschbaumer, S. Poisel

If sizable portions of the thoracic spine are to be exposed in addition to the thoracolumbar junction and the lumbar spine, Hodgson's approach may be combined with a second thoracotomy.

3.2.1 Principal Indication

- Mostly long-curve scoliosis

3.2.2 Choice of Side of Approach

This approach generally can be applied to the right as well as to the left side.

3.2.3 Choice of Level of Thoracotomy

Entry will generally be made at least one intercostal space higher than the most cranially situated vertebra to be reached. The intercostal thoracotomy can then be combined with the typical approach to the thoracolumbar spine according to Hodgson with resection of the 10th rib.

Example: Thoracotomy in sixth intercostal space, resection of 10th rib: T7–L5 approach.

3.2.4 Positioning and Incision

Depending on the side of the approach, the patient is placed on the right or left side. The skin incision begins near the midline, continues forward along the sixth rib for example, and then curves in a caudal direction slightly anteriorly to the anterior axillary line. About three fingerbreadths medial to the anterior iliac spine, it is extended into the right upper and lower abdomen, depending on the exposure desired (**Fig. 3.18**). Now a skin–subcutaneous tissue flap is dissected in a caudal and posterior direction until the 10th rib becomes visible (**Fig. 3.19**). Hereafter, the procedure initially conforms to the typical approach according to Hodgson (see Section 3.1.4, **Fig. 3.3ff**).

The latissimus dorsi and serratus anterior are transected as far caudally as possible (see **Figs. 2.32** and **2.33**), and then the external oblique is divided in the direction of its fibers. Subsequently, the deep layers of the abdominal muscles are dissected. The peritoneum is exposed and retracted medially with a cotton applicator, in this case from the right lateral and posterior abdominal wall. Owing to the anatomy of the liver, the possibility of stripping peritoneum from the underside of the diaphragm on the right side is very limited. The posterior aspect of the right liver lobe is fused with the diaphragm over an approximately palm-sized area. Resection of the 10th rib is followed typically by thoracotomy. After exposure of the 10th costal cartilage, the diaphragm is transected fairly closely to the rib, and the liver with the central portions of the diaphragm is thus progressively retracted medially. This provides an increasingly satisfactory approach to the more posteriorly located segments of the diaphragm (**Fig. 3.20**). After tagging with sutures, the right diaphragmatic crus is transected. Next the retroperitoneal tissue and the parietal pleura over the spine are split in customary fashion, the segmental vessels are ligated, and the inferior vena cava is retracted to the left (**Fig. 3.21**). The spine can thus be exposed from L5, and possibly from the sacrum, to at least T11.

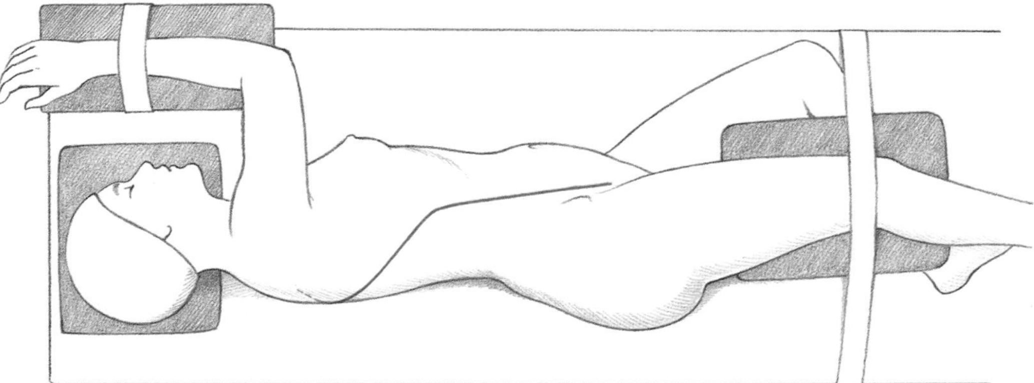

Fig. 3.18 Approach to thoracolumbar spine with two-fold thoracotomy. Positioning and incision.

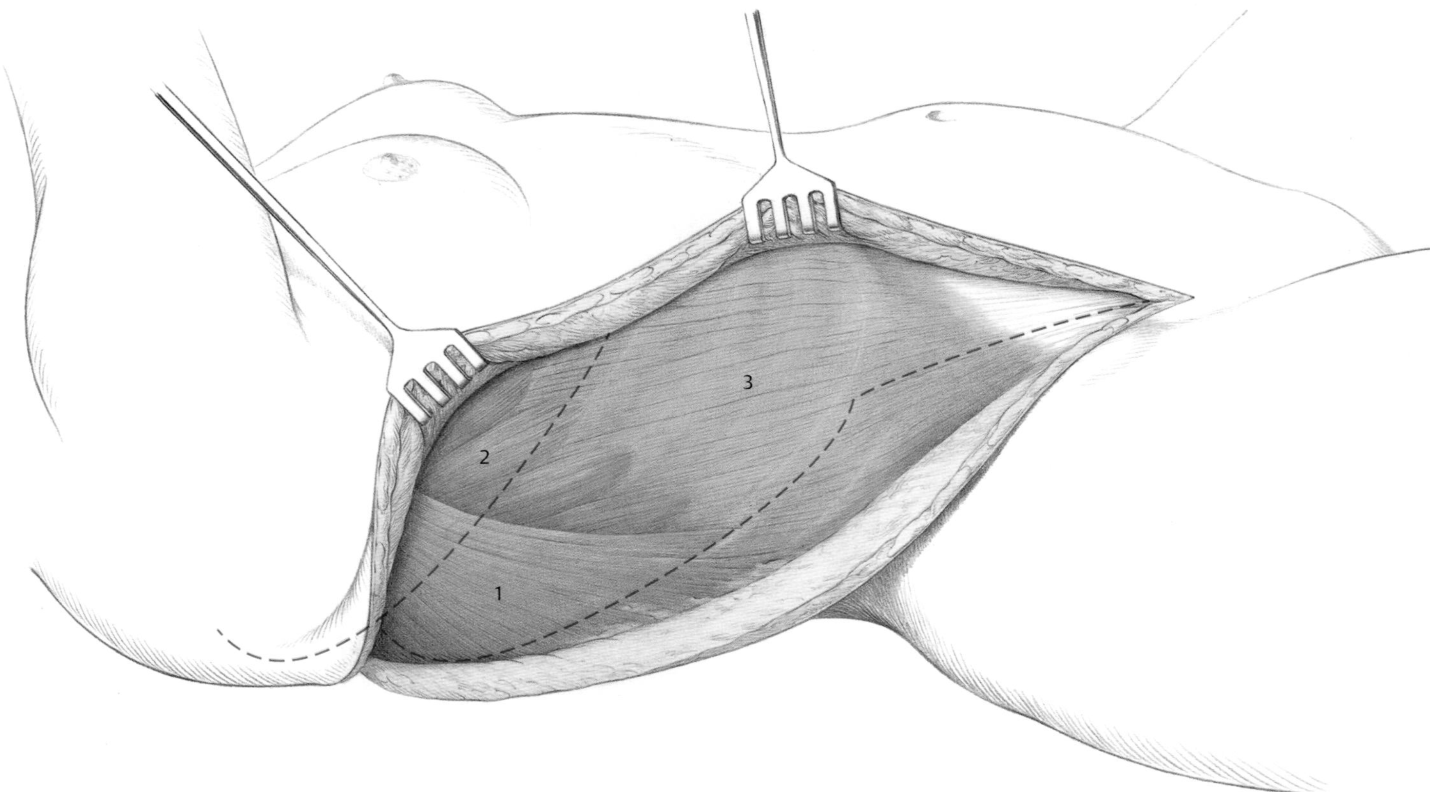

Fig. 3.19 Exposure of the operative field after incision of the skin and subcutaneous tissue. The latissimus dorsi is transected as far caudally as possible in accordance with the standard thoracolumbar approach (the caudal dashed line). For intercostal thoracotomy (the cranial dashed line), the cranial portion of the latissimus dorsi is folded upward.

1 Latissimus dorsi
2 Serratus anterior
3 External oblique

Fig. 3.20 Operative site after resection of the 10th rib. Transection of the diaphragm including the right diaphragmatic crus and exposure of the right retroperitoneal space. ►

1 Latissimus dorsi
2 Serratus anterior
3 Psoas major
4 Quadratus lumborum
5 Diaphragm
6 Diaphragm, right crus
7 Inferior vena cava
8 Sympathetic trunk
9 Greater splanchnic nerve
10 Iliohypogastric nerve
11 Genitofemoral nerve
12 Inferior lobe of the right lung
XI, XII Ribs

Fig. 3.21 Operative site with exposure of the caudal segment of the thoracic spine and lumbar spine after ligation and transection of the segmental vessels. The lower margin of the liver and the inferior vena cava are visible. ►

1 Medial arcuate ligament
2 Lateral arcuate ligament
3 Sympathetic trunk
4 Greater splanchnic nerve
5 Inferior vena cava
6 Lumbar arteries and veins
7 Posterior intercostal arteries and veins
8 Liver

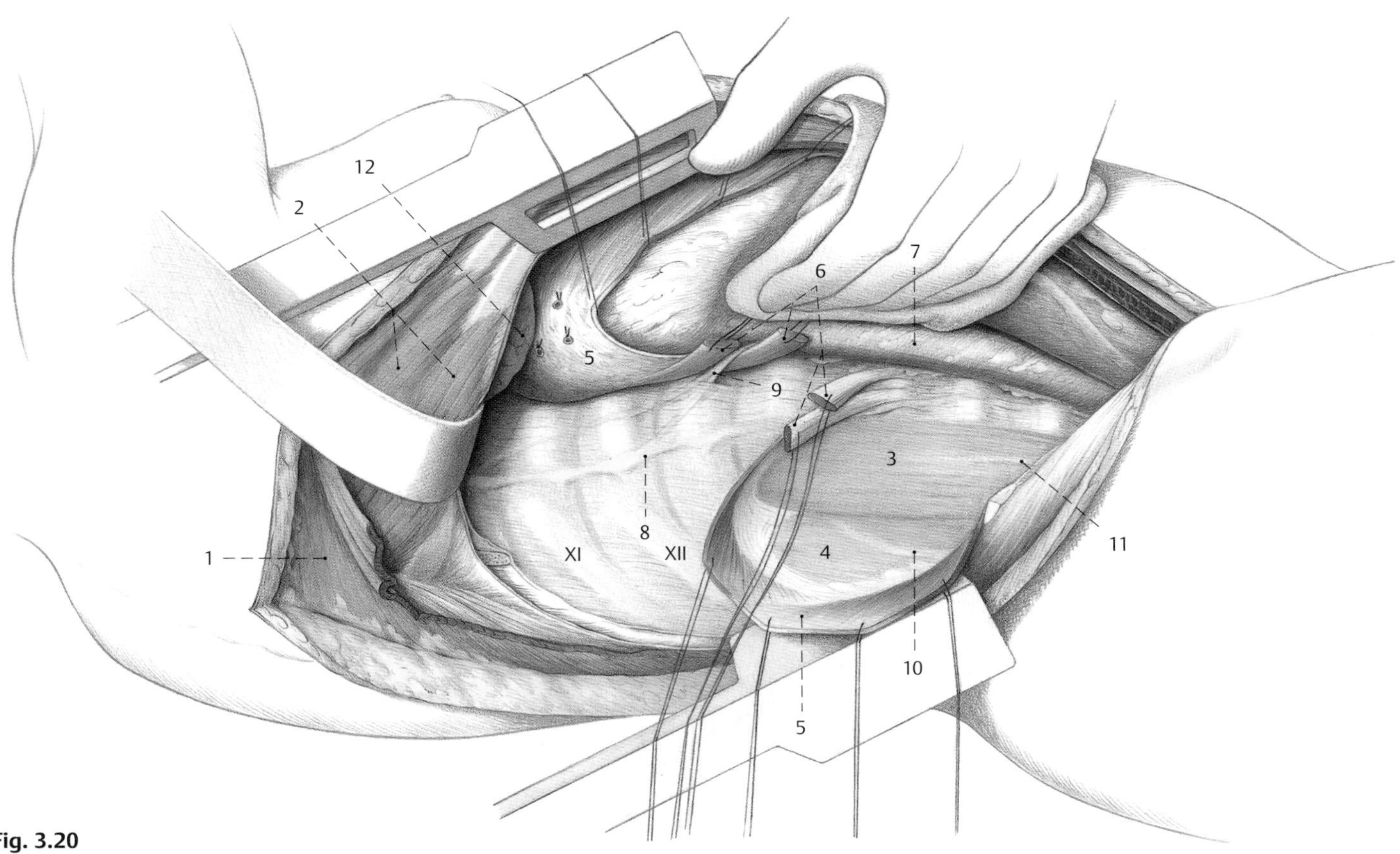

Fig. 3.20

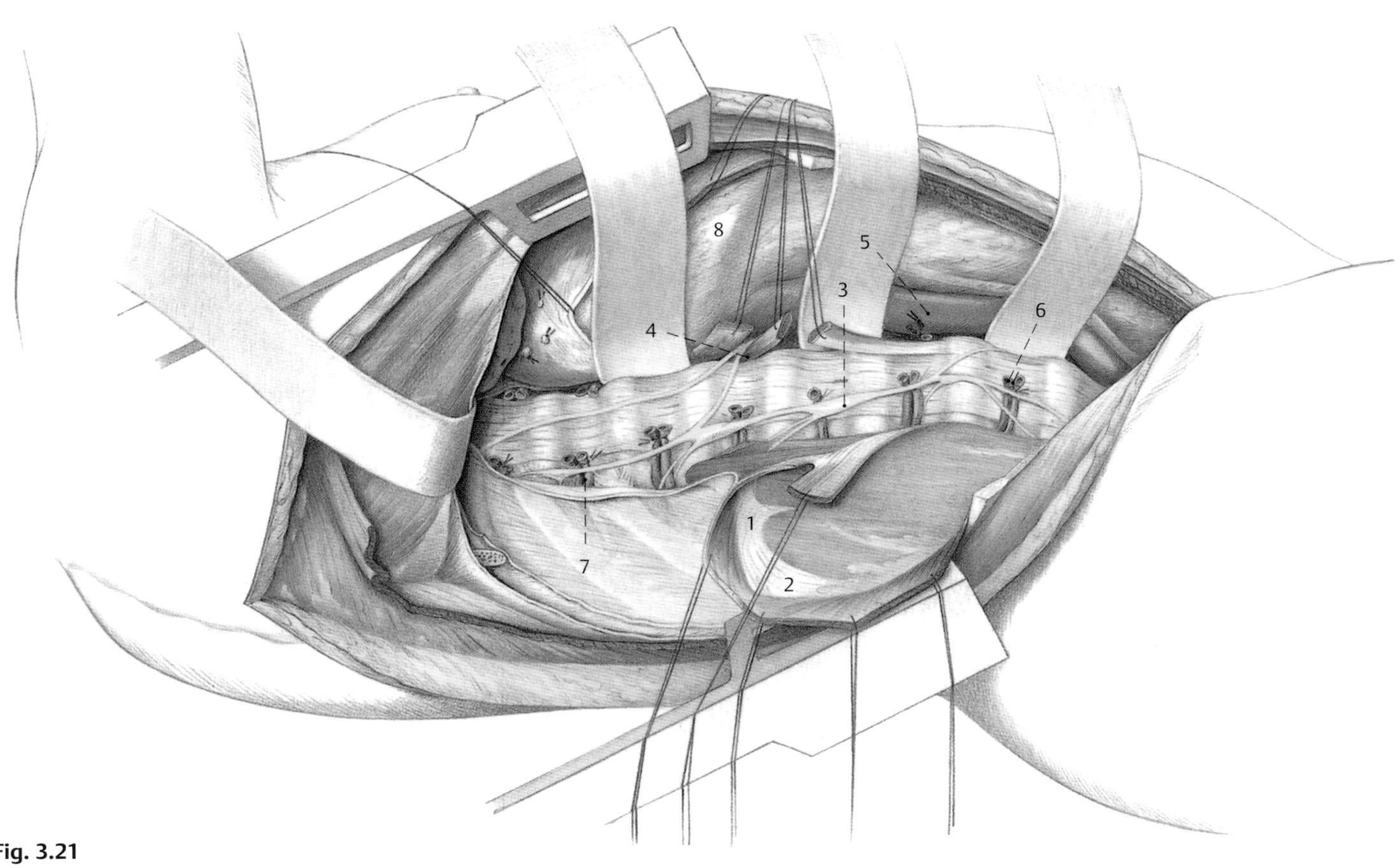

Fig. 3.21

After this part of the procedure, the cranial portion of the transected latissimus dorsi is retracted upward, and an intercostal thoracotomy is performed in the sixth intercostal space (see **Fig. 3.19**; see also Section 2.1.6, **Fig. 2.7**). The intercostal muscles are transected, the thoracic cavity is opened, and a rib spreader is inserted (**Fig. 3.22**). The splitting of the parietal pleura begun in the area of the thoracolumbar junction is continued over the spine in a cranial direction. Further exposure of the spine is performed in typical fashion following ligation and transection of the segmental vessels. Depending on the necessary operative steps, the ribs located between the intercostal thoracotomy and the thoracolumbar approach (generally three or four) may be mobilized in a cranial or caudal direction so that the desired vertebrae may be reached.

3.2.5 Wound Closure

The intercostal thoracotomy is closed in the customary manner with pericostal sutures (see **Fig. 2.21**). Otherwise, standard wound closure, as in Hodgson's approach to the thoracolumbar spine, is performed (see **Figs. 3.16** and **3.17**).

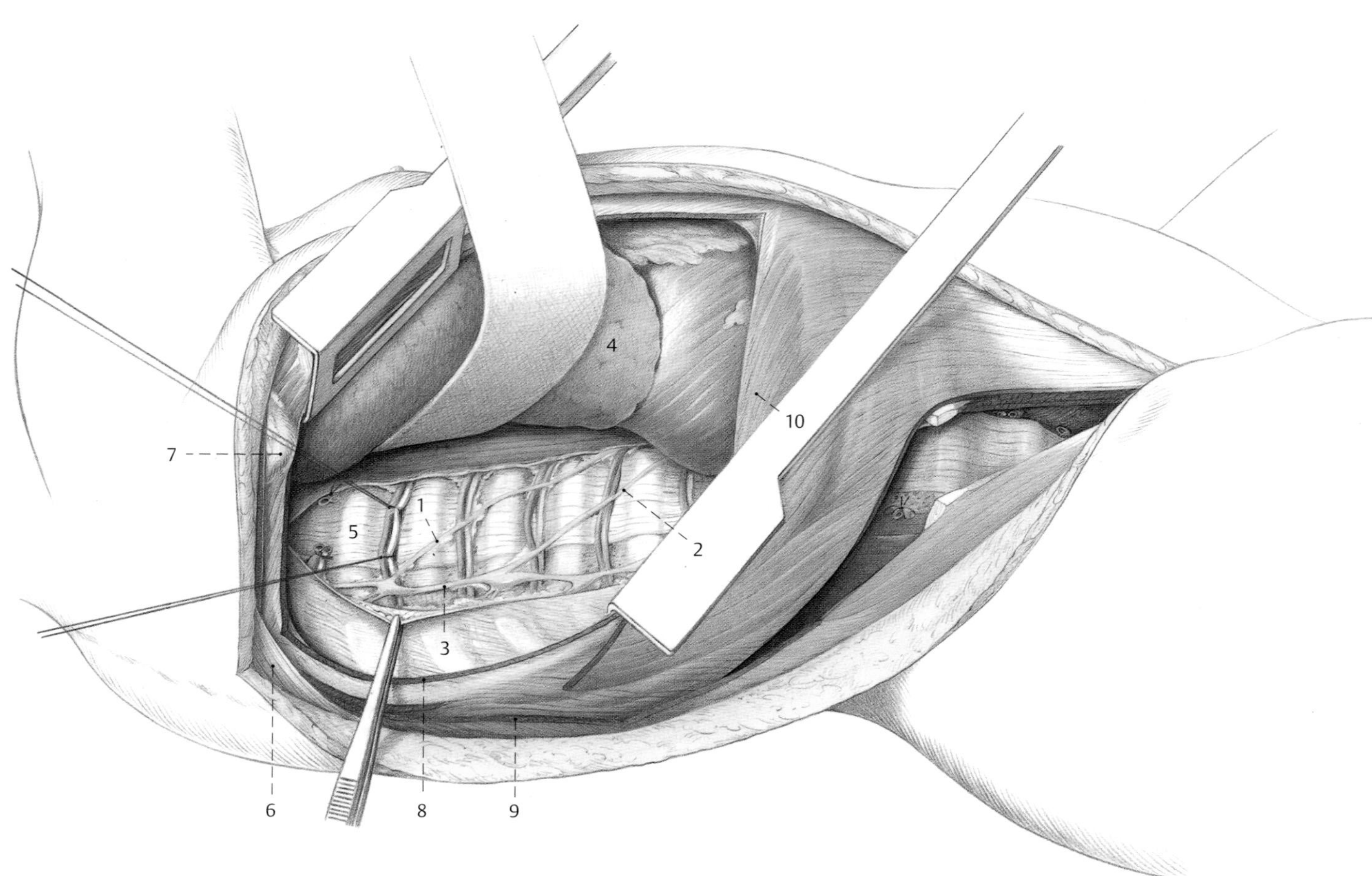

Fig. 3.22 Appearance after intercostal thoracotomy in the sixth intercostal space. Exposure of the thoracic spine; the thoracolumbar approach is seen in the right margin of the figure.

1 Greater splanchnic nerve
2 Lesser splanchnic nerve
3 Sympathetic trunk
4 Lung
5 Anterior longitudinal ligament
6 Trapezius
7 Inferior angle of the scapula
8 Internal intercostal muscles
9 Latissimus dorsi
10 Serratus anterior

3.3 Retroperitoneal Extrapleural Approach to Thoracolumbar Spine T11–L5 According to Mirbaha

R. Bauer, F. Kerschbaumer, S. Poisel

3.3.1 Principal Indications

- Kyphosis
- Tumors
- Spondylitis

For clear exposure of several vertebrae in the region of the thoracolumbar junction, the transpleural approach according to Hodgson is generally preferred. The extrapleural approach according to Mirbaha should be used when only one or two spinal segments have to be reached in the area of the thoracolumbar junction.

Generally speaking, this approach to the thoracolumbar junction can be made from the right as well as from the left side. Insofar as the side of the approach is not dictated by the underlying disease (e.g., the scoliotic component in thoracolumbar kyphosis, tumor extension, etc.), the left-sided approach is preferable. Since we have described Hodgson's transpleural retroperitoneal approach from the left, the retropleural approach will be described, for didactic reasons, from the right.

3.3.2 Positioning and Incision

(**Fig. 3.23**)

The patient is placed on the left side and the right arm is moved above the head so that it is outside the operative field. The skin incision is made along the spinous processes of T9–T11 and continued anteriorly along the 12th rib as far as approximately a fingerbreadth above the anterior iliac spine. An overview extending to L2 is thus obtained. If more caudally situated lumbar vertebrae need to be exposed as well, the skin incision may be extended obliquely (segmental nerves!) in a caudal direction (see **Fig. 3.2**).

The following muscles are transected (**Fig. 3.24**): latissimus dorsi and the external oblique and then, one layer deeper, serratus posterior inferior. Following dissection—in some cases mere elevation may be sufficient—of iliocostalis, the lumbocostal ligament, a strong fascial band between the quadratus lumborum, psoas, and intrinsic back muscles, is exposed. Now the 12th rib can be seen. Subsequently, the deep abdominal muscle layers (internal oblique and transverse muscles) are transected, exposing the peritoneum (**Fig. 3.25**). This is now mobilized from the lateral abdominal wall and retracted medially. In this manner, the upper lumbar spine is exposed retroperitoneally. The peritoneum is then detached from the inferior surface of the diaphragm. Strong fibers of Henle's ligament are detached from the costal process of L1 with the topmost portion of quadratus lumborum. Using a small cotton ball swab, the pleura is now cautiously retracted in a proximal direction from the anterior aspect of the quadratus lumborum (**Fig. 3.26**). Next the 12th rib is exposed subperiosteally and the medial portion is resected. Then the bed of the 12th rib is incised in the middle, and the lower half is retracted caudally together with the quadratus lumborum (**Fig. 3.27**). The subcostal nerve should be spared. The pleura is now further mobilized cranially with the aid of a cotton ball. After the pleura and peritoneum have been stripped from it (**Fig. 3.28**), the diaphragm is transected above the lumbocostal arch (arcuate ligament) in a manner permitting reunion. The right diaphragmatic crus is likewise transected after tagging with sutures (**Fig. 3.29**).

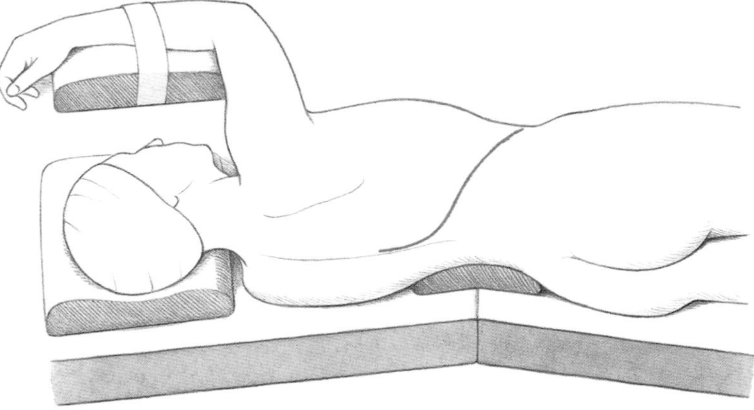

Fig. 3.23 Extrapleural retroperitoneal Mirbaha approach. Positioning and incision.

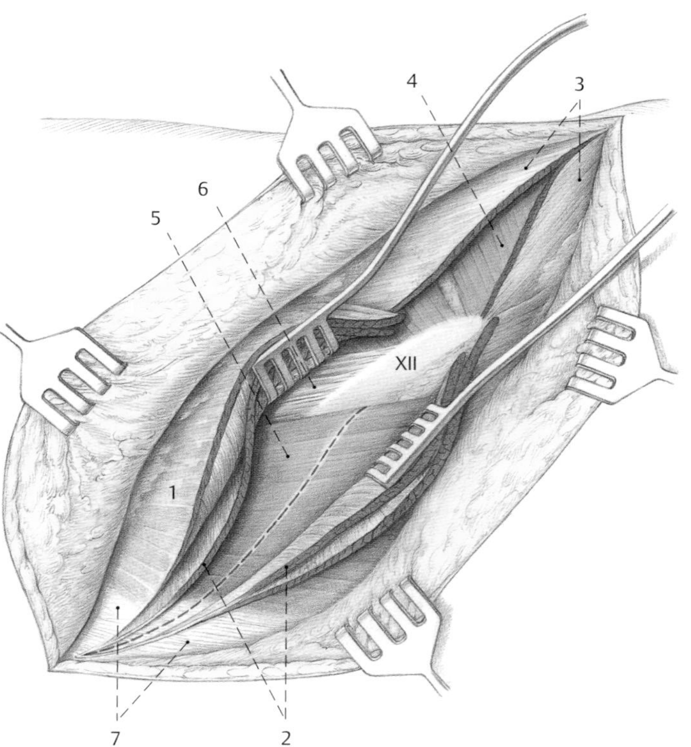

Fig. 3.24 Operative site after transection of the latissimus dorsi and external oblique as well as serratus posterior inferior. Iliocostalis (intrinsic back muscle) is divided along the dashed line.

1 Latissimus dorsi
2 Serratus posterior inferior
3 External oblique
4 Internal oblique
5 Iliocostalis
6 External intercostal muscle
7 Thoracolumbar fascia, superficial layer
XII Rib

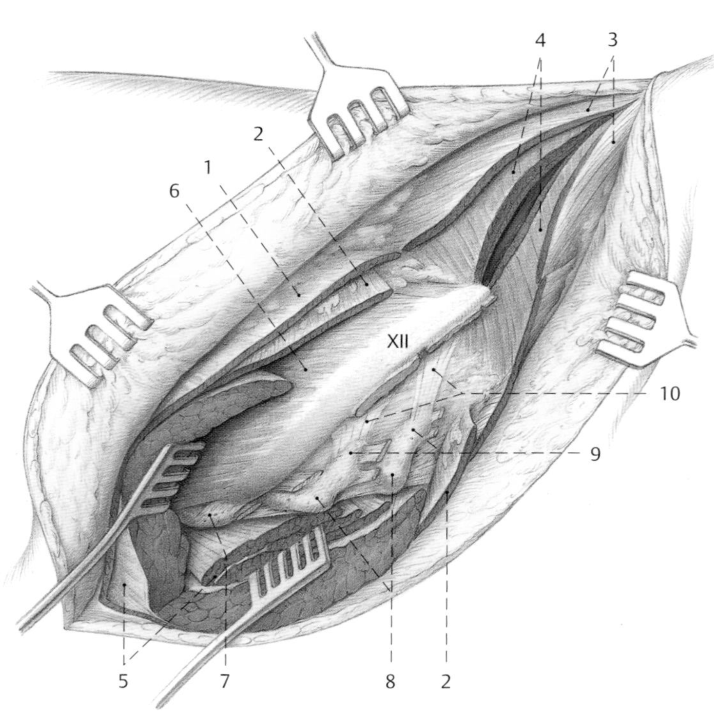

Fig. 3.25 Operative site after transection of the intrinsic back muscles and deep abdominal muscle layers.

1 Latissimus dorsi
2 Serratus posterior inferior
3 External oblique
4 Internal oblique
5 Intrinsic back muscles
6 External intercostal muscle
7 Transverse process of T12
8 Mamillary processes of L1 and L2
9 Costal processes of L1 and L2
10 Lumbocostal ligament
XII Rib

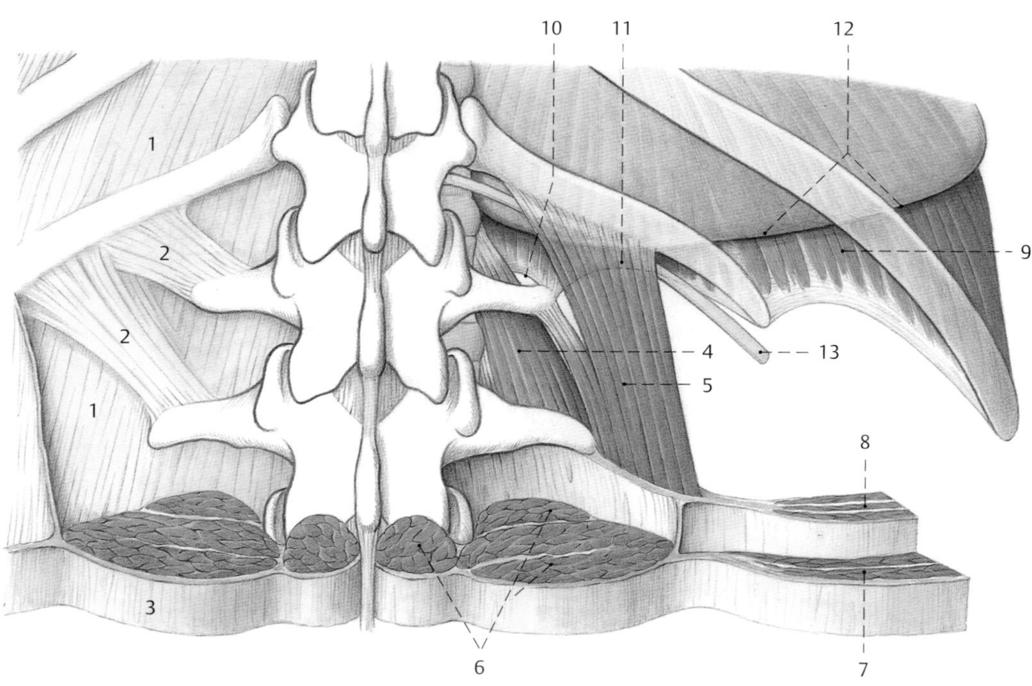

Fig. 3.26 Schematic representation of the thoracolumbar approach from the posterior. Special importance is attached to the relation between the following structures: 12th rib, diaphragmatic origins, medial and lateral arcuate ligament, quadratus lumborum, lumbocostal (Henle's) ligament and pleural border.

1 Thoracolumbar fascia, deep layer
2 Lumbocostal ligament
3 Thoracolumbar fascia, superficial layer
4 Psoas major
5 Quadratus lumborum
6 Intrinsic back muscles
7 Latissimus dorsi and serratus posterior inferior
8 Lateral abdominal muscles
9 Diaphragm, costal part
10 Medial arcuate ligament
11 Lateral arcuate ligament
12 Costodiaphragmatic recess
13 Subcostal nerve

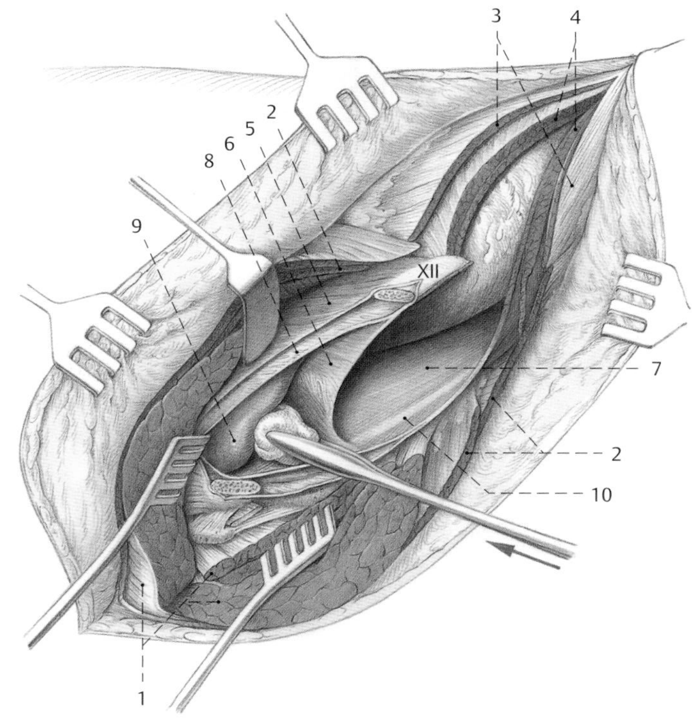

Fig. 3.27 Operative site after partial resection of the 12th rib. The parietal pleura is retracted cranially with a cotton applicator (see arrow).

1 Intrinsic back muscles
2 Latissimus dorsi and serratus posterior inferior
3 External oblique
4 Internal oblique and transversus abdominis
5 External intercostal muscle
6 Diaphragm
7 Psoas major
8 Periosteum of the 12th rib
9 Costodiaphragmatic recess with lung
10 Subcostal nerve
XII Cartilage of the 12th rib

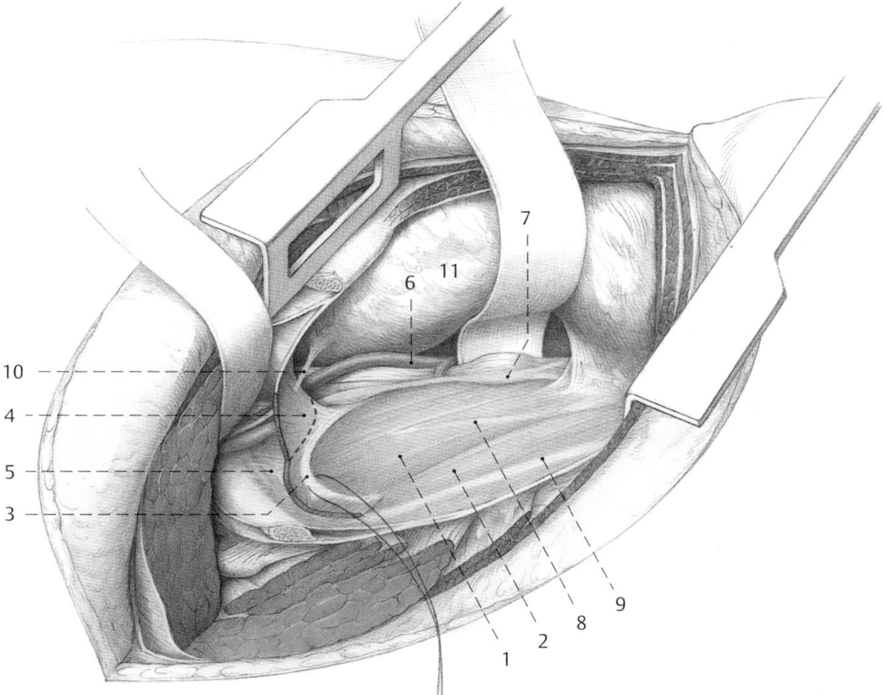

Fig. 3.28 The right retroperitoneal space is exposed. The diaphragm is transected along the dashed line above the lateral arcuate ligament.

1 Psoas major
2 Quadratus lumborum
3 Medial arcuate ligament
4 Diaphragm
5 Subcostal vessels
6 Ascending lumbar vein
7 Sympathetic trunk
8 Ilioinguinal nerve
9 Subcostal nerve
10 Greater splanchnic nerve
11 Parietal peritoneum with preperitoneal fat

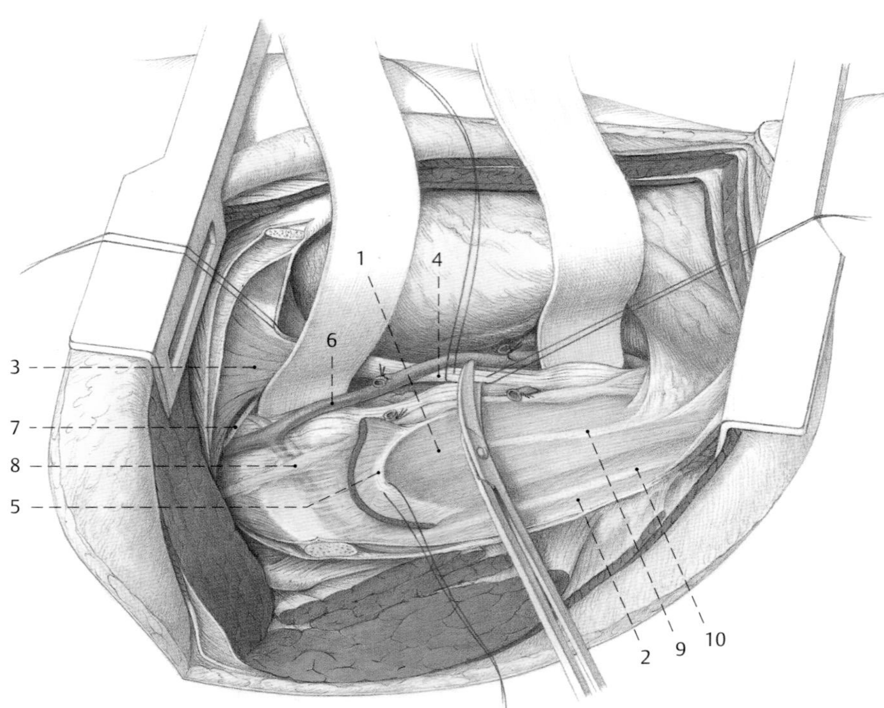

Fig. 3.29 Operative site after transection of the diaphragm. The right diaphragmatic crus is likewise transected after tagging with sutures.

1 Psoas major
2 Quadratus lumborum
3 Diaphragm
4 Diaphragm, right medial crus
5 Medial arcuate ligament
6 Ascending lumbar vein
7 Greater splanchnic nerve
8 Sympathetic trunk
9 Ilioinguinal nerve
10 Subcostal nerve

3.3.3 Exposure of the Vertebrae

The vertebral bodies are exposed in conventional fashion. The retroperitoneal tissue and the parietal pleura at the thoracolumbar junction are split, and the segmental vessels are exposed and transected following the application of ligatures. If the approach is to be enlarged in a cranial direction, the parietal pleura can readily be further retracted in this direction and the medial half of the 11th rib resected (**Fig. 3.30**).

With a sufficiently long incision, L5 or the cranial segment of the sacrum can be reached by this approach.

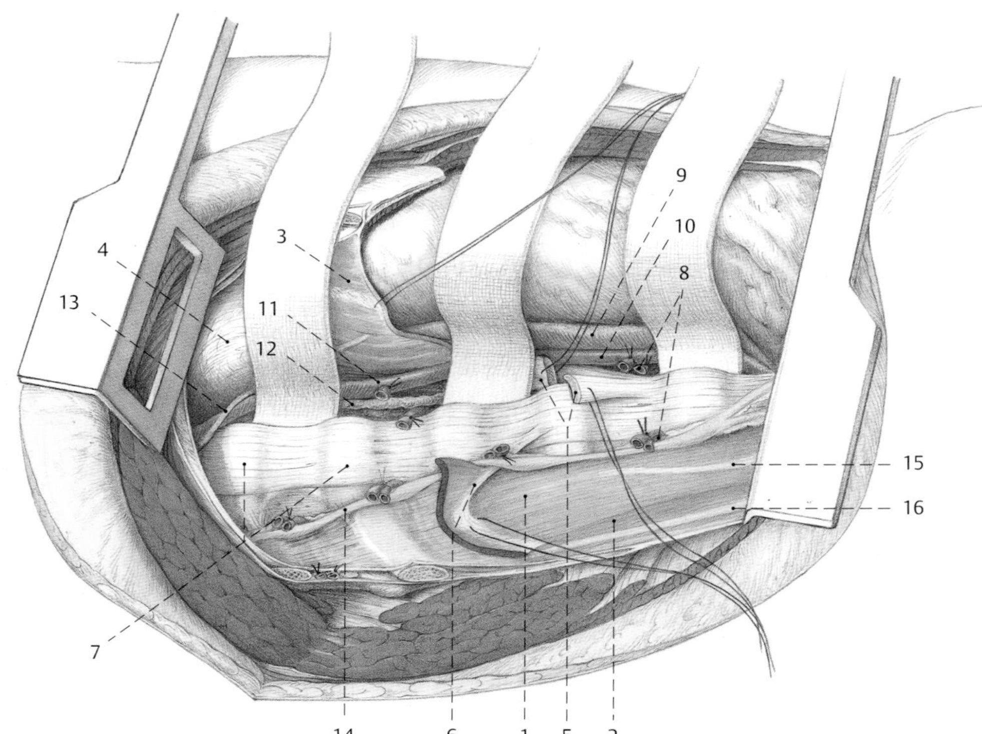

Fig. 3.30 Operative site with exposure of the vertebral bodies at the thoracolumbar junction after transection of the segmental vessels and additional resection of the 11th rib.

1 Psoas major
2 Quadratus lumborum
3 Diaphragm
4 Diaphragm, tendinous center
5 Diaphragm, right crus
6 Medial arcuate ligament
7 Anterior longitudinal ligament
8 Lumbar vessels
9 Inferior vena cava
10 Ascending lumbar vein
11 Azygos vein
12 Thoracic duct
13 Greater splanchnic nerve
14 Sympathetic trunk
15 Ilioinguinal nerve
16 Subcostal nerve

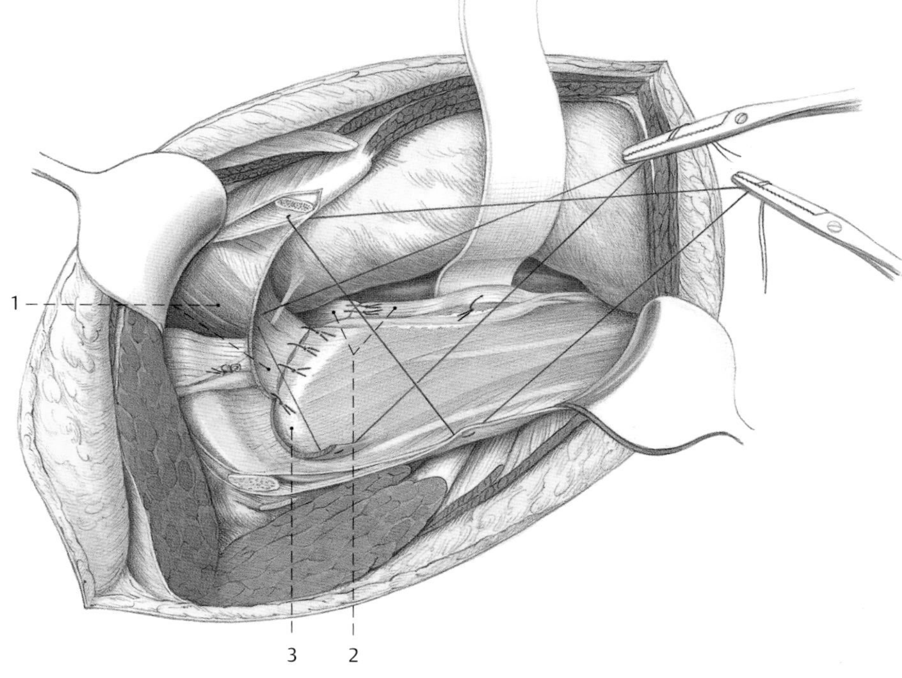

Fig. 3.31 Wound closure. After suture of the right diaphragmatic crus, the right half of the diaphragm is united by means of interrupted sutures tied extrapleurally.

1 Diaphragm
2 Diaphragm, right medial crus
3 Medial arcuate ligament

3.3.4 Wound Closure

The diaphragmatic crus is reattached with interrupted sutures, followed by appropriate suture of the diaphragm above the lumbocostal arch. The presence of retaining sutures facilitates apposition (**Fig. 3.31**). Finally, the quadratus lumborum is reattached to the cranial half of the periosteum of the 12th rib. The abdominal muscles are sutured in layers, and iliocostalis as well as serratus posterior inferior and latissimus dorsi are sutured (**Fig. 3.32**).

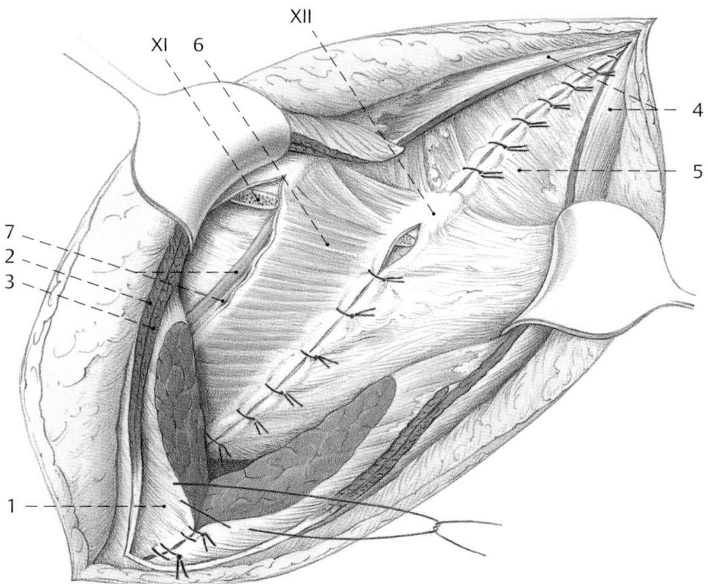

Fig. 3.32 Suture of the deep abdominal muscle layers and reattachment of quadratus lumborum to the periosteum of the 12th rib. Suture of the intrinsic back muscles.

1 Intrinsic back muscles
2 Latissimus dorsi
3 Serratus posterior inferior
4 External oblique
5 Internal oblique
6 Intercostal muscles
7 Intercostal vessels
XI, XII Ribs

4 Lumbar Spine and Lumbosacral Junction

4.1 Retroperitoneal Approach to the Lumbar Spine L2–L5

R. Bauer, F. Kerschbaumer, S. Poisel

4.1.1 Principal Indications

- Kyphosis
- Tumors
- Spondylitis

Generally, this approach to the lumbar spine can be made from the right as well as from the left side. Insofar as the side of the approach is not dictated by the underlying disease (e.g., the scoliotic component in thoracolumbar kyphosis, tumor extension, etc.), the left-sided approach is used.

4.1.2 Positioning and Incision

The patient is placed on the right side. If conditions warrant, the table may be tilted in the lumbar region, and a kidney rest may be applied. In this way, the distance between the costal arch and the iliac crest is increased. To stabilize the position, the patient's right leg is flexed at the hip and knee, while the left leg remains relatively extended. To avoid pressure points, a cushion is placed between the two legs. Straps are used to secure the patient (**Fig. 4.1**).

If an approach to L2 is needed, it is best to resect the 12th rib. An alternative is a subcostal flank incision. The skin incision begins near the midline at the level of the spinous process of T11, continues along the 12th rib, and then extends obliquely forward to the vicinity of the rectus sheath. Depending on the desired area of exposure, it may be extended caudad lateral to the rectus sheath.

Now the latissimus dorsi is dissected transversely to the direction of its fibers, and the external oblique is in part divided parallel to the direction of its fibers (**Fig. 4.2**). On the next deeper plane, serratus posterior inferior is transected in the posterior region of the wound and, more anteriorly, the internal oblique together with the transversus abdominis (**Fig. 4.3**).

Transection of the deep abdominal muscle layers provides access to the retroperitoneal space. The kidney and the ureter are retracted to the right. Now quadratus lumborum becomes visible (**Fig. 4.4**). At this point, the intrinsic back muscles are divided at the level of the 12th rib as indicated by the dashed line, the periosteum over the 12th rib is incised, and the peripheral portion of the rib is resected (**Fig. 4.5**). Opening of the pleural cavity is thus avoided (**Fig. 4.6**; see also **Fig. 3.26**). Subsequently, the periosteum of the rib bed is split in the middle, and the cranial half is retracted upward together with the diaphragm that is attached here. Care should be taken to preserve the 11th and 12th intercostal nerves (subcostal nerve). Finally, a thoracic retractor is applied (**Fig. 4.7**). **Fig. 4.8** presents the anatomical site.

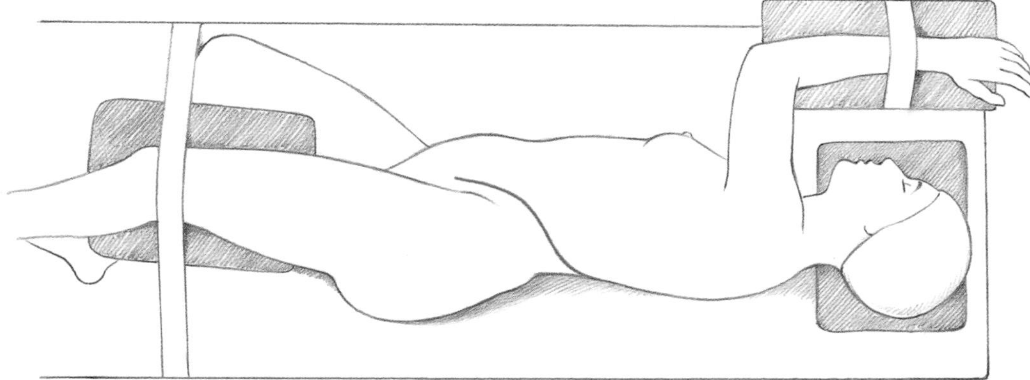

Fig. 4.1 Retroperitoneal approach to the lumbar spine. Positioning and incision.

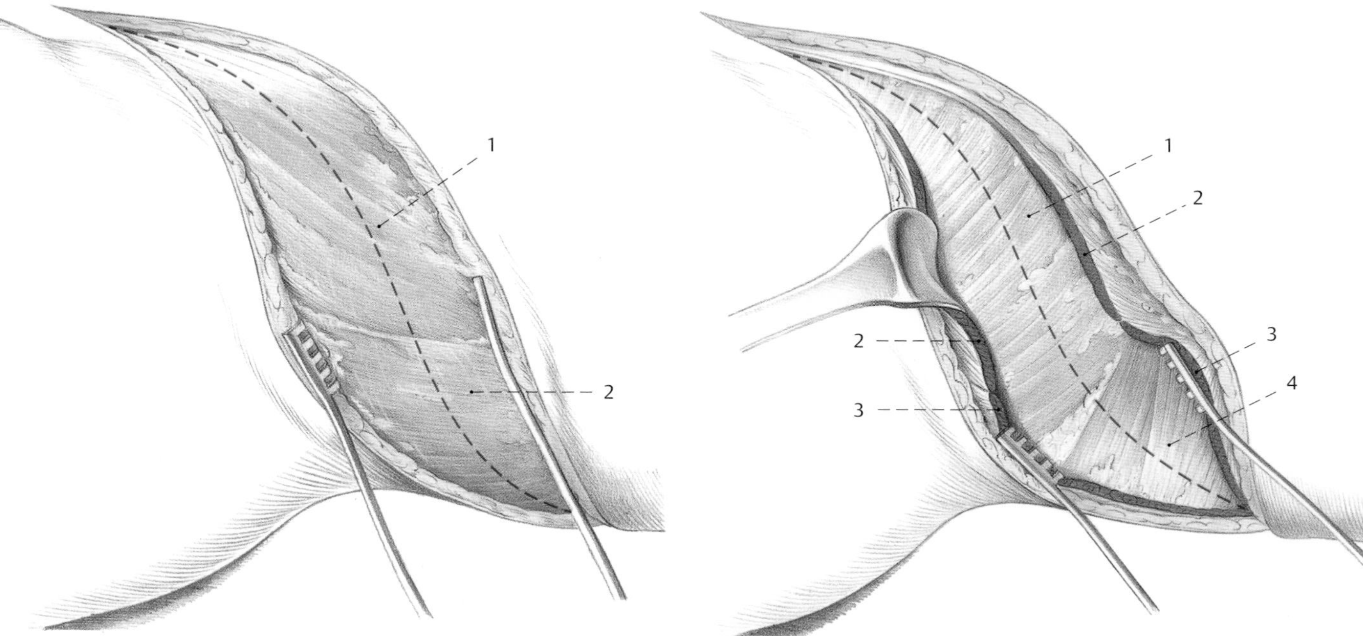

Fig. 4.2 Transection of the latissimus dorsi and external oblique.

1 External oblique
2 Latissimus dorsi

Fig. 4.3 Transection of serratus posterior inferior and the deep abdominal muscle layers.

1 Internal oblique
2 External oblique
3 Latissimus dorsi
4 Serratus posterior inferior

Fig. 4.4 Appearance after transection of the abdominal muscles. The iliocostalis has been transected (curved dashed line) and the periosteum of the 12th rib incised (straight dashed line).

1 External oblique
2 Internal oblique
3 Transversus abdominis
4 Latissimus dorsi
5 Serratus posterior inferior
6 Quadratus lumborum
7 Iliocostalis
8 Preperitoneal fat

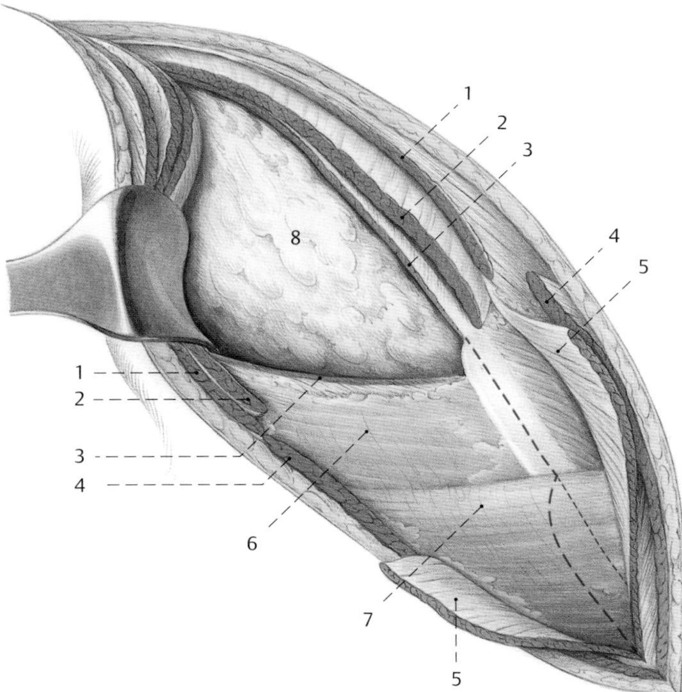

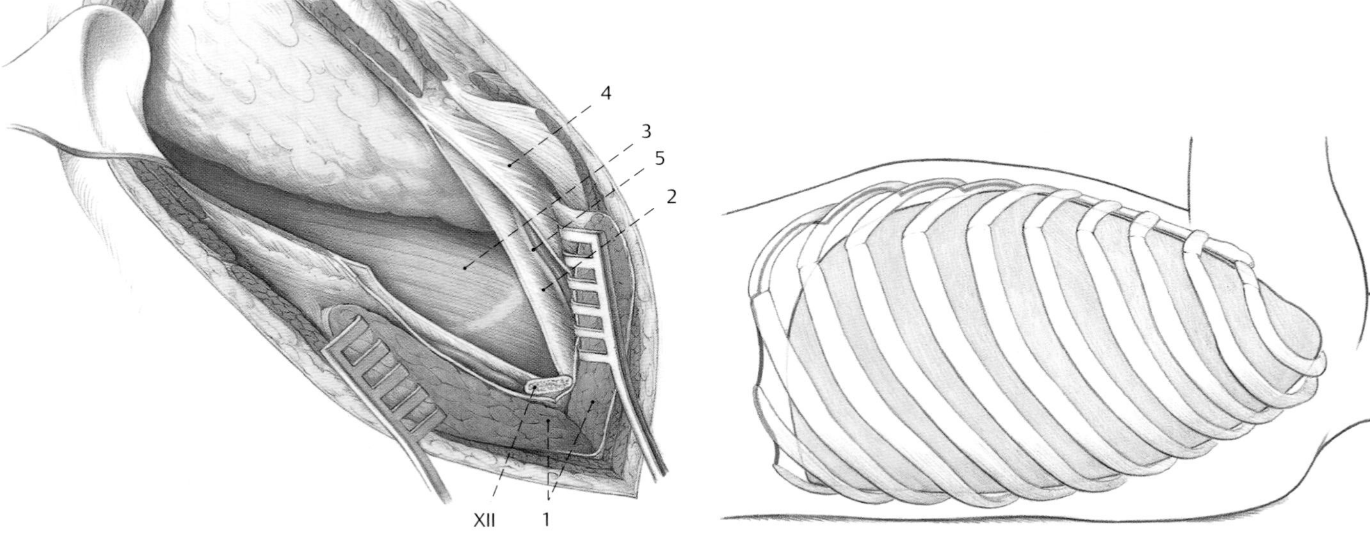

Fig. 4.5 Appearance after resection of the 12th rib and division of the periosteal rib bed.

1 Iliocostalis
2 Diaphragm
3 Quadratus lumborum
4 External intercostal muscle
5 Intercostal vein and nerve
XII Rib

Fig. 4.6 Schematic representation of the pleural border (blue), the origin of the diaphragm (red), and the course of the ribs.

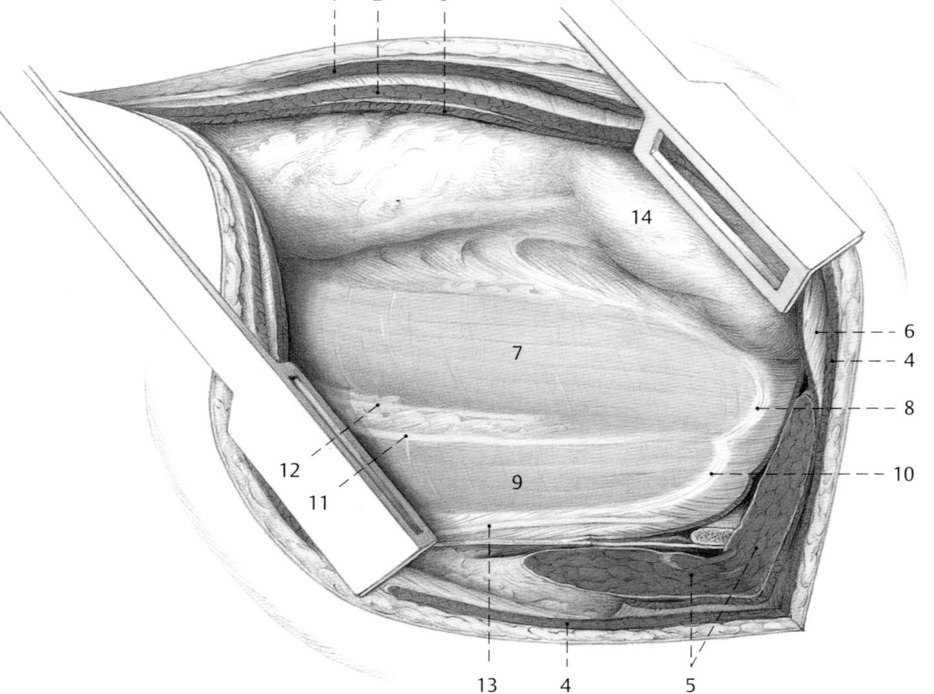

Fig. 4.7 Operative site after insertion of the thoracic retractor.

1 External oblique
2 Internal oblique
3 Transversus abdominis
4 Latissimus dorsi
5 Iliocostalis
6 Serratus posterior inferior
7 Psoas major
8 Medial arcuate ligament
9 Quadratus lumborum
10 Lateral arcuate ligament
11 Iliohypogastric nerve
12 Ilioinguinal nerve
13 Subcostal nerve
14 Perirenal fat capsule

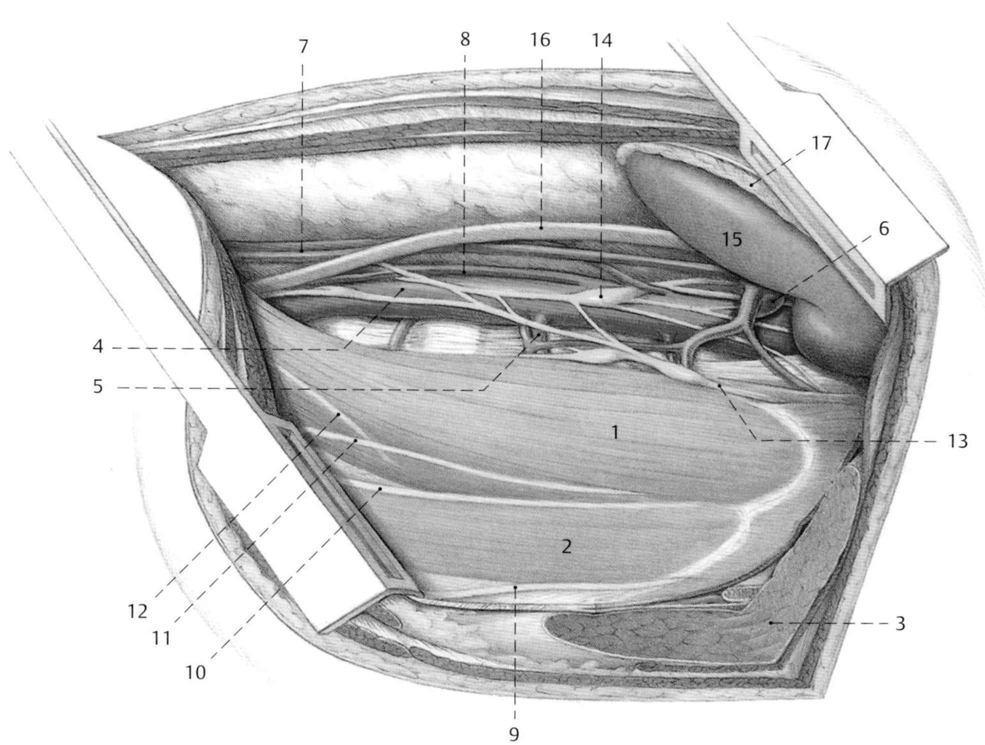

Fig. 4.8 Anatomical site in the retroperitoneal approach to the lumbar spine.

1 Psoas major
2 Quadratus lumborum
3 Iliocostalis
4 Abdominal aorta
5 Lumbar artery and vein
6 Renal vein
7 Spermatic vessels
8 Inferior mesenteric artery
9 Subcostal nerve
10 Iliohypogastric nerve
11 Ilioinguinal nerve
12 Genitofemoral nerve
13 Sympathetic trunk
14 Inferior mesenteric ganglion
15 Left kidney
16 Ureter
17 Perirenal fat capsule

4.1.3 Exposure of the Vertebrae

The retroperitoneal tissue overlying the lumbar spine is split longitudinally, the sympathetic trunk being left laterally. The segmental vessels are exposed in customary fashion and are transected in the midline if possible. Vertebral bodies and intervertebral disks are then accessible over the entire circumference (**Fig. 4.9**).

4.1.4 Wound Closure

To begin with, the bed of the 12th rib is sutured in the peripheral area. Further wound closure is effected in layers, largely in conformity with the procedure used for the extrapleural retroperitoneal approach according to Mirbaha (see Section 3.3.4, **Fig. 3.32**).

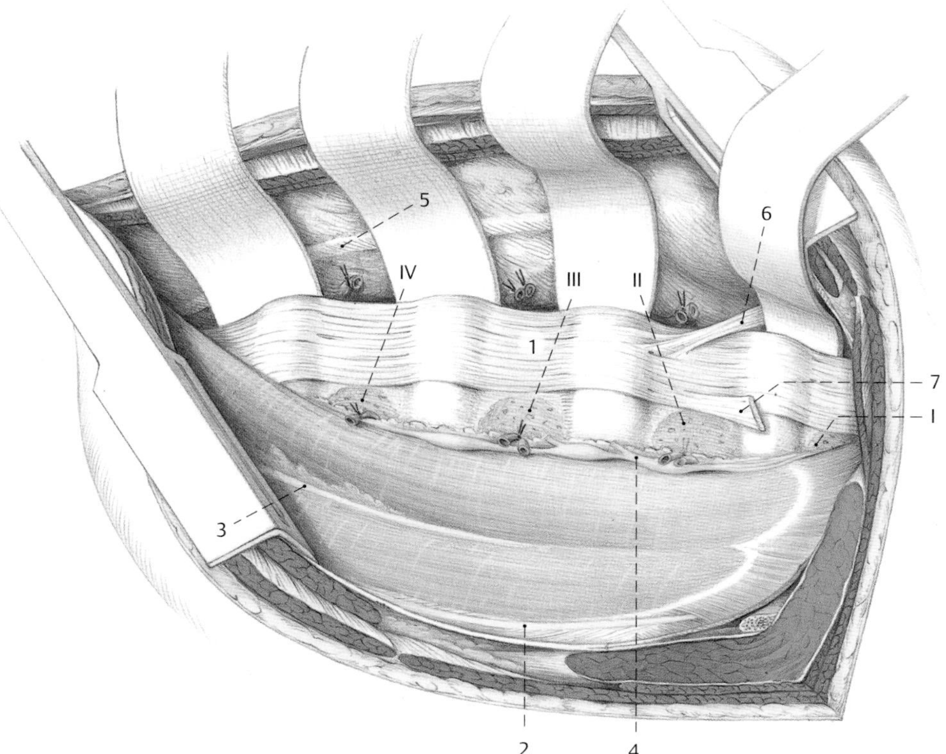

Fig. 4.9 Operative site after transection of the segmental vessels.

1 Anterior longitudinal ligament
2 Subcostal nerve
3 Ilioinguinal nerve
4 Sympathetic trunk
5 Ureter
6 Right crus
7 Left crus
I–IV Vertebrae

4.2 Transperitoneal Approach to the Lumbosacral Junction L4–S1

R. Bauer, F. Kerschbaumer, S. Poisel

4.2.1 Principal Indications

- Spondylolisthesis
- Presacral osteochondrosis
- Tumors

4.2.2 Positioning and Incision

The patient is placed supine with a bolster under the lumbar spine. The operating table is angulated in the middle, producing a hyperlordosis that facilitates the approach to the promontory. Lowering of the legs at the same time reduces venous reflux.

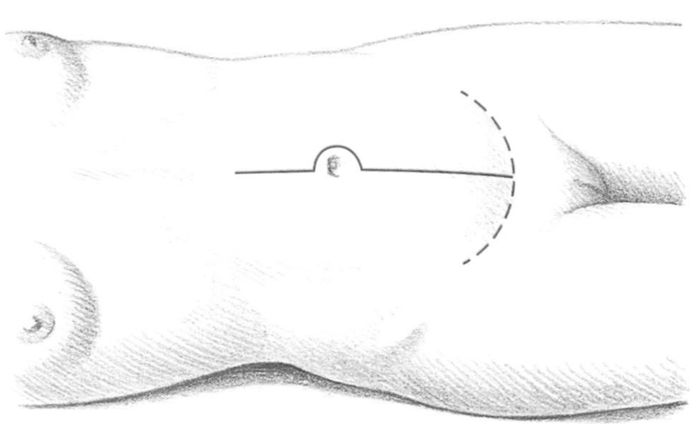

Fig. 4.10 Transperitoneal approach to the lumbosacral junction. The skin incision may be made in the midline; the alternative is a Pfannenstiel incision two fingerbreadths above the symphysis.

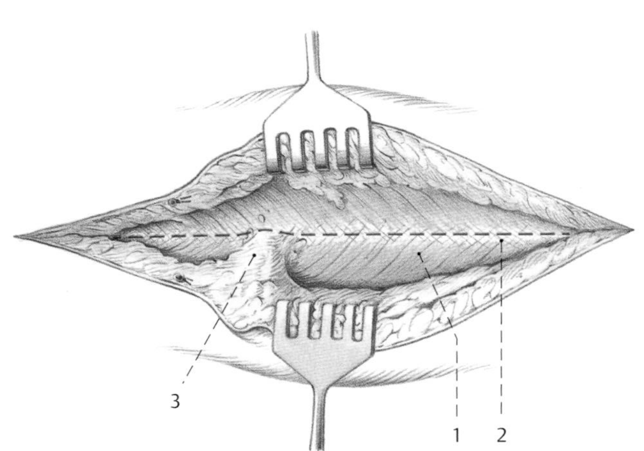

Fig. 4.11 Operative site after incision of the skin and subcutaneous tissue; the linea alba is divided in the midline with a scalpel.

1 Rectus abdominis
2 Linea alba
3 Umbilicus

A midline laparotomy curving to the left of the umbilicus is performed in the usual manner (**Fig. 4.10**). The skin incision begins two to three fingerbreadths above the umbilicus and ends three fingerbreadths above the symphysis. Following dissection of the subcutaneous tissue, the linea alba is exposed and divided in the midline with a scalpel. The subjacent peritoneum is now lifted with two forceps, incised with a scalpel, and then split longitudinally with scissors (**Figs. 4.11** and **4.12**).

4.2.3 Exposure of the Vertebrae

The wound is distracted with large laparotomy hooks, and the greater omentum is retracted upward. The loops of the small intestine and the root of the mesentery are retracted upward by an assistant with the aid of a fairly large wet sponge. The right and left mesocolon are likewise retracted with wet sponges, and the sigmoid, located caudally and to the left, is retracted downward by means of a spatula.

The parietal peritoneum is now incised in a slightly oblique direction, from two fingerbreadths proximal to the bifurcation of the aorta to two fingerbreadths distal to the promontory (**Fig. 4.13**). When splitting the peritoneum, care should be taken not to damage any branches of the subjacent superior hypogastric plexus. When in doubt, incision of the posterior peritoneal layer may be preceded by infiltration of the subjacent tissue with saline solution. This causes the peritoneum to rise, while the superior hypogastric plexus remains attached to the vessels.

Using closed scissor blades and cotton applicators, the peritoneum is now bilaterally mobilized in a lateral direction and may be snared with a retaining suture. The retroperitoneal

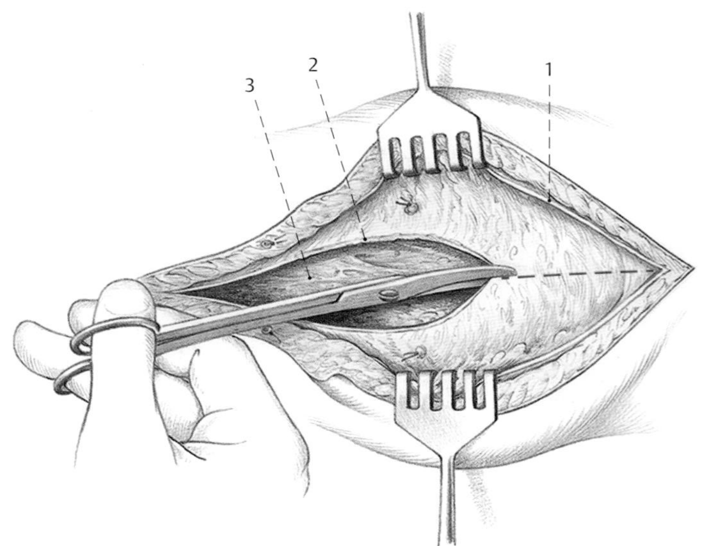

Fig. 4.12 Splitting of peritoneum with scissors.

1 Linea alba
2 Parietal peritoneum
3 Greater omentum

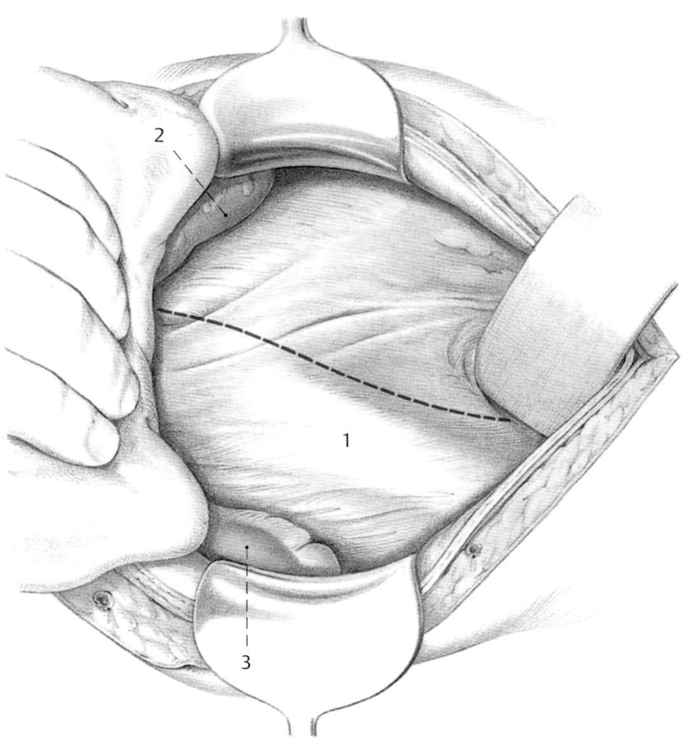

Fig. 4.13 Operative site after opening of the abdomen. The posterior peritoneal layer is transected along the dashed line.

1 Parietal peritoneum
2 Sigmoid colon
3 Cecum

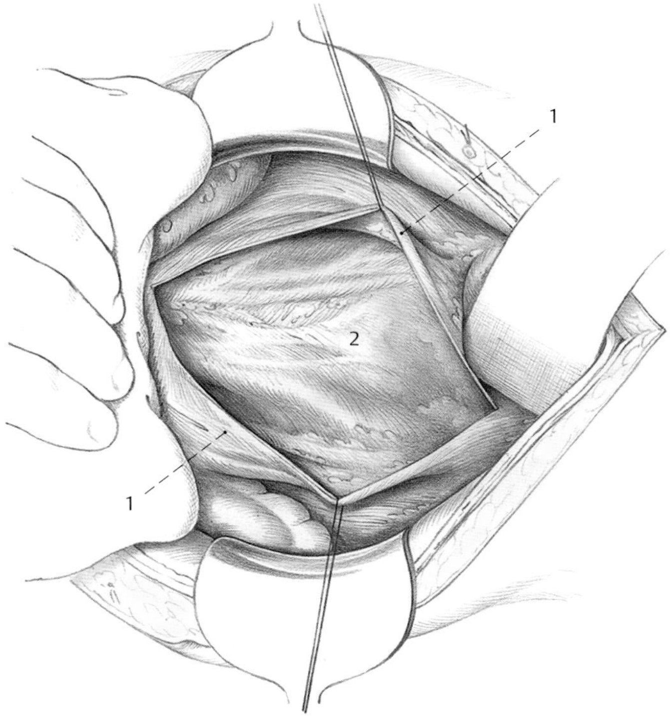

Fig. 4.14 Blunt dissection of the peritoneum in a lateral direction and snaring with stay sutures. The superior hypogastric plexus is revealed.

1 Parietal peritoneum
2 Superior hypogastric plexus

vessels and the superior hypogastric plexus are covered by a fatty connective tissue layer, which must be bluntly opened to the right of the midline over the right common iliac artery. This tissue with the superior hypogastric plexus, which runs caudad over the promontory in front of the aortic bifurcation and is somewhat to the left of the midline, is now bluntly dissected with the aid of cotton applicators toward the left in one layer, freeing it from the aortic bifurcation (**Figs. 4.13** and **4.14**). The promontory is now readily visible, and the median sacral artery and the median sacral vein, which is not always present, can now be ligated. If necessary for better mobilization, the aorta and the right and left common iliac arteries may be snared from below. Subsequently, the vena cava, which is located behind the arteries, and the left common

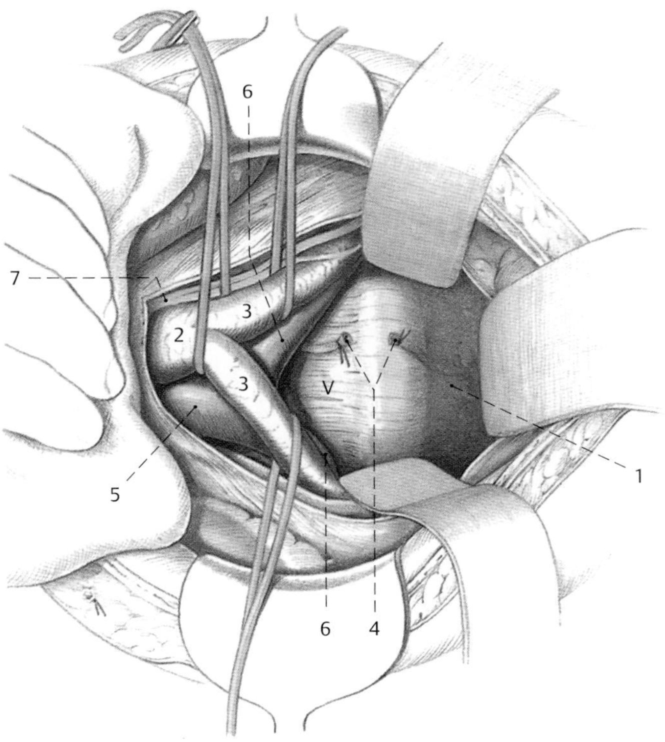

Fig. 4.15 Exposure of the promontory and caudal half of the fifth lumbar vertebra and upper half of the first sacral vertebra following transection of the median sacral artery, snaring of the aorta and left and right common iliac artery, and retraction of the left and right common iliac veins.

1 Sacrum
2 Abdominal aorta
3 Common iliac artery
4 Median sacral artery
5 Inferior vena cava
6 Common iliac vein
7 Superior hypogastric plexus
V Lumbar vertebra

iliac vein are cautiously retracted craniad from the promontory. Flexible spatulas or Harmon retractors may now be applied on both sides of the presacral intervertebral disk to protect the major vessels of the pelvis (**Fig. 4.15**).

Through appropriately cautious dissection of the left common iliac vein and the inferior vena cava, exposure of the intervertebral disk L4–L5 can also be achieved in most cases using this approach. If the bifurcation of the aorta and venous confluence is located more caudally, dissection between the aorta and vena cava (Louis) has been found useful for exposure of the third and fourth intervertebral disks. In this case, it is first necessary to pass below the aorta, snare it, and retract it toward the left, after which the fourth lumbar vascular bundle should be and ligated. The inferior vena cava can now be dissected free, toward the right, using cotton applicators, so that the fourth and, if necessary, the third intervertebral disk as well can be exposed between two Harmon retractors (**Fig. 4.16**).

4.2.4 Anatomical Site

(**Fig. 4.17**)

The following anatomical structures lie between the parietal peritoneum, on the one hand, and the fifth lumbar vertebra and the promontory, on the other hand.

The superior hypogastric plexus lies in reticular fashion on the anterior aspect of the aorta, the promontory, and the left common iliac artery. It is responsible for the sympathetic innervation of the genitourinary system and receives its main branches from the lumbar sympathetic trunk ganglia. The appearance and situation of this nerve plexus vary. Behind the nerve plexus is the bifurcation of the aorta, generally at the level of the fourth vertebra or the L4–L5 intervertebral disk. On the left side of the aorta is the inferior mesenteric artery, which arises from the anterior aspect of the aorta at approximately the level of the third lumbar vertebra.

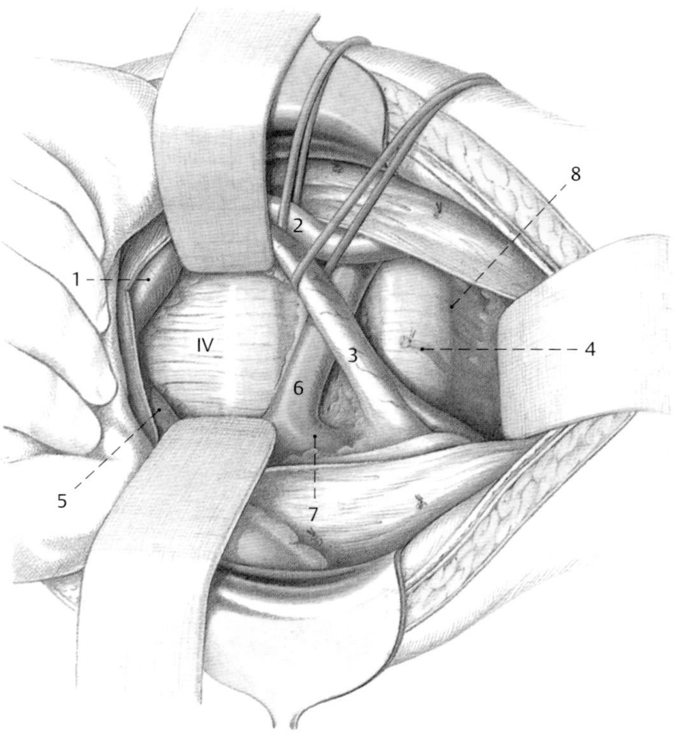

Fig. 4.16 Exposure of the fourth lumbar vertebra and L4–L5 intervertebral disk between the aorta and the inferior vena cava following ligation and transection of the fourth segmental vascular bundle.

1 Abdominal aorta
2 Left common iliac artery
3 Right common iliac artery
4 Median sacral artery
5 Inferior vena cava
6 Left common iliac vein
7 Right common iliac vein
8 Promontory
IV Lumbar vertebra

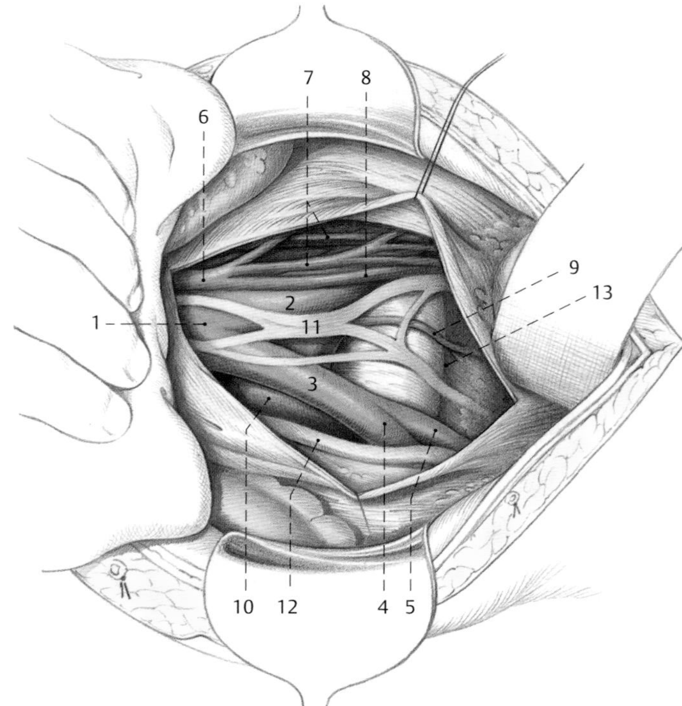

Fig. 4.17 Anatomical site anterior to the fifth lumbar vertebra and promontory.

1 Abdominal aorta
2 Left common iliac artery
3 Right common iliac artery
4 External iliac artery
5 Internal iliac artery
6 Inferior mesenteric artery
7 Sigmoid vessels
8 Superior rectal artery
9 Median sacral artery
10 Right common iliac vein
11 Superior hypogastric plexus
12 Right ureter
13 Promontory

The two ureters cross the iliac arteries, descending from lateral to medial at the level of the origin of the internal iliac artery. The confluence of the left and right common iliac veins is located on the right side caudally and behind the bifurcation of the aorta. In most cases, the level of the venous confluence corresponds to the fifth lumbar vertebra or the L4–L5 intervertebral disk. In exceptional cases, the venous confluence may be located higher than the aortic bifurcation. The median sacral artery and, as a rule, the median sacral vein are found in the midline over the promontory.

4.2.5 Wound Closure

The parietal peritoneum is closed with a continuous absorbable suture. The wet sponges are now removed so that the loops of the small intestine and the root of the mesentery resume their normal positions. Before downward retraction of the greater omentum, it should be ensured that there has been no torsion of the mesentery root. The linea alba and the transversalis fascia in the lower wound area are now grasped with Mikulicz clamps and elevated, and the peritoneum is closed with a continuous absorbable suture. Closure of the rectus sheath with nonabsorbable material is followed by conventional closure of the skin and subcutaneous tissue.

4.2.6 Dangers

After opening of the parietal peritoneum, dissection of the aorta and the left and right common iliac artery may entail injury to the superior hypogastric plexus. This injury may result in retrograde ejaculation in males. If dissection is carried too far in the lateral direction, there is a risk of damaging the ureters. They cross the iliac arteries at the level of origin of the internal iliac artery. The ureter is generally adherent to the parietal peritoneum and is identifiable by the fact that it undergoes contractions upon palpation with the fingers. Another danger is damage to the great vessels, notably the left common iliac vein or the inferior vena cava. Deep-seated ectopic kidneys or horseshoe kidneys can hamper or prevent a transperitoneal approach. It is therefore advisable before the operation to obtain a urogram and perform computed tomography in addition to angiography to determine the level of the aortic bifurcation.

4.2.7 Note

The transperitoneal approach to the lumbosacral intervertebral disk can be accomplished fairly rapidly if the patient is appropriately prepared (good bowel evacuation, preoperative liquid diet). Since partial damage to the superior hypogastric plexus cannot be ruled out even with careful dissection, this approach should be used in men only if a posterior or lateral extraperitoneal approach is not feasible.

4.3 Minimally Invasive Lateral Approach to the Lumbar Spine L2–L5

F. Kandziora

4.3.1 Principal Indications

- Scoliosis
- Kyphosis
- Vertebral body fractures
- Tumors
- Diskitis and spondylodiskitis
- Degenerative spinal disease, especially degenerative lumbar scoliosis

4.3.2 Positioning

(**Fig. 4.18**)

The patient is placed on the right side in a stable position as access is usually obtained from the left side. In exceptional cases, for example spondylodiskitis with a right-sided psoas abscess, the approach can be from the right. It should be possible to bend the operating table to open up the space between the iliac crest and the lowermost rib. The greater trochanter should be centered over the axis of the table hinge. Unintentional scoliotic flexion of the spine due to angling of the operating table must be avoided, especially when instrumentation is planned, so as not to risk fixation of the spine in an incorrect position. The patient's hip should be flexed to approximately 30° to relax the psoas and make it easier to retract.

4.3.3 Localization

Exact lateral positioning of the patient is required preoperatively (**Fig. 4.18**). The position is confirmed by radiographs in two planes. The C-arm must be freely mobile around the patient. Depending on the pathology, the skin incision is planned in the line of the skin creases. In the case of disk pathology (**Fig. 4.18**), the anterior and posterior borders and the superior and inferior end plates of the mobile segment are drawn on the skin. The planned skin incision is then slightly oblique from anterocaudal to posterocranial over the intervertebral disk space (**Fig. 4.18**).

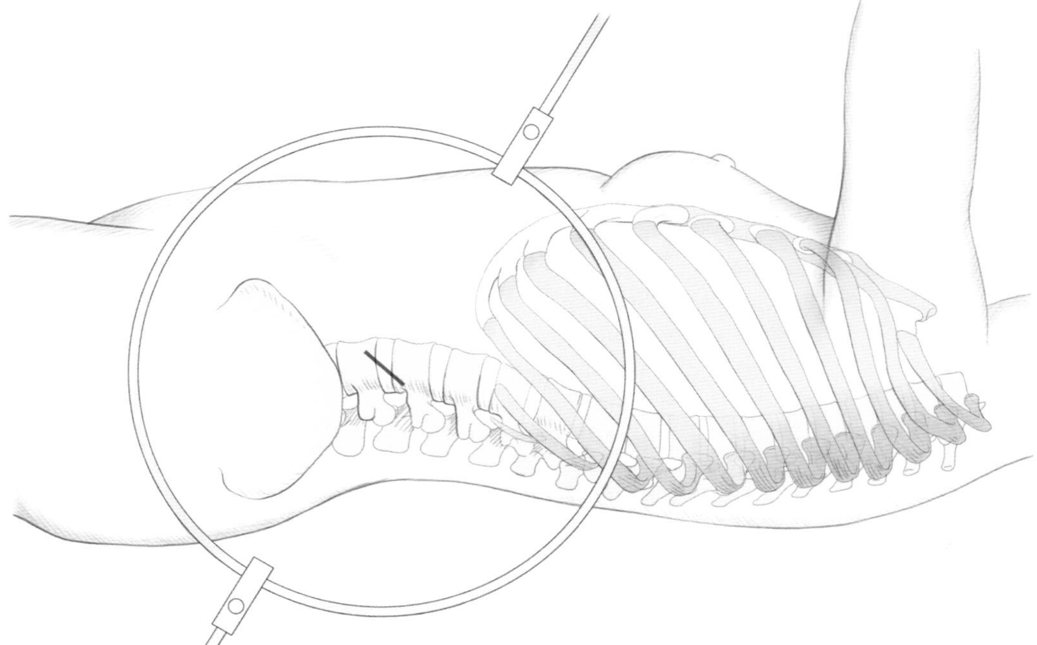

Fig. 4.18 The patient is in the strict right lateral decubitus position with the retractor system preassembled. The image converter projection of the spine is drawn on the skin, and the skin incision is marked.

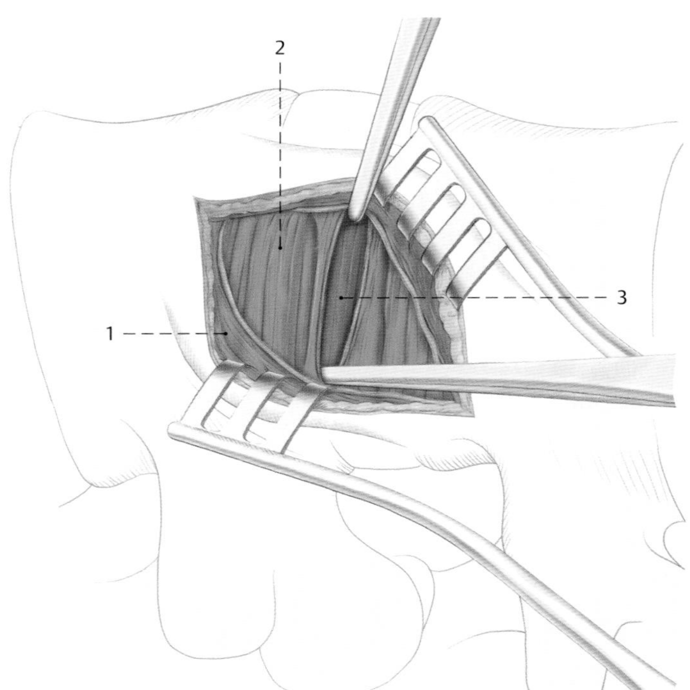

Fig. 4.19 Pushing apart the abdominal muscle layers in the line of their fibers.

1 External oblique
2 Internal oblique
3 Transversus abdominis

Because of the vascular anatomy (the course of the left common iliac vein), lateral exploration in a caudal direction is usually possible only as far as the cranial surface of L5. The diaphragm is the cranial limit of this approach. When disease extends over a long distance, the minimally invasive lateral approach to the lumbar spine can be combined with a purely thoracoscopic or minimally invasive, thoracoscopy-assisted approach to the thoracolumbar junction (see Section 2.4). "Minimally invasive" exposure of T10–T11 to L5 is possible by "slitting" the diaphragm in this combination.

4.3.4 Incision

The length of the skin incision depends on the underlying pathology and the extent of the spine to be exposed. An incision of 4–8 cm usually suffices (**Fig. 4.18**). The skin incision is followed by division of the subcutaneous fat and exposure of the fascia of the external oblique. After opening the fascia with a scalpel, the three muscle layers of external oblique, internal oblique, and transversus abdominis are forced apart bluntly in the line of their fibers with Langenbeck retractors or forceps (**Fig. 4.19**). After division of the posterior parts of the fascia of the transversus abdominis, the peritoneum is exposed bluntly (**Fig. 4.20**). This is then pushed medially and anteriorly from the lateral abdominal wall with a cotton applicator (**Fig. 4.21**) to expose the psoas (**Fig. 4.22**). Once the psoas has been exposed, two modifications of the approach are possible.

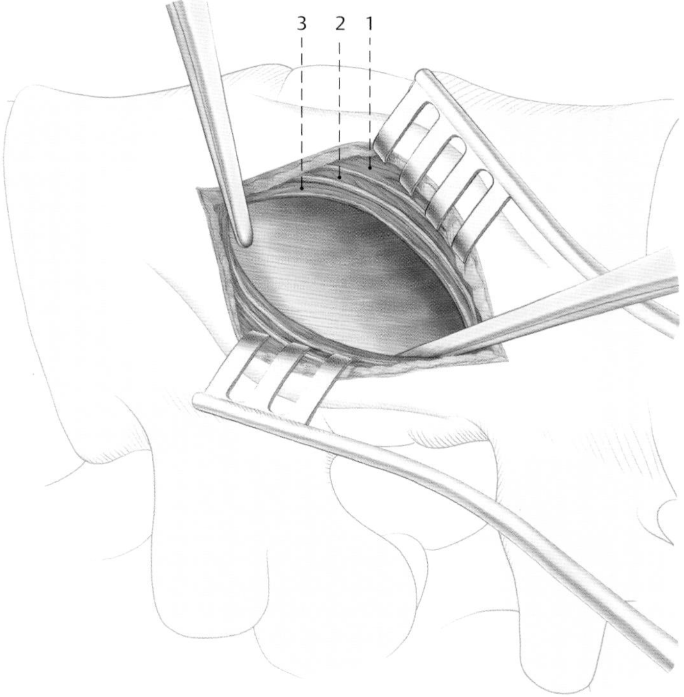

Fig. 4.20 Division of the posterior parts of the fascia of transversus abdominis and exposure of the peritoneum.

1 External oblique
2 Internal oblique
3 Transversus abdominis

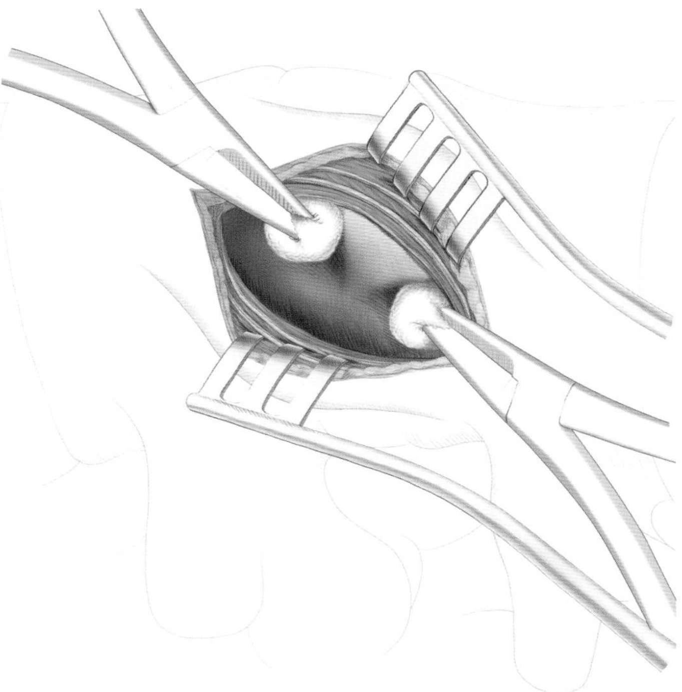

Fig. 4.21 Bluntly pushing the peritoneum away from the abdominal wall.

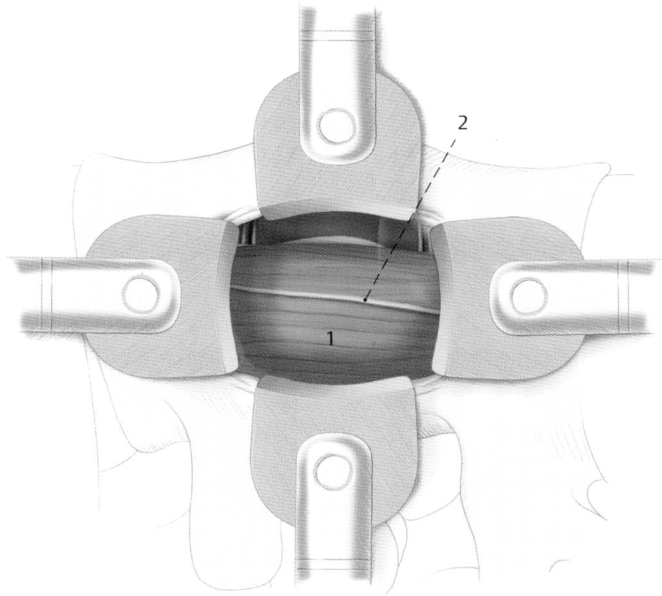

Fig. 4.22 Exposure of the psoas, maintaining the exposure with retractors.

1 Psoas
2 Genitofemoral nerve

Transpsoas Approach

In the transpsoas approach, the longitudinal fibers of the psoas are pushed apart. Because of the nerve roots that run in the psoas, it is generally recommended to do this with neuromonitoring. Support by specialist neuromonitoring staff and appropriate additional equipment are offered by the industry.

Classic Approach

(**Figs. 4.23** and **4.24**)

The retroperitoneal tissue is exposed anteriorly beyond the psoas. The intervertebral disks are exposed between the sympathetic trunk and anterior psoas border. The vessels and sympathetic trunk are retracted medially. The intersegmental vessels are divided in the usual way and also retracted anteriorly and posteriorly. In addition, the psoas is retracted posteriorly from the lateral parts of the vertebral bodies, beginning at the intervertebral disk space.

With both variants, half of the circumference of the vertebral bodies can be exposed (**Figs. 4.23** and **4.24**). The achieved exposure should be maintained by a self-retaining retractor system in both the transpsoas and the classic approach.

4.3.5 Wound Closure

The muscle fascia of the transversus abdominis is closed. The abdominal muscles are reapproximated selectively and in layers with interrupted sutures.

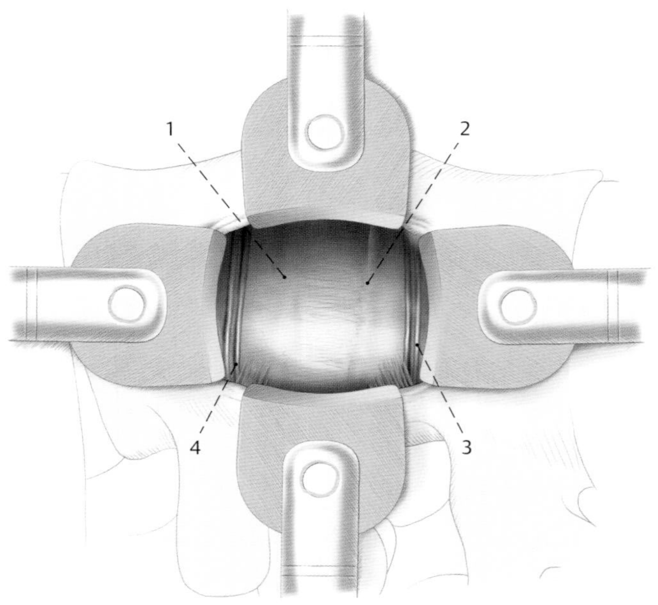

Fig. 4.23 Classic approach. The intervertebral disk space is exposed after posterior retraction of the psoas.

1 Fourth lumbar vertebra
2 Third lumbar vertebra
3 Posterior intercostal artery
4 Anterior external vertebral venous plexus

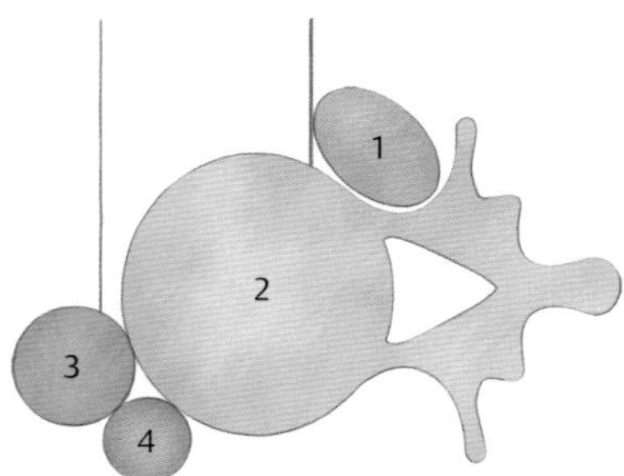

Fig. 4.24 Schematic drawing of the final exposure in the classic approach.

1 Psoas
2 Vertebral body
3 Aorta
4 Vena cava

Spine, Posterior Approaches

5 Cervical Spine

5.1 Posterior Approach to the Cervical Spine and Occipitocervical Junction

R. Bauer, F. Kerschbaumer, S. Poisel

5.1.1 Principal Indications

- Occipitocervical instability
- Degenerative changes
- Trauma
- Tumors

5.1.2 Positioning and Incision

The patient is placed in the prone position with a cushion under the chest. The head rests on a padded U-shaped brace and is slightly flexed (**Fig. 5.1**). When necessary (fracture-dislocations, cervicooccipital instability in rheumatoid arthritis), cranial traction may be applied. Extensive shaving of the back of the neck and head is required. The median skin incision is begun two fingerbreadths above the external occipital protuberance and continued as far as the tip of the seventh spinous process (vertebra prominens).

After splitting of the subcutaneous tissue, self-retaining wound retractors are inserted, and hemostasis is performed. Using a diathermy scalpel, a median incision is now made through the nuchal fascia onto the nuchal ligament. At this point, the trapezius, which is coherent with the fascia, can be bilaterally mobilized, and the wound retractor can be moved to the plane that is next deepest (**Fig. 5.2**).

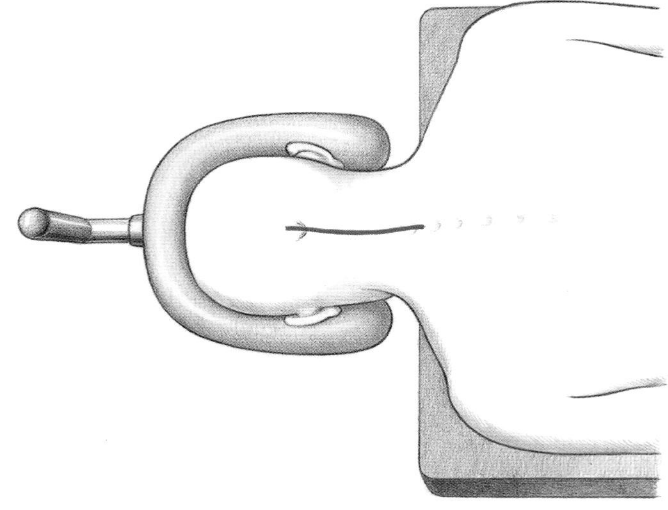

Fig. 5.1 Posterior approach to the cervical spine with occipitocervical junction. Positioning and incision.

5.1.3 Exposure of the Spine

The nuchal ligament is transected in the midline and incised as far as the tips of the spinous processes. The muscle layer that has been transected in the midline is retracted with the wound retractor. The deep muscle layer is then detached from the spinous processes using the diathermy scalpel. The dissection is effected near the bone, from cranial to caudal, beginning at the spinous process of the second cervical vertebra. If

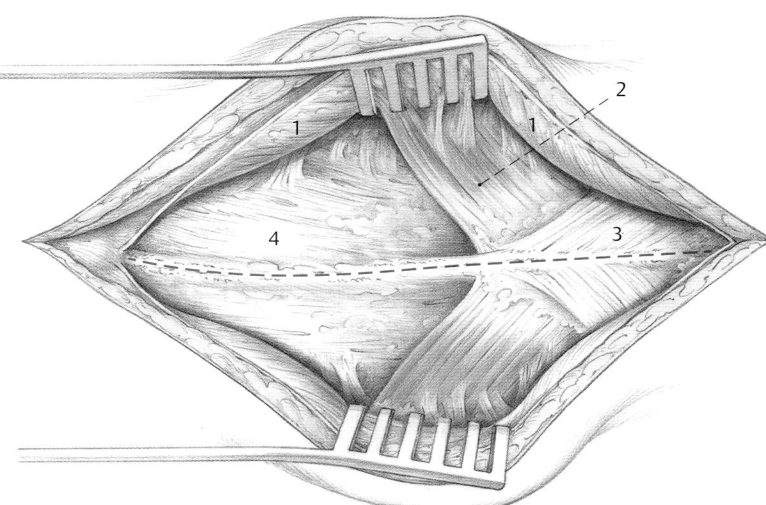

Fig. 5.2 Operative site after transection of the nuchal fascia and insertion of self-retaining retractors. Dissection is now performed in the midline to the spinous processes (dashed line).

1 Trapezius
2 Splenius capitis
3 Rhomboid minor
4 Semispinalis capitis

necessary (occipitocervical fusion), the muscles taking origin from, or attached to, the occiput (trapezius, semispinalis capitis) may be detached by a T-shaped dissection (**Fig. 5.3**). With the use of a sharp raspatory, the short rotator and multifidus muscles are now detached—moving in a caudal direction from the second spinous process—from the spinous processes and the articular processes, and subperiosteal exposure is performed as far as the lateral boundary of the facet joints. Hemostasis is effected by the application of gauze swabs. Subsequently, that portion of the squamous part of the occipital bone which is caudal to the external occipital protuberance is exposed subperiosteally with a sharp raspatory. This invariably leads to bleeding from the suboccipital venous plexus, which can be stopped by electrocoagulation.

Now the posterior tubercle of the atlas, located deeply in the midline, is palpated with the fingertip. The muscle originating here (rectus capitis posterior minor) is detached on both sides, and, using the raspatory, the arch of the atlas is subperiosteally exposed on both sides for about 1.5 cm (**Fig. 5.4**). The tip of the raspatory should remain in continuous contact with the bone so that injury to the vertebral artery can be avoided. The vertebral artery, after passing through the transverse foramen of the atlas, runs bilaterally in a medial direction in the groove for the vertebral artery, the ridge of which becomes visible and palpable upon careful exposure (**Fig. 5.5**). More laterally, the posterior branch of the second cervical nerve, the main branch of which is the greater occipital nerve, emerges between the first and second cervical vertebrae. This nerve should also be spared. The wound retractors are inserted into the deepest muscle layer and opened wider. The vertebral arches, the ligamenta flava, and the atlantooccipital membrane are uncovered with curettes and small raspatories. The interspinal ligaments are removed as a rule if posterior fusion is desired (**Fig. 5.6**).

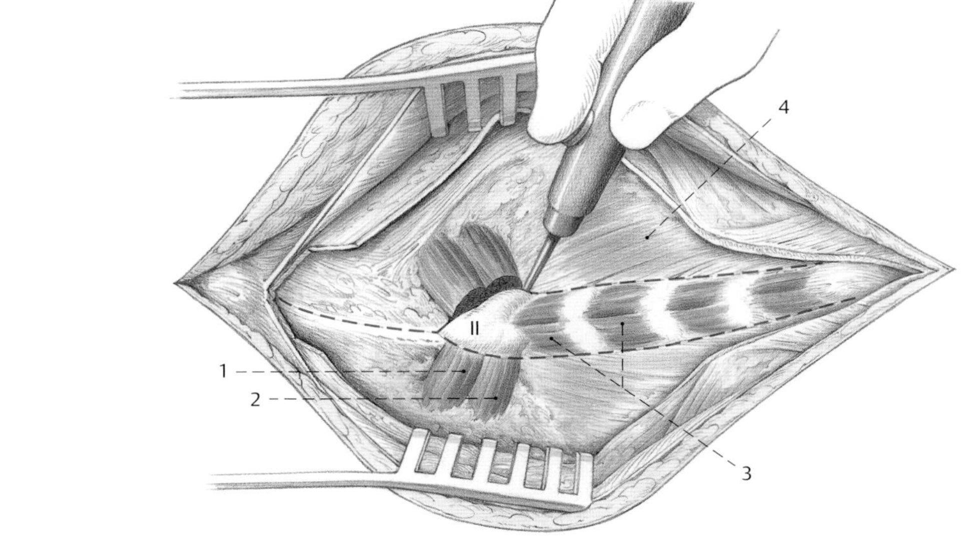

Fig. 5.3 Dissection of the medial and deep layers of the nuchal muscles close to the bone, beginning at the spinous process of the second cervical vertebra, and proceeding in a caudal direction.

1 Rectus capitis posterior major
2 Obliquus capitis inferior
3 Interspinal muscles
4 Semispinalis cervicis
II Spinous process of the axis

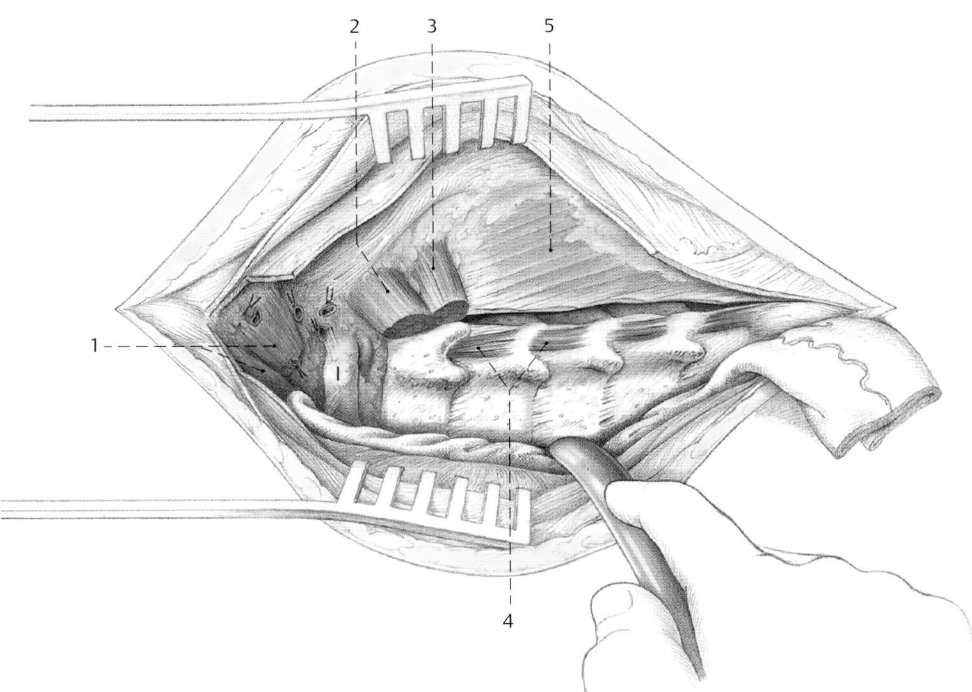

Fig. 5.4 Subperiosteal retraction of the deep nuchal muscles with a raspatory as far as the facet joints. Tamponade with gauze swabs. Ligation or electrocoagulation of the suboccipital venous plexus. Caution: subperiosteal dissection of the atlantal arch should not extend beyond 1.5 cm laterally from the midline to avoid damage to the vertebral artery.

1 Rectus capitis posterior minor
2 Rectus capitis posterior major
3 Obliquus capitis inferior
4 Interspinal muscles
5 Semispinalis cervicis
I Posterior arch of the atlas

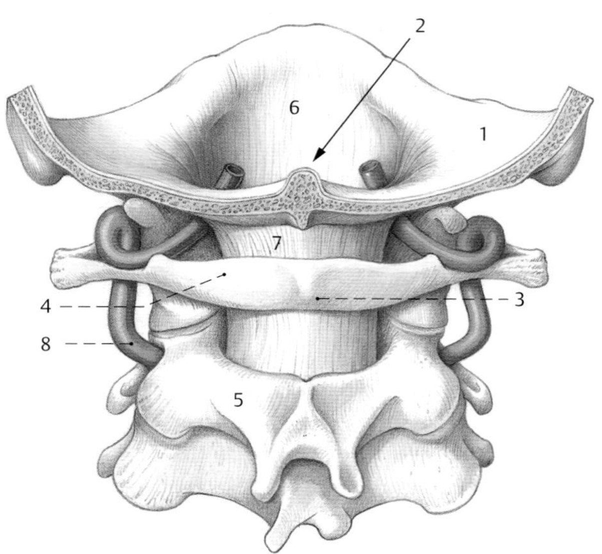

Fig. 5.5 Schematic representation of the occipitocervical junction from the rear, showing the course of the vertebral artery.

1 Squamous part of the occipital bone
2 Foramen magnum
3 Posterior tubercle of the atlas
4 Posterior arch of the atlas
5 Spinous process of the axis
6 Tectorial membrane
7 Posterior atlantooccipital membrane
8 Vertebral artery

5.1.4 Dangers

If the first and second vertebral arches are dissected too far in a lateral direction, the vertebral artery or the suboccipital and greater occipital nerves may be injured. In rheumatoid arthritis, the posterior arch of the first cervical vertebra is very thin and may be damaged by the raspatory if too much pressure is applied.

5.1.5 Anatomical Site

(**Figs. 5.7** and **5.8**)

The muscles of the neck are classified as follows:

- Trapezius
- Rhomboid minor
- Intrinsic back muscles
  - Splenius capitis and splenius cervicis
  - Semispinalis capitis and semispinalis cervicis
  - Multifidus muscles
  - Rotator muscles (inconstant), interspinal muscles
  - Short cervical muscles:
    - Rectus capitis posterior (major and minor)
    - Obliquus capitis (superior and inferior)

The posterior branch of the second spinal nerve (cutaneous branch: greater occipital nerve) exits in a posterior direction between the first and second cervical vertebrae. It becomes subcutaneous one fingerbreadth distal to the tendinous arch between the trapezius and the sternocleidomastoid muscle, and supplies the skin of the occiput. The posterior ramus of the third spinal nerve emerges between the second and third cervical vertebrae. Its cutaneous branch, the third occipital nerve, is inconstant and also supplies the skin of the occiput. The vertebral artery passes from the transverse foramen of the atlas in a medial direction behind the atlantooccipital joint and then runs through the atlantooccipital membrane into the foramen magnum and thence into the cranial cavity.

5.1.6 Wound Closure

The wound is closed by suture of the muscles and the nuchal ligament.

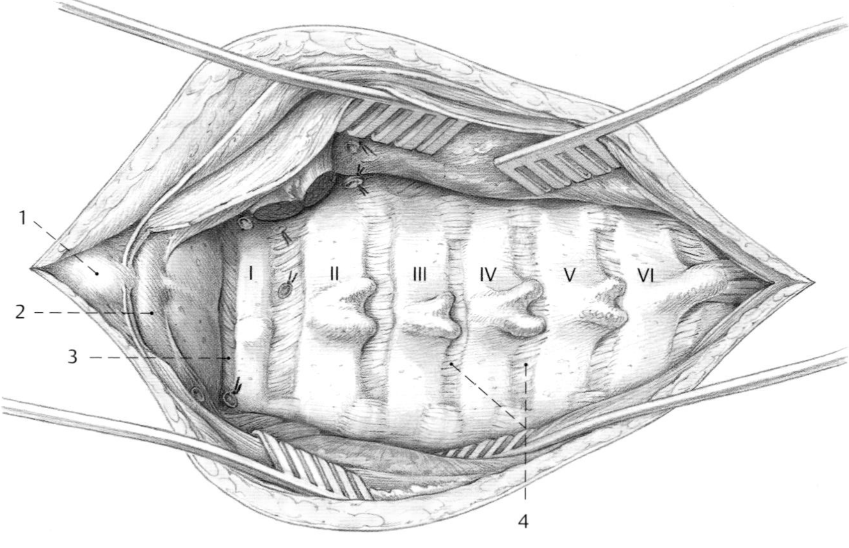

Fig. 5.6 Exposure of the cervical spine from the occiput to the sixth cervical vertebra.

1 External occipital protuberance
2 Superior nuchal line
3 Posterior atlantooccipital membrane
4 Ligamenta flava
I–VI Cervical vertebrae

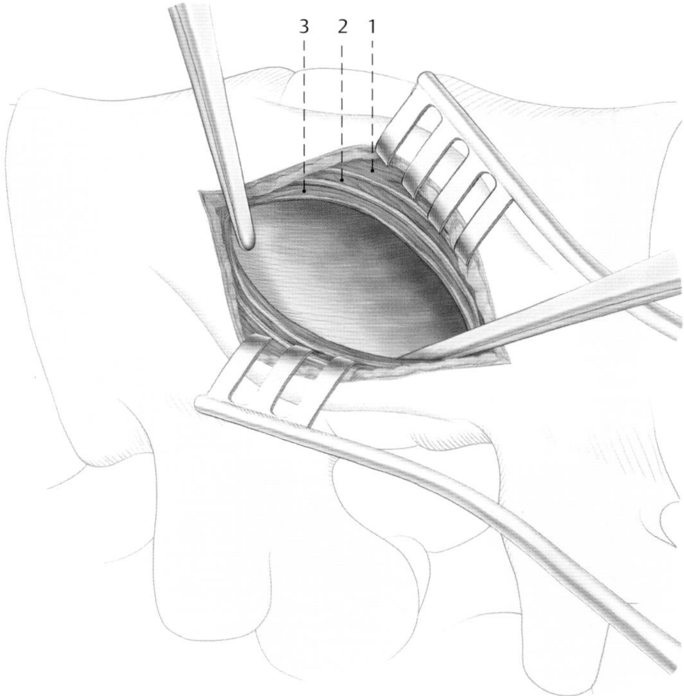

Fig. 4.20 Division of the posterior parts of the fascia of transversus abdominis and exposure of the peritoneum.

1 External oblique
2 Internal oblique
3 Transversus abdominis

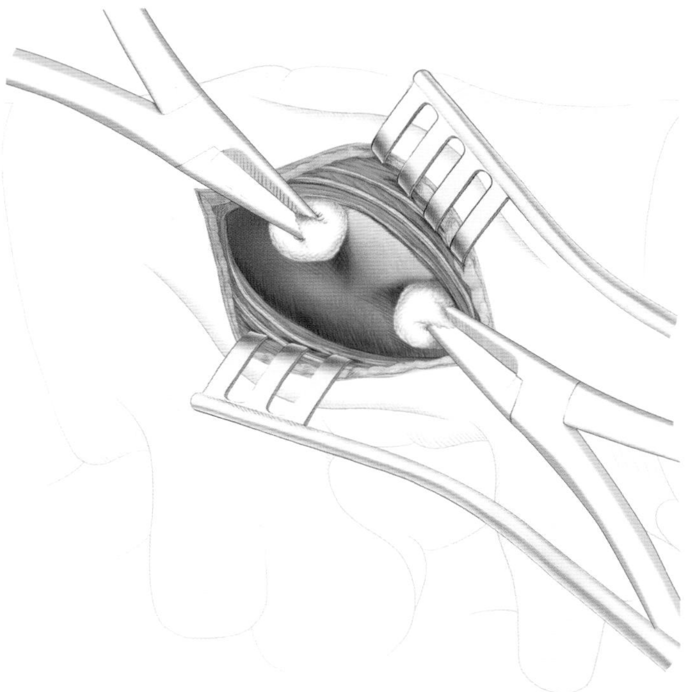

Fig. 4.21 Bluntly pushing the peritoneum away from the abdominal wall.

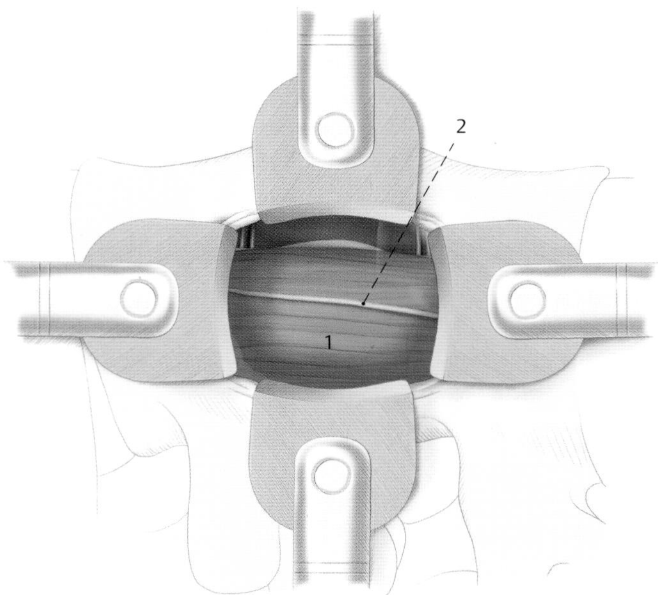

Fig. 4.22 Exposure of the psoas, maintaining the exposure with retractors.

1 Psoas
2 Genitofemoral nerve

Transpsoas Approach

In the transpsoas approach, the longitudinal fibers of the psoas are pushed apart. Because of the nerve roots that run in the psoas, it is generally recommended to do this with neuromonitoring. Support by specialist neuromonitoring staff and appropriate additional equipment are offered by the industry.

Classic Approach

(**Figs. 4.23** and **4.24**)

The retroperitoneal tissue is exposed anteriorly beyond the psoas. The intervertebral disks are exposed between the sympathetic trunk and anterior psoas border. The vessels and sympathetic trunk are retracted medially. The intersegmental vessels are divided in the usual way and also retracted anteriorly and posteriorly. In addition, the psoas is retracted posteriorly from the lateral parts of the vertebral bodies, beginning at the intervertebral disk space.

With both variants, half of the circumference of the vertebral bodies can be exposed (**Figs. 4.23** and **4.24**). The achieved exposure should be maintained by a self-retaining retractor system in both the transpsoas and the classic approach.

4.3.5 Wound Closure

The muscle fascia of the transversus abdominis is closed. The abdominal muscles are reapproximated selectively and in layers with interrupted sutures.

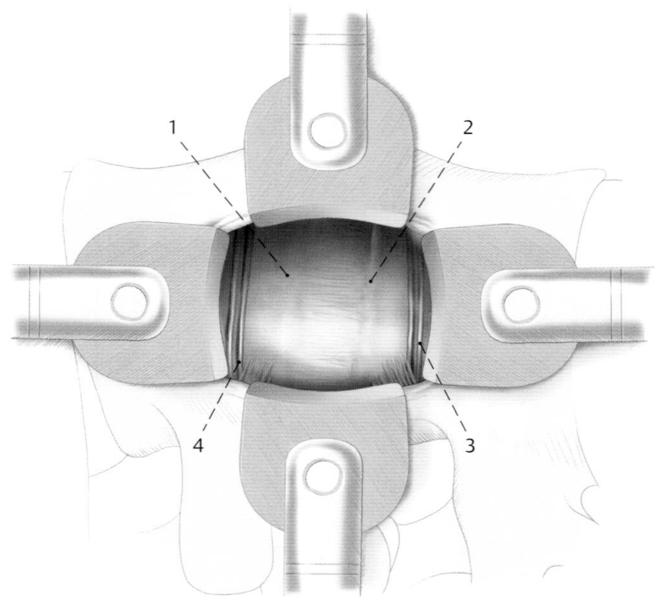

Fig. 4.23 Classic approach. The intervertebral disk space is exposed after posterior retraction of the psoas.

1 Fourth lumbar vertebra
2 Third lumbar vertebra
3 Posterior intercostal artery
4 Anterior external vertebral venous plexus

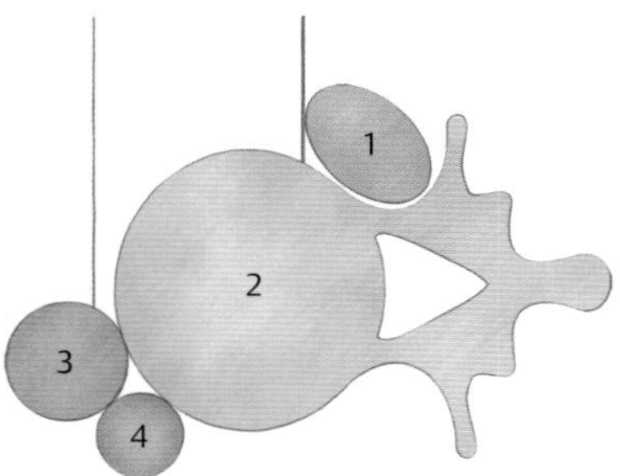

Fig. 4.24 Schematic drawing of the final exposure in the classic approach.

1 Psoas
2 Vertebral body
3 Aorta
4 Vena cava

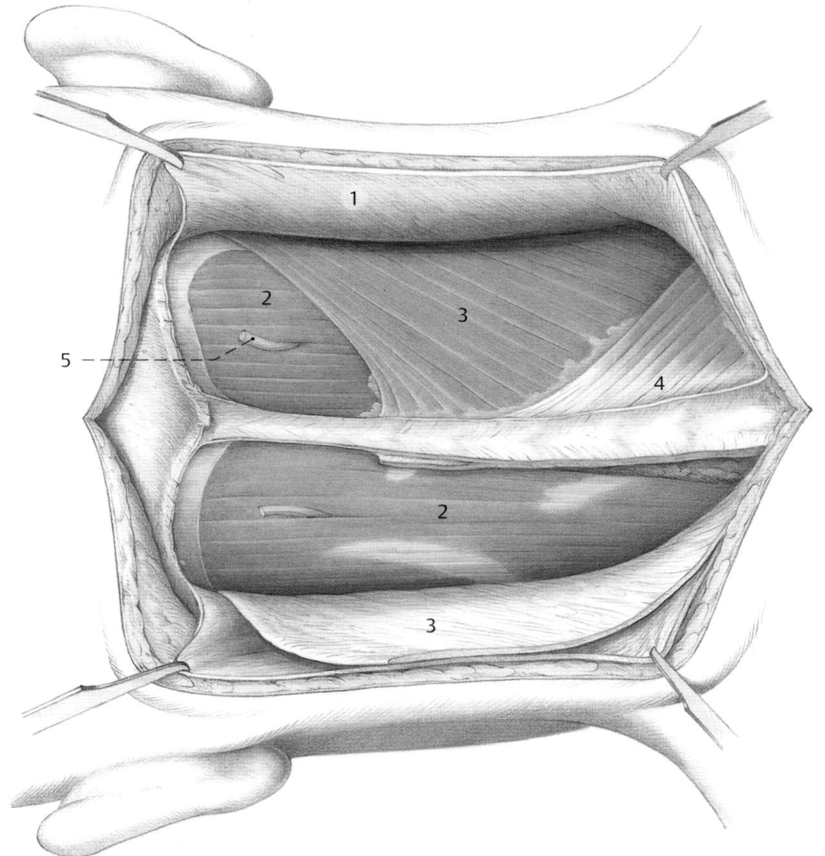

Fig. 5.7 Anatomical site of the superficial and middle layers of the nuchal muscles.

1 Trapezius
2 Semispinalis capitis
3 Splenius capitis
4 Rhomboid minor
5 Greater occipital nerve

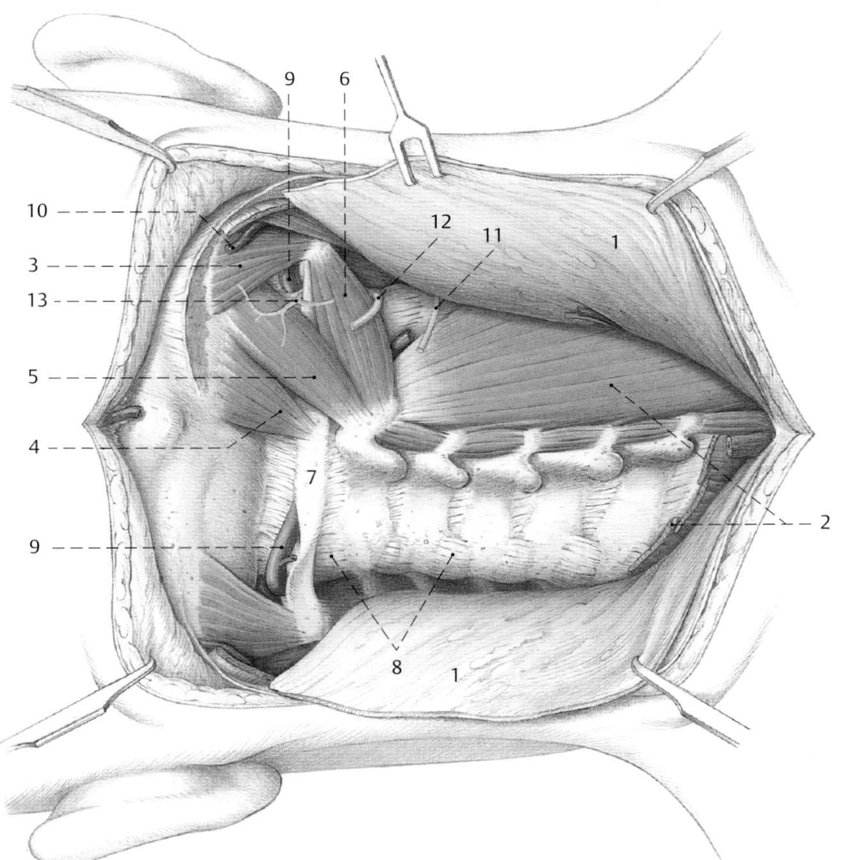

Fig. 5.8 Anatomical site of the deep layers of the nuchal muscles.

1 Semispinalis capitis
2 Semispinalis cervicis
3 Obliquus capitis superior
4 Rectus capitis posterior minor
5 Rectus capitis posterior major
6 Obliquus capitis inferior
7 Posterior arch of the atlas
8 Articular processes of the vertebrae
9 Vertebral artery
10 Occipital artery
11 Third occipital nerve
12 Greater occipital nerve
13 Suboccipital nerve

6 Thoracic and Lumbar Spine

6.1 Costotransversectomy T3–T10

R. Bauer, F. Kerschbaumer, S. Poisel

6.1.1 Principal Indications

- Retropleural abscess in spondylitis
- Biopsy
- Tumors
- Vertebral body fractures

6.1.2 Choice of Side of Approach

Approach is possible from both sides and depends on the site of the lesion.

6.1.3 Positioning and Incision

The operation may be performed with the patient in the prone or semilateral position. For exposure of the vertebral bodies alone, the semilateral position affords a better view toward the anterior direction. For the approach to the upper region of the thoracic spine, the arm on the affected side is maximally abducted to move the scapula as far away from the midline as possible (**Fig. 6.1**).

Two types of skin incision are possible:
- A straight paramedian incision about three fingerbreadths lateral to the spinous processes.
- A T-shaped incision, which provides a better overview.

The transverse portion of the incision is at the level of the vertebra to be exposed (intraoperative markings are made by means of image converter or X-ray), while the longitudinal incision is made over the tips of the spinous processes and is approximately 15 cm long. Transection of the skin and subcutaneous tissue is followed by mobilization of the two skin flaps in the cranial and caudal directions. The superficial muscular layer (trapezius) is divided transversely (**Fig. 6.2**). Using a diathermy scalpel, the intrinsic muscles of the back are now detached near the bone from the spinous processes, in keeping with the skin incision. Cranial and caudal to the transverse incision, the intrinsic muscles of the back are dissected free from the vertebral arches and transverse processes with a raspatory. The longissimus muscle is then transversely dissected and retracted upward and downward (**Fig. 6.3**). The rib leading to the diseased vertebral body is thus identified.

The periosteum over this rib is split with cutting diathermy and carefully retracted with the raspatory. To begin with, the inferior border of the rib is exposed subperiosteally from lateral to medial. The upper border of the rib is exposed subperiosteally by dissecting from medial to lateral until the rib has been exposed subperiosteally over its entire circumference. Now a rib raspatory is used to continue the subperiosteal exposure laterally (8–10 cm) until the desired width of exposure has been obtained. The subperiosteal exposure in the medial direction extends to the costotransverse joint. Using rib shears, the rib is first transected laterally, the costotransverse joint is then opened with a scalpel, and the transverse process is exposed subperiosteally as far as the lamina. The transverse process may then be separated at its base with a narrow chisel and removed with rongeurs. The rib, already laterally detached, is lifted out of the wound area, and the periosteum underlying the rib is now carefully stripped with a raspatory as far as the costovertebral joint, sparing the neurovascular bundle caudal to the rib. Removal of the rib is accomplished by rotary motions on the rib and simultaneous retraction of the costovertebral joint capsule. Careless manipulation can lead to bleeding from the segmental vessels. Generally, three ribs are resected.

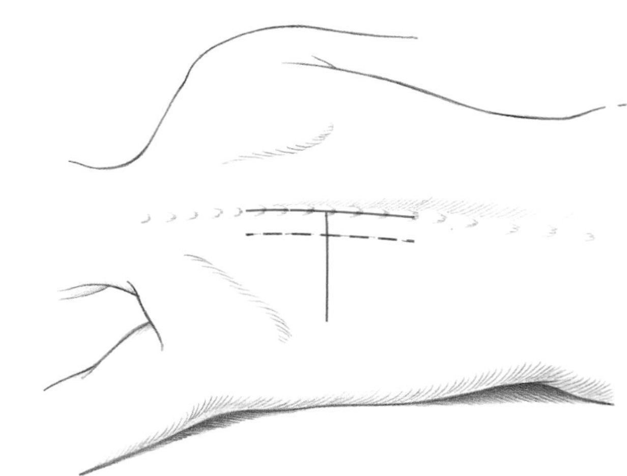

Fig. 6.1 Costotransversectomy. A prone or semilateral position is used, with the arm abducted. The skin incision is T-shaped with the transverse portion over the diseased vertebral body or longitudinal (dashed line) three fingerbreadths from the midline.

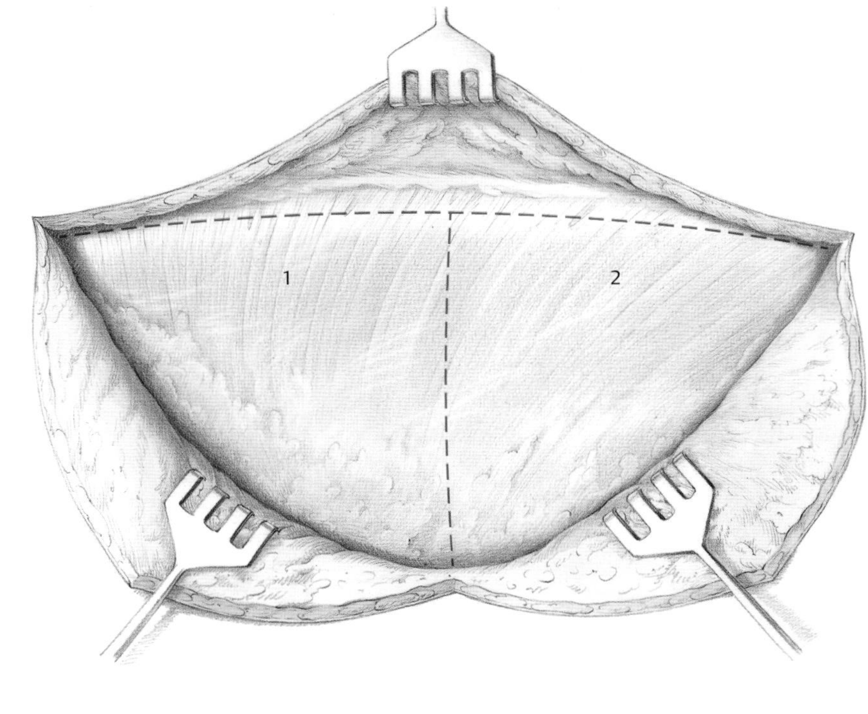

Fig. 6.2 Operative site after transection of the skin and subcutaneous tissue. T-shaped incision of the posterior muscles (dashed lines).

1 Trapezius, transverse part
2 Trapezius, ascending part

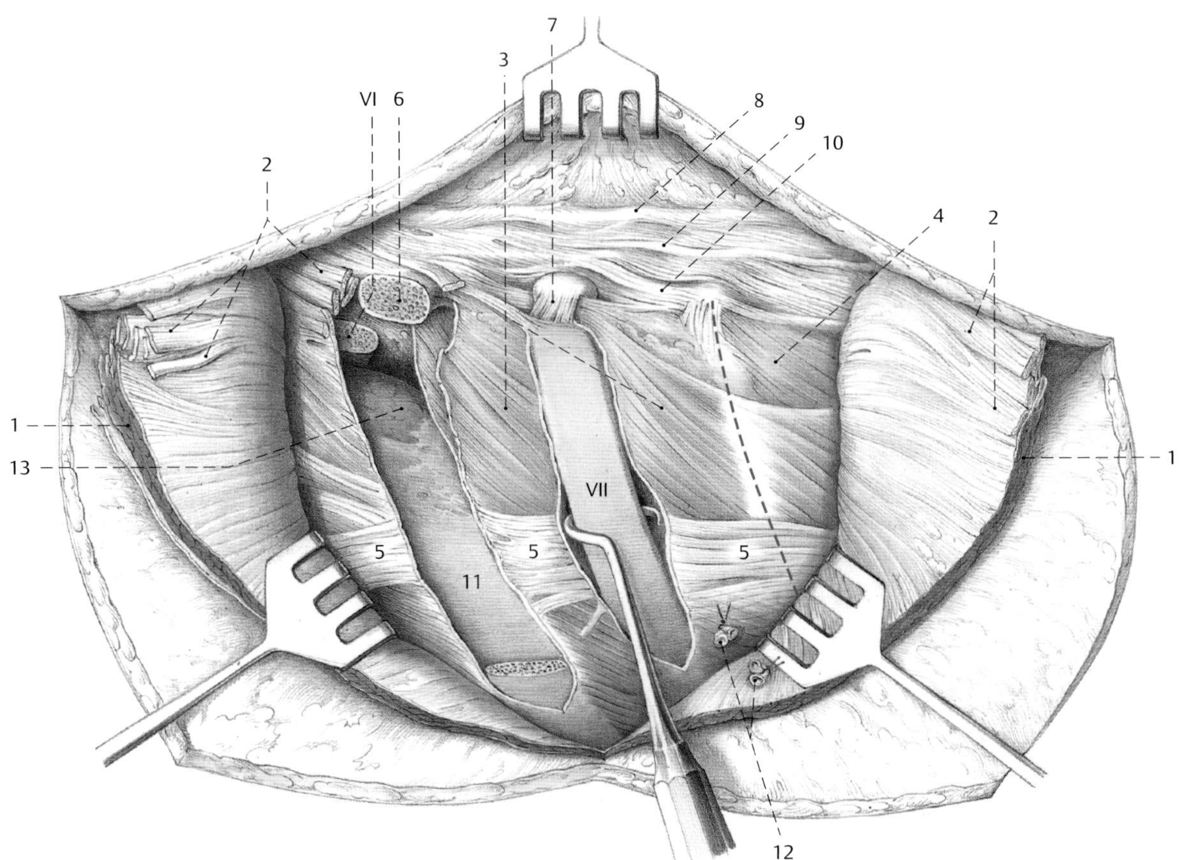

Fig. 6.3 After craniad and caudad dissection of the muscle flaps, the costal periosteum is split and the rib is exposed subperiosteally over a length of 8–10 cm. After opening of the costotransverse joint capsule and removal of the transverse process at the base, the rib is transected laterally with rib cutters, lifted out of the wound, and exarticulated following careful detachment of the costovertebral joint capsule.

1 Trapezius
2 Longissimus
3 External intercostal muscles
4 Semispinalis
5 Iliocostalis
6 Transverse process of the sixth thoracic vertebra
7 Costotransverse ligament
8 Supraspinal ligament
9 Interspinal ligament
10 Intertransverse ligament
11 Periosteum of the fifth rib
12 Intercostal vessels, lateral cutaneous branches
13 Parietal pleura
VI, VII Ribs

6.1.4 Exposure of the Vertebrae

The endothoracic fascia underlying the costal periosteum and the parietal pleura are carefully retracted from the anterior aspect of the vertebral bodies and intervertebral disks with cotton applicators, preserving the neurovascular bundles. The remains of the intercostal muscles lying between the resected ribs are dissected free from the segmental vessels (**Fig. 6.4**). If necessary, the intercostal vessels may be ligated and transected anterior to the vertebral body, but the segmental nerves should be preserved if possible as, beginning at T6, they supply the abdominal muscles. After retraction of the parietal pleura from the anterior aspect of the vertebral bodies, flexible spatulas may be introduced so that two to three vertebral bodies are revealed laterally from behind (**Fig. 6.5**).

6.1.5 Wound Closure

Before wound closure, positive pressure breathing should be employed to make certain that the parietal pleura has not been injured. If it has, a suction drain must be introduced. Wound closure is effected by reapproximation, in layers, of the divided muscles.

6.1.6 Note

Costotransversectomy was formerly considered to be the standard approach, particularly for the surgical treatment of tuberculous spondylitis. This approach has nowadays been largely supplanted by thoracotomy, which provides a better overview. Costotransversectomy is indicated, above all, when thoracotomy is precluded for medical or technical reasons, or when tumors involving both posterior vertebral structures and the vertebral body have to be resected in a single session. This approach has also been described for the internal fixation of vertebral fractures when anterior decompression of the vertebral canal is required at the same time.

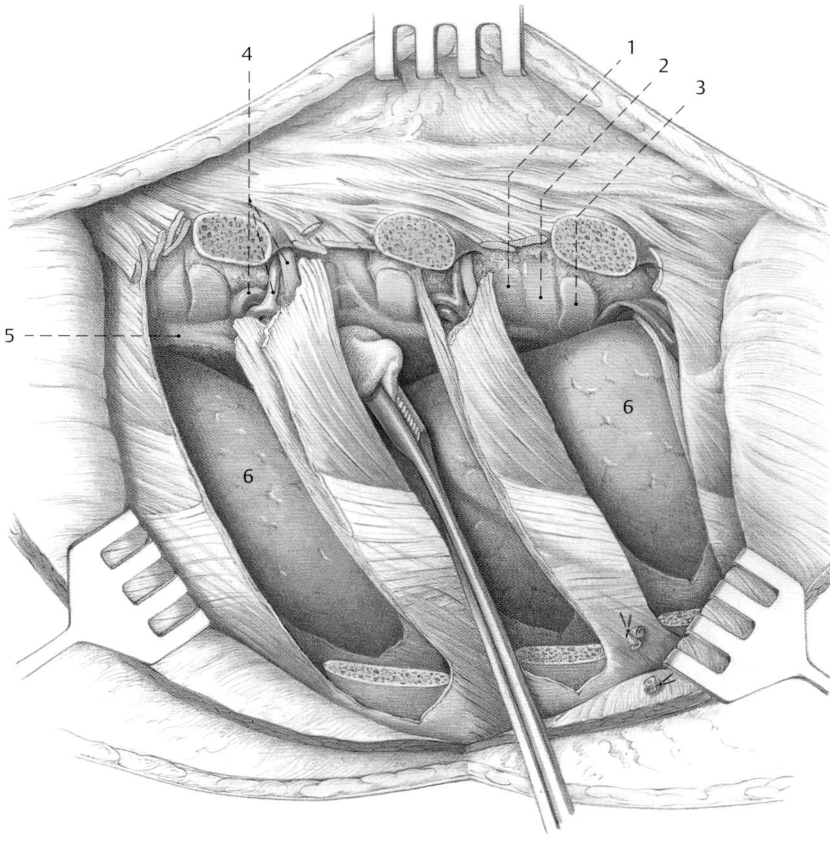

Fig. 6.4 Blunt dissection of the endothoracic fascia and parietal pleura beneath the rib bed, from the lateral and anterior aspects of the thoracic vertebrae, and from the intervertebral disks.

1 Inferior costal facet
2 Intervertebral disk
3 Superior costal facet
4 Intercostal artery, vein, and nerve
5 Sympathetic trunk
6 Lung with parietal pleura

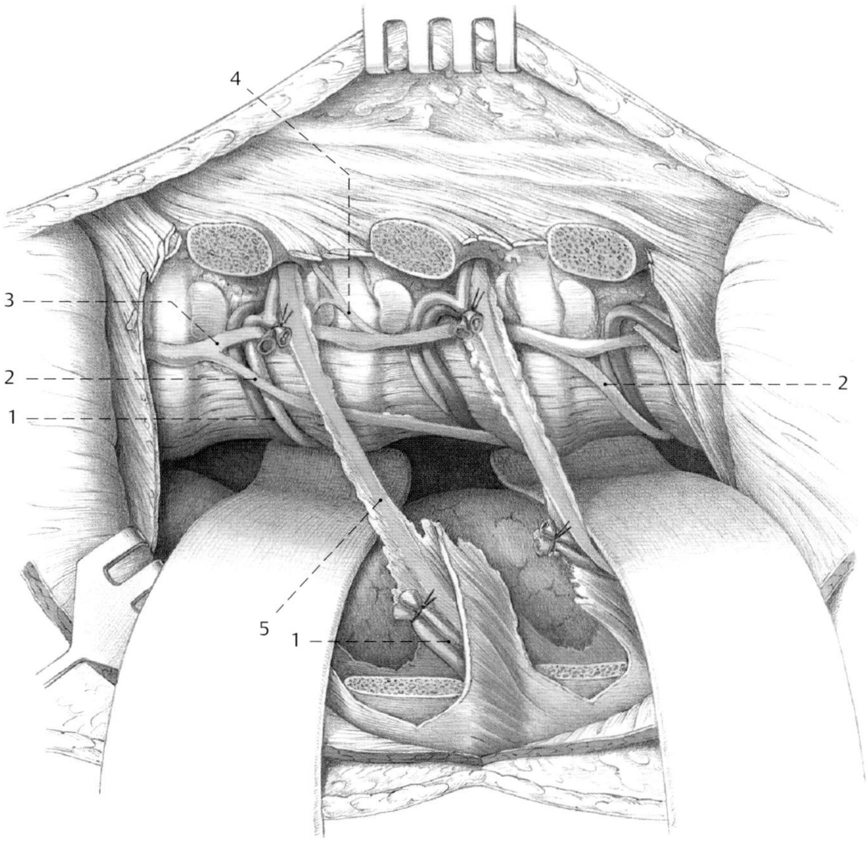

Fig. 6.5 Exposure of the intercostal neurovascular bundles by dissection of the intercostal muscles. If necessary, the intercostal vessels may be ligated and transected. The intercostal nerves should be spared.

1 Intercostal vessels
2 Greater splanchnic nerve
3 Sympathetic trunk
4 Communicating branch
5 Intercostal nerve

6.2 Posterior Approach to the Thoracic and Lumbar Spine

R. Bauer, F. Kerschbaumer, S. Poisel

6.2.1 Principal Indications

- Scoliosis
- Kyphosis
- Fractures
- Tumors

6.2.2 Positioning and Incision

The patient is placed prone with bolsters under the chest and under both iliac crests, or is placed on special supports, for example a Relton-Hall frame (**Fig. 6.6**). Care should be taken not to compress the abdomen, so that venous congestion and hence increased venous hemorrhage during the operation may be prevented. A straight midline incision is made, even in scoliosis. If fusion is to be performed, the incision should be one to two segments longer than the intended length of fusion (**Fig. 6.7**). Subsequently, the subcutaneous tissue is dissected as far as the fascia, and wound retractors are inserted.

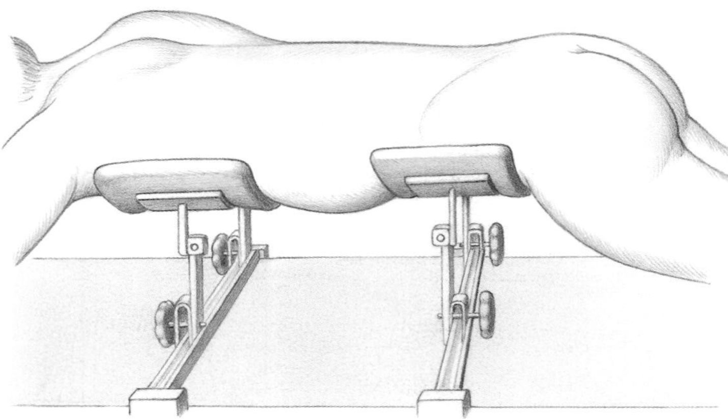

Fig. 6.6 Posterior approach to the thoracic and lumbar spine. Positioning on a Relton-Hall frame.

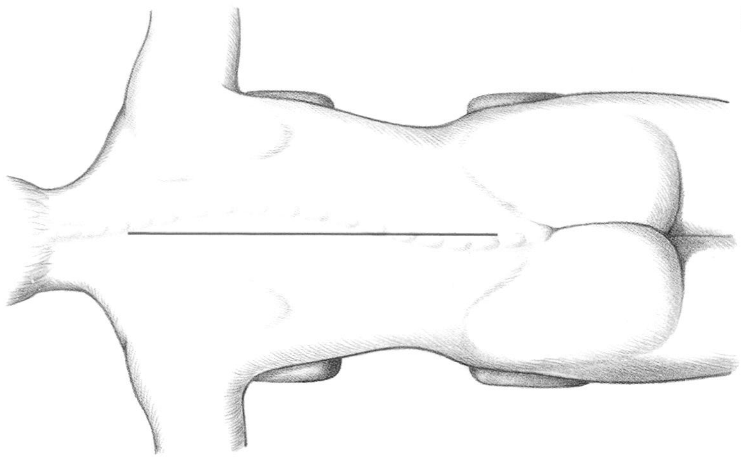

Fig. 6.7 Incision.

6.2.3 Exposure of the Thoracic Spine

In children and adolescents, the cartilaginous spinous process apophyses are split in the midline in longitudinal direction, together with the interspinal ligaments (**Fig. 6.8**). The apophyses with the adhering periosteum can easily be retracted with a raspatory to the base of the spinous processes or to the vertebral arches. In adult patients, the fascia has to be detached with a diathermy scalpel near the bone on both sides of the spinous process. Retraction of the muscle in operations for scoliosis is usually begun on the side of the concavity (**Fig. 6.9**). The dissection is carried out from caudal to cranial.

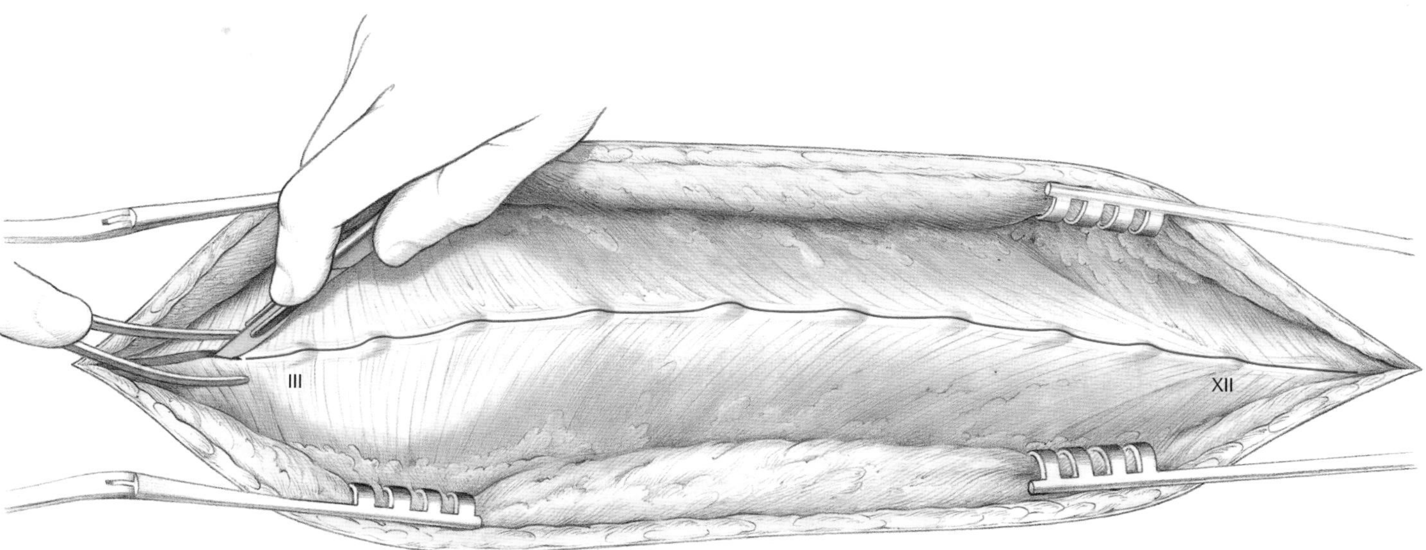

Fig. 6.8 In adolescents and children, the cartilaginous spinous process apophyses and interspinal ligaments are incised in the midline and retracted laterally with the periosteum.

III–XII Spinous processes

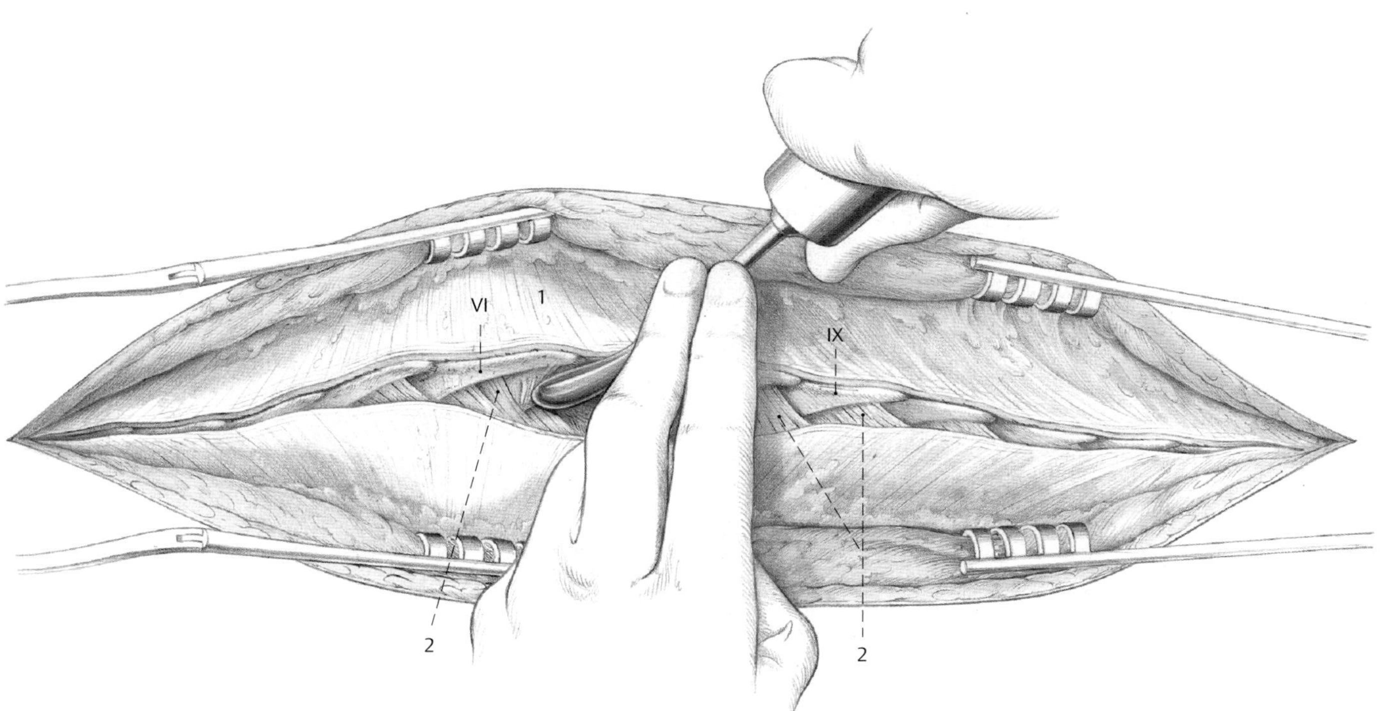

Fig. 6.9 Subperiosteal exposure with a raspatory down to the base of the spinous processes.

1 Trapezius
2 Multifidus muscles
VI, IX Spinous processes

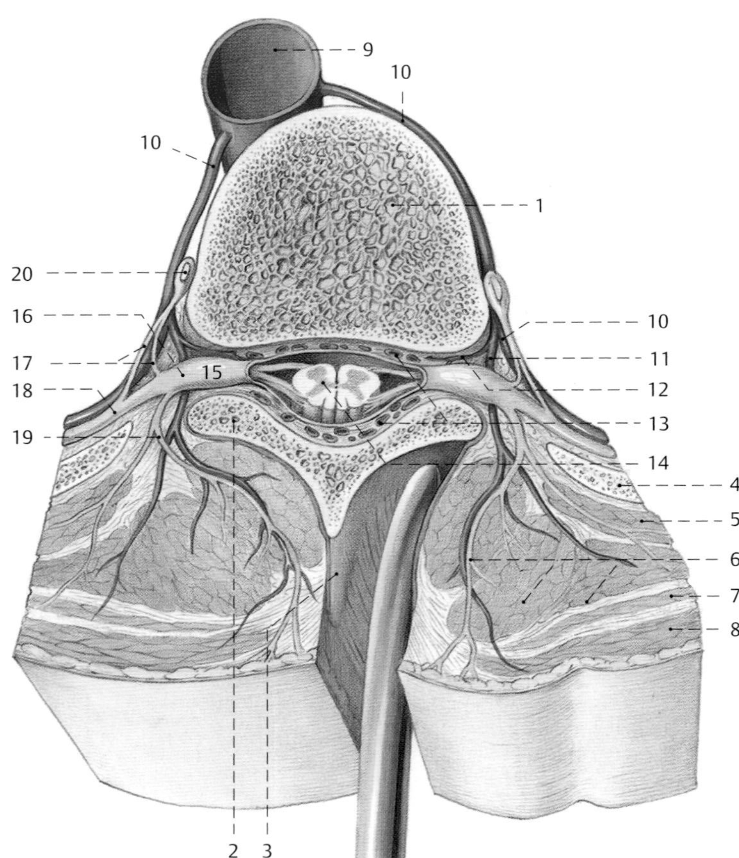

Fig. 6.10 Cross-section in the region of the thoracic spine; subperiosteal dissection.

1 Vertebral body
2 Lamina of the vertebral arch
3 Spinous process
4 Rib
5 External oblique muscle of the abdomen
6 Intrinsic back muscles
7 Serratus posterior inferior
8 Trapezius
9 Thoracic aorta
10 Posterior intercostal arteries
11 Posterior branch
12 Spinal branch
13 Anterior and posterior internal vertebral venous plexus
14 Spinal medulla
15 Spinal ganglion
16 Spinal nerve
17 Communicating branches
18 Anterior ramus
19 Posterior ramus
20 Sympathetic trunk

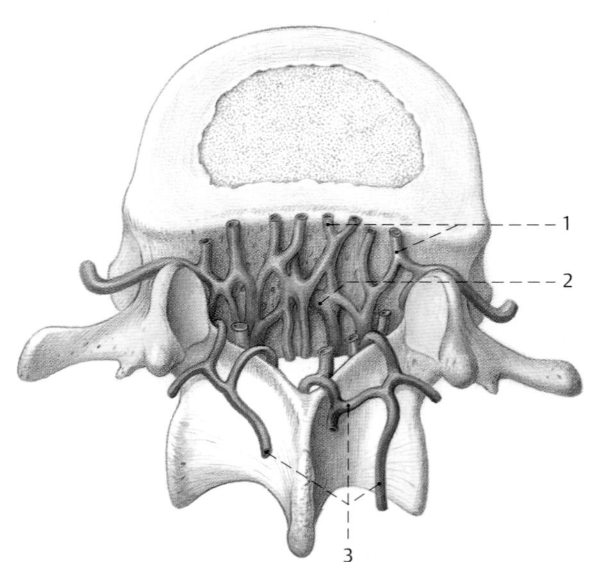

Fig. 6.11 Schematic representation of the vertebral venous plexus.

1 Anterior internal vertebral venous plexus
2 Basivertebral vein
3 Posterior external vertebral venous plexus

The exposure should be strictly subperiosteal so that the neurovascular supply of the muscles may be spared and hemorrhage avoided (**Fig. 6.10**).

There may be severe bleeding from the posterior external vertebral venous plexus (**Fig. 6.11**), which must be stopped by electrocoagulation or tamponade.

The subperiosteal exposure is continued laterally as far as the ends of the transverse processes. When the concave side has been exposed, it is tamponaded with gauze swabs, and the same procedure is then followed on the contralateral side.

When the spinalis and semispinalis muscles have been stripped, the multifidus and rotator muscles are dissected free.

Particularly in adult patients, sharp dissection of the tendons with a scalpel may be necessary in some cases (**Figs. 6.12** and **6.13**).

If vertebral fusion is planned, the joint capsules of the segments involved, as well as all remnants of the tendon insertions between the spinous processes, and the interspinal ligaments need to be removed. This is done by dissecting the capsules of the vertebral joints from craniomedial to caudolateral, using a Cobb elevator (**Fig. 6.14**).

For anatomical orientation, the 12th thoracic and the first lumbar vertebra can be used. The 12th thoracic vertebra has a regressive transverse process that overlies a readily mobile 12th rib. The first lumbar vertebra has a nonmobile costal process. The joint between the 11th and the 12th thoracic vertebrae is positioned frontally, similar to the other thoracic facet joints, whereas the T12–L1 joint is situated sagittally, similar to the lumbar facet joints. These locational characteristics apply in approximately 90% of the cases. In the presence of anatomical uncertainties (such as lumbar ribs), a lateral radiograph may be obtained intraoperatively to determine the location.

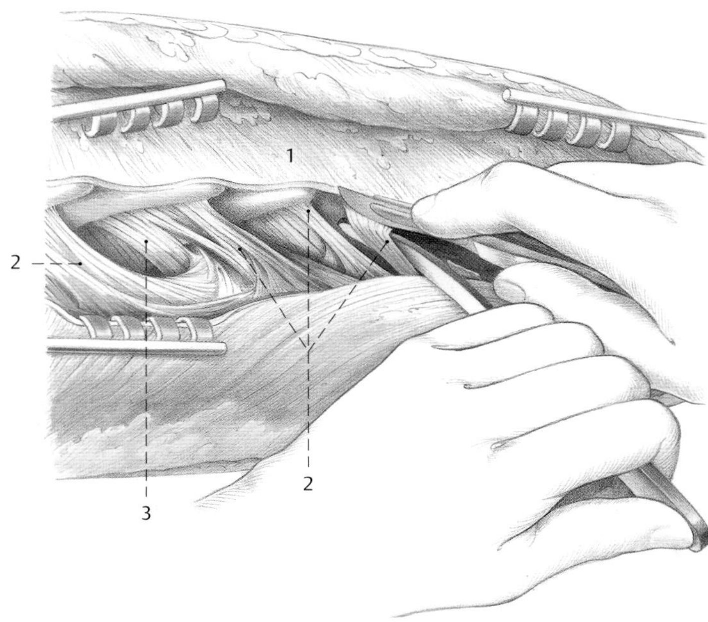

Fig. 6.12 Dissection of semispinalis and multifidus from the lower edge of the spinous processes. In part, this dissection is done sharply with a scalpel.

1 Trapezius
2 Semispinalis
3 Multifidus

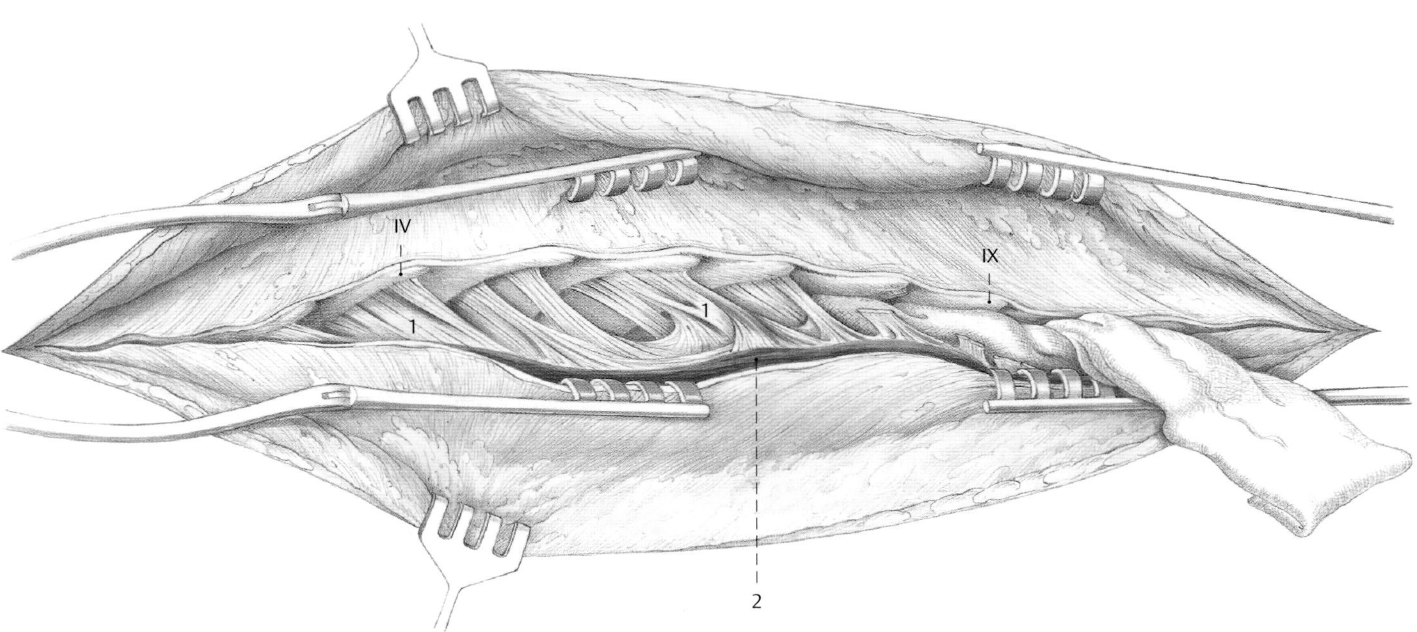

Fig. 6.13 Tamponade of the wound with a gauze swab and insertion of retractors into the muscle. The dissection is performed on the thoracic spine from caudal to cranial.

1 Multifidus muscles
2 Spinalis
IV–IX Spinous processes

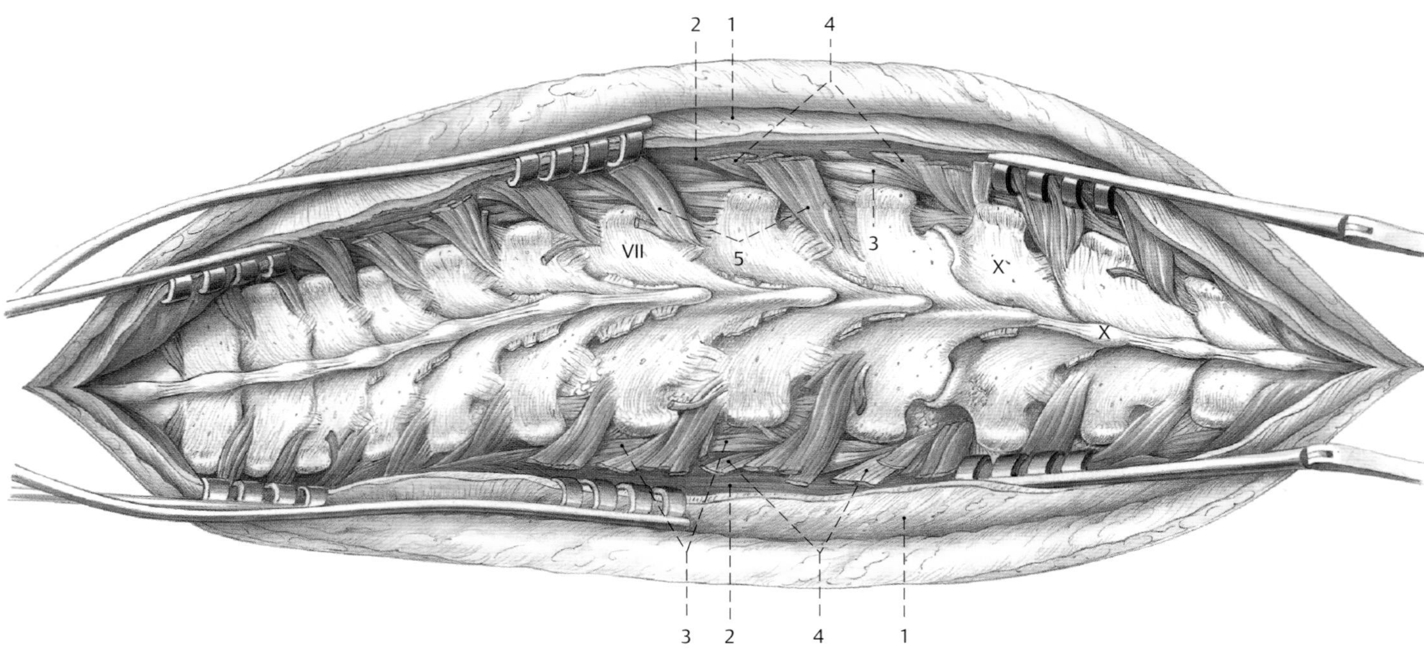

Fig. 6.14 Operative site after subperiosteal exposure of the posterior vertebral elements. At the level of the ninth and 10th thoracic vertebrae the capsules of the facet joints were removed bilaterally.

1 Trapezius
2 Spinalis
3 Semispinalis
4 Multifidus
5 Rotator muscles
VII, X Thoracic vertebrae

6.2.4 Exposure of the Lumbar Spine

(**Fig. 6.15**)

Exposure of the lumbar spine is accomplished from the posterior side in the same manner as for exposure of the thoracic spine, but the dissection is carried out from cranial to caudal. As far as possible, the muscles and tendons are stripped from the spinous processes subperiosteally; in children and adolescents, the joint capsules may be dissected in the same plane. The costal process to the end of which the dissection should be performed lies laterally and slightly anteriorly and caudally to the upper articular process. Retraction of the muscles requires more force in this region than for the thoracic spine. Dissection can be facilitated by propping up the Cobb elevator like a lever on the tip of the intact spinous process. The remaining muscle is removed from the transverse processes with a gauze swab. The retractors are now placed more deeply and are distracted until the posterior vertebral elements are exposed as far as the ends of the costal processes. Now the spinous processes are cleared of soft tissue, especially on the inferior edges, and the joint capsules are removed. The latter can be detached most readily with a scalpel and forceps (**Fig. 6.16**). The anatomical orientation of the lumbar spine is easy to determine. There is no ligamentum flavum caudal to S1 (except in cases of anomaly), the spinous process of L5 is clearly larger than that of S1, and the lumbosacral joint generally is the last one. In the presence of spina bifida or vertebral arch fractures, the elevator may enter the vertebral canal if the dissection is not performed with sufficient care.

6.2.5 Wound Closure

Wound closure is effected in two layers by suture of the paraspinal muscles and the overlying fascia. In children and adolescents, the split spinous process apophyses are readily united by sutures.

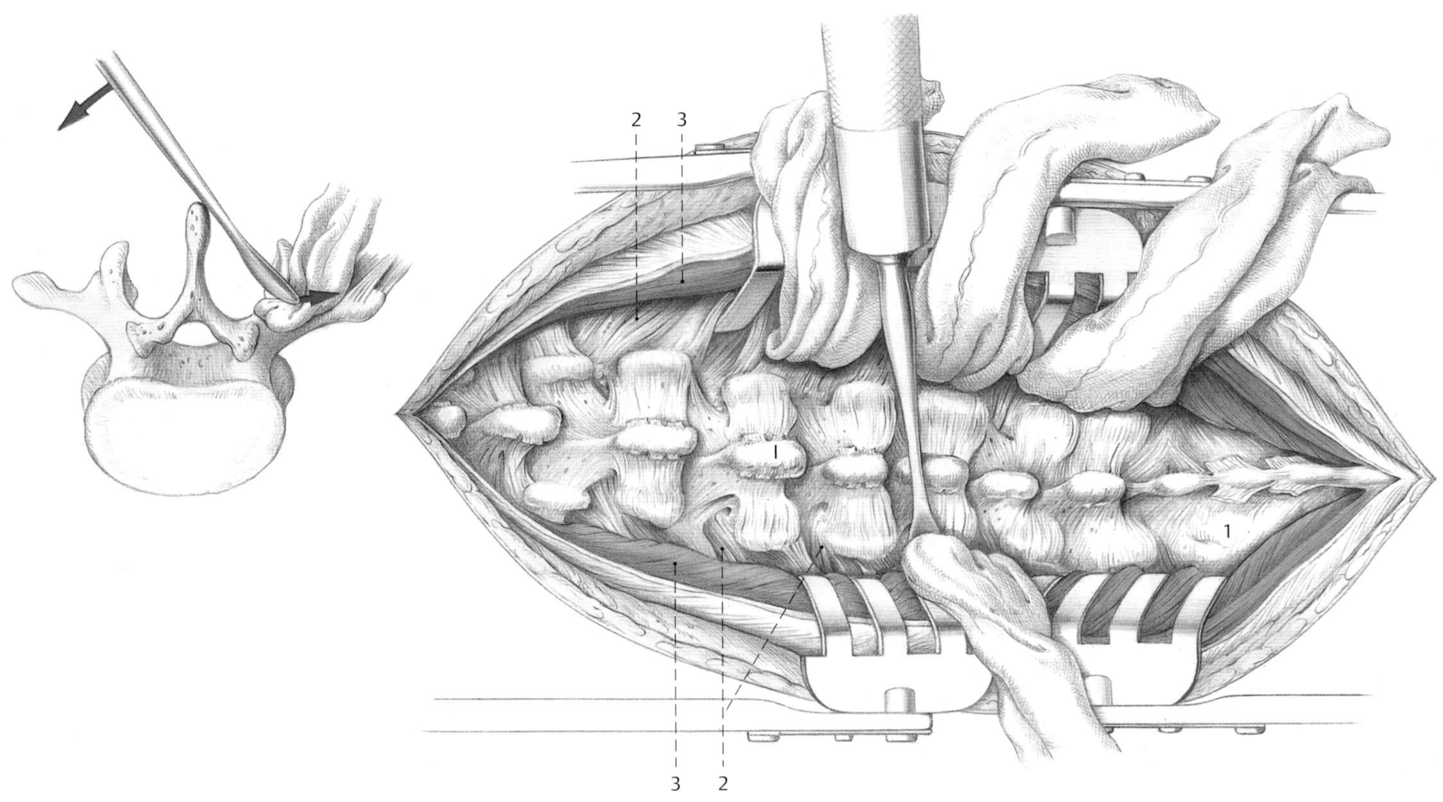

Fig. 6.15 Exposure of the lumbar spine from the posterior. Subperiosteal exposure of the spinous processes and vertebral arches to the area of the joints and as far as the base of the transverse processes. At this site, gauze swabs are introduced for the remaining exposure to the tip of the transverse process (inset).

1 Sacrum
2 Multifidus
3 Longissimus
I Spinous process

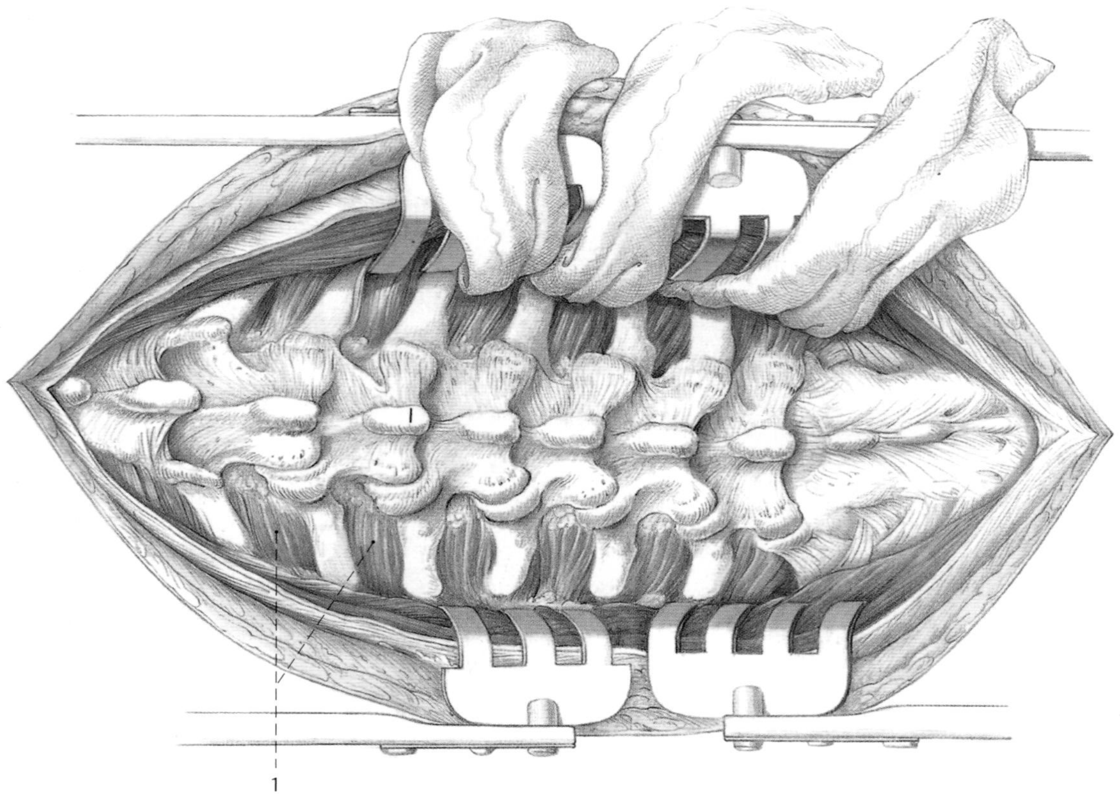

Fig. 6.16 Exposure of the lumbar spine and lumbosacral junction from posterior.

1 Multifidus
I Lumbar vertebra

6.3 Paraspinal Approach to the Lumbosacral Junction According to Wiltse

R. Bauer, F. Kerschbaumer, S. Poisel

6.3.1 Principal Indications

- Spondylolisthesis

6.3.2 Positioning and Incision

(**Fig. 6.17**)

The patient is placed in the prone position on a Relton-Hall frame (see **Fig. 6.6**).

Two paramedian skin incisions are made about three fingerbreadths lateral to the spinous processes. One skin incision may in some cases be extended somewhat inferolaterally if it should become necessary to remove bone graft material from the posterior part of the ilium. The fascia of the iliocostalis muscle is exposed and split longitudinally in the outer third.

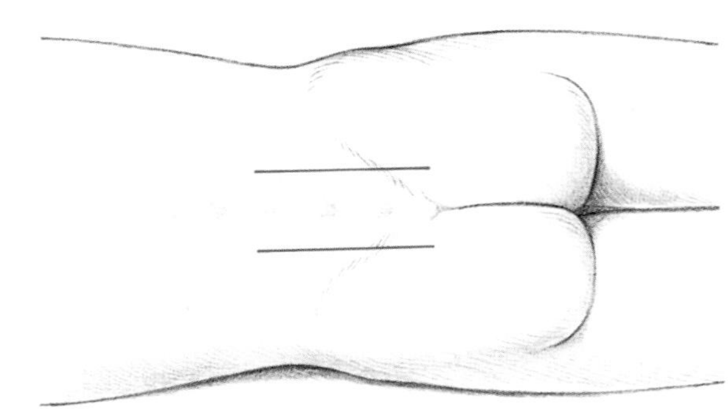

Fig. 6.17 Paraspinal approach to the lumbar spine according to Wiltse. Skin incision.

6.3.3 Exposure of the Posterolateral Vertebral Elements

(**Fig. 6.18**)

Following blunt dissection through the iliocostalis muscle, the L5–S1 facet joint can first be palpated with the finger. This joint is visualized after medial and lateral retraction of the muscle with a Cobb elevator. The muscle is split further cranially and caudally as needed. Next, the ala of the sacrum, the inferior and superior articular processes of L5, as well as the costal process of L5 are exposed subperiosteally. For better visualization of the articular processes, the L5–S1 joint capsule is removed. If necessary, the vertebral arch of L5, which is generally very mobile in spondylolysis, and the ligamentum flavum can be exposed further after mediad retraction of the muscle. This also makes laminectomy or foraminotomy possible. In spondylolysis, fibrous scar tissue is found in the area of the interarticular portion and may have to be removed by cutting. In posterolateral fusion of L5–S1 according to Wiltse, opening of the L4–L5 facet joint should be avoided.

Too deep a dissection between the ala of the sacrum and the costal process of L5 can lead to injury to the fifth lumbar spinal nerve.

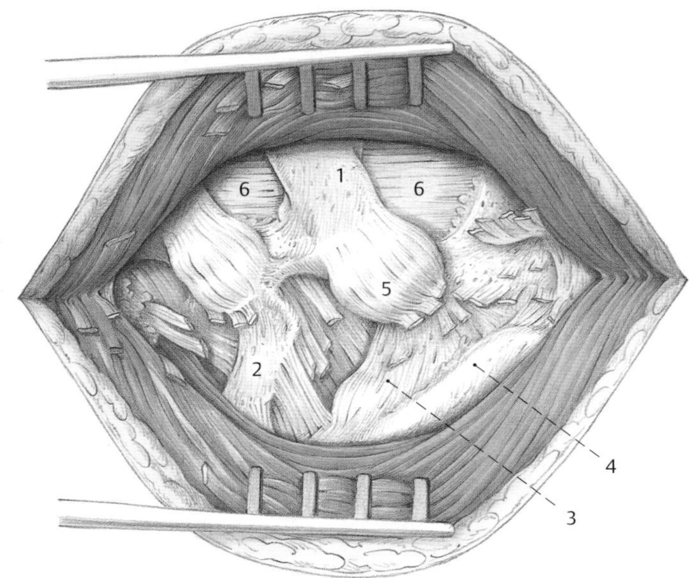

Fig. 6.18 Appearance after longitudinal splitting of the fascia and muscle. Exposure of the L4–L5 and L5–S1 facet joints as well as of the costal process of the fifth lumbar vertebra and the ala of the sacrum. The soft tissue overlying the ligamentum flavum has been removed.

1 Lamina of the fifth lumbar vertebra
2 Costal process of the fifth lumbar vertebra
3 Ala of sacrum
4 Iliac crest
5 Articulation between the fifth lumbar and first sacral vertebrae
6 Ligamenta flava

6.3.4 Wound Closure

Wound closure is effected by suture of iliocostalis and the overlying fascia.

6.4 Short Posterior Approach to the Lumbar Spine for Laminotomy and Removal of an Intervertebral Disk

R. Bauer, F. Kerschbaumer, S. Poisel

6.4.1 Principal Indications

- Disk prolapse
- Vertebral stenosis

6.4.2 Positioning and Incision

The operation may be performed with the patient placed in a lateral position or in the knee–elbow position with the lumbar spine rendered kyphotic (**Fig. 6.19**). The skin incision is generally made over the fourth and fifth spinous processes and is approximately 10 cm in length (**Fig. 6.20**). The thoracolumbar fascia is opened in the midline with a diathermy scalpel, and the paraspinal muscles are subsequently retracted with a raspatory, subperiosteally if possible, as far as the facet joints. Following hemostasis and tamponade with gauze swabs, self-retaining retractors are introduced. Then all the soft tissues overlying the ligamentum flavum are removed (**Fig. 6.21**).

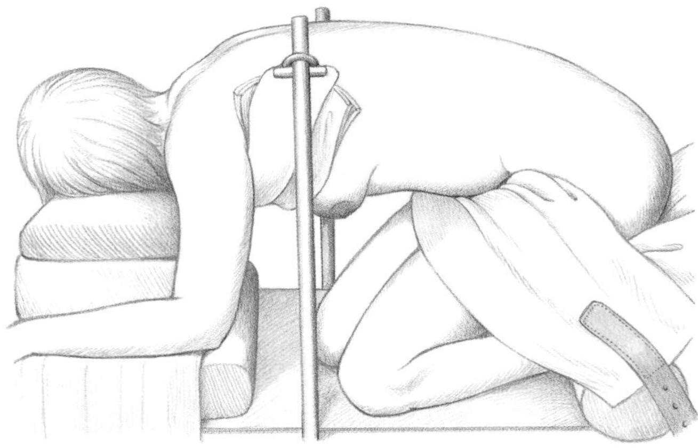

Fig. 6.19 Short posterior approach to the lumbar spine (laminotomy). The patient is in the knee–elbow position.

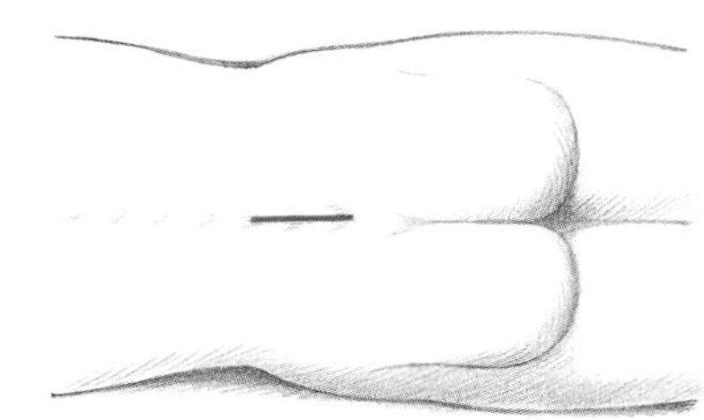

Fig. 6.20 Skin incision in the midline, 10 cm long.

6.4.3 Exposure of the Vertebral Canal

The inferior border of the next higher vertebral arch is removed with Leksell forceps or a Hajek punch. The ligamentum flavum is then grasped with forceps and, using a scalpel, is incised in the midline from cranial to caudal, separated from the upper edge of the next vertebra, and removed (**Fig. 6.22**). With the aid of a dissector and small cotton swabs, the epidural fat is removed, exposing the dura and nerve root. The nerve root may be cautiously retracted in a medial direction with a cotton swab or root hook so that the posterolateral portion of the intervertebral disk becomes visible (**Fig. 6.23**).

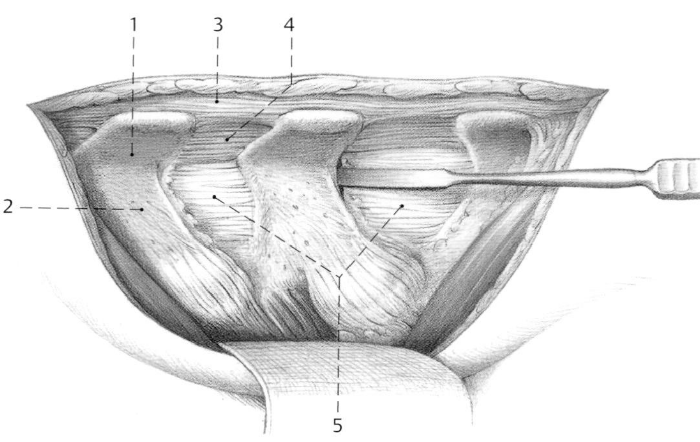

Fig. 6.21 Operative site after retraction of the paraspinal muscles and exposure of the vertebral arches, ligamentum flavum, and facet joints. Retraction of the ligamentum flavum from the vertebral arch.

1 Spinous process
2 Lamina
3 Supraspinal ligament
4 Interspinal ligament
5 Ligamenta flava

6.4.4 Wound Closure

The wound is closed by suture of the divided muscle and fascia.

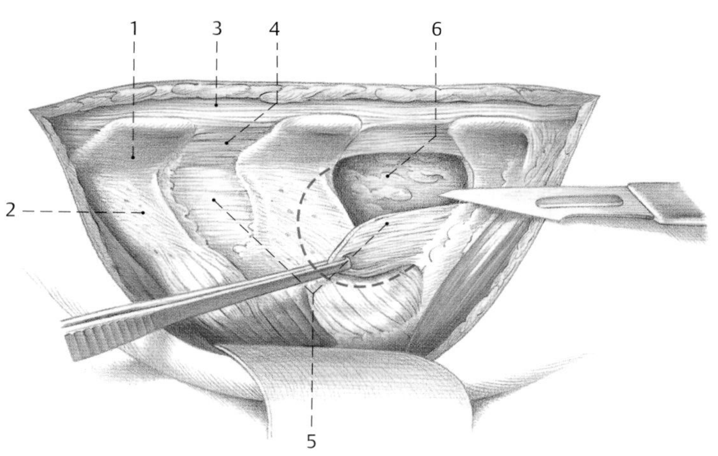

Fig. 6.22 Resection of the ligamentum flavum. The extent of the laminotomy is shown by the dashed line.

1 Spinous process
2 Lamina
3 Supraspinal ligament
4 Interspinal ligament
5 Ligamenta flava
6 Epidural fat

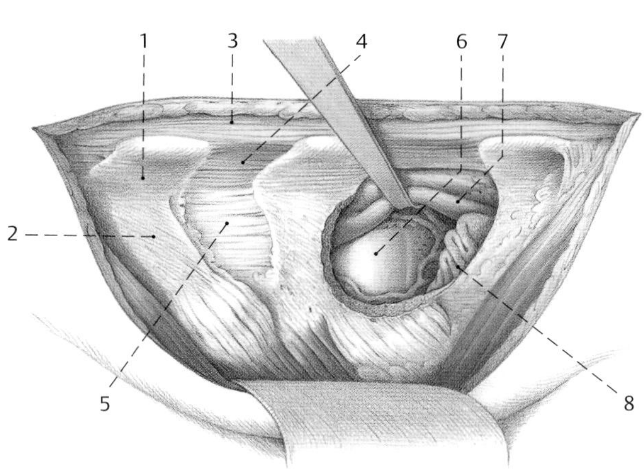

Fig. 6.23 Operative site after laminotomy. Removal of the ligamentum flavum and medial third of the facet joint for exposure of the nerve root, lateral recess, and intervertebral disk.

1 Spinous process
2 Lamina
3 Supraspinal ligament
4 Interspinal ligament
5 Ligamenta flava
6 Intervertebral disk
7 Root of the spinal nerve
8 Swab

Further Reading: Spine

[1] Adachi B. Das Arteriensystem der Japaner. Kyoto: Kaiserlich-japanische Universität zu Kyoto; 1928

[2] Bauer R. Die operative Behandlung der Skoliose. Bern: Huber; 1979

[3] Bauer R. Der vordere Zugang zur Wirbelsäule. Stuttgart: Thieme; 1983

[4] Beisse R. Endoscopic surgery on the thoracolumbar junction of the spine. Eur Spine J 2010;19(Suppl 1):S52–S65

[5] Bertagnoli R, Vazquez RJ. The Anterolateral TransPsoatic Approach (ALPA): a new technique for implanting prosthetic disc-nucleus devices. J Spinal Disord Tech 2003;16(4):398–404

[6] Bühren V, Beisse R, Potulski M. Minimally invasive ventral spondylodesis in injuries to the thoracic and lumbar spine [in German]. Chirurg 1997;68(11):1076–1084

[7] Cauchoix J, Binet JP. Anterior surgical approaches to the spine. Ann R Coll Surg Engl 1957;21(4):237–243

[8] Cauchoix J, Binet JP, Evrard J. Les voies d'abord inhabituelles dans l'abord des corps vertebraux, cervicaux et dorsaux. Ann Chir 1957;74:1463

[9] Colletta AJ, Mayer PJ. Chylothorax: an unusual complication of anterior thoracic interbody spinal fusion. Spine 1982;7(1):46–49

[10] Cordier P, Devos L, Deleroix A. Essai de classification des variations du système azygos intrathoracique. C R Assoc Anat 1938;33:100–118

[11] Crock HV, Yoshizawa H. The Blood Supply of the Vertebral Column and the Spinal Cord in Man. Berlin: Springer; 1977

[12] Denck H. Eingriffe an der Brustwand. In: Breitner B, ed. Chirurgische Operationslehre. Munich: Urban & Schwarzenberg; 1981

[13] Dommisse GF. Some factors in the management of fractures and fracture-dislocations of the spine at lumbo-dorsal level. The significance of the blood supply of the spine. Reconstr Surg Traumatol 1972;13:108–123

[14] Dommisse GF. The blood supply of the spinal cord. A critical vascular zone in spinal surgery. J Bone Joint Surg Br 1974;56(2):225–235

[15] Dwyer AF, Newton NC, Sherwood AA. An anterior approach to scoliosis. A preliminary report. Clin Orthop Relat Res 1969;62(62):192–202

[16] Dwyer AF. Experience of anterior correction of scoliosis. Clin Orthop Relat Res 1973;(93):191–206

[17] Eisenstein S, O'Brien JP. Chylothorax: a complication of Dwyer's anterior instrumentation. Br J Surg 1977;64(5):339–341

[18] Fang HSY, Ong GB. Direct anterior approach to the upper cervical spine. J Bone Joint Surg Am 1962;44:1588–1604

[19] Fey B. L'abord du rein par voie thoracoabdominale. Arch Urol 1925;5:169

[20] Freebody D, Bendall R, Taylor RD. Anterior transperitoneal lumbar fusion. J Bone Joint Surg Br 1971;53(4):617–627

[21] Goldstein LA, Dickerson RC. Atlas of Orthopaedic Surgery. St. Louis: Mosby; 1981

[22] Hellinger J. Der transoropharyngeale Zugang zu C1 und C2 [in German]. Beitr Orthop Traumatol 1981;28(1):25–31

[23] Henry AK. Extensile Exposure. 2nd ed. Edinburgh: Livingstone; 1957

[24] Hodge WA, DeWald RL. Splenic injury complicating the anterior thoracoabdominal surgical approach for scoliosis. A report of two cases. J Bone Joint Surg Am 1983;65(3):396–397

[25] Hodgson AR, Stock FE. Anterior spinal fusion a preliminary communication on the radical treatment of Pott's disease and Pott's paraplegia. Br J Surg 1956;44(185):266–275

[26] Hodgson AR. Approach to the cervical spine C 3 –C 7. Clin Orthop Relat Res 1965a;39(39):129–134

[27] Hodgson AR. Correction of fixed spinal curves. J Bone Joint Surg Am 1965b;47:1221–1227

[28] Hodgson AR, Yau ACMC. Anterior surgical Approaches to the Spinal Column. In: Apley AG, ed. Recent Advances in Orthopedics. London: Churchill; 1969

[29] Hughes FA. Resection of the 12th rib in the surgical approach to the renal fossa. J Urol 1949;61(2):159–162

[30] Kirkaldy-Willis WH, Thomas TG. Anterior approaches in the diagnosis and treatment of infections to the vertebral bodies. J Bone Joint Surg Am 1965;47:87–110

[31] Lagevarianten KS. Lage- und Formveränderungen der Pars thoracalis des Ductus thoracicus. Fortschr Röntgenstr 1975;122 (1):1–5

[32] Louis R. Surgery of the Spine. Berlin: Springer; 1983

[33] McAfee PC, Regan JJ, Geis WP, Fedder IL. Minimally invasive anterior retroperitoneal approach to the lumbar spine. Emphasis on the lateral BAK. Spine 1998;23(13):1476–1484

[34] Mayer HM. A new microsurgical technique for minimally invasive anterior lumbar interbody fusion. Spine 1997;22(6):691–699, discussion 700

[35] Mayer HM. The ALIF concept. Eur Spine J 2000;9(Suppl 1):S35–S43

[36] Mayer HM. Microsurgical Anterior Approach to T5 -T10 (mini-TTA). In: Mayer HM, ed. Minimally Invasive Spine Surgery: a Surgical Manual. Berlin: Springer; 2005:129–137

[37] Mirbaha MM. Anterior approach to the thoraco-lumbar junction of the spine by a retroperitoneal-extrapleural technic. Clin Orthop Relat Res 1973;(91):41–47

[38] Moe JH, Winter RB, Bradford DS, Lonstein JE. Scoliosis and Other Spinal Deformities. Philadelphia: Saunders;1978

[39] Nagamatsu G. Dorso-lumbar approach to the kidney and adrenal with osteoplastic flap. J Urol 1950;63(4):569–581

[40] Nanson EM. The anterior approach to upper dorsal sympathectomy. Surg Gynecol Obstet 1957;104(1):118–120

[41] Pimenta L. Lateral endoscopic transpsoas retroperitoneal approach for lumbar spine surgery. VIII Brazilian Society Congress on Spine Pathology, May 2001; Belo Horizonte, Brazil

[42] Platzer W. Atlas der topographischen Anatomie. Stuttgart: Thieme; 1982

[43] Platzer W. Bewegungsapparat. 4th ed. Stuttgart: Thieme; 1984. Taschenatlas der Anatomie; Band 1

[44] Riley LH Jr. Surgical approaches to the anterior structures of the cervical spine. Clin Orthop Relat Res 1973;(91):16–20

[45] Riseborough EJ, Herndon JH. Scoliosis and Other Deformities of the Axial Skeleton. Boston: Little Brown; 1975

[46] Rosenthal D, Rosenthal R, de Simone A. Removal of a protruded thoracic disc using microsurgical endoscopy. A new technique. Spine 1994;19(9):1087–1091

[47] Salcman M, Jamaris J, Leveque H, Ducker TB. Transoral cervical corpectomy with the aid of the microscope. Spine 1979;4 (3):209–212

[48] Seddon HK. Pott's Paraplegia. In: Platt H, ed. Modern Trends in Orthopedics. London: Butterworth; 1956

[49] Southwick WO, Robinson RA. Surgical approaches to the vertebral bodies in the cervical and lumbar regions. J Bone Joint Surg Am 1957;39-A(3):631–644

[50] Verbiest H. Anterolateral operations for fractures and dislocations in the middle and lower parts of the cervical spine. Report of a series of forty-seven cases. J Bone Joint Surg Am 1969;51 (8):1489–1530

[51] Whitesides TE Jr, Kelly RP. Lateral approach to the upper cervical spine for anterior fusion. South Med J 1966;59(8):879–883

[52] Wiltse LL, Bateman JG, Hutchinson RH, Nelson WE. The paraspinal sacrospinalis-splitting approach to the lumbar spine. J Bone Joint Surg Am 1968;50(5):919–926

[53] Wiltse LL. The paraspinal sacrospinalis-splitting approach to the lumbar spine. Clin Orthop Relat Res 1973;(91):48–57

Pelvis and Lower Extremity

7 Pelvis: Pelvic Ring

7.1 Approach to the Symphysis and Anterior Pelvis

F. Stuby, K. Weise

7.1.1 Principal Indications

- Symphysis rupture
- Medial pubic bone fractures
- Symphysiodesis

7.1.2 Positioning and Incision

The operation is performed with the patient placed supine on a standard or carbon operating table. The leg on the injured side is draped to allow free movement, and the genital area must also be covered by sterile drapes. Depending on the injury pattern, the incision is either an extension of the vertical lower abdominal laparotomy incision or—in the case of isolated pelvic fractures—a transverse Pfannenstiel-type incision approximately one fingerbreadth above the usually palpable pubic tubercle (**Fig. 7.1**). After the subcutaneous tissue has been divided, the linea alba is sought and split lengthwise (**Fig. 7.2**). The bladder is then palpated cautiously and retracted cranially (**Fig. 7.3**). Extra caution is required in revision surgery to avoid bladder injury because adhesions may be present. The muscle bellies of rectus abdominis are retracted laterally on both sides. The attachment to the pubic tubercle is often partially avulsed on one side. Complete division of the rectus abdominis is not usually necessary. The symphysis and medial parts of the pubic rami can now usually be visualized readily from the cranial aspect. The bladder can be retracted in posterosuperior direction with a broad spatula.

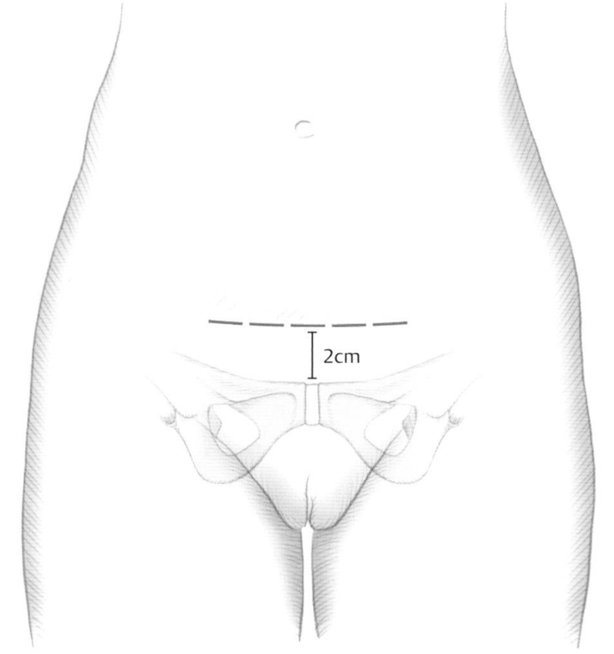

Fig. 7.1 Approach to the symphysis and anterior pelvis, incision.

7.1.3 Wound Closure

During wound closure, the rectus abdominis is reattached with transosseous sutures, and the linea alba is closed securely to avoid the development of a hernia.

7.1.4 Dangers

Possible complications of this approach include bladder and peritoneal injuries and postoperative hernias.

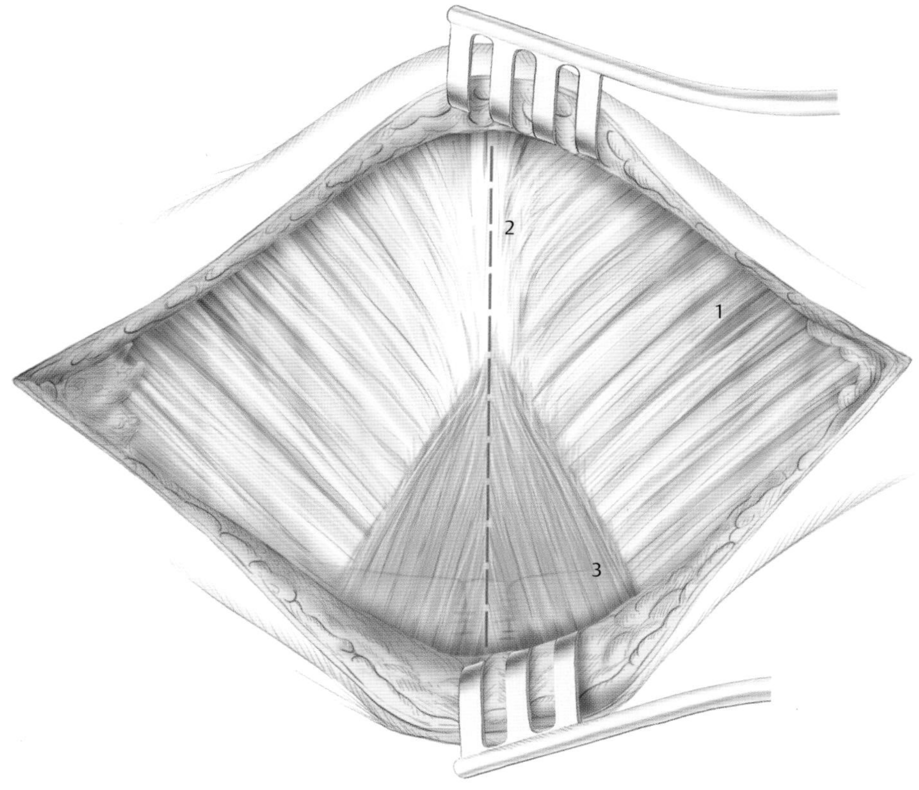

Fig. 7.2 Exposure of the linea alba and rectus abdominis.

1 Rectus abdominis
2 Linea alba
3 Pyramidalis

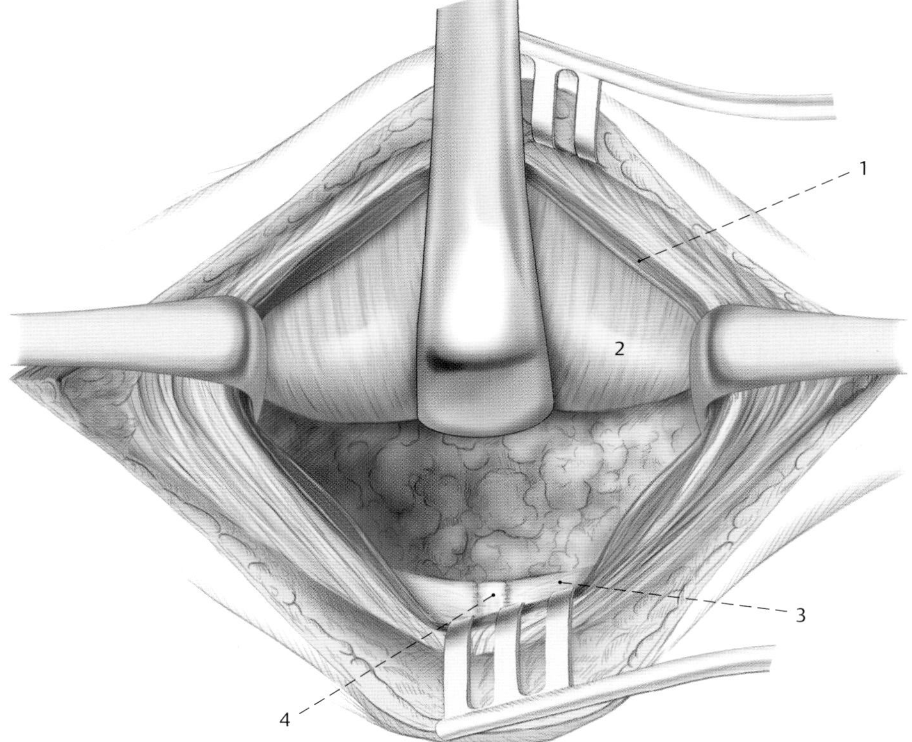

Fig. 7.3 Exposure of the symphysis with the bladder retracted cranially.

1 Rectus abdominis
2 Bladder
3 Superior pubic ramus
4 Symphysis

7.2 Anterior Approach to the Posterior Pelvis

F. Stuby, K. Weise

7.2.1 Principal Indications

- Pelvic ring fractures involving the ala of the ilium
- Rupture of the sacroiliac joint
- Revision surgery of the posterior pelvis
- Arthrodesis of the sacroiliac joint

7.2.2 Positioning and Incision

The operation is performed with the patient placed supine on a standard or extension operating table. The leg on the injured side is draped to allow free movement. The anterior superior iliac spine and iliac crest are marked.

The approach consists of the first window of the ilioinguinal approach (**Fig. 7.4**).

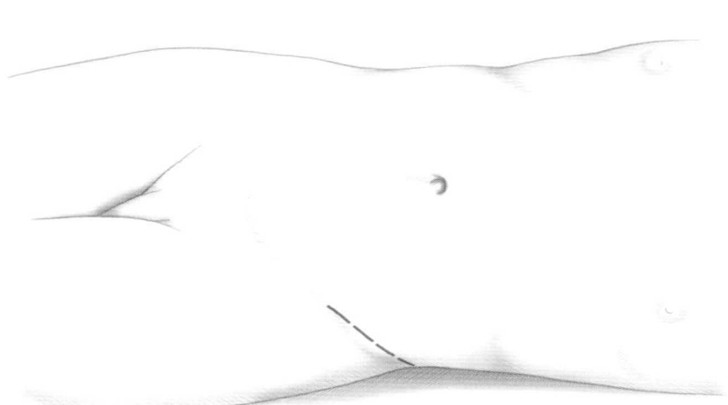

Fig. 7.4 Anterior approach to the posterior pelvis (first window of the ilioinguinal approach), incision on the left side.

The incision extends along the iliac crest from its furthest end to the anterior superior iliac spine (**Fig. 7.5**). For complete ilioinguinal access, the incision is extended to the symphysis. The tendinous attachment of the external oblique fascia on the iliac crest is divided somewhat lateral to the crest (**Fig. 7.6**). Dissection then continues subperiosteally on the inside of the ala of the ilium into the iliac fossa as far as the linea terminalis and the anterior ligaments of the sacroiliac joint. Bleeding from the nutrient channels of the ala of the ilium may occur and must be controlled with bone wax. The iliacus is retracted anteromedially with wide Hohmann retractors. The sacroiliac joint and lateral parts of the sacrum can now be exposed (**Fig. 7.7**). The lumbosacral trunk runs approximately 15–20 mm medial to the sacroiliac joint directly on the anterior surface of the sacrum and should be spared during dissection (**Fig. 7.8**). If dissection is strictly subperiosteal, the risk of injuring the lumbosacral trunk can be minimized.

7.2.3 Wound Closure

The wound is closed in layers with reattachment of the external oblique fascia to the iliac crest.

7.2.4 Dangers

Possible complications of this approach are bleeding from the nutrient channels of the ala of the ilium, injuries to the lumbosacral trunk, especially the L5 root, which courses on the anterior surface of the lateral sacrum, and also a hernia if the fascia is incompletely reattached.

Injury to the lateral cutaneous nerve of the thigh may also occur.

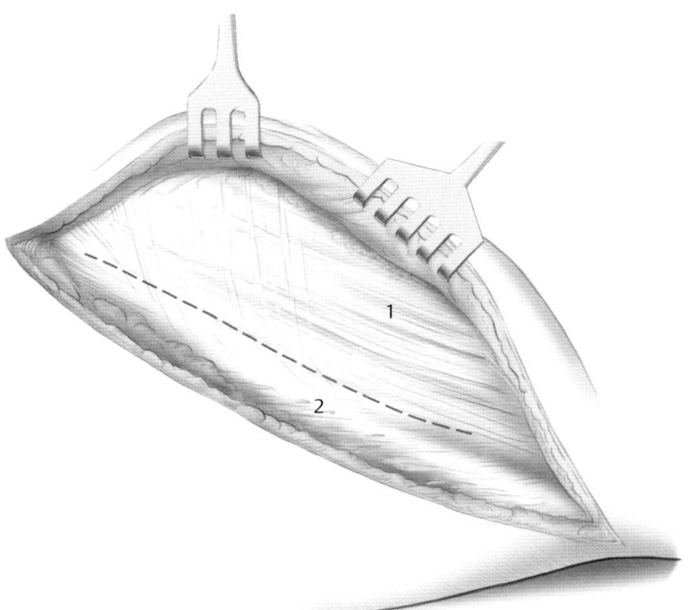

Fig. 7.5 Exposure of the fascial junction of the external oblique with the iliac crest and incision directly over the iliac crest.

1 Aponeurosis of external oblique
2 Left iliac crest

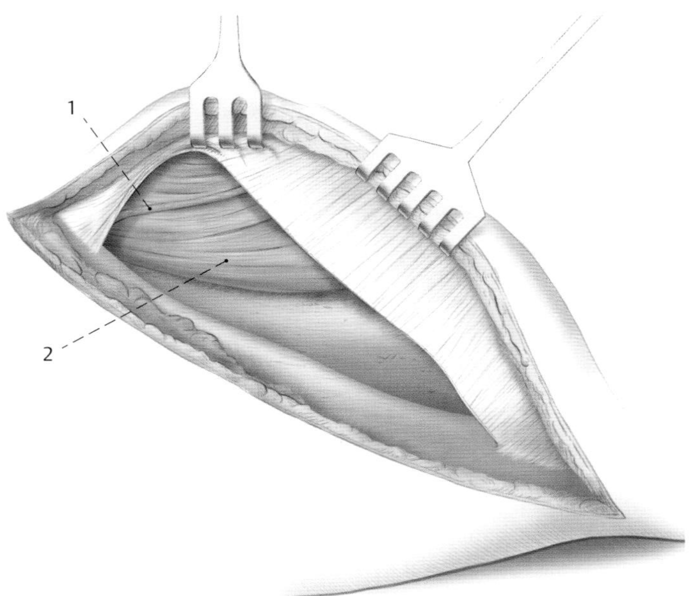

Fig. 7.6 After incising the fascia of the external oblique, the iliacus is pushed subperiosteally from the inside of the ala of the ilium.

1 Lateral cutaneous nerve of the thigh
2 Iliacus

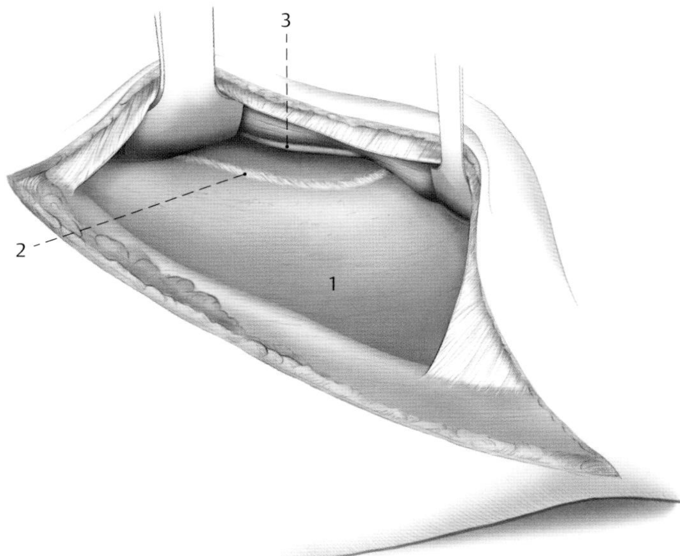

Fig. 7.7 Further elevation of the periosteum until the anterior part of the sacroiliac joint and the lumbosacral trunk are exposed.

1 Iliac fossa
2 Sacroiliac joint
3 Lumbosacral trunk

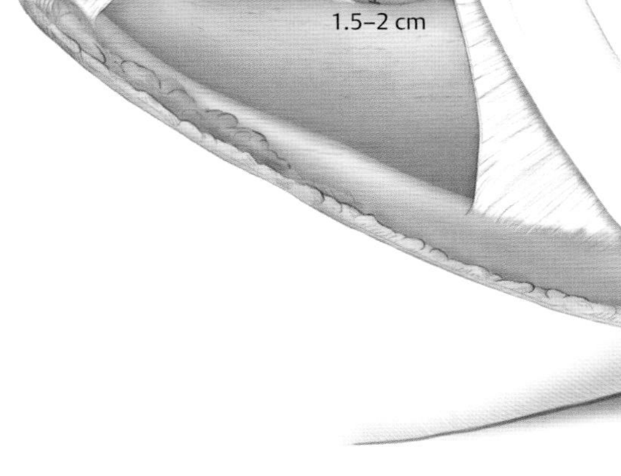

Fig. 7.8 Safe zone of the lateral sacrum anterior to screw placement, sparing the L5 lumbosacral trunk.

7.3 Posterior Approach to the Sacrum

F. Stuby, K. Weise

7.3.1 Principal Indications

- Fractures of the sacrum with narrowing of the spinal canal
- Neurologic signs of nerve compression
- Sacral instability
- Spinopelvic dissociation

7.3.2 Positioning and Incision

The operation is performed with the patient placed prone on a standard or carbon operating table (**Fig. 7.9**). Depending on fracture type, for bilateral exposure the incision is in the midline over the spinous processes of the sacrum from S1 to S4 as far as the anal cleft (**Fig. 7.10**). The lumbosacral fascia is then dissected off the spinous processes, and the multifidus is divided sharply from the posterior surface of the sacrum. A proximally pedicled muscle flap is now raised, tapered distally, and can be elevated proximally (**Fig. 7.11**). Dissection continues cranially to the transverse process of L5.

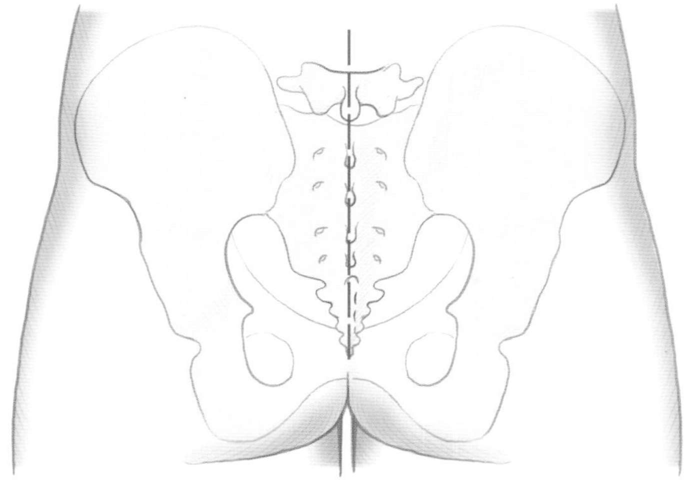

Fig. 7.9 Posterior approach to the sacrum, incision.

7.3.3 Wound Closure

The fascia of the elevated muscle flap is reattached, and the wound is closed in layers.

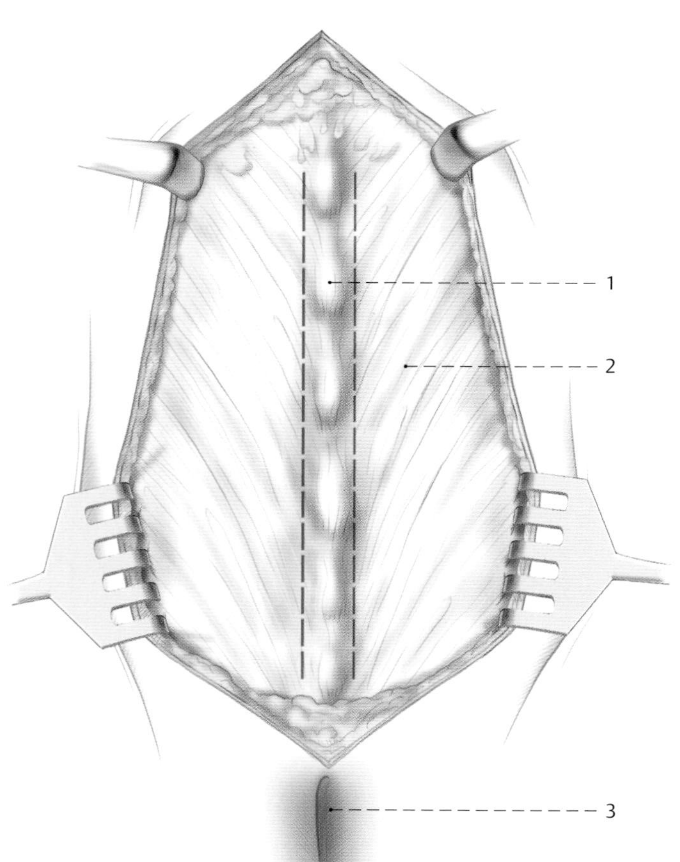

Fig. 7.10 Incision of the fascia of multifidus on either side of the spinous processes.

1 Spinous process
2 Lumbosacral fascia
3 Anal cleft

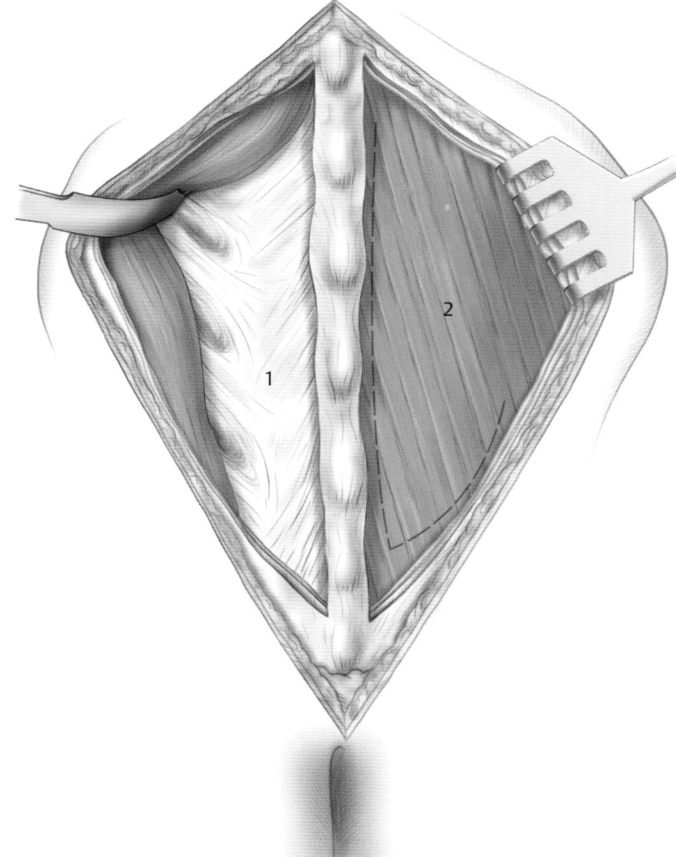

Fig. 7.11 Retraction of multifidus from the posterior surface of the sacrum after division of the muscle.

1 Posterior surface of the sacrum
2 Multifidus lumborum

7.4 Lateral Minimally Invasive Approach for Trans-sacroiliac Screw Placement

F. Stuby, K. Weise

7.4.1 Principal Indications

- Lateral fractures of the sacrum with instability of the pelvis
- Sacroiliac joint rupture
- Transforaminal fractures of the sacrum without significant dislocation

7.4.2 Positioning and Incision

The patient should be given laxatives preoperatively so that the sacrum is not obscured by air on radiography.

The operation should be performed on a carbon table with the patient placed prone or supine. If supine positioning is chosen, it is advisable to place a square cushion beneath the sacrum.

Good radiographic imaging of the pelvis, including views of the ala, obturator, and inlet and outlet, should be ensured prior to sterile draping. If imaging in all required planes is not possible, the positioning should be altered accordingly.

Only then is the affected site prepped, extending far posteriorly. With dislocated fractures, the leg on the affected side should remain mobile.

The anterior superior iliac spine, the greater trochanter, and the extended femoral axis are then marked (**Fig. 7.12**). The image converter is then directed laterally, and the correct incision site is found on the lateral projection of S1 (**Fig. 7.13**). The lateral surface of the ala of the ilium is then reached by blunt dissection at the level of S1. A relatively shallow depression can usually be palpated here with the tip of the instrument. The Kirschner guide wire can then be introduced under image converter control (inlet/outlet).

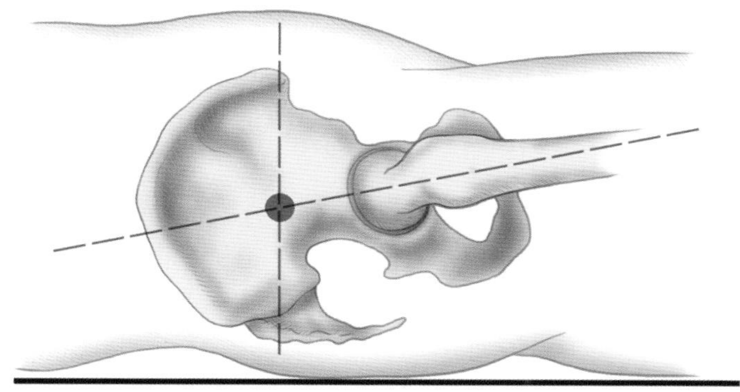

Fig. 7.12 Minimally invasive approach for the posterior pelvis, showing the reference lines for finding the correct incision site, sagittal plane.

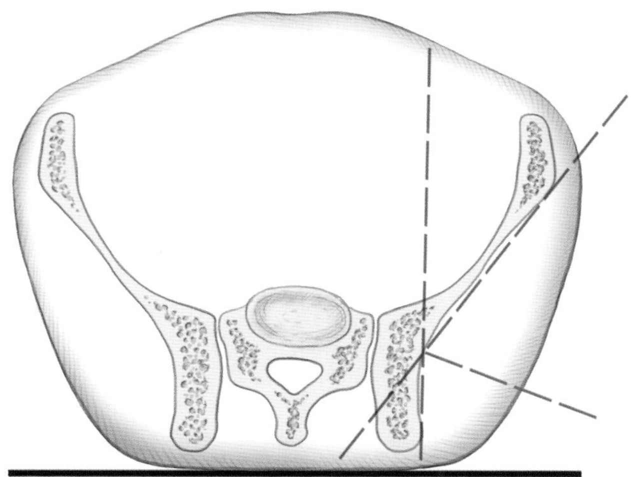

Fig. 7.13 Reference lines for finding the correct incision site, axial plane.

7.5 Approach to the Ischium and Pubis

R. Bauer, F. Kerschbaumer, S. Poisel

7.5.1 Principal Indications

- Tumors
- Osteomyelitis
- Pelvic osteotomies
- Fractures

7.5.2 Positioning and Incision

The patient is placed in lithotomy position with the thigh abducted and flexed. In this approach, waterproof draping of the perineal region and shaving of pubic hair are especially important.

The curved skin incision begins two fingerbreadths cranial to the palpable pubic tubercle and runs somewhat laterally to the anterior border of the inferior pubic ramus as far as the ischial tuberosity (**Fig. 7.14**).

After the subcutaneous tissue has been split, the skin flap is dissected distally so that the layer between the adductors and gluteus maximus can be recognized. Gluteus maximus is now bluntly retracted in a posterior direction. Injury to the spermatic cord in the proximal and superior wound regions must be avoided (**Fig. 7.15**).

7.5.3 Exposure of the Ischium and Pubis

Proceeding from anterior to posterior, the periosteum over the pubis and ischium is incised. Then the adductor muscles, together with obturator externus and, in the posterior wound angle, the ischiocrural muscles, are retracted with a raspatory. The medial portion of the superior pubic ramus, the inferior pubic ramus, the ischial tuberosity, the ischium, and the obturator membrane are now exposed (**Fig. 7.16**). In the upper and medial wound regions, the adductor muscles (pectineus) should be dissected sparingly and retracted not too far from the obturator membrane to avoid injury to the obturator vessels and nerves.

If the inner aspect of the inferior pubic ramus is to be exposed as well, the dissection should also be subperiosteal on the posterior aspect of the inferior pubic ramus from medial to lateral, using the raspatory. In this step, the ischiocavernosus and transverse perineal muscles are detached (**Fig. 7.16**).

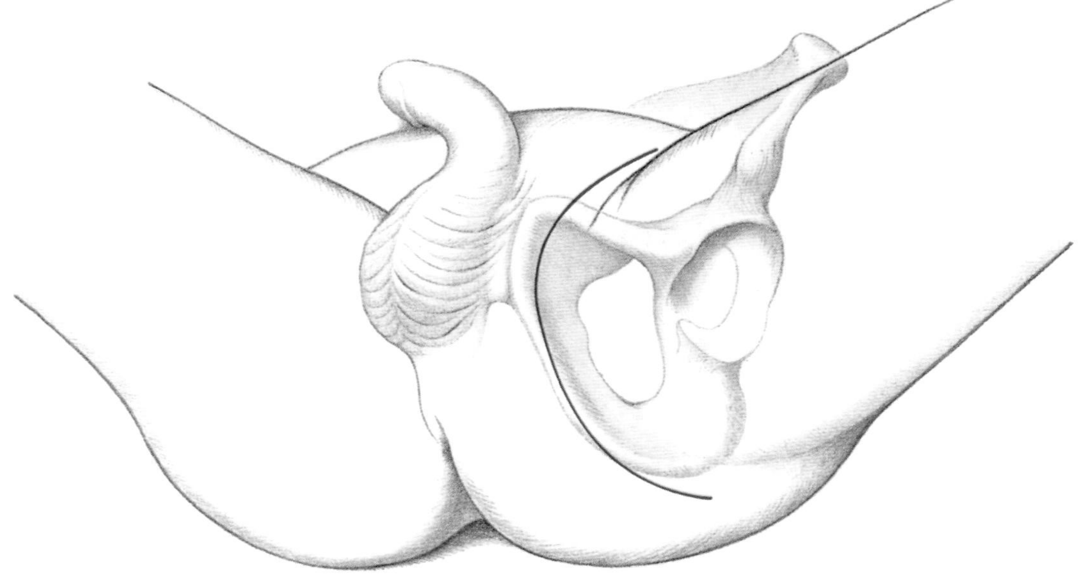

Fig. 7.14 Approach to the pubis and ischium. Lithotomy position. Incision (left side).

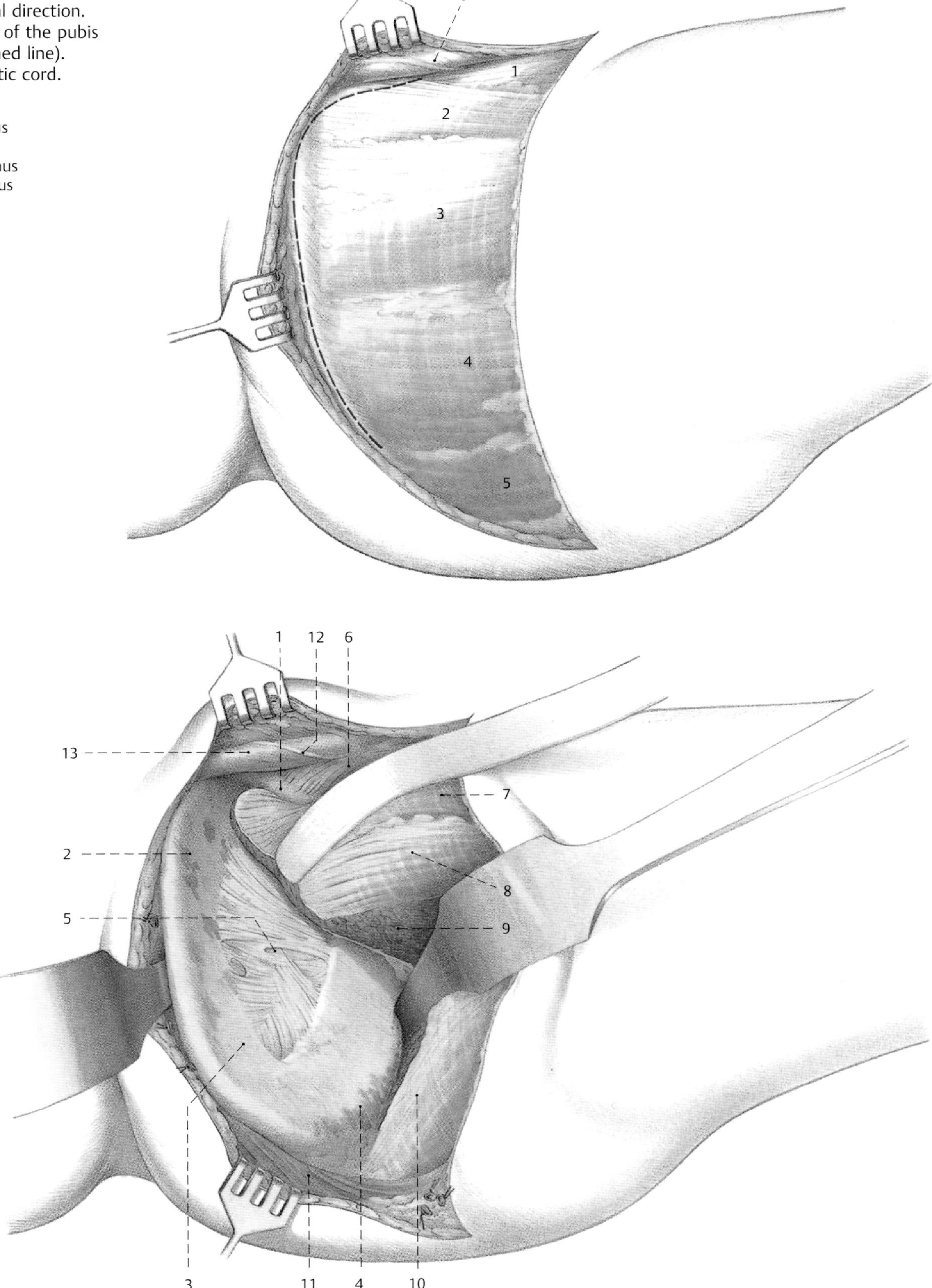

Fig. 7.15 Dissection of the skin flap in a distal direction. Periosteal incision of the pubis and ischium (dashed line). Avoid the spermatic cord.

1 Pectineus
2 Adductor longus
3 Gracilis
4 Adductor magnus
5 Gluteus maximus
6 Spermatic cord

Fig. 7.16 Appearance after detachment of the adductor muscles from the pubis and ischium, and the ischiocrural muscles from the ischial tuberosity. The adductor muscles must not be further mobilized proximally or medially (because of the vessels and obturator nerve).

1 Superior pubic ramus
2 Inferior pubic ramus
3 Ramus of the ischium
4 Ischial tuberosity
5 Obturator membrane
6 Pectineus
7 Adductor longus
8 Gracilis
9 Obturator externus and adductor brevis
10 Adductor magnus
11 Gluteus maximus
12 Ilioinguinal nerve
13 Spermatic cord

7.5.4 Anatomical Site

(Fig. 7.17)

The following anatomical structures may be damaged during exposure of the pubic bone and ischium:

- When dissecting the inner aspect of the superior pubic ramus, a vascular connection between the obturator and epigastric vessels, which occurs as a variation, the so-called corona mortis, may be injured, and this can lead to major hemorrhage. If possible, the Hohmann elevator should therefore be inserted medially below the insertion of the inguinal ligament.
- In the proximal wound region, insufficiently careful dissection can cause injury to the spermatic cord.
- Retraction of the adductor muscles in the medial area of the pubis must not be carried too far since the obturator nerve as well as the obturator vessels may otherwise be overstretched or transected.
- Exposure of the inner aspect of the inferior pubic ramus should be strictly subperiosteal to avoid damage to the pudendal vessels and the pudendal nerve.
- Exposure of the lesser sciatic foramen should likewise be done strictly subperiosteally as the sciatic nerve courses closely behind it.

7.5.5 Wound Closure

In wound closure, less abduction of the leg is useful for better periosteal or transosseous reattachment of the detached adductor muscles.

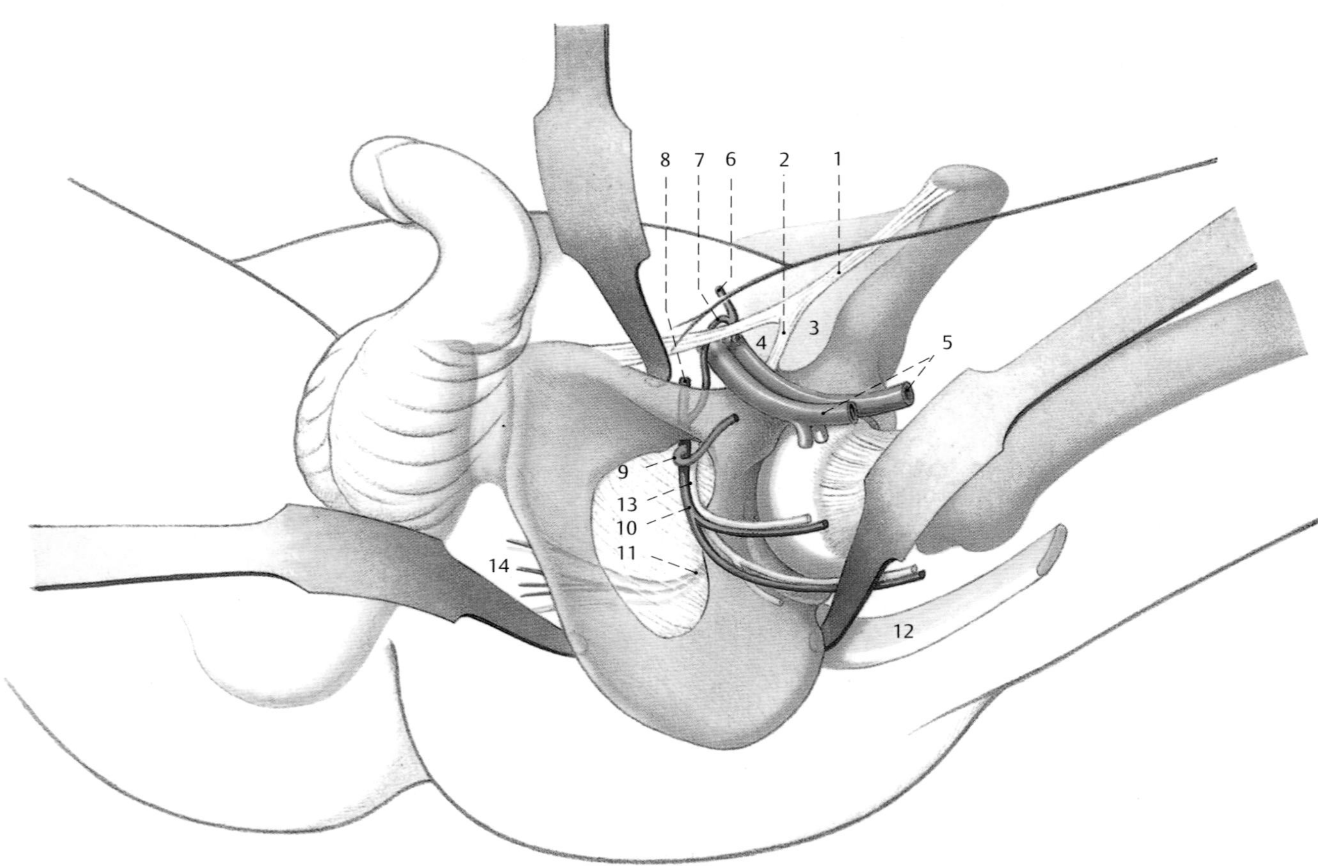

Fig. 7.17 Anatomical site. The Hohmann retractors may be placed at the designated locations after cautious subperiosteal dissection.

1 Inguinal ligament
2 Iliopectineal arch
3 Lacuna of muscles
4 Lacuna of vessels
5 Femoral artery and vein
6 Inferior epigastric artery
7 "Corona mortis"
8 Obturator artery
9 Anterior branch of the obturator artery
10 Posterior branch of the obturator artery
11 Internal pudendal artery
12 Sciatic nerve
13 Obturator nerve
14 Pudendal nerve

8 Pelvis: Acetabulum

8.1 Ilioinguinal Approach According to Letournel

R. Bauer, F. Kerschbaumer, S. Poisel, F. Stuby, K. Weise

8.1.1 Principal Indications

- Fractures of the acetabulum (anterior wall, anterior column, transverse fractures, combined fractures, two-column fractures)
- Pelvic ring fractures with sacroiliac joint rupture, fractures of the ala of the ilium
- Tumors
- Osteomyelitis

8.1.2 Positioning and Incision

The patient is placed in the supine position on a standard or extension table if indicated. If intraoperative three-dimensional radiographs or navigation are planned, a carbon table should be used. The leg on the affected side is draped to allow free movement. The anterior superior iliac spine and iliac crest are marked.

The approach consists of three windows, which, by sequential retraction of the soft tissues, provide good exposure of the inside of the ala of the ilium, the quadrilateral surface, and the superior pubic ramus as far as the symphysis (**Fig. 8.1**).

To open the first window, which is also used for anterior stabilization of sacroiliac instability, the incision is made from the posterior portion of the iliac crest as far as the anterior superior iliac spine. For full ilioinguinal access, the incision is continued as far as the symphysis. The tendinous attachment of the external oblique fascia is now divided on the iliac crest just lateral to the anterior superior iliac spine (**Fig. 8.2**). The iliac fossa is exposed subperiosteally from the internal surface of the pelvis as far as the linea terminalis and anterior sacroiliac ligaments (**Fig. 8.3**). The sacroiliac joint and lateral parts of the sacrum can now be exposed; the lumbosacral trunk runs approximately 15–20 mm medial to the sacroiliac joint directly on the surface of the sacrum and should be spared during dissection. The risk of damaging the lumbosacral trunk can be minimized by strictly subperiosteal dissection.

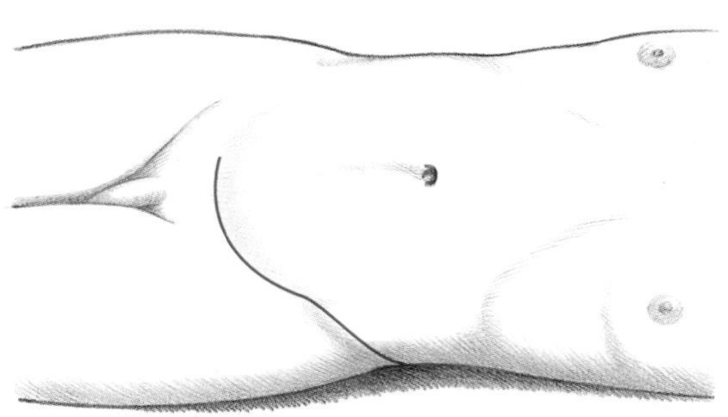

Fig. 8.1 Ilioinguinal approach according to Letournel. Positioning and incision (left side).

Dissection of the second window starts at the anterior superior iliac spine by opening the fascia of the external oblique muscle, with exposure of the spermatic cord or uterine ligament, which is snared together with the ilioinguinal nerve (**Fig. 8.4**). The posterior wall of the inguinal canal is now opened with division of the common origin of the internal oblique, transversus abdominis, and transversalis fascia from the inguinal ligament. A strip of inguinal ligament approximately 1 cm wide should remain to facilitate subsequent reapproximation and anatomical closure of the inguinal canal. The lateral femoral cutaneous nerve, which must be spared, is exposed laterally. The vascular space is then carefully dissected. The iliopectineal arch is exposed by bluntly retracting the vessels medially and the iliopsoas and femoral nerve laterally, and it can be divided sharply as far as its attachment to the iliopubic eminence. The iliopsoas is now snared (**Fig. 8.5**).

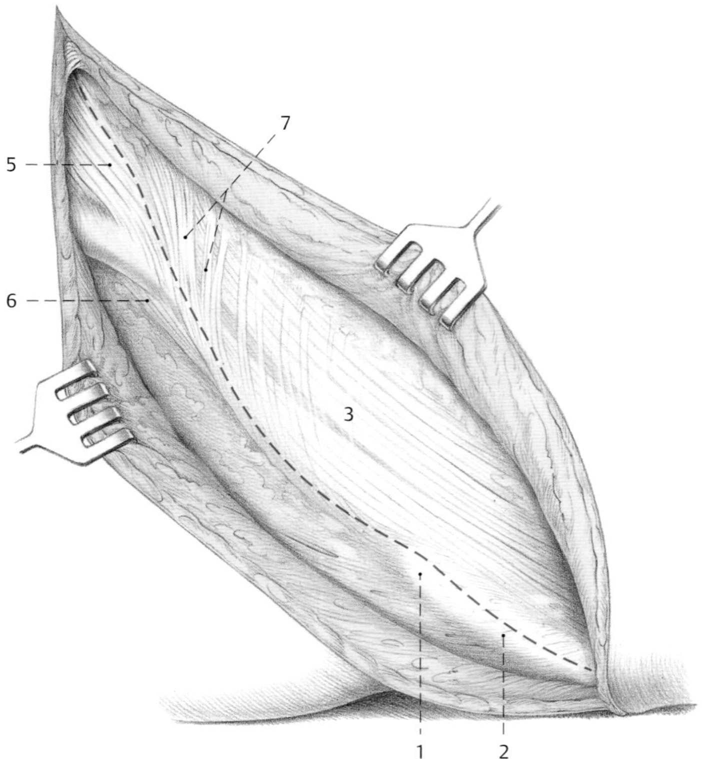

Fig. 8.2 Division of the aponeurosis of the external oblique and detachment of the abdominal muscles from the iliac crest along the dashed line.

1 Anterior superior iliac spine
2 Iliac crest
3 Aponeurosis of external oblique
4 Spermatic cord
5 Medial crus
6 Lateral crus
7 Intercrural fibers

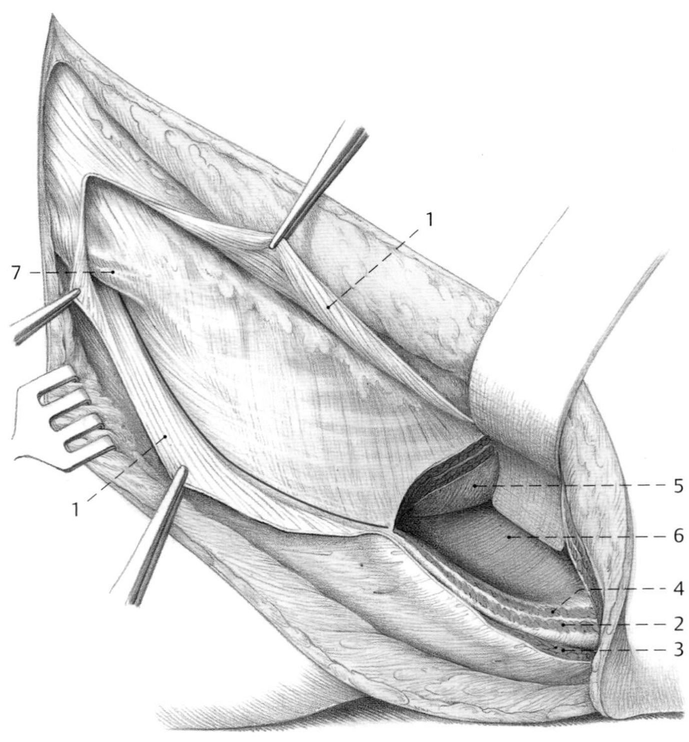

Fig. 8.3 Subperiosteal exposure of the internal iliac fossa and detachment of the deep abdominal muscles from the inguinal ligament.

1 Aponeurosis of external oblique
2 Internal oblique
3 External oblique
4 Transversus abdominis
5 Iliacus
6 Iliac fossa
7 Spermatic cord

Fig. 8.4 Snaring of the spermatic cord with a Penrose drain, and transection and dissection of the iliopectineal arch between the vascular and muscle compartments.

1 Psoas major
2 Iliacus
3 Iliopectineal arch
4 Spermatic cord
5 Iliac fossa
6 External iliac artery and vein
7 Superficial circumflex iliac artery and vein
8 Iliohypogastric nerve
9 Femoral nerve
10 Lateral femoral cutaneous nerve

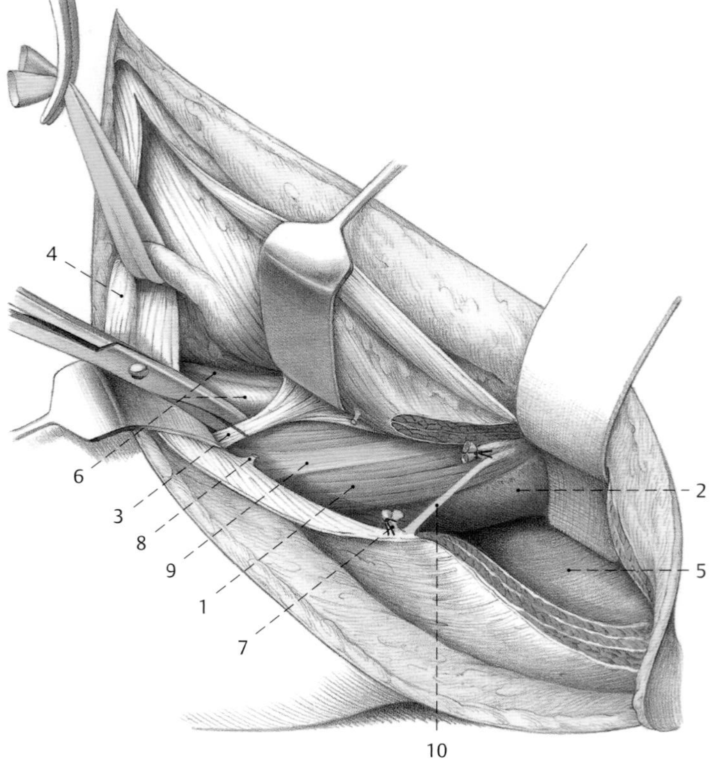

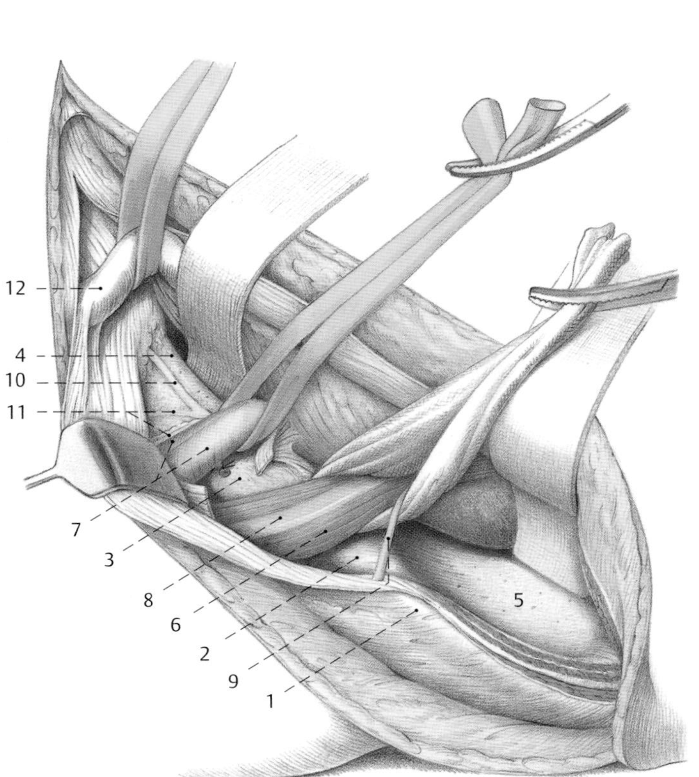

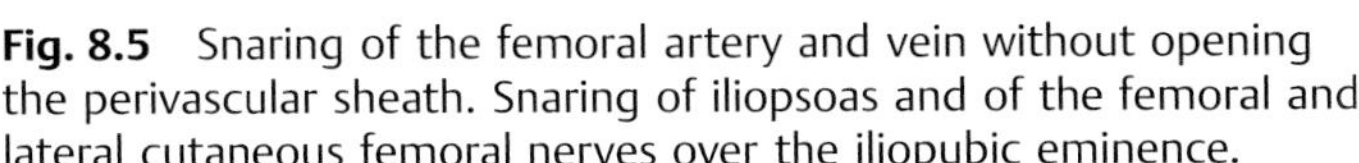
Fig. 8.5 Snaring of the femoral artery and vein without opening the perivascular sheath. Snaring of iliopsoas and of the femoral and lateral cutaneous femoral nerves over the iliopubic eminence.

1 Anterior superior iliac spine
2 Anterior inferior iliac spine
3 Iliopubic eminence
4 Pecten pubis
5 Iliac fossa
6 Psoas major
7 External iliac artery and vein
8 Femoral nerve
9 Lateral femoral cutaneous nerve
10 Genital branch of the genitofemoral nerve
11 Femoral branch of the genitofemoral nerve
12 Spermatic cord

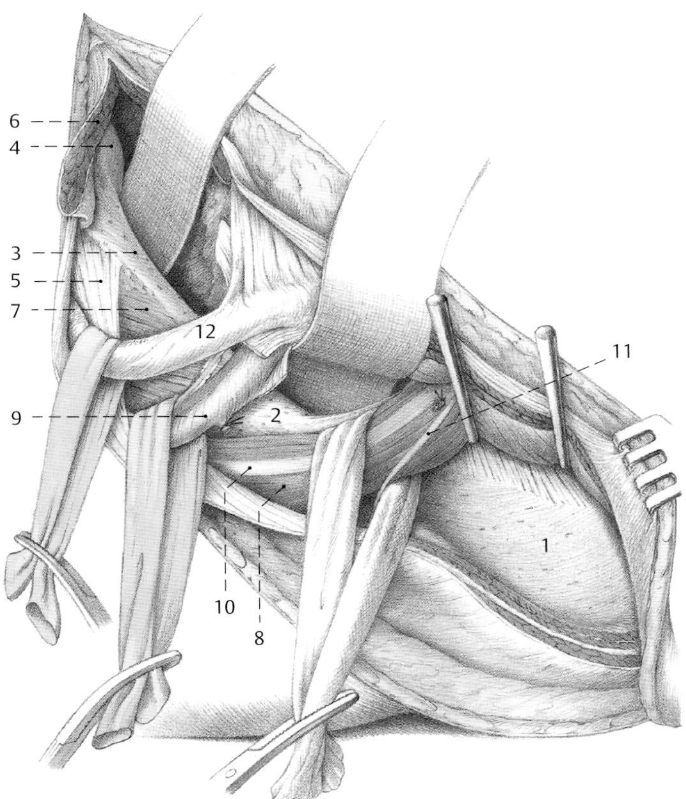

Fig. 8.6 Exposure of the symphysis following the transection of rectus abdominis and insertion of flexible spatulas. Introduction of two Steinmann nails into the ala of the sacrum.

1 Iliac fossa
2 Iliopubic eminence
3 Pecten pubis
4 Pubic symphysis
5 Inguinal ligament
6 Rectus abdominis
7 Pectineus
8 Psoas major
9 External iliac artery and vein, femoral branch of the genitofemoral nerve
10 Femoral nerve
11 Lateral femoral cutaneous nerve of the thigh
12 Spermatic cord

The third window is located between the snared vessels and the lateral border of rectus abdominis. Adequate exposure of the medial pubic ramus is achieved by careful dissection and retraction of rectus abdominis. There may be anastomoses between the external iliac or inferior epigastric artery and the obturator artery ("corona mortis"), which should be ligated prior to bone exposure.

If dissection of the symphysis is required, this is done by splitting the linea alba, if possible without dividing the attachment of the rectus abdominis (**Fig. 8.6**).

According to von Lanz and Wachsmuth, the obturator artery arises from the inferior epigastric artery in 22–28 %, from the external iliac artery in 1–2 %, from the internal iliac artery in 45 %, and from the inferior gluteal artery in 10 % of cases.

8.1.3 Anatomical Site

(**Fig. 8.7**)

The following anatomical structures lie between the split aponeurosis of the external oblique muscle and the anterior pelvic bone as seen from lateral to medial: iliacus, the lateral femoral cutaneous nerve, the femoral nerve, psoas major, psoas minor, the genitofemoral nerve, the iliopectineal arch, the femoral vessels, and the spermatic cord with the ilioinguinal nerve. Located behind the symphysis, which is revealed at the medial angle of the wound, is the bladder. Craniad dissection of the peritoneum exposes the fifth lumbar vertebra, the promontory, and the iliac vessels and testicular vessels.

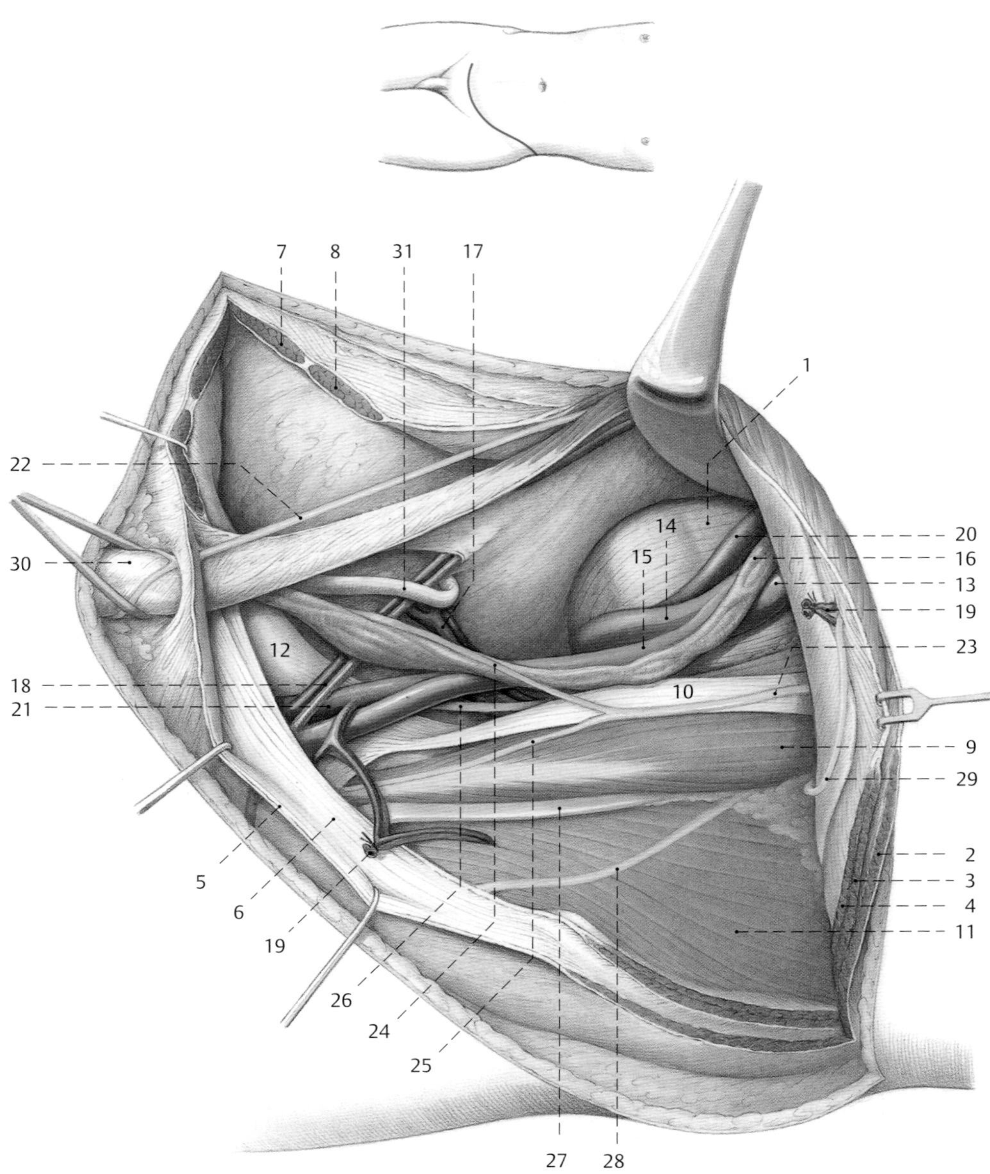

Fig. 8.7 Anatomical site of the ilioinguinal approach.

1 Fifth lumbar vertebra
2 External oblique
3 Internal oblique
4 Transversus abdominis
5 Aponeurosis of external oblique
6 Aponeurosis of internal oblique
7 Pyramidalis
8 Rectus abdominis
9 Psoas major
10 Psoas minor (var.)
11 Iliacus
12 Pecten pubis
13 Common iliac artery
14 Internal iliac artery
15 External iliac artery
16 Testicular vessels
17 Superior vesical vessels
18 Inferior epigastric vessels
19 Superficial circumflex iliac vessels
20 Common iliac vein
21 External iliac vein
22 Ilioinguinal nerve
23 Genitofemoral nerve
24 Genital branch of the genitofemoral nerve
25 Femoral branch of the genitofemoral nerve
26 Obturator nerve
27 Femoral nerve
28 Lateral femoral cutaneous nerve of the thigh
29 Iliohypogastric nerve
30 Spermatic cord
31 Vas deferens

8.1.4 Wound Closure

Anatomical wound closure is required to avoid a postoperative hernia. Rectus abdominis is reattached with subsequent reconstruction of the posterior wall of the inguinal canal using an absorbable continuous suture (**Fig. 8.8**). Adequate patency of the internal inguinal ring is essential. The iliopectineal arch does not have to be reconstructed. Finally, the aponeurosis of the external oblique is reattached, and the wound is closed (**Fig. 8.9**).

8.1.5 Dangers

Frequent complications of this approach are bleeding from the nutrient channels, hemorrhage from the corona mortis, injury to the lateral femoral cutaneous nerve, and hernia if the inguinal region is not reconstructed in full. However, many other complications are possible because of the extensive dissection. If the operation is prolonged and the vessels are manipulated extensively, medical prophylaxis for thrombosis warrants particular attention.

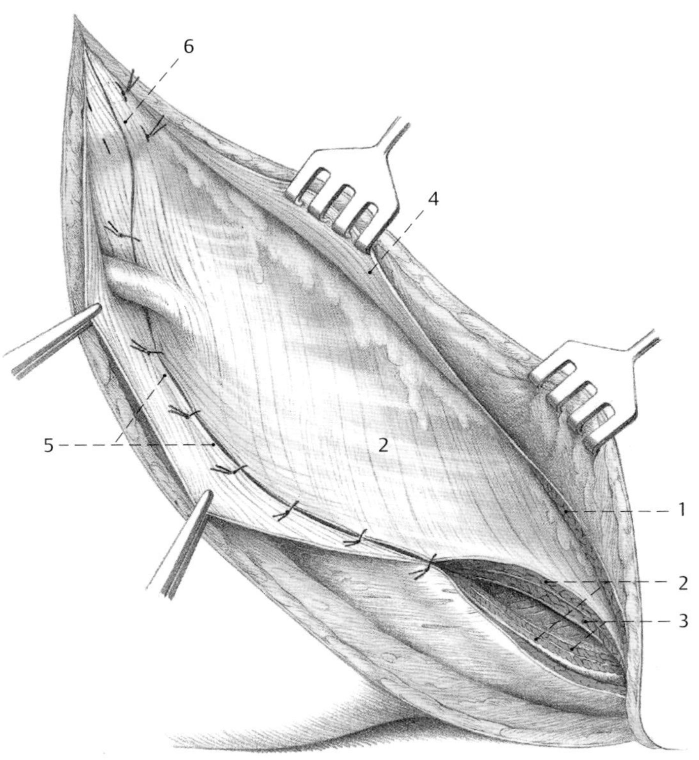

Fig. 8.8 Suture of the posterior wall of the inguinal canal and rectus abdominis.

1 External oblique
2 Internal oblique
3 Transversus abdominis
4 Aponeurosis of the external oblique
5 Inguinal ligament
6 Rectus sheath (anterior layer)

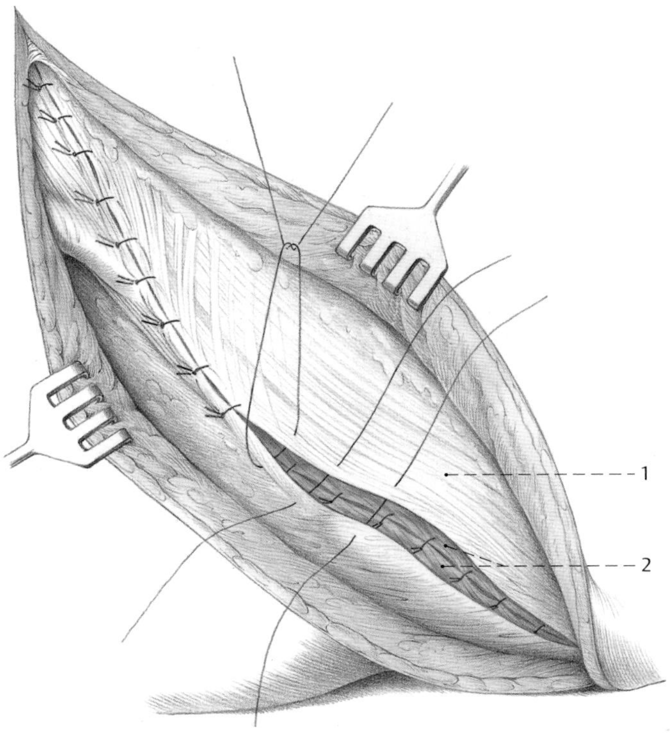

Fig. 8.9 Suture of abdominal muscles stripped off the iliac crest and of the aponeurosis of the external oblique.

1 Aponeurosis of the external oblique
2 Internal oblique

8.2 Posterior Approach to the Hip According to Kocher-Langenbeck

R. Bauer, F. Kerschbaumer, S. Poisel, F. Stuby, K. Weise

8.2.1 Principal Indications

- Acetabular fractures involving the posterior column, posterior wall and transverse fractures, in combination with the anterior approach in the case of two-column fractures
- Removal of intra-articular bone fragments

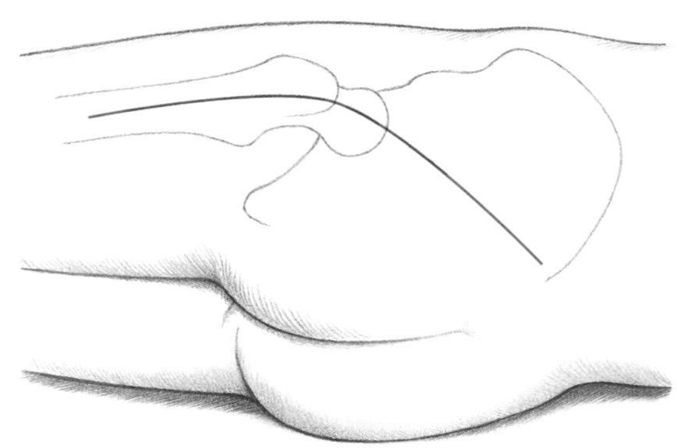

Fig. 8.10 Posterior approach to the hip. Positioning and incision.

8.2.2 Positioning and Incision

The operation can be performed with the patient placed in the prone or lateral decubitus position. In both cases, the leg is draped to allow free movement. The skin incision begins slightly caudal to the palpable greater trochanter, follows the femoral axis cranially, and then curves posteriorly above the trochanter, aiming for the posterior superior iliac crest. After the fascia lata has been exposed, it is split longitudinally somewhat posterior to the trochanter (**Fig. 8.10**).

Gluteus maximus is split in the line of its fibers until the gluteal neurovascular bundle becomes visible. This must be spared as the inferior gluteal nerve innervates the anterior part of gluteus maximus.

The trochanteric bursa is now excised, and the sciatic nerve is then identified, most easily where it courses over quadratus femoris. The nerve does not have to be snared but must be spared throughout the operation. Tension on the nerve can be reduced by flexing the knee. After identifying the pelvitrochanteric muscles ("short external rotators"), these are divided approximately 1–2 cm from their origin on the trochanter (**Fig. 8.11**). The medial circumflex femoral artery must always be spared. It is located at the superior border of quadratus femoris. The tendon ends are snared and dissected from the hip joint capsule to the sciatic notch (**Fig. 8.12**). The posterior joint capsule is now incised, and the femoral head is exposed. To improve visualization, a Schanz screw can be inserted in the femoral neck through the innominate tubercle to allow iatrogenic dislocation.

8.2.3 Wound Closure

The short external rotators are fixed to the posterior border of gluteus medius during wound closure. This is followed by suture of the iliotibial tract and complete wound closure.

Fig. 8.11 With the leg internally rotated, the pelvitrochanteric muscles (short external rotators) are tenotomized.

1 Inferior gemellus
2 Superior gemellus
3 Obturator internus
4 Piriformis
5 Gluteus minimus
6 Gluteus medius
7 Gluteus maximus
8 Quadratus femoris
9 Vastus lateralis
10 Fascia lata
11 Sciatic nerve

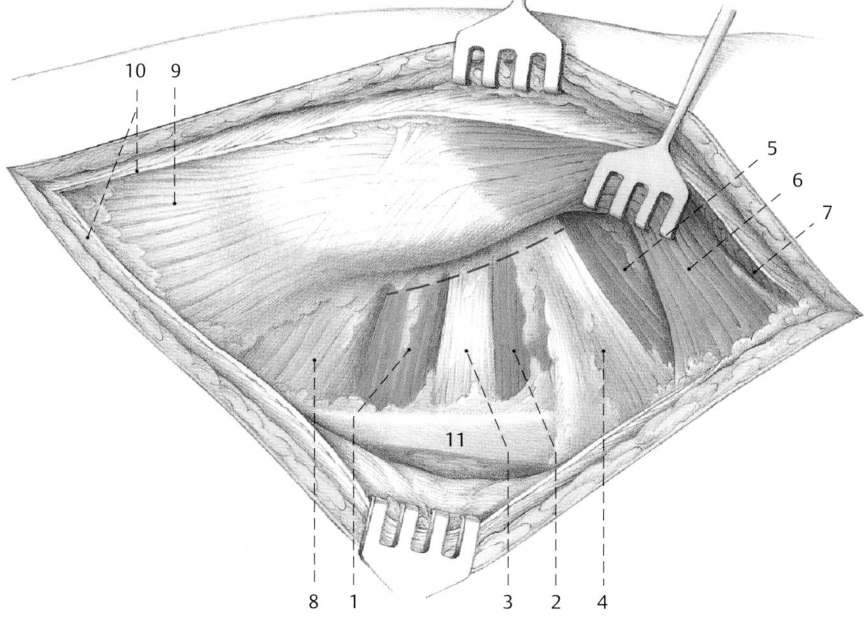

Fig. 8.12 A T-shaped opening is made in the hip joint after the short external rotators have been retracted posteriorly.

1 Hip joint capsule
2 Greater trochanter
3 Gluteus maximus
4 Gluteus medius
5 Gluteus minimus
6 Piriformis, gemelli, obturator internus, obturator externus
7 Quadratus femoris
8 Vastus lateralis

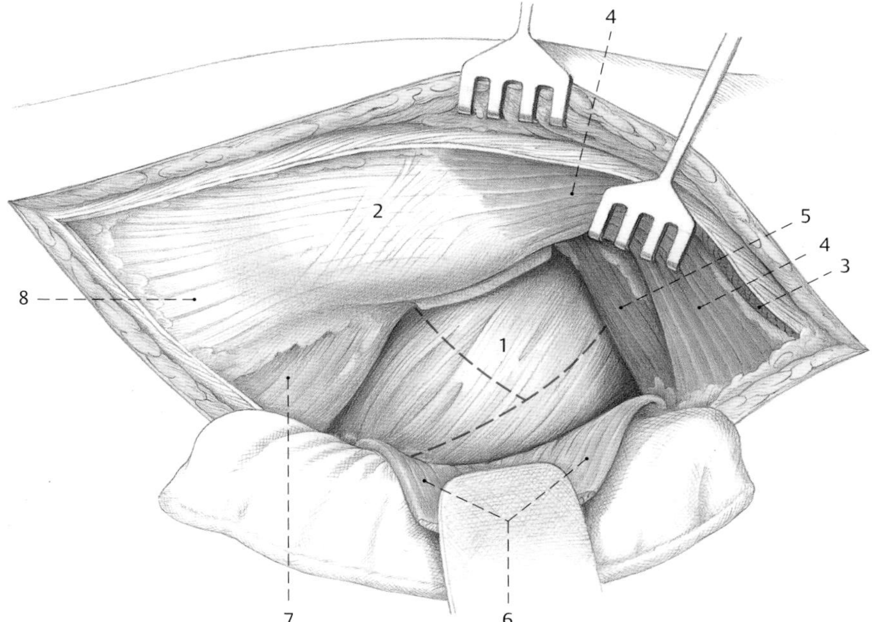

8.2.4 Dangers

Possible complications of this approach include injuries to the sciatic nerve, injuries to the medial circumflex femoral artery with resulting reduced perfusion of the femoral head, and injuries to the inferior gluteal nerve with resulting atrophy of gluteus maximus.

8.2.5 Extension by Stepped Trochanter Osteotomy

If greater exposure of the hip is necessary, stepped trochanter osteotomy (trochanter flip according to Mercati) can be performed.

The origin of vastus lateralis on the trochanter is exposed (**Fig. 8.13**). A shallow, stepped, sagittal osteotomy is now performed. With the leg abducted, further mobilization is achieved both cranially, medial to gluteus medius, and distally and medially beneath vastus lateralis. The entire muscle chain can then be retracted medially when the hip is flexed (**Fig. 8.14**). Using a Schanz screw in the innominate tubercle, the femoral head can now be elevated out of the joint through a circular capsulotomy. This allows almost complete exposure of the acetabular joint surface (**Fig. 8.15**).

Two small screws suffice for reattaching the osteomized cortical fragments.

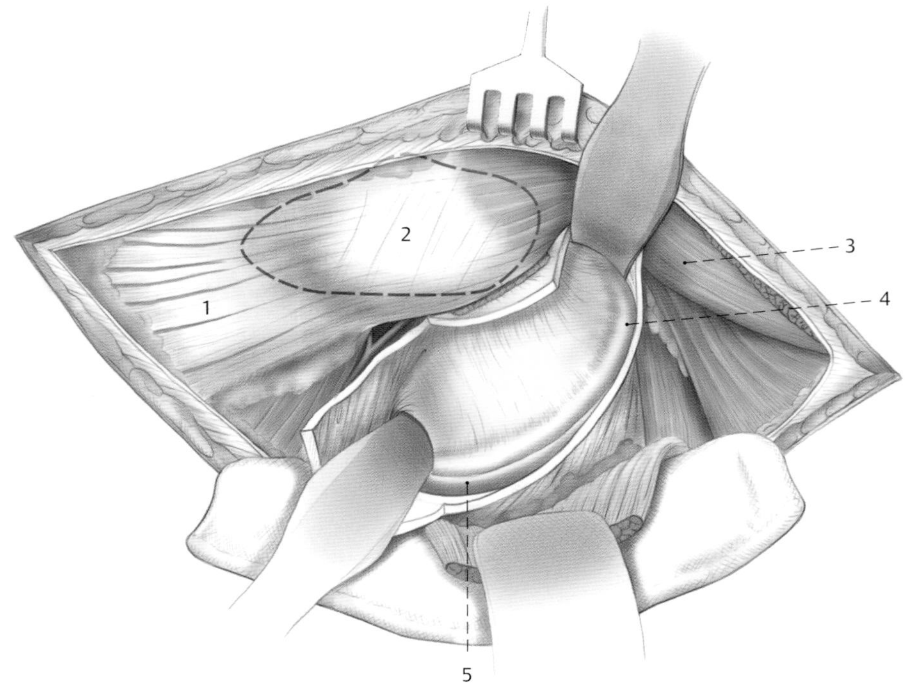

Fig. 8.13 With the hip opened, two Hohmann retractors can be passed around the femoral neck for better exposure. If necessary, an osteotomy of the greater trochanter can be performed (dashed line).

1 Vastus lateralis
2 Greater trochanter
3 Gluteus medius
4 Femoral head
5 Acetabular rim

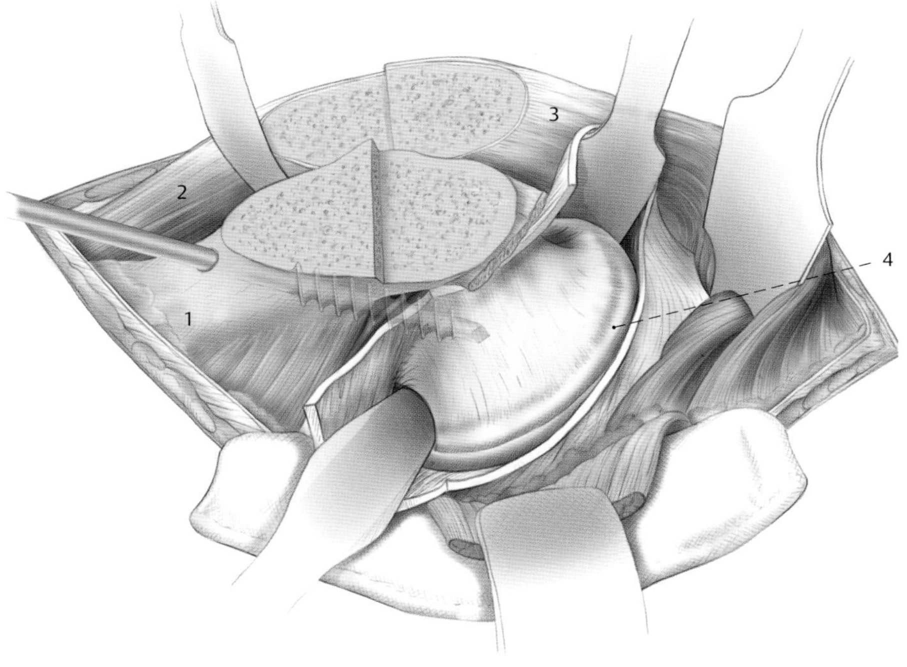

Fig. 8.14 After stepped osteotomy, the entire bone fragment with the origin of gluteus medius and vastus lateralis is dislocated anteriorly.

1 Femoral shaft
2 Vastus lateralis
3 Gluteus medius
4 Femoral head

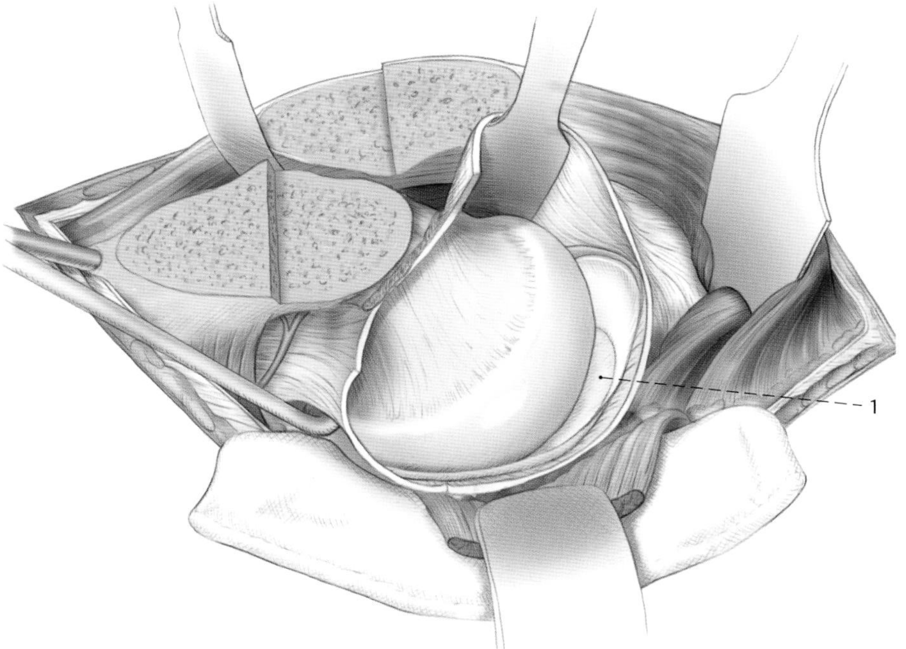

Fig. 8.15 Partial surgical hip dislocation with relatively complete inspection of the joint is possible with caudolateral traction via a Schanz screw inserted into the femoral neck from the innominate tubercle.

1 Acetabulum

8.3 Anterior Limited Approach According to Stoppa

F. Stuby, K. Weise

8.3.1 Principal Indications

- Acetabular fractures with central protrusion and fracture of the quadrilateral surface
- Lateral pubic ramus fractures
- Compound acetabular fractures in elderly patients (often in combination with the first window of the Letournel ilioinguinal approach)

8.3.2 Positioning and Incision

The operation is performed with the patient placed supine on a standard or carbon table; the leg is draped to allow free movement. Good radiographic imaging of the pelvis, including views of the ala, obturator, and inlet and outlet, should be ensured prior to sterile draping.

The skin incision runs horizontally about two fingerbreadths above the palpable symphysis, and is made slightly longer on the injured side. If a vertical lower abdominal laparotomy has already been performed in polytrauma patients or for previous surgery, this incision can also be used.

Following dissection through the subcutaneous tissue, the linea alba is sought and split between the vertical bellies of rectus abdominis. After exposing the symphysis, the bladder is retracted in a posterosuperior direction in the retropubic space and the muscle on the injured side is divided transversely somewhat proximal to its attachment (**Fig. 8.16**). The

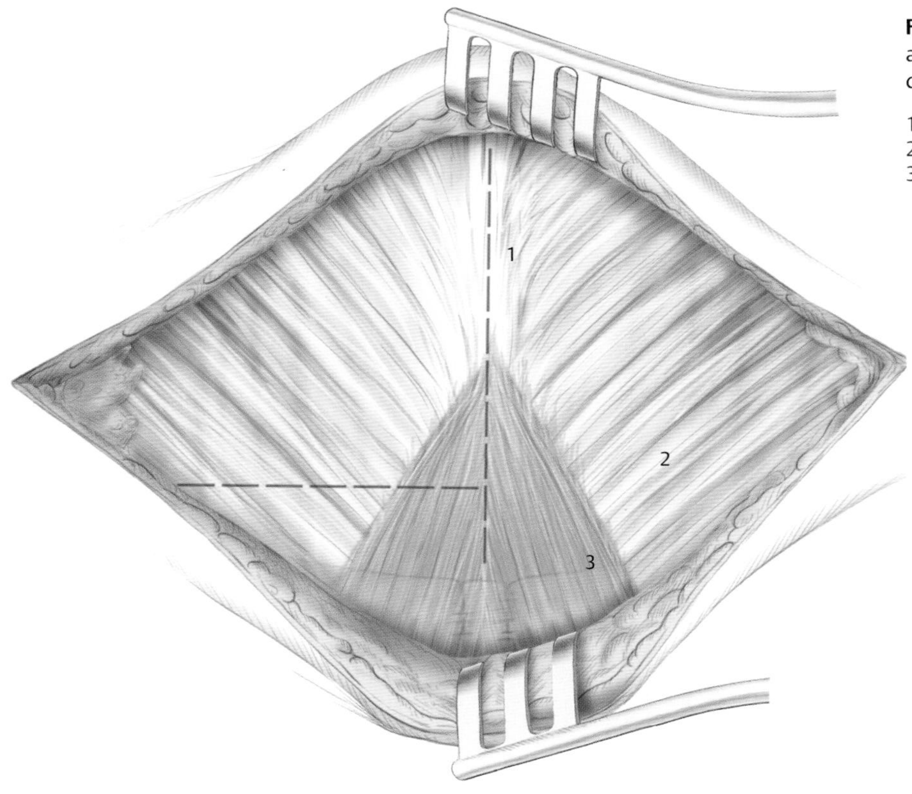

Fig. 8.16 The Stoppa approach extended by an additional horizontal incision of the rectus abdominis on the injured side.

1 Linea alba
2 Rectus abdominis
3 Pyramidalis

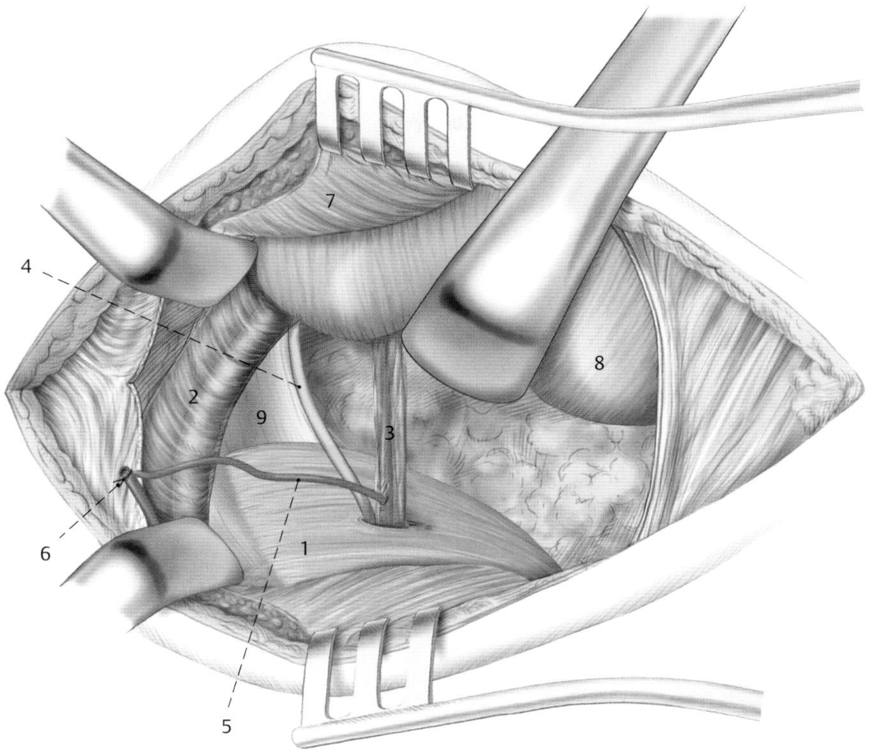

Fig. 8.17 After further dissection, the external iliac, internal iliac, and obturator vessels are exposed and spared.

1 Obturator internus
2 External iliac artery and vein
3 Obturator artery and vein
4 Obturator nerve
5 "Corona mortis"
6 Inferior epigastric artery
7 Rectus abdominis
8 Bladder
9 Quadrilateral surface

femoral vessels are now retracted in a cranial direction so that the lateral part of the superior pubic ramus is exposed. Dissection into the pelvis continues between the preperitoneal fat and the obturator internus.

The presence of an anastomosis between the obturator artery and the external iliac or inferior epigastric artery ("corona mortis") should be sought. If present, this should be ligated prior to further exposure of the quadrilateral surface (**Fig. 8.17**). The ischial spine and greater sciatic notch are then exposed as far as the sacroiliac joint with a raspatory.

8.3.3 Wound Closure

After placing a deep Redon drain, the rectus abdominis is reattached, and the fascia in the linea alba is reconstructed. Reconstruction of the inguinal canal is not necessary (cf. ilioinguinal approach).

8.3.4 Dangers

Possible complications of this approach are hemorrhage from the corona mortis, bladder injuries, injury to the peritoneum, and hernia if fascial closure is incomplete.

8.4 Transiliac Approach According to Judet

R. Bauer, F. Kerschbaumer, S. Poisel

8.4.1 Principal Indications

- Exposure of the sacroiliac joint
- Lateral exposure of L5 and S1
- Exposure of nerve roots L5–S2

8.4.2 Positioning and Incision

The patient is placed in a lateral position. The main incision is made in the midline between the anterior and posterior superior iliac spines, beginning approximately 10 cm cranial to the iliac crest and ending 15 cm caudal to it (**Fig. 8.18**). After splitting of the subcutaneous tissue and insertion of retractors, the gluteal muscles are detached from their sacral and iliac origins along a curved line (**Fig. 8.19**). For exposure of the gluteal surface, retraction of the gluteal muscles has to be rigorously subperiosteal. Next the greater sciatic foramen is subperiosteally exposed with a curved raspatory (**Fig. 8.20**), care being taken to avoid injury to the superior gluteal artery. Following the introduction of a curved spatula into the greater sciatic foramen, the iliac crest is subperiosteally exposed in the area of the lumbocostal trigone, and subsequently the internal iliac fossa is exposed subperiosteally with the aid of a raspatory. A straight osteotomy through the iliac bone may now be performed with a chisel or oscillating saw along the line drawn in **Fig. 8.21**.

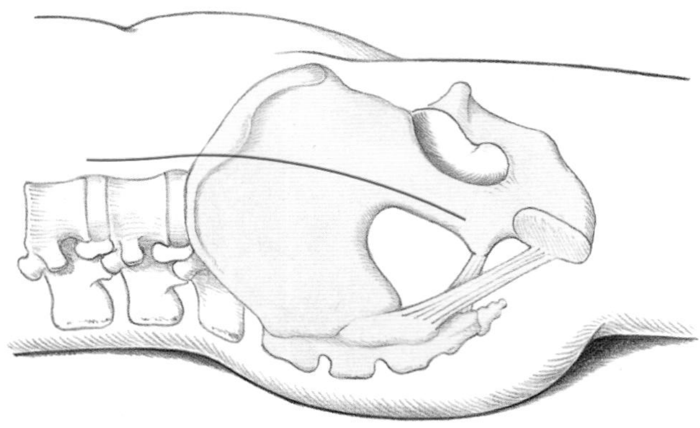

Fig. 8.18 Transiliac approach according to Judet. Incision (right side).

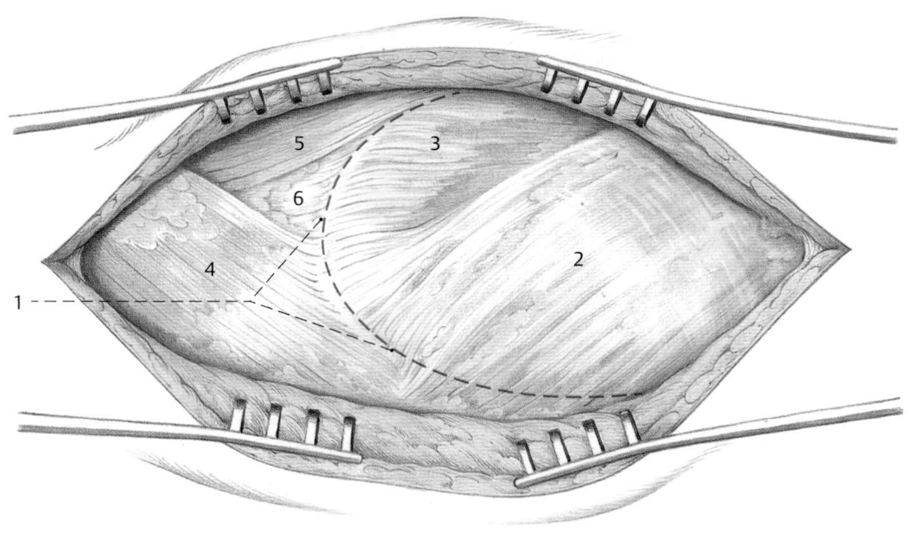

Fig. 8.19 Detachment of the gluteal muscles from the ilium and sacrum along the dashed line.

1 Iliac crest
2 Gluteus maximus
3 Gluteus medius
4 Latissimus dorsi
5 External oblique
6 Lumbosacral trigone

Fig. 8.20 Subperiosteal detachment of the gluteal muscles from the outer wall of the ilium. Exposure of the greater sciatic foramen.

1 Gluteal surface
2 Greater sciatic foramen
3 Gluteus maximus
4 Gluteus medius
5 External oblique
6 Latissimus dorsi
7 Superior gluteal vessels

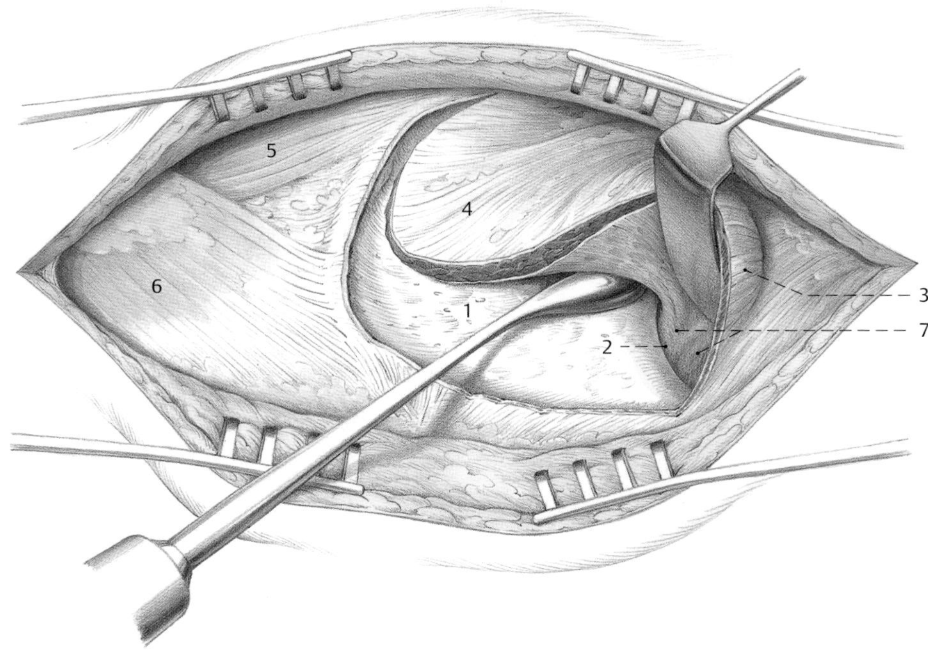

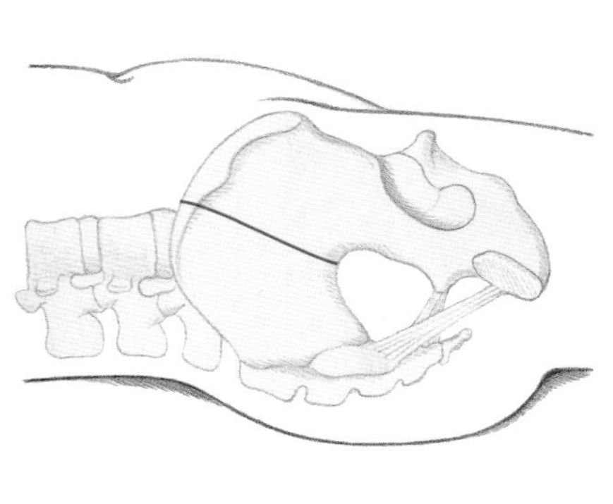

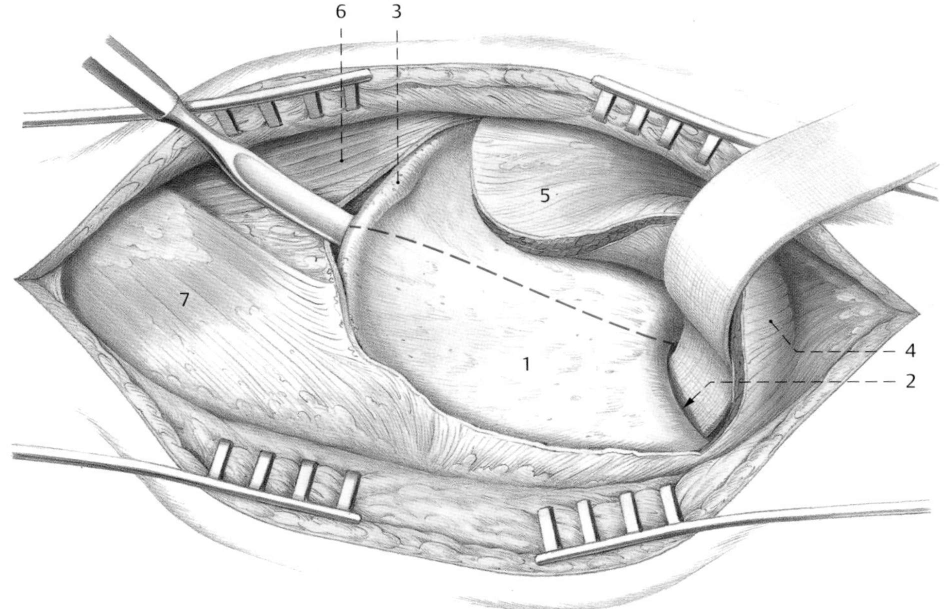

Fig. 8.21 Following exposure of the greater sciatic foramen, a spatula is inserted to protect the superior gluteal vessels. This is followed by subperiosteal exposure of the iliac fossa. Straight transection of the ilium along the dashed line (also see detail).

1 Gluteal surface
2 Greater sciatic foramen
3 Iliac crest
4 Gluteus maximus
5 Gluteus medius
6 External oblique
7 Latissimus dorsi

8.4.3 Exposure of the Sacroiliac Joint

A Cobb elevator is introduced into the iliac fossa via the osteotomy cleft. With the aid of the raspatory, the anterior portion of the ilium is retracted medially so that the posterior portion can be grasped with bone-holding forceps and retracted laterally. Using the raspatory, the anterior portion of the sacroiliac joint capsule is subperiosteally retracted, and the posterior iliac fragment is turned up laterally (**Fig. 8.22**).

After dissection and partial transection of parts of iliacus and blunt retraction of psoas major, the fifth lumbar vertebra, the presacral intervertebral disk, and the superior portions of the first sacral vertebra are revealed. Further, the anterior branches of the first and fifth lumbar and first and second sacral nerves can be visualized. Lying in the depth of the wound, covered by connective tissue, are the internal iliac artery and vein, and the superior gluteal artery and vein. The auricular surface is likewise readily visible (**Fig. 8.22**).

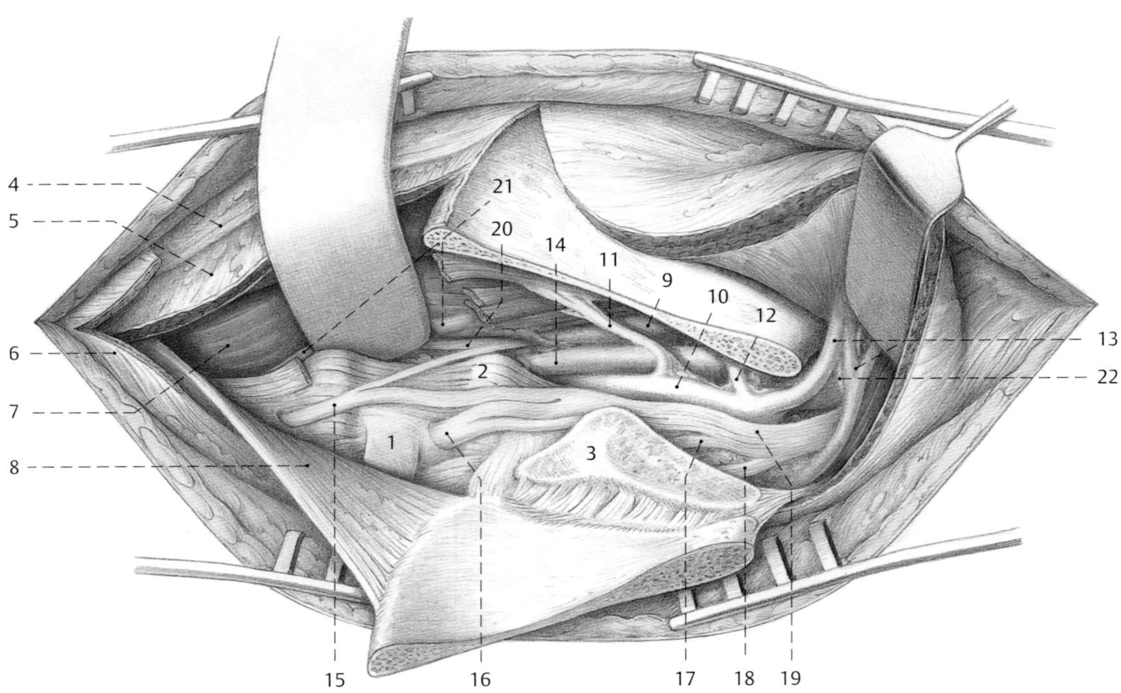

Fig. 8.22 Operative site after opening of the anterior sacroiliac joint capsule and upward reflection of the posterior iliac fragment. Some fibers of the iliacus muscle have been transected, and psoas major has been retracted in a medial direction. Exposure of the articular surface of the sacrum (auricular surface), the spinal nerves L4–S2, and the lateral surface of L5 and S1.

1 Fifth lumbar vertebra
2 Promontory
3 Auricular surface
4 External oblique
5 Internal oblique
6 Latissimus dorsi
7 Psoas major
8 Quadratus lumborum
9 External iliac artery
10 Internal iliac artery
11 Iliac branch of the iliolumbar artery (var.)
12 Lumbar branch of the iliolumbar artery (var.)
13 Superior gluteal artery and vein
14 External iliac vein
15 Anterior ramus of L4
16 Anterior ramus of L5
17 Anterior ramus of S1
18 Anterior ramus of S2
19 Sacral plexus
20 Obturator nerve
21 Femoral nerve
22 Superior gluteal nerve

8.4.4 Anatomical Site

(**Fig. 8.23**)

With appropriate dissection, the transiliac approach allows exposure of the following anatomical structures, descending from cranial to caudal:

The femoral nerve and the obturator nerve can be exposed by retraction or partial resection of a portion of psoas major. Behind these nerves lies the division into the external and internal iliac arteries. The corresponding veins are situated between or posterior to the arteries. The intervertebral foramina as well as the spinal nerves of L4–S3 become visible in this order from cranial to caudal. The inferior gluteal artery as well as the superior gluteal artery with the accompanying veins are found in the caudal portion of the wound area. The spinal nerves and the lumbosacral plexus are located directly anterior to the opened sacroiliac joint.

8.4.5 Wound Closure

Following reduction of both iliac fragments, two plates applied from the outside provide for stable fixation. The detached gluteal muscles are resutured at their origin.

8.4.6 Dangers

Careless dissection of the greater sciatic foramen may cause injury to the superior gluteal artery.

8.4.7 Note

Before lifting up the posterior iliac fragment, the anterior sacroiliac joint capsule needs to be detached with precision since the iliac bone otherwise cannot be properly reflected upward.

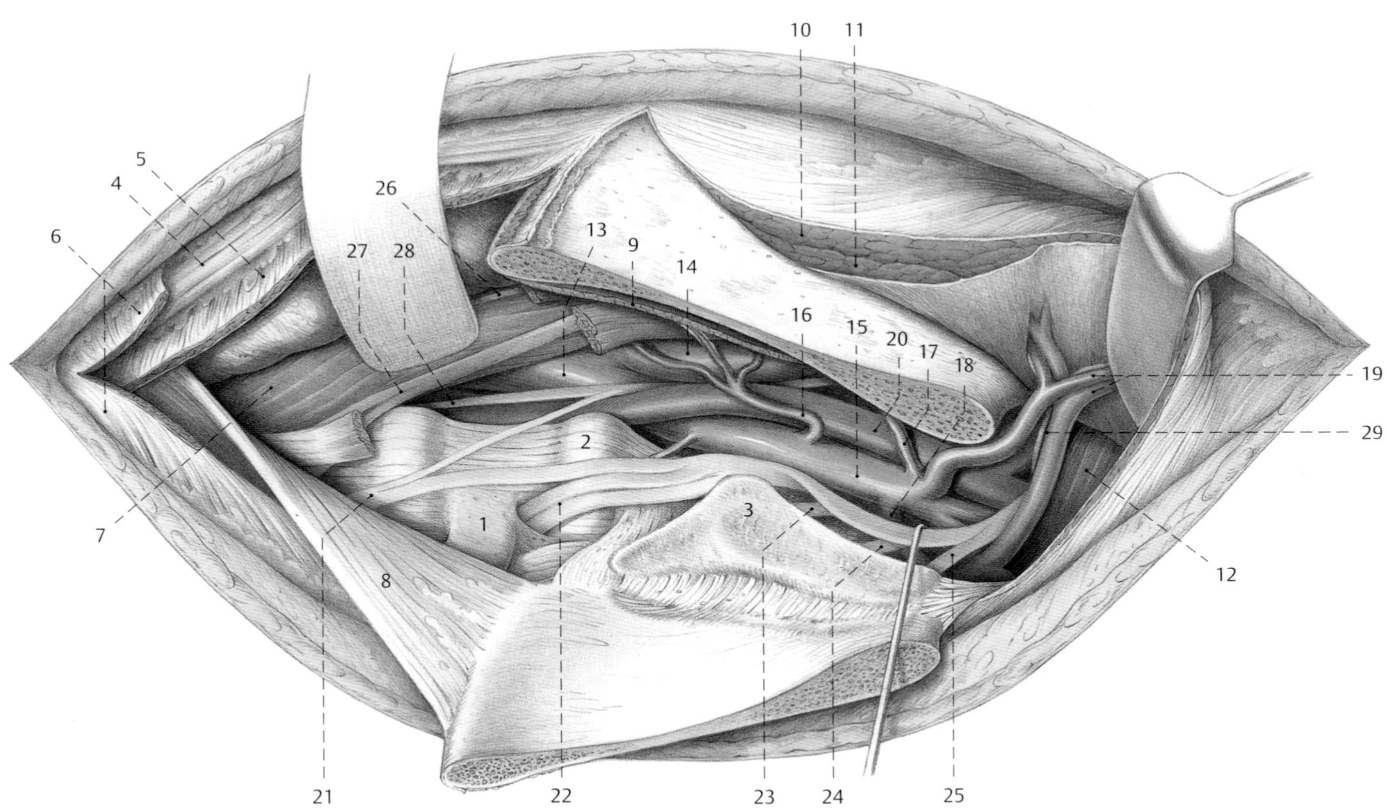

Fig. 8.23 Anatomical site of the transiliac approach.

1 Fifth lumbar vertebra
2 Promontory
3 Auricular surface
4 External oblique
5 Internal oblique
6 Latissimus dorsi
7 Psoas major
8 Quadratus lumborum
9 Iliacus
10 Gluteus medius
11 Gluteus minimus
12 Piriformis
13 Common iliac artery
14 External iliac artery
15 Internal iliac artery
16 Iliac branch of iliolumbar artery (var.)
17 Lumbar branch of iliolumbar artery (var.)
18 Lateral sacral artery
19 Superior gluteal artery and vein
20 External iliac vein
21 Anterior branch of L4
22 Anterior branch of L5
23 Anterior branch of S1
24 Anterior branch of S2
25 Anterior branch of S3
26 Genitofemoral nerve
27 Femoral nerve
28 Obturator nerve
29 Superior gluteal nerve

8.5 Approach to the Acetabulum According to Judet

R. Bauer, F. Kerschbaumer, S. Poisel

8.5.1 Principal Indications

- Fractures of the pelvic bones
- Tumors
- Osteomyelitis

8.5.2 Positioning and Incision

The patient is customarily placed on their side. Optionally, a semilateral or supine position may be used. The skin incision is begun in the posterior third of the iliac crest and then runs in an arc to the anterior superior iliac spine and continues from here 20 cm distally in a straight line (**Fig. 8.24**). After division of the subcutaneous tissue, the iliotibial tract is split over the tensor of fascia lata, avoiding injury to the lateral cutaneous nerve of the thigh (**Fig. 8.25**).

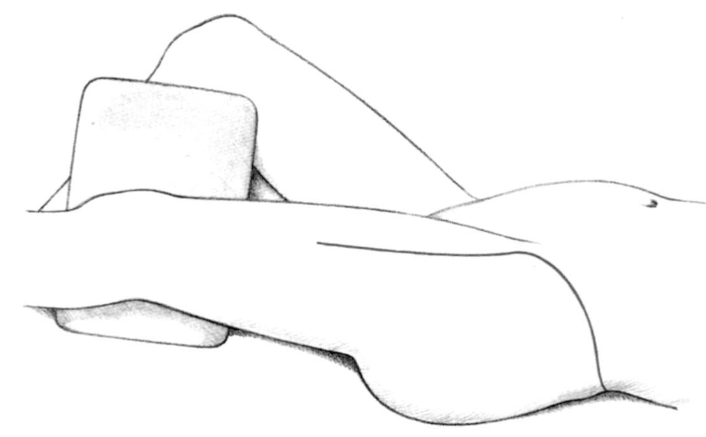

Fig. 8.24 Judet approach. Positioning and incision.

The layer between sartorius and the tensor of fascia lata is now bluntly dissected, and both muscles are retracted (**Fig. 8.26**). Subsequently, the tensor of fascia lata and the gluteal muscles are subperiosteally detached from the outer surface of the ilium (**Fig. 8.27**). Following exposure of the hip joint capsule from in front, first gluteus medius and gluteus

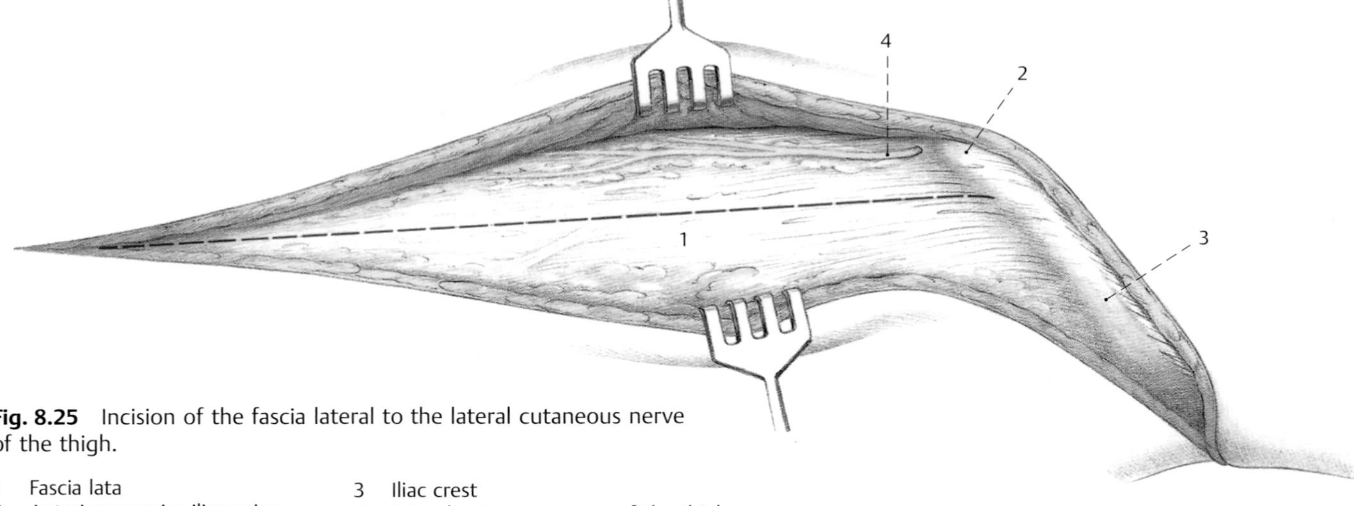

Fig. 8.25 Incision of the fascia lateral to the lateral cutaneous nerve of the thigh.

1 Fascia lata
2 Anterior superior iliac spine
3 Iliac crest
4 Lateral cutaneous nerve of the thigh

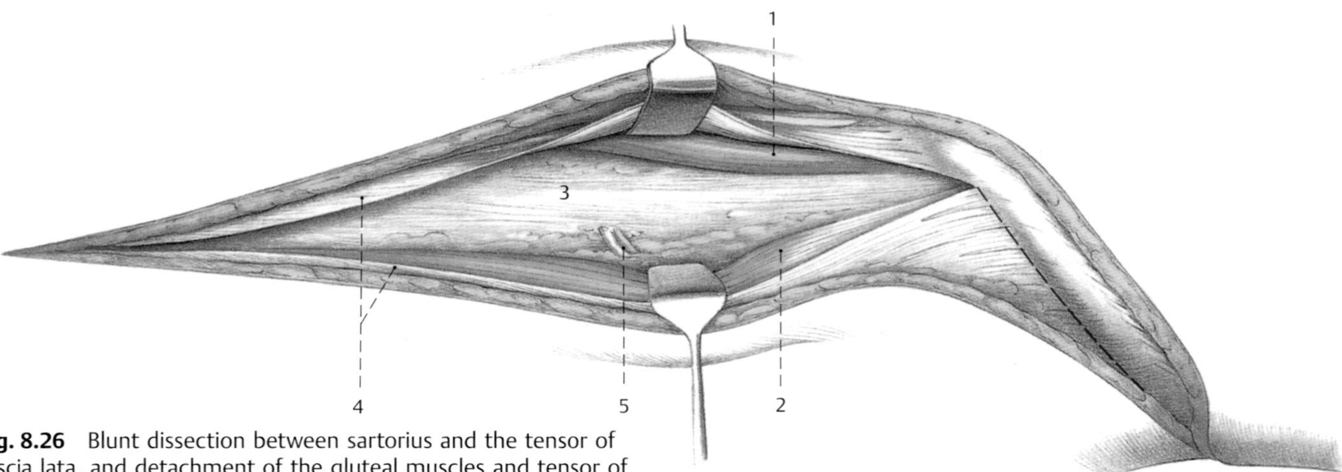

Fig. 8.26 Blunt dissection between sartorius and the tensor of fascia lata, and detachment of the gluteal muscles and tensor of fascia lata from the iliac crest (dashed line).

1 Sartorius
2 Tensor of fascia lata
3 Rectus femoris
4 Fascia lata
5 Ascending branch of the lateral circumflex femoral artery

minimus, and then piriformis are sharply transected close to their insertion into the greater trochanter (**Fig. 8.28**). This corresponds to R. Judet's original method. However, if possible, a stepped trochanter osteotomy should be performed.

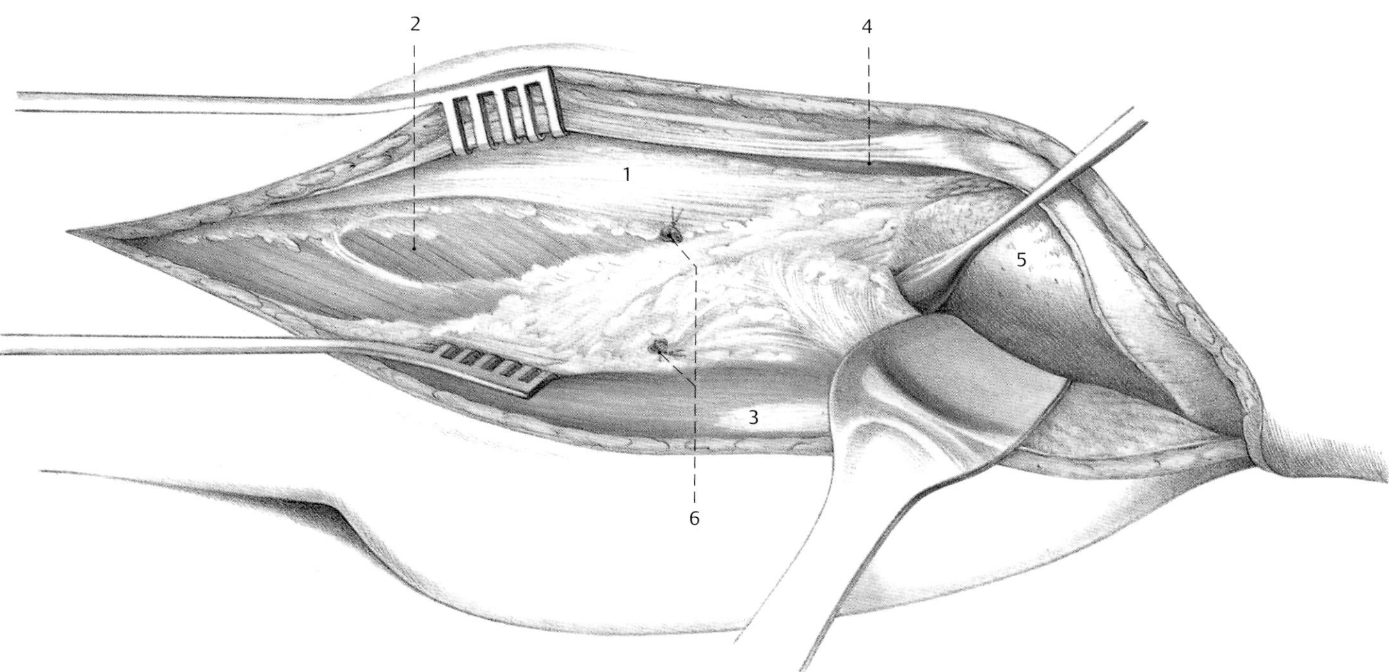

Fig. 8.27 Subperiosteal retraction of the gluteal muscles and tensor of fascia lata from the external aspect of the ilium, and exposure of the anterior portion of the hip joint capsule.

1 Rectus femoris
2 Vastus intermedius
3 Tensor of fascia lata
4 Sartorius
5 Ala of ilium, gluteal surface
6 Ascending branch of the lateral circumflex femoral artery

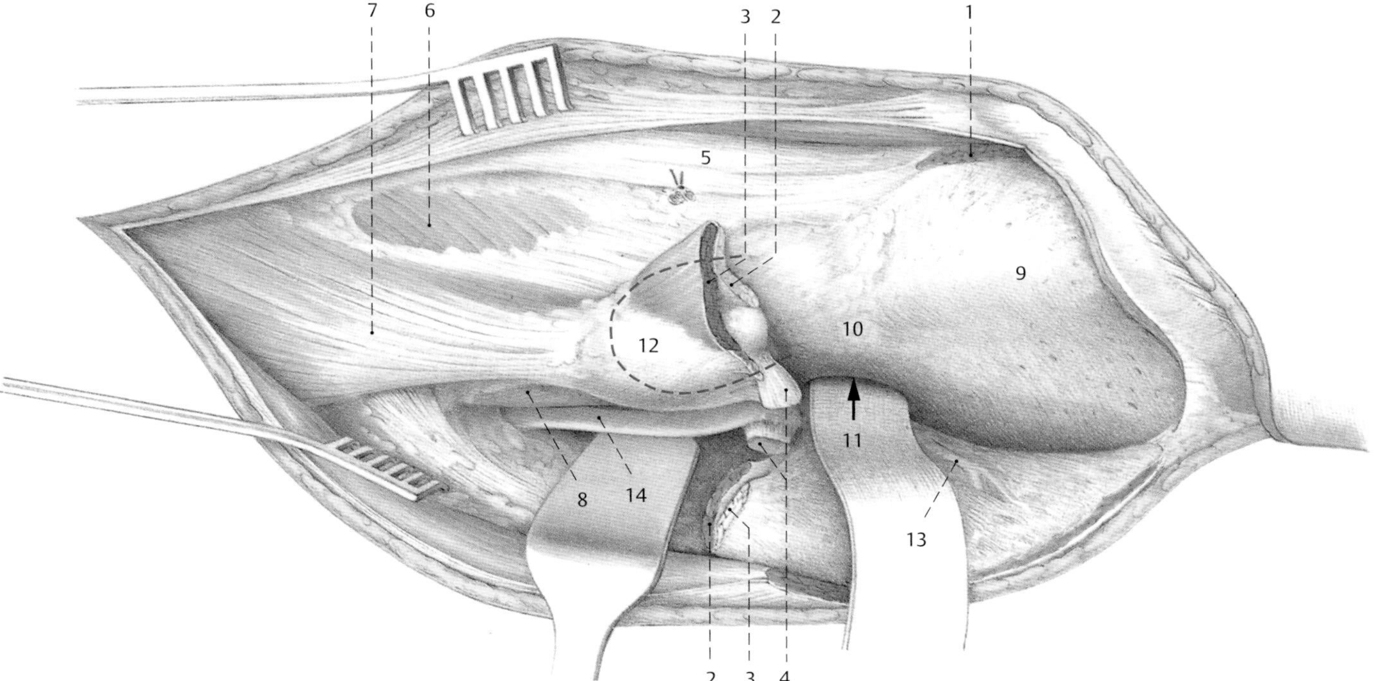

Fig. 8.28 Operative site after detachment of gluteus medius, gluteus minimus, and piriformis from the greater trochanter or optional trochanter osteotomy (dashed line).

1 Tensor of fascia lata
2 Gluteus minimus
3 Gluteus medius
4 Piriformis
5 Rectus femoris
6 Vastus intermedius
7 Vastus lateralis
8 Biceps femoris, long head
9 Ala of ilium
10 Body of ilium
11 Greater sciatic foramen
12 Greater trochanter
13 Superior gluteal vessels
14 Sciatic nerve

8.5.3 Exposure of the Pelvic Bone

The leg is now maximally rotated internally, and then the short external rotator muscles are also sharply transected. The internal rotation of the leg increases the distance to the sciatic nerve and thus lessens the chance of injury to it. The acetabular rim and the posterior pelvic bone, from the ilium to the ischium, are now exposed (**Fig. 8.29**).

If exposure of the iliac fossa and the anterior pelvic bone is required, the surgeon changes sides. The abdominal muscles and iliacus are detached from the iliac crest, and with the aid of a raspatory the iliac fossa is subperiosteally dissected as far as the greater sciatic foramen. Flexible spatulas are then inserted into the greater sciatic foramen (**Fig. 8.30**). This allows clear exposure of the iliac fossa and the gluteal surface, as well as of the anterior and posterior pelvic bone as far as the ischial tuberosity.

8.5.4 Wound Closure

Exact reattachment of the gluteal muscles to the greater trochanter and the iliac crest, as well as suture of the detached abdominal and iliacus muscles to the iliac crest, are necessary.

8.5.5 Dangers

When transecting the short external rotators (see **Fig. 8.29**), care should be taken to avoid damage to the branch of the medial circumflex femoral artery that supplies the head of the femur.

8.5.6 Note

This approach should be used only in exceptional cases inasmuch as the extensive bilateral denudation of the ilium and ischium compromises the vascular supply of these bones.

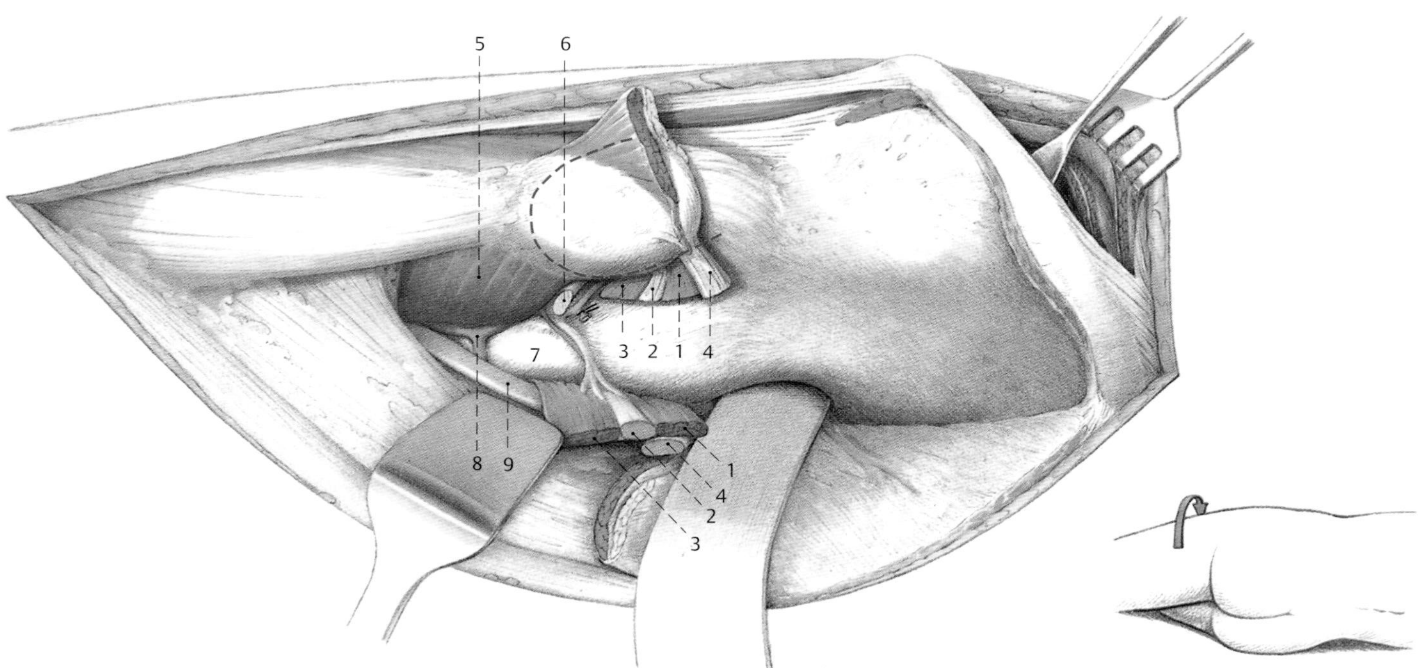

Fig. 8.29 Following maximal internal rotation of the leg (see detail), the short external rotators are divided approximately 1 cm posterior to the greater trochanter. Injury to the branch of the medial circumflex femoral artery supplying the head of the femur must be avoided. Exposure of the posterior pelvis as far as the ischial tuberosity. Detachment of the abdominal and iliacus muscles is shown in the upper right-hand corner. If required: trochanteric osteotomy.

1 Superior gemellus
2 Obturator internus
3 Inferior gemellus
4 Piriformis
5 Quadratus femoris
6 Tendon of obturator externus
7 Ischial tuberosity
8 Medial circumflex femoral artery, deep branch
9 Sciatic nerve

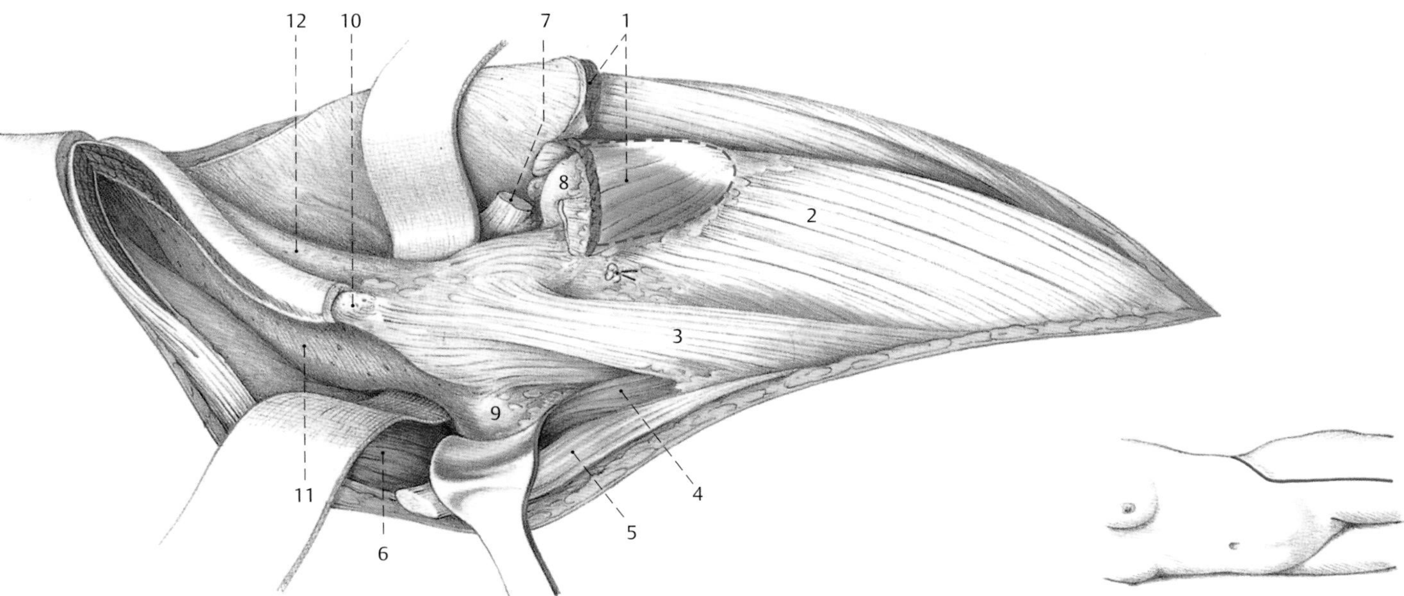

Fig. 8.30 Operative site after subperiosteal detachment of the iliacus muscle from the inner aspect of the ilium. Insertion of spatulas into the sciatic foramen, exposure of the ilium from inside and outside and of the proximal portions of the anterior pelvic bone. Alternatively: trochanteric osteotomy.

1 Gluteus medius
2 Vastus lateralis
3 Rectus femoris
4 Iliopsoas
5 Sartorius
6 Iliacus
7 Piriformis
8 Greater trochanter
9 Iliopubic eminence
10 Anterior superior iliac spine
11 Ala of ilium, iliac fossa
12 Ala of ilium, gluteal surface

9 Hip Joint

9.1 Posterior Approach to the Hip Joint with Dislocation According to Ganz

F. Kerschbaumer

9.1.1 Principal Indications

- Femoroacetabular impingement
- T-fracture of the acetabulum
- Transverse acetabular fractures involving the posterior wall
- Pipkin fractures
- Osteochondritis dissecans of the hip
- Intra-articular therapy of cartilage and bone damage due to femoral head necrosis
- Hip resurfacing arthroplasty

9.1.2 Positioning and Incision

We recommend placing the patient in the lateral position with the symphysis and sacrum supported and the operated leg on a foam pad. The incision, approximately 30 cm in length, is the same as the one described by Gibson for the posterolateral approach and curves posteriorly with the hip flexed. The fascia lata is split distally, and the incision is extended proximally and posteriorly into the aponeurosis of gluteus maximus. The leg is then extended, and self-retaining retractors or a Charnley frame can be inserted (**Fig. 9.1**). The posterior part of gluteus medius and its relation to the piriformis tendon can be exposed by incising the trochanteric bursa and dissecting it posteriorly.

The approach is continued according to the guidelines published by Ganz (2001). Unlike the classic posterolateral approach, in the Ganz technique the blood supply of the femoral head is spared by preserving the vessels supplying it, includ-

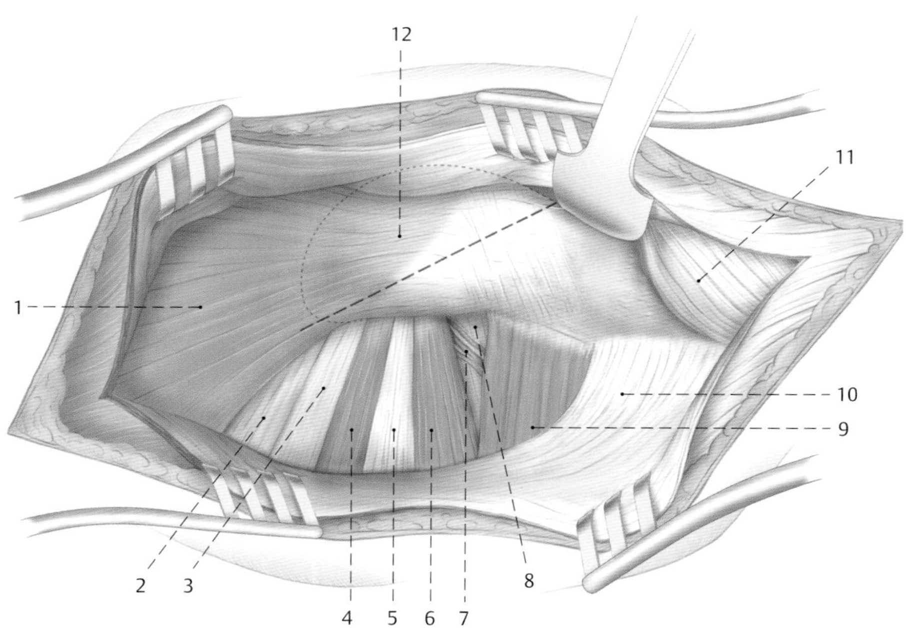

Fig. 9.1 The trochanteric osteotomy should be shallow and level or oblique (dashed line). The posterior corner of the greater trochanter is left, to spare the piriform fossa. The tendon of vastus lateralis is first divided from the femur and undermined with a Hohmann elevator.

1 Gluteus medius
2 Gluteus minimus
3 Piriformis
4 Superior gemellus
5 Obturator internus
6 Inferior gemellus
7 Medial circumflex femoral artery and vein
8 Obturator externus
9 Quadratus femoris
10 Tendon of gluteus maximus
11 Vastus lateralis
12 Greater trochanter

ing the short external rotators. The vastus lateralis muscle is first retracted in anterior direction, anterior to the attachment of the gluteus maximus tendon, and a Hohmann elevator is passed beneath it. A shallow trochanteric osteotomy, either level or oblique, is then performed with saw and osteotome. The posterior tip of the trochanter is left intact to protect the vessels. The trochanter is then separated from the femur and dislocated in anterior direction, preserving its muscle connection to gluteus medius and vastus lateralis (**Fig. 9.2**). To do this, it is necessary to divide residual fibers of gluteus minimus from the posterior angle of the trochanter with a scalpel. With this osteotomy technique, the piriform fossa should not be touched. This renders the hip joint capsule, including its cranial boundary, readily visible. A Hohmann elevator can now be inserted over the anterior acetabular rim with the thigh slightly flexed. It should be noted that the medial circumflex femoral artery and vein run proximally beneath the quadratus femoris muscle and over obturator externus, and subsequently flow subsynovially into the capsule and femoral head (**Fig. 9.2**).

The blood supply of the femoral head is also provided by more distal vessels and by anterior branches of the lateral circumflex femoral artery. The leg is now extended and maximally externally rotated (**Fig. 9.3**). This provides visualization of the entire anterior, superior, and also inferior parts of the hip joint capsule. The capsule is now incised along the posterior and superior rim of the acetabulum, continued parallel to the more cranial iliofemoral ligament and then in a caudal direction as far as the psoas tendon. In the event of posterior acetabular

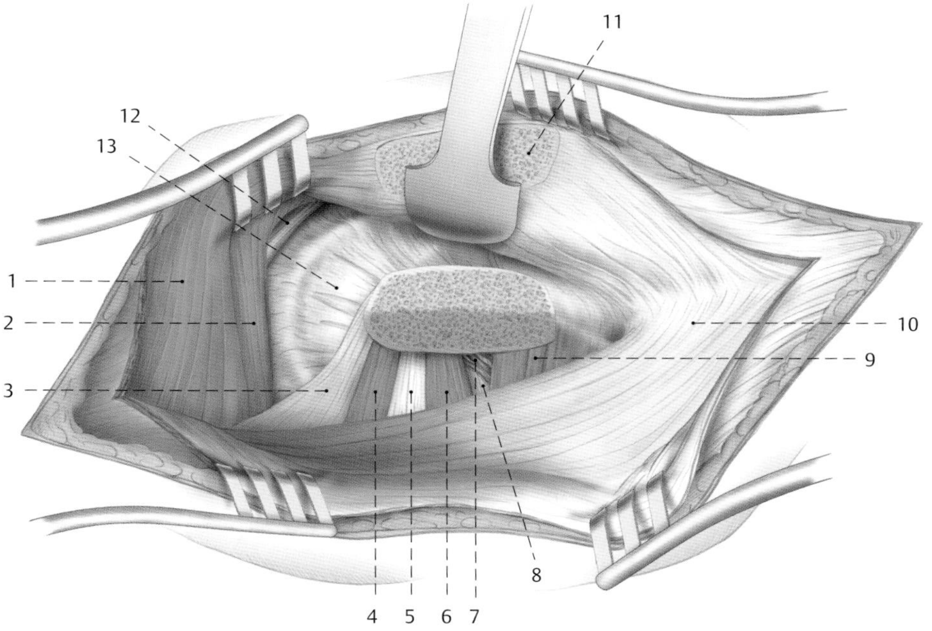

Fig. 9.2 After trochanteric osteotomy, the musculotendinous connection between the gluteal and vastus muscles and the trochanter fragment is dislocated anteriorly. A Hohmann elevator is inserted at the anterior acetabular rim with the thigh slightly flexed.

1 Gluteus medius
2 Gluteus minimus
3 Piriformis
4 Superior gemellus
5 Obturator internus
6 Inferior gemellus
7 Medial circumflex femoral artery/vein
8 Obturator externus
9 Quadratus femoris
10 Tendinous insertion of gluteus maximus
11 Trochanter fragment
12 Reflected head of rectus femoris
13 Right hip joint capsule

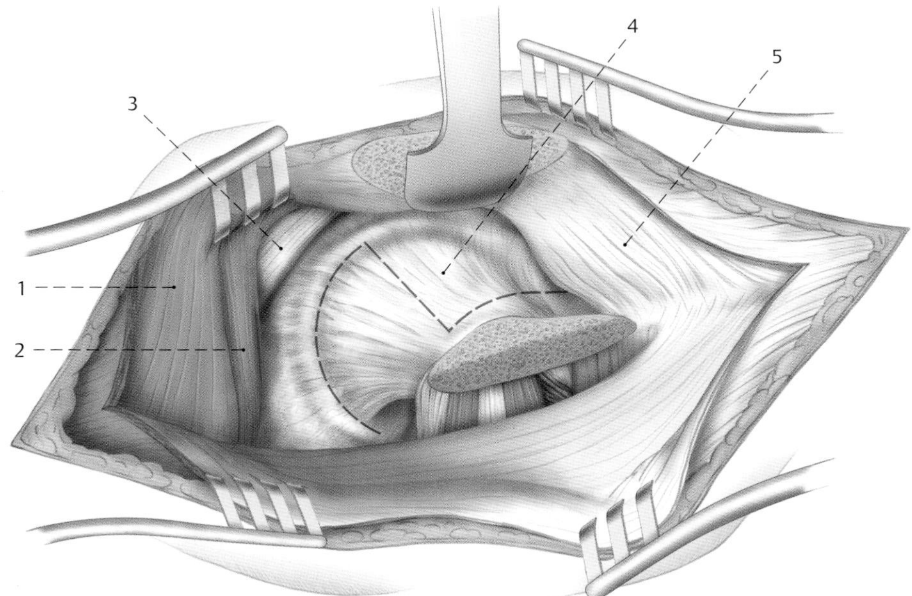

Fig. 9.3 The dashed line shows the direction of incision of the hip joint capsule according to the Ganz technique. At this time, the leg should be extended and maximally externally rotated. If necessary, a second Hohmann elevator can be introduced between the joint capsule and psoas tendon. Note the intact external rotators and vessels.

1 Gluteus medius
2 Gluteus minimus
3 Reflected head of rectus femoris
4 Right hip joint capsule
5 Vastus lateralis

pathology (acetabular rim fractures or injuries to the posterior pelvic column), the capsule incision can be extended posteriorly with the leg internally rotated.

It is also possible to notch the tendinous insertion of the piriformis muscle without endangering the vascular supply of the femoral head. The hip is now dislocated with the leg cautiously flexed and externally rotated (**Fig. 9.4**). The lower leg is placed in a sterile bag. A Hohmann elevator can now be inserted anterior to the labrum with a second one posteriorly, giving complete exposure of the entire circumference of the acetabulum (**Fig. 9.5**). Should exposure of the acetabular roof be necessary, the reflected head of rectus femoris can be detached and another Hohmann retractor can be inserted in the ilium beneath gluteus minimus.

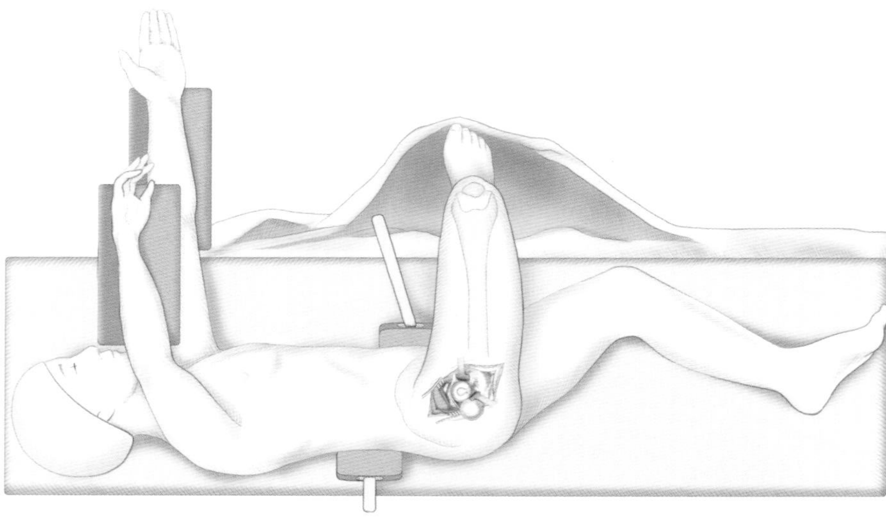

Fig. 9.4 The femoral head is dislocated gently with the thigh externally rotated and flexed, and the lower leg is placed in a sterile bag at the edge of the table.

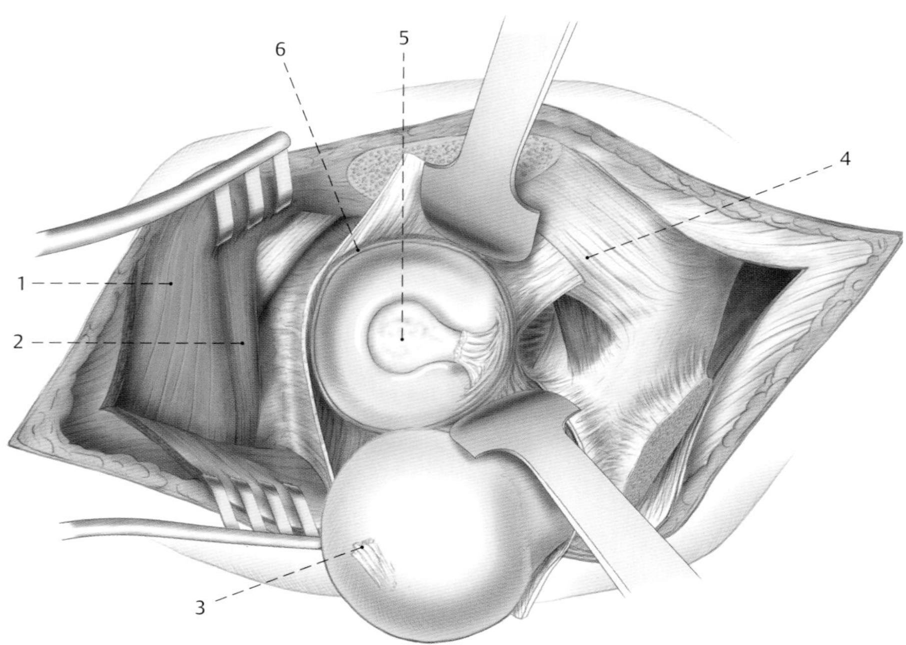

Fig. 9.5 After the introduction of anterior and posterior Hohmann retractors, the entire circumference of the acetabulum is clearly exposed along with the femoral head. If necessary, the acetabular roof can be exposed after detachment of the reflected head and retraction of gluteus minimus with another Hohmann retractor.

1 Gluteus medius
2 Gluteus minimus
3 Incision of the ligament of the head of femur
4 Vastus lateralis
5 Acetabular fossa
6 Acetabular labrum

9.1.3 Wound Closure

After reduction of the hip in extension and internal rotation, the capsule is sutured with braided absorbable size 1 suture material. The musculotendinous combination of the greater trochanter, vastus lateralis, gluteus medius, and gluteus minimus is replaced and fixed to the original osteotomy with two size 3.5 or 4.5 cortical screws.

9.1.4 Dangers

Trochanteric pseudarthrosis has been described as a potential postoperative complication. Heterotopic periarticular ossification may occur, especially after acetabular fractures. If the femoral head and neck are skeletized excessively, vascular injury in the form of partial femoral head necrosis is possible.

9.2 Posterior Minimally Invasive Approach

F. Kerschbaumer

9.2.1 Principal Indication

- Hip arthroplasty

The lateral decubitus position is the same as that used for the usual Gibson posterolateral approach. The pelvis is stabilized by supports both posteriorly at the level of the lumbosacral junction and anteriorly at the symphysis. Both thighs are flexed approximately 45°, and the leg to be operated on is placed on a foam pad and is freely mobile. Because of the relatively short skin incision, I recommend marking it on the skin beforehand, if necessary using an image converter. Two-thirds of the incision should be proximal to the tip of the trochanter. Depending on the patient's size, the length of the incision is 7–12 cm (**Fig. 9.6**).

Following the skin incision, the subcutaneous tissue is elevated from the fascia over gluteus maximus with a pad or abdominal sponge, and a wound spreader is inserted (**Fig. 9.7**). To protect the skin, it is advisable to place pads between the skin and the jaws of the retractor. In this way, the skin window can be shifted proximally and distally by traction and pressure on the self-retaining retractor to allow a sufficiently long incision of the gluteus maximus and adjacent fascia lata over the greater trochanter.

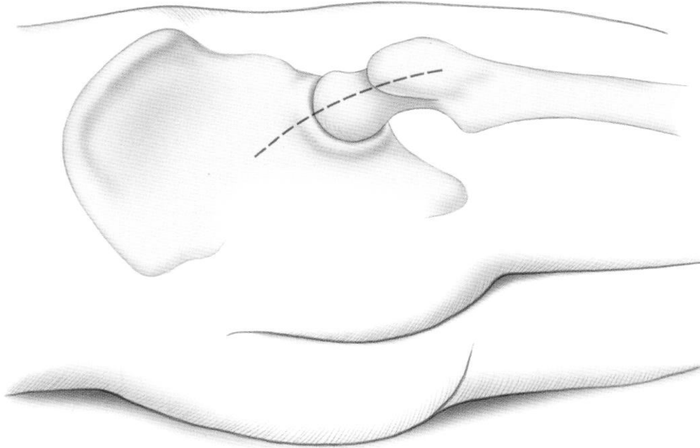

Fig. 9.6 The skin incision is approximately 7–12 cm long, two-thirds proximal and one-third distal to the tip of the trochanter. The incision runs posterolaterally in the line of the anterior fibers of gluteus maximus.

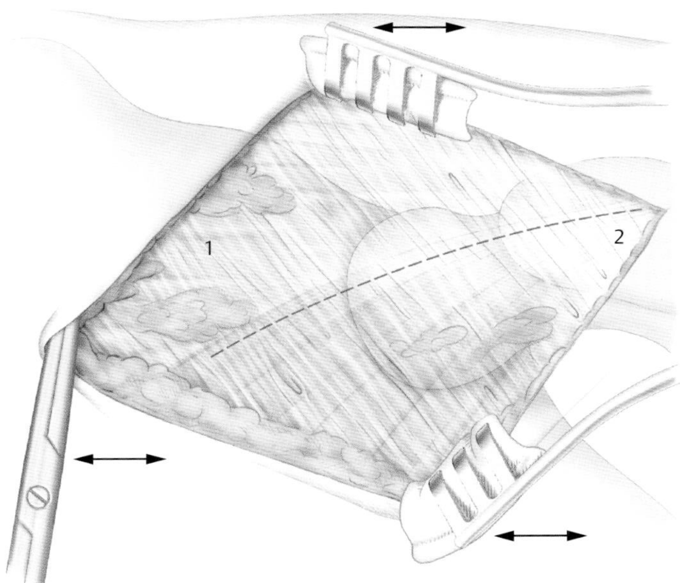

Fig. 9.7 Subcutaneous dissection window over the fascia of gluteus maximus, which can be moved proximally and distally if necessary. Note the protective pads under the retractors to avoid pressure injury to the skin.

1 Aponeurosis of gluteus maximus
2 Iliotibial tract

The leg is then maximally extended and internally rotated by the second assistant (**Fig. 9.8**). The self-retaining retractor is reinserted more deeply into gluteus maximus and opened. The trochanteric bursa, which covers the external rotators and adjacent gluteal muscles, is now dissected and retracted posteriorly (**Fig. 9.9**). At this point, the position of the sciatic nerve should be located by palpation.

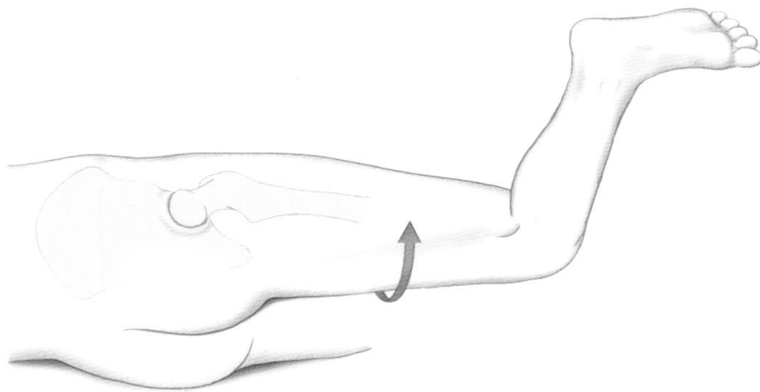

Fig. 9.8 The hip is extended and internally rotated to allow dissection of the hip capsule and exposure of the external rotators.

9.2.2 Exposure of the Hip Joint

The piriformis tendon is the key to atraumatic exposure of the joint capsule. First, the gluteus medius is cautiously retracted proximally with a Langenbeck retractor, and the roundish white tendon of piriformis is then detached as far distally as possible in the trochanteric fossa. It should be noted that the form of the piriformis muscle is quite variable, and it is often fused with the neighboring gluteus minimus. In these cases, the boundaries of piriformis must be defined by palpation alone, and it must be divided from gluteus minimus. The whitish joint capsule is now exposed. Gluteus minimus, which covers the capsule, is dissected off it carefully with a narrow raspatory, extending the hip slightly again so that an angled Hohmann elevator can be inserted (**Fig. 9.9**).

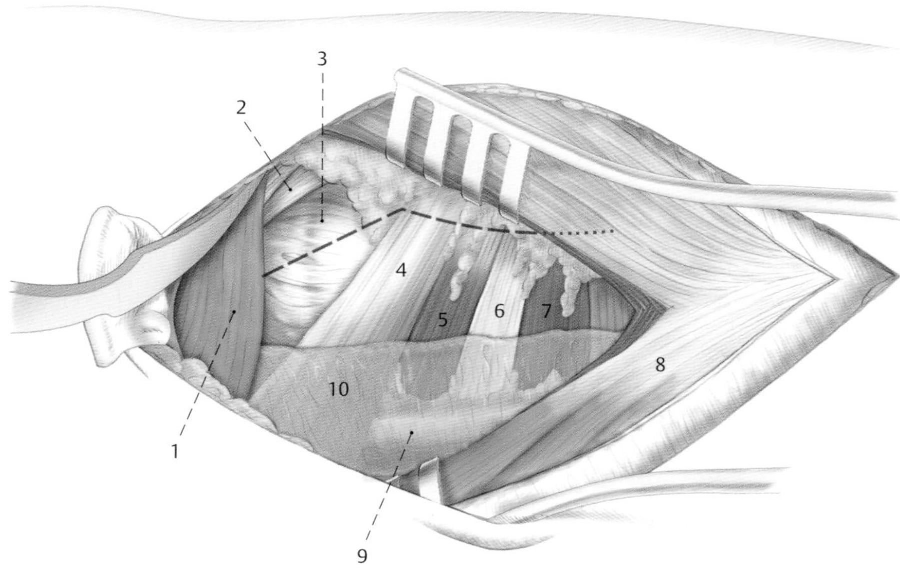

Fig. 9.9 Gluteus minimus is cautiously retracted cranially with a curved Hohmann retractor without injuring the muscle fibers. The joint capsule and the tendons of the external rotators are then incised from proximal to distal close to the bone in the piriform fossa. The upper border of quadratus femoris is the distal limit of this incision.

1 Gluteus minimus
2 Reflected head of rectus femoris
3 Hip joint capsule
4 Piriformis
5 Superior gemellus
6 Obturator internus
7 Inferior gemellus
8 Gluteus maximus
9 Sciatic nerve
10 Trochanteric bursa dissected and retracted posteriorly

The joint capsule and adjacent rotators are now divided from proximal to distal by a slightly curved incision that ends distally at the upper border of quadratus femoris. Further flexion and internal rotation of the hip expose the medial circumflex femoral artery and accompanying veins lying on the tendon of obturator externus, which is beneath quadratus femoris. The vessels must be ligated and divided. The obturator externus tendon is divided (**Fig. 9.10**). The self-retaining retractor can now be inserted at a deeper level. A Hohmann retractor is placed cranially over the femoral neck, and the neck and head of the femur are now exposed (**Fig. 9.11**). The femoral neck osteotomy can now be performed in situ with a narrow and relatively short oscillating saw, the direction of which depends on the caput-collum-diaphyseal angle of the femur. In coxa vara, the superior part of the osteotomy should be divided with a chisel. Alternatively, it is possible to dislocate the femoral head prior to the osteotomy and then divide the femoral neck (**Fig. 9.11**).

9.2.3 Exposure of the Acetabulum

To expose the acetabulum, two Hohmann retractors are usually inserted in the anterior and posteroinferior positions (**Fig. 9.12**). The inferior joint capsule is now dissected off the underlying obturator externus with blunt dissecting scissors, and the capsule is then split radially as far as the transverse ligament. If necessary, a third Hohmann retractor can be placed distally in the obturator foramen (**Fig. 9.12**). Sponges must be placed beneath all retractors throughout the operation to protect the skin from pressure injury. The operation table is now tilted by approximately 20° toward the surgeon to provide optimal exposure and illumination of the acetabulum.

9.2.4 Wound Closure

For wound closure, the assistant holds the thigh extended with the knee flexed and the leg internally rotated to approximately 30° initially. Starting proximally, the capsule is closed together with the adherent musculotendinous layer with three or four sutures. To ensure that the capsule is watertight, the sutures are tied with the thigh slightly externally rotated. This allows reconstruction of the ischiocrural ligament and prevention of postoperative dislocation. If the leg has a pronounced externally rotated deformity preoperatively, we do not reattach the piriformis tendon (**Fig. 9.13**). A subfascial drain is placed, and the wound is closed in layers.

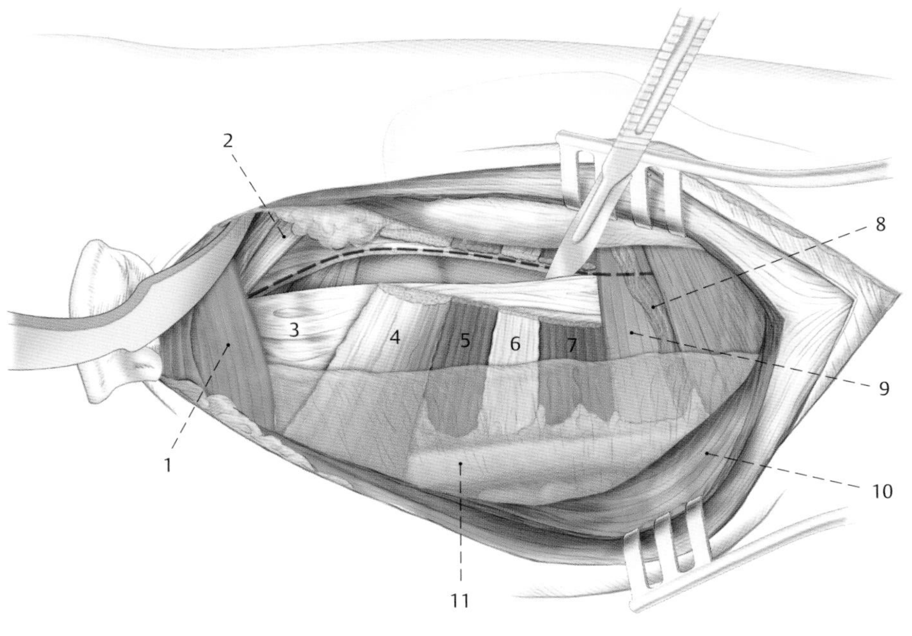

Fig. 9.10 Flexion and further internal rotation of the hip exposes the medial circumflex femoral artery and the obturator externus muscle beneath it. The vessels are ligated, and the obturator externus tendon is divided.

1 Gluteus minimus
2 Reflected head of rectus femoris
3 Joint capsule
4 Piriformis
5 Superior gemellus
6 Obturator internus
7 Inferior gemellus
8 Medial circumflex femoral artery with accompanying veins
9 Obturator externus
10 Gluteus maximus
11 Sciatic nerve

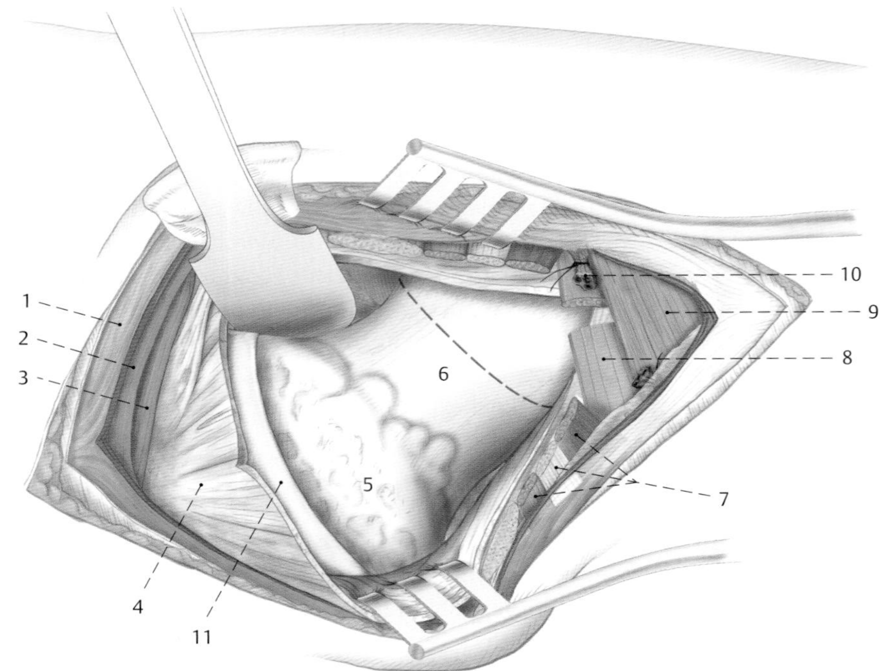

Fig. 9.11 Osteotomy of the femoral neck can be performed before or after dislocation of the femoral head. Osteotomy prior to dislocation is less traumatic to the muscles, especially with stiff joints and in muscular patients.

1 Gluteus maximus
2 Gluteus medius
3 Gluteus minimus
4 Joint capsule
5 Head of femur
6 Neck of femur
7 Triceps coxae (superior gemellus, obturator internus, inferior gemellus)
8 Obturator externus
9 Quadratus femoris
10 Medial circumflex femoral artery
11 Acetabular labrum

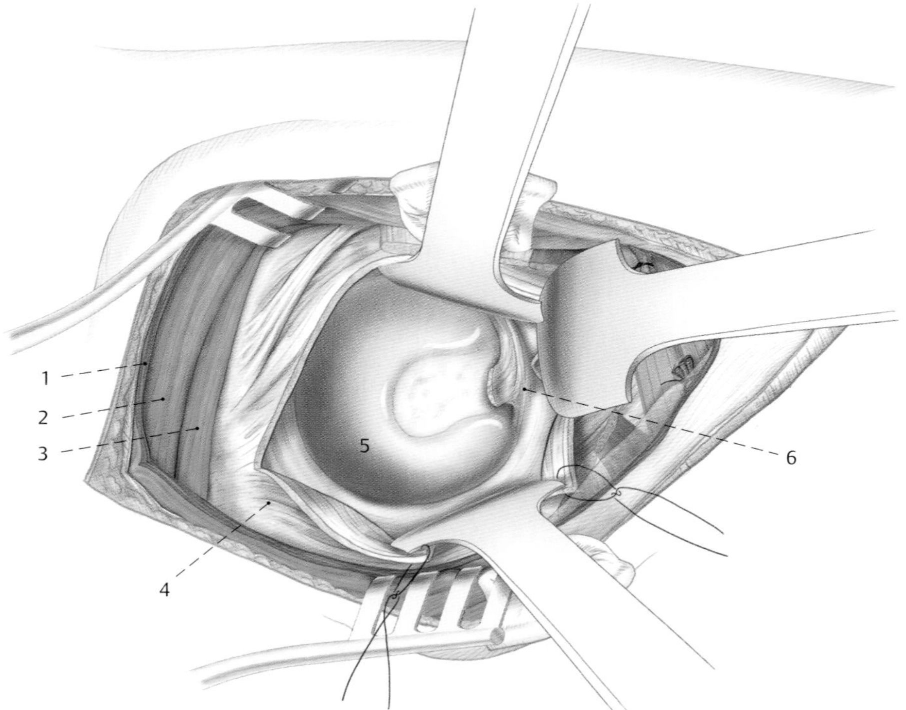

Fig. 9.12 Exposure of the acetabulum after radial incision of the inferior part of the joint capsule as far as the transverse ligament. The tip of the anterior Hohmann retractor is placed on top of the iliopubic eminence, thereby pushing the femur forward. If possible, only two Hohmann retractors should be used, but an additional one can be placed distally in the obturator foramen if visualization is poor.

1 Gluteus maximus
2 Gluteus medius
3 Gluteus minimus
4 Joint capsule
5 Lunate surface
6 Transverse ligament of the acetabulum

9.2.5 Dangers

The sciatic nerve is not normally at risk in primary operations. However, the level of nerve division is variable, and when it is at a high level the fibular part may perforate the piriformis muscle and therefore run further laterally than usual. For this reason, palpation at the start of the operation is recommended. In revision surgery, scarring may also cause the sciatic nerve to be in abnormal position. In my opinion, the described minimally invasive approach is unsuitable for revision operations.

Deliberate exposure and ligature or coagulation of the medial circumflex femoral vessels is important to avoid postoperative bleeding. During inferior dissection and incision of the joint capsule, the close relation of the capsule, obturator externus, and medial circumflex femoral artery should be noted.

To avoid postoperative dislocation, I recommend closing the joint capsule and preserving it, together with the attached rotator muscles.

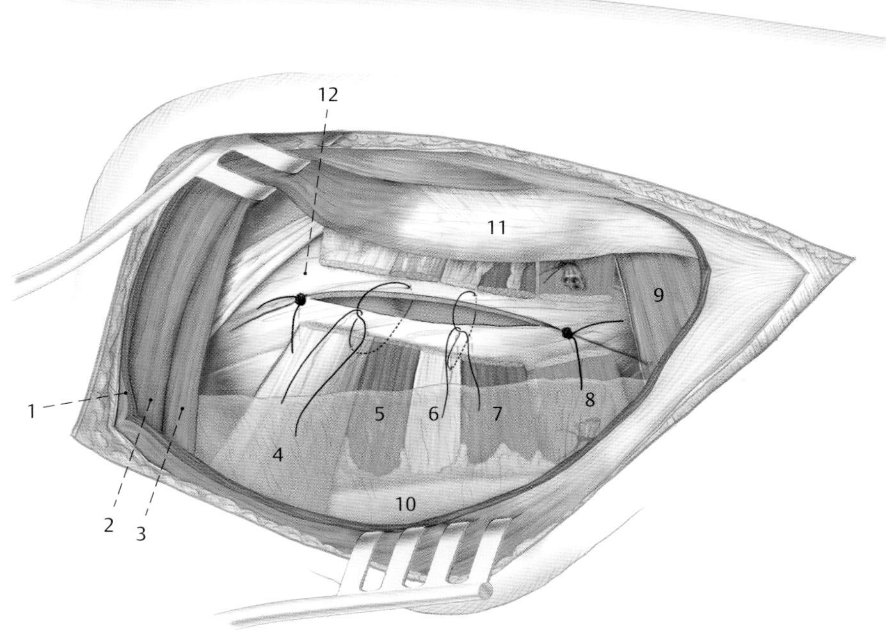

Fig. 9.13 With this approach, the joint capsule is preserved and is closed with the attached muscle at the end of the operation. To tie the sutures, the thigh is extended and externally rotated. This corrects and closes any "soft spot" between the ischiofemoral and iliofemoral ligaments to guard against dislocation.

1 Gluteus maximus
2 Gluteus medius
3 Gluteus minimus
4 Piriformis
5 Superior gemellus
6 Obturator internus
7 Inferior gemellus
8 Obturator externus
9 Quadratus femoris
10 Sciatic nerve
11 Greater trochanter
12 Joint capsule

9.3 Transgluteal Approach According to Bauer

R. Bauer, F. Kerschbaumer, S. Poisel

9.3.1 Principal Indications

- Total joint replacement
- Femoral neck fractures
- Femoral neck osteotomies
- Juvenile slipped femoral capital epiphysis
- Hip joint synovectomy

9.3.2 Positioning and Incision

The patient is placed in the supine position with a pad under the buttocks. The incision corresponds to the slightly curved one shown in **Fig. 9.24**. After splitting the subcutaneous tissue and the fascia lata parallel to the skin incision, the gluteus medius and minimus and vastus lateralis are divided in their anterior third in line with their fibers (**Fig. 9.14**).

It should be ensured that the tendoperiosteal tissue between the gluteus medius and vastus lateralis on the front of the greater trochanter is carefully stripped from the bone in one layer. This detachment is best accomplished by diathermy.

9.3.3 Exposure of the Hip Joint Capsule

The anterior portions of the joint capsule are dissected free with a Cobb elevator. A curved Hohmann elevator is inserted between the origin of the rectus muscle and the anterior acetabular wall. A cranially placed Hohmann elevator intervenes between the joint capsule and gluteus minimus, and another is placed distally between iliopsoas and the joint capsule. If necessary, a second anterior Hohmann elevator may be inserted somewhat distal to the large curved elevator. The incision of the hip joint capsule is T-shaped (**Fig. 9.15**). After broad opening of the joint capsule near the acetabulum, two Hohmann elevators may be inserted between the capsule and the femoral neck. No damage to the femoral head circulation is likely to result from this procedure (**Fig. 9.16**).

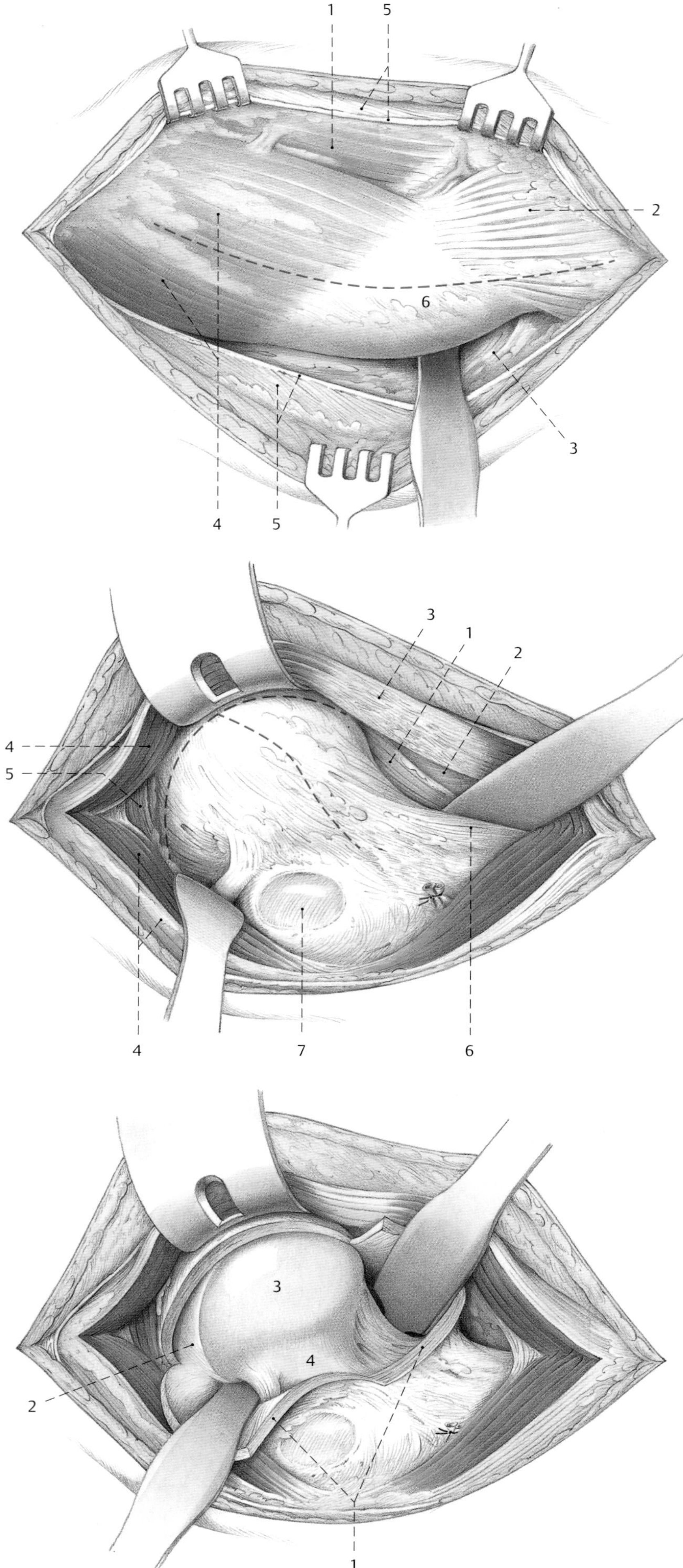

Fig. 9.14 Transgluteal approach to the hip joint. Incision of gluteus medius and vastus lateralis at the border between the middle and anterior thirds of the muscle (right leg).

1 Tensor of fascia lata
2 Vastus lateralis
3 Gluteus maximus
4 Gluteus medius
5 Fascia lata
6 Greater trochanter

Fig. 9.15 The muscle layer composed of the gluteus medius and minimus, the tendoperiosteal tissue at the greater trochanter, and the vastus lateralis is retracted in an anterior direction. Following exposure of the hip joint capsule, Hohmann retractors are placed. A T-shaped incision is made in the hip joint capsule.

1 Iliopsoas
2 Vastus intermedius
3 Vastus lateralis
4 Gluteus medius
5 Gluteus minimus
6 Iliofemoral ligament
7 Trochanteric bursa of gluteus minimus

Fig. 9.16 Appearance after opening the hip joint capsule. Hohmann elevators are inserted behind the neck of the femur, and the leg is maximally externally rotated and adducted.

1 Joint capsule
2 Acetabular labrum
3 Head of femur
4 Neck of femur

9.3.4 Anatomical Site

As shown in **Fig. 9.17**, one of the advantages of the transgluteal approach is that the superior gluteal nerve is protected against undue retractor pressure by the wide muscular coat of gluteus minimus (cf. **Fig. 9.28**). The course of the superior gluteal nerve has been better revealed by detaching the gluteus medius muscle from the iliac crest and greater trochanter. Other advantages of this approach are clear exposure of the femoral neck, the upper parts of the hip joint capsule, and the femoral neck resection plane for total hip replacement.

9.3.5 Wound Closure

(**Fig. 9.18**)

The wound is closed by apposition of the muscles split in line of their fibers (gluteus medius and minimus and vastus lateralis). The fascioperiosteal plate is firmly sutured in the region of the greater trochanter.

9.3.6 Note

The transgluteal approach is routinely employed by the authors for total hip replacement. In this approach, osteotomy of the greater trochanter seldom proves necessary.

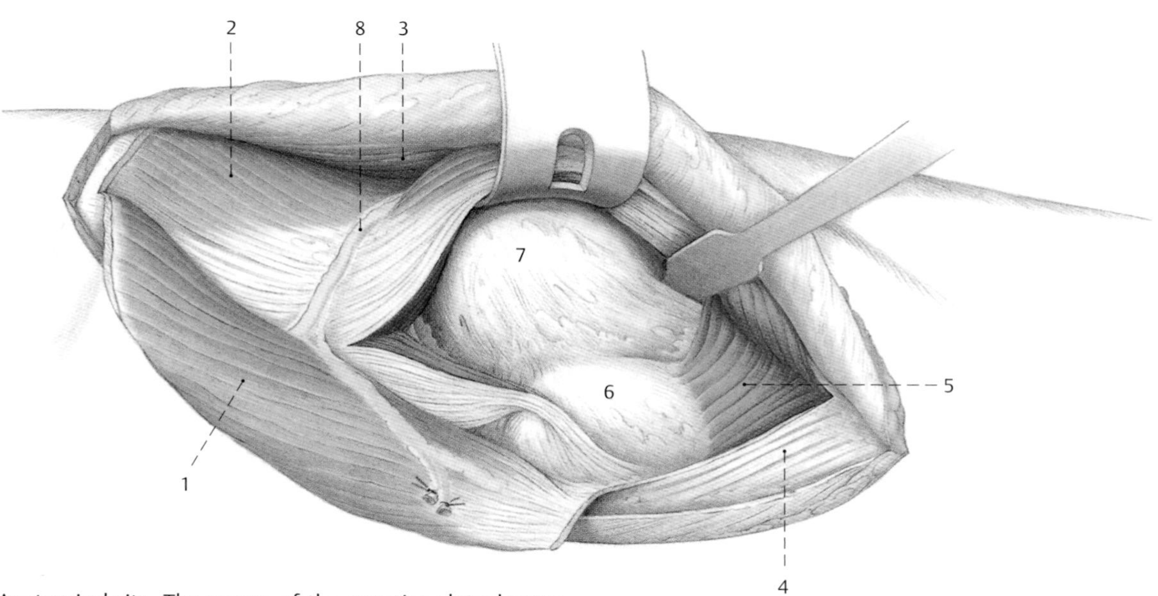

Fig. 9.17 Anatomical site. The course of the superior gluteal nerve in the transgluteal approach. Gluteus medius was partly severed at the iliac crest and the greater trochanter, and retracted posteriorly.

1 Gluteus medius
2 Gluteus minimus
3 Tensor of fascia lata
4 Vastus lateralis
5 Vastus intermedius
6 Greater trochanter
7 Head of femur
8 Superior gluteal nerve

Fig. 9.18 Closure of the muscle with interrupted sutures.

1 Gluteus medius
2 Tensor of fascia lata
3 Vastus lateralis

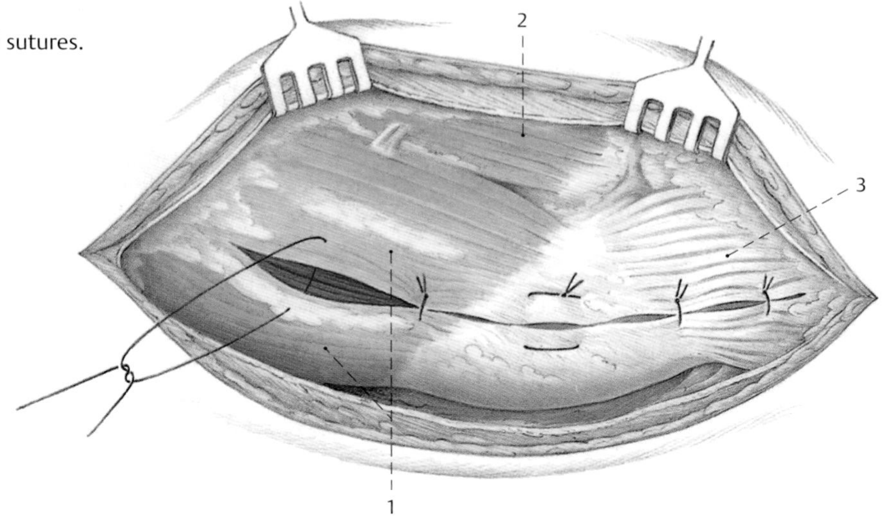

9.4 Minimally Invasive Transgluteal Approach

A. Roth

9.4.1 Principal Indications

- Total joint replacement
- Hemiarthroplasty
- Femoral neck fractures
- Femoral neck osteotomies
- Juvenile slipped femoral capital epiphysis
- Hip joint synovectomy

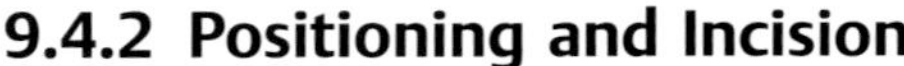

9.4.2 Positioning and Incision

The patient is placed in the supine or lateral decubitus position. If the supine position is chosen, part of the buttock on the operated side projects over the edge of the table so that the soft tissues can shift posteriorly and the trochanter region is covered with as thin a layer of soft tissue as possible.

The skin incision is made over the greater trochanter parallel to the axis of the leg and is 5–11 cm in length. The distal limit of the incision is projected on the inferior border of the acetabulum (**Fig. 9.19**). The relation of the trochanter to the acetabulum on X-ray can be used to assist orientation.

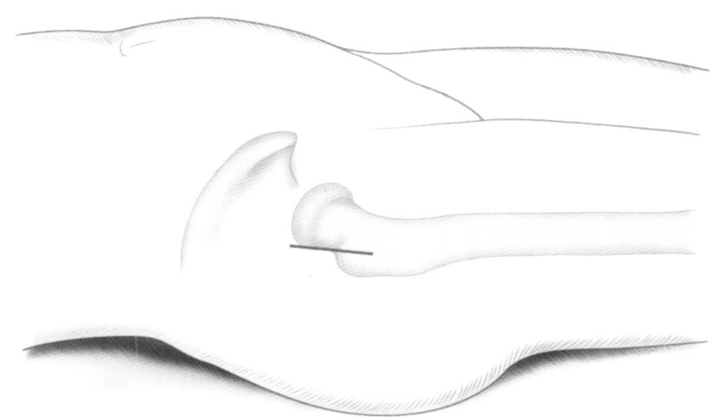

Fig. 9.19 Minimally invasive transgluteal approach. Positioning and incision in relation to the acetabulum.

The iliotibial tract is incised parallel to the skin incision. This incision can be extended by up to 2 cm subcutaneously, deviating approximately 15° anteriorly at the distal end and 15° posteriorly at the proximal end (**Fig. 9.20**).

The bursa is incised parallel to the skin incision from the tip of the trochanter extending distally over the vastus lateralis. The insertion of gluteus medius is then divided from the trochanter tip (**Fig. 9.21**). Subperiosteal dissection continues as far as the capsule, detaching the tendon of gluteus minimus, which remains joined with gluteus medius.

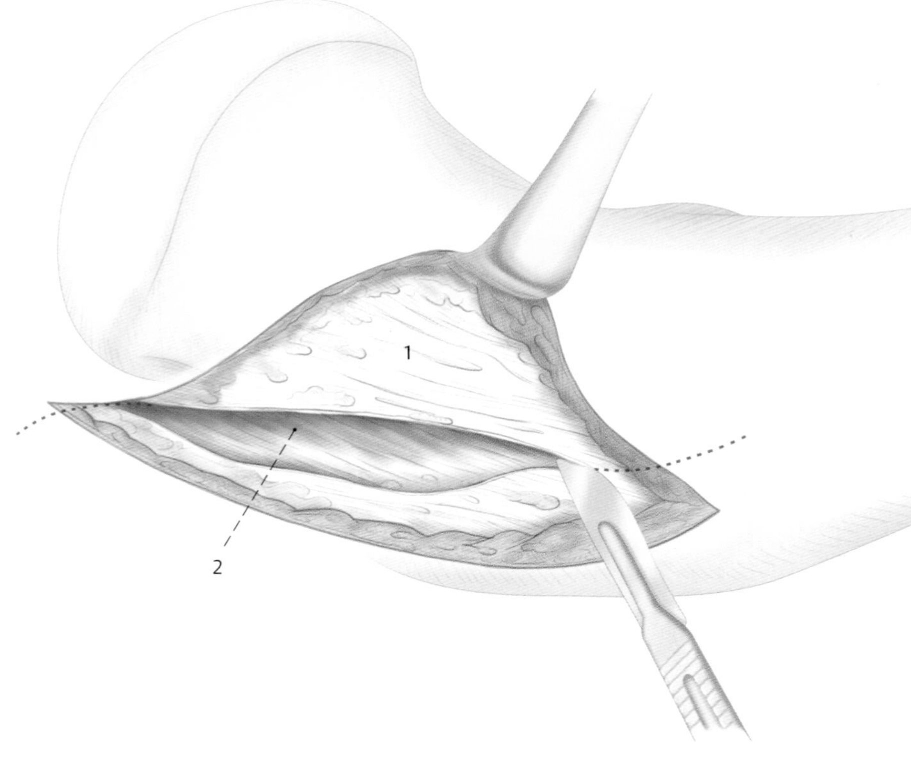

Fig. 9.20 Splitting of the fascia lata parallel to the skin incision at the level of the innominate tubercle. The incision is extended up to 2 cm subcutaneously, curving slightly in a distal anterior and proximal posterior direction.

1 Fascia lata (iliotibial tract)
2 Gluteus medius

9.4.3 Exposure of the Hip Joint Capsule

The anterior portions of the joint capsule are dissected free with a Cobb elevator. A curved narrow Hohmann elevator is inserted anteriorly between the origin of rectus femoris and the anterior margin of the acetabulum. A straight or curved Hohmann elevator protects the cranial part of the joint capsule. Another Hohmann elevator may be inserted between iliopsoas and the joint capsule (**Fig. 9.22**).

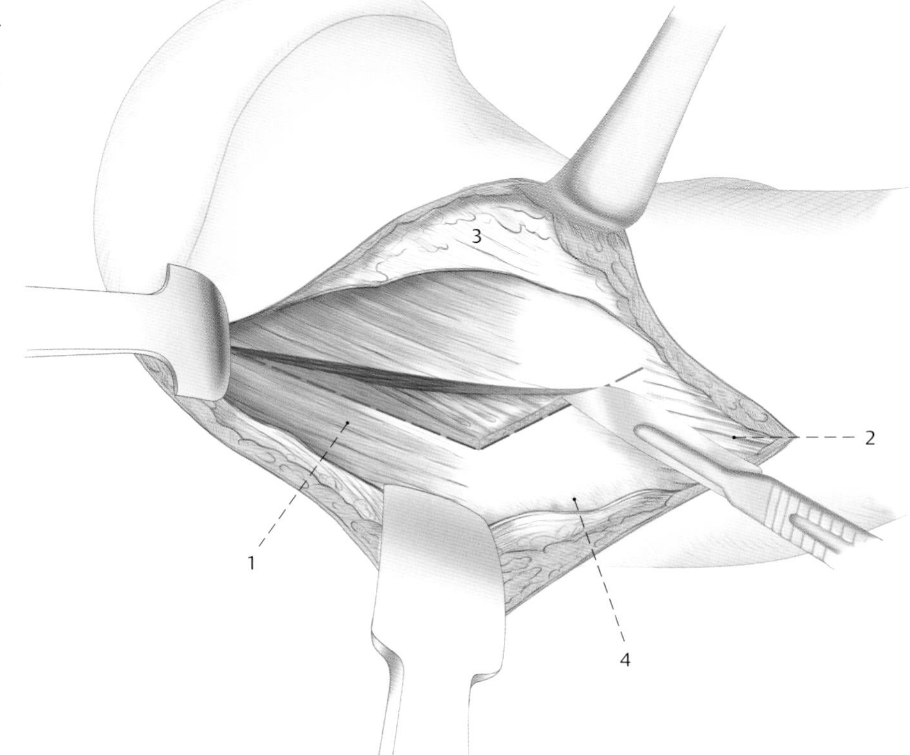

Fig. 9.21 Incision of the tendinous insertion of gluteus medius close to the trochanter. The incision begins at the trochanter tip and curves slightly distally. Dissection continues to the joint capsule with division of the tendon of gluteus minimus.

1 Gluteus medius
2 Vastus lateralis
3 Fascia lata
4 Greater trochanter

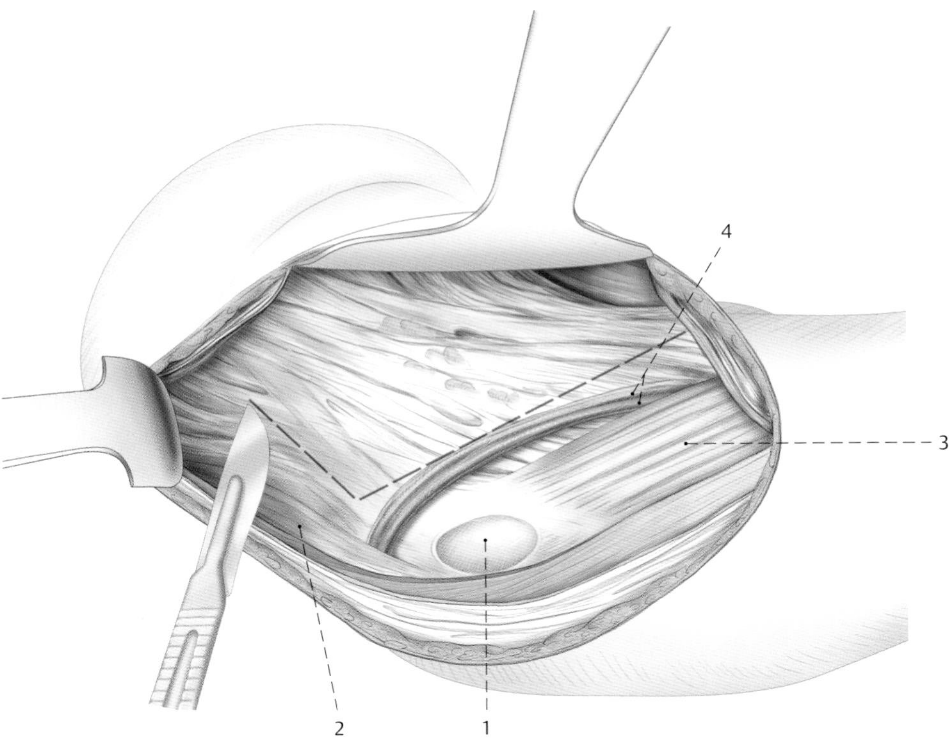

Fig. 9.22 Exposure of the joint capsule, protecting it with Hohmann elevators. L-shaped incision or inverted T-shaped incision of the joint capsule and subsequent resection.

1 Trochanteric bursa
2 Gluteus medius
3 Vastus lateralis
4 Lateral circumflex femoral artery and vein

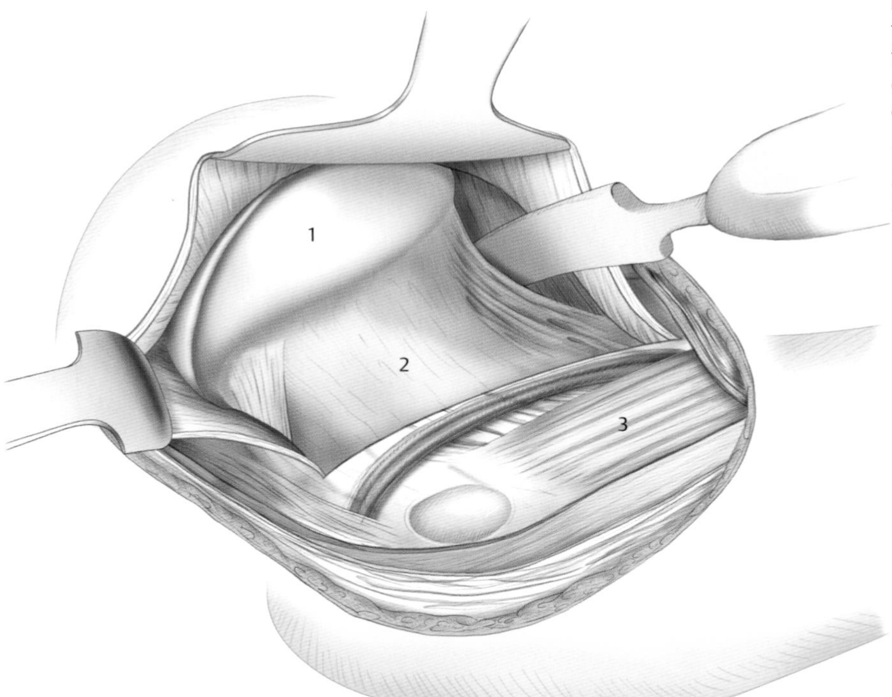

Fig. 9.23 Insertion of a Hohmann retractor on the anterior border of the acetabulum. The leg is flexed approximately 20°. The capsule is dissected distally as far as the lesser trochanter with a Cobb elevator.

1 Head of femur
2 Neck of femur
3 Vastus lateralis

An L-shaped incision is made in the right hip joint capsule (or a reverse L-shaped incision in the left joint capsule); the joint capsule is then elevated anteriorly. If necessary, the capsule is mobilized far medially in the direction of the lesser trochanter using a Cobb elevator (**Fig. 9.23**).

9.4.4 Wound Closure

The capsule can be closed superiorly by an interrupted suture. The muscles are reattached using side-to-side suture of the gluteal muscles to the remaining tendon stump on the greater trochanter. Two or three full-thickness sutures are placed to reinforce the tendon of gluteus minimus. The iliotibial tract is closed with absorbable interrupted sutures.

9.4.5 Dangers

Injury can occur to the superior gluteal nerve by an incision too far proximally when dividing gluteus medius above the tip of the trochanter.

9.4.6 Note

When arthroplasty is performed through this approach, angled instruments must be used for implantation, and the iliotibial tract is not dislocated behind the greater trochanter.

9.5 Anterolateral Approach to the Hip Joint

R. Bauer, F. Kerschbaumer, S. Poisel, A. Roth

9.5.1 Principal Indications

- Total joint replacement
- Hemiarthroplasty
- Femoral neck fractures
- Juvenile slipped femoral epiphysis
- Synovectomy
- Femoral neck osteotomies

9.5.2 Positioning and Incision

The patient is placed supine with a small pad under the buttocks. The skin incision begins approximately 2–3 cm below and a handbreadth posterior to the anterior superior iliac spine and runs laterally in distal direction over the greater trochanter (**Fig. 9.24**). The incision curves slightly toward the trochanter and then continues in a straight line for a few centimeters along the lateral thigh. After dividing the subcutaneous tissue, the junction between the tensor of fascia lata and the gluteal muscles beneath the fascia can be seen. The fascia lata is incised parallel to the skin incision, from distal to proximal (**Fig. 9.25**). The incision should be made between the muscular portions of the tensor of fascia lata and the gluteus maximus. The space between the gluteal muscles and tensor of fascia lata is then dissected bluntly. The posterior portion of the fascia is retracted with a Hohmann elevator, while a Langenbeck retractor is used for retraction of the anterior portion. A vascular bundle is usually found on the anterior border of gluteus medius, which passes to the tensor of fascia lata and must be coagulated, or ligated and transected (**Fig. 9.26**).

The leg is flexed and externally rotated, and Hohmann retractors are inserted to expose the hip joint capsule.

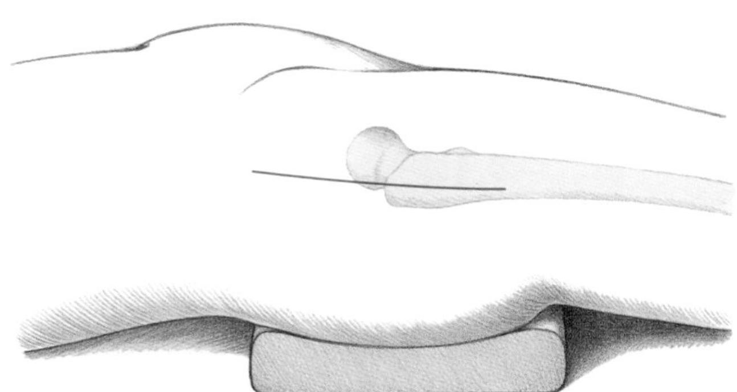

Fig. 9.24 Anterolateral approach to the hip joint. Positioning and incision.

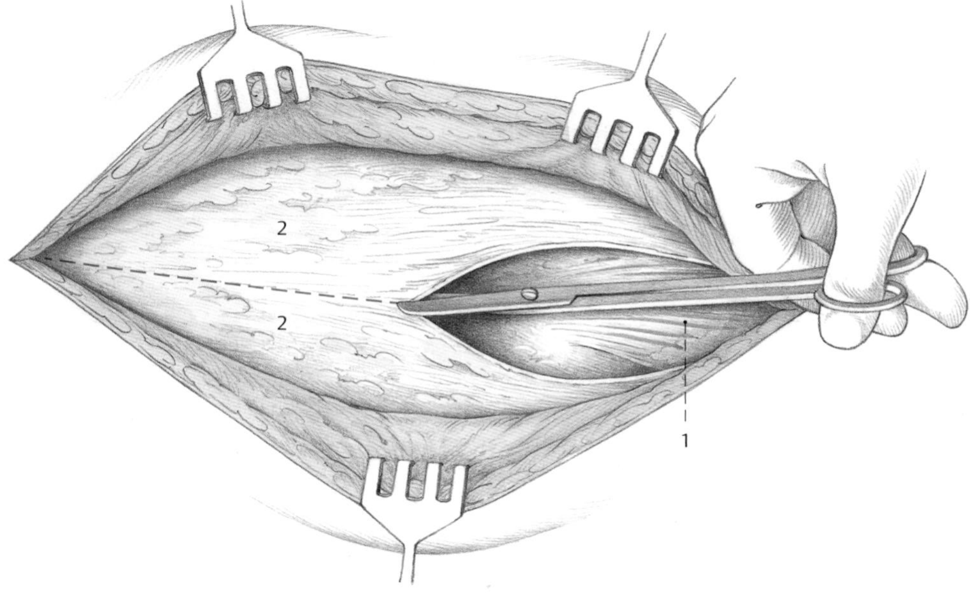

Fig. 9.25 Splitting of fascia lata parallel to the skin incision between the tensor of fascia lata and gluteus maximus.

1 Vastus lateralis
2 Fascia lata (iliotibial tract)

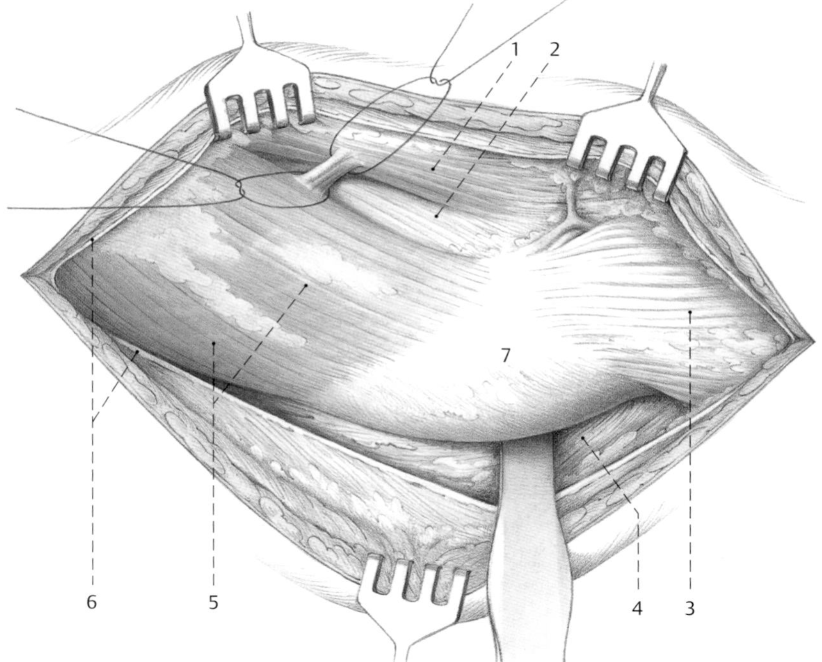

Fig. 9.26 Retraction of fascia lata and dissection between the tensor of fascia lata and gluteus medius. Ligature or electrocoagulation of the vessels regularly found here.

1 Tensor of fascia lata
2 Gluteus minimus
3 Vastus lateralis
4 Gluteus maximus
5 Gluteus medius
6 Fascia lata
7 Greater trochanter

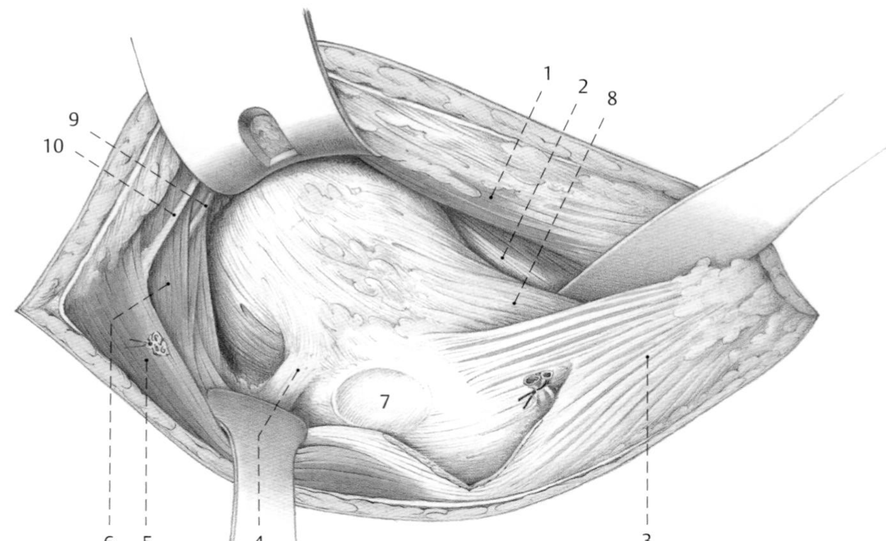

Fig. 9.27 Exposure of the anterior hip joint capsule and placement of Hohmann retractors in the anterior, inferior, and superior positions. Caution: the upper approach is limited by the superior gluteal nerve, which runs transversely.

1 Rectus femoris
2 Iliopsoas
3 Vastus lateralis
4 Piriformis
5 Gluteus medius
6 Gluteus minimus
7 Trochanteric bursa
8 Iliofemoral ligament
9 Superior gluteal vessels
10 Superior gluteal nerve

9.5.3 Exposure of the Hip Joint Capsule

The anterior portion of the hip joint capsule is dissected free of fascia and muscles with a Cobb elevator. Using the elevator, the plane between the head of the rectus femoris muscle and the anterior wall of the acetabulum is exposed, and a wide curved Hohmann elevator is inserted (**Fig. 9.27**). Then the layer between the joint capsule and iliopsoas is dissected, and a pointed Hohmann elevator is placed here. The tendinous insertion of gluteus medius and minimus onto the greater trochanter is incised distally for a short distance until the underlying bursa becomes visible. After dissection of the proximal portions of the capsule with a raspatory, a straight Hohmann elevator can be inserted at this site as well. A T-shaped opening can be made in the hip joint capsule (see **Figs. 9.15** and **9.16**). Dislocation of the femoral head is now possible in adduction and external rotation.

9.5.4 Wound Closure

During wound closure, reinsertion of the detached portions of gluteus medius and minimus is important.

9.5.5 Dangers

(**Figs. 9.28, 9.29, 9.30, 9.31**)

Part of the superior gluteal nerve runs transversely in far proximal location (roughly 5 cm above the tip of the greater trochanter) between gluteus medius and the tensor of fascia lata, which it supplies. The nerve can be damaged by traction or transected at this point, which interferes with the function of the tensor of fascia lata (**Fig. 9.28**).

The position of the posterior Hohmann elevator and its distance from the sciatic nerve are shown in **Figs. 9.29** and **9.30**. Distal placement of the elevator and simultaneous maximal external rotation of the leg can entail damage to the sciatic nerve.

The position of the Hohmann elevator at the anterior border of the acetabulum and its proximity to the neurovascular bundle are shown in **Fig. 9.31**. Excessive pull on the middle, anteriorly placed elevator may cause tensile damage to the femoral nerve, particularly if this elevator is not placed below the muscles but with its tip lying in the muscle. Improper positioning of this elevator can also cause damage to the femoral artery or the deep femoral artery. Too deep a placement of the distal Hohmann elevator or placement in muscle distally entails the risk of injury to the medial circumflex femoral artery.

9.5.6 Note

The free edge of gluteus medius is directly adherent to the tensor of fascia lata, especially proximally, and is firmly joined to this muscle by an intermuscular aponeurosis toward the anterior superior iliac spine. At about the level of the trochanter, the two muscles are again separate. Directly anterior to the greater trochanter, there is an angle between gluteus medius, vastus intermedius, and the tensor of fascia lata, which is filled with loose connective tissue or fat. This region provides a direct approach to the proximal femur and femoral neck region.

Partial division of gluteus medius and minimus from the greater trochanter is recommended to avoid damaging the gluteal muscles by traction on the retractors. If adequate exposure of the hip joint capsule is not possible through this approach, a further incision can be made in the gluteal muscle at the greater trochanter or else, in rare cases, trochanteric osteotomy may be performed (Charnley approach).

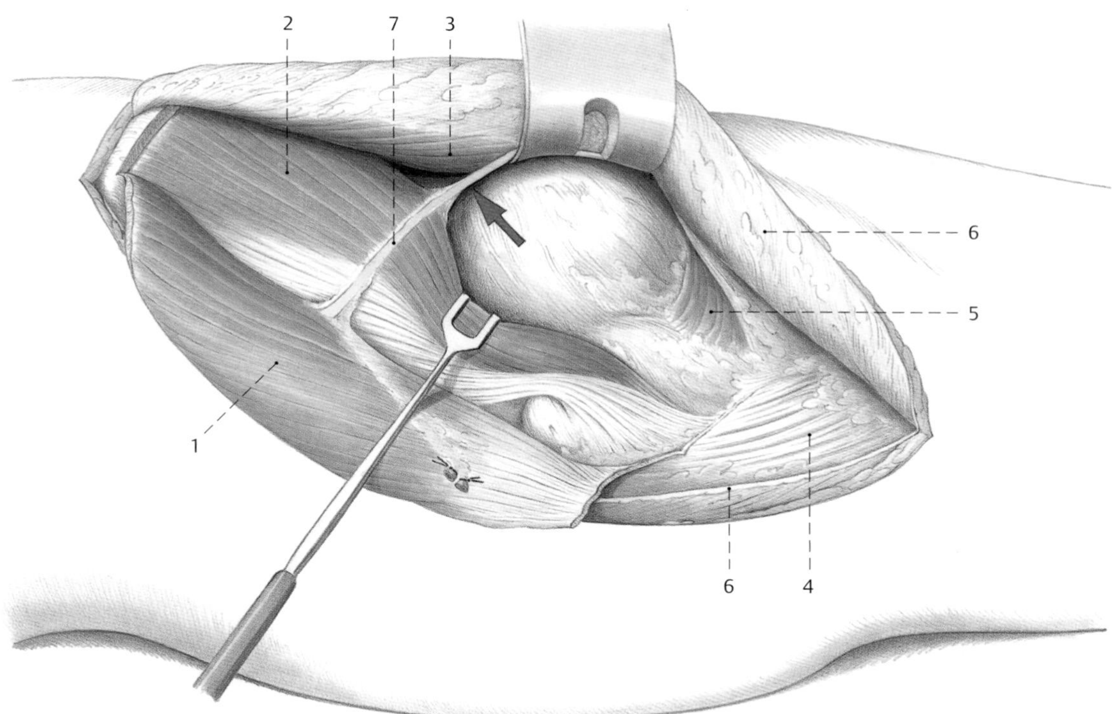

Fig. 9.28 Anatomical site. The gluteus medius has been separated at the iliac crest and the greater trochanter, and retracted to reveal the course of the superior gluteal nerve. The red arrow marks the site where the nerve may be damaged during the operation.

1 Gluteus medius
2 Gluteus minimus
3 Tensor of fascia lata
4 Vastus lateralis
5 Vastus intermedius
6 Fascia lata
7 Superior gluteal nerve

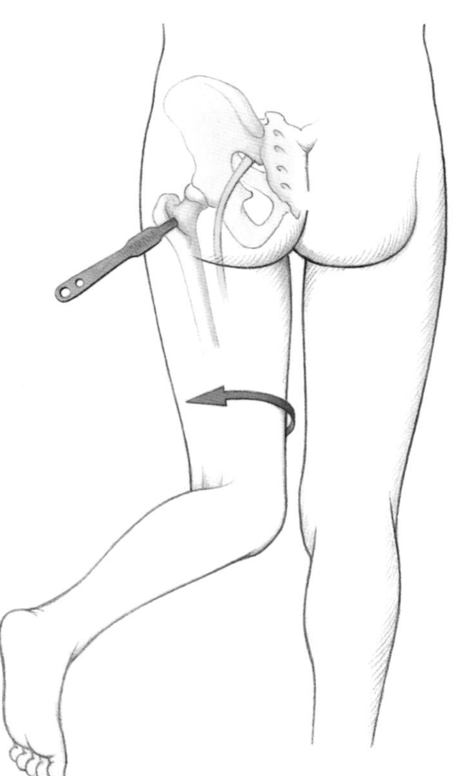

Fig. 9.29 Schematic representation of the position of the posterior Hohmann retractor in relation to the sciatic nerve during internal rotation (relatively great distance).

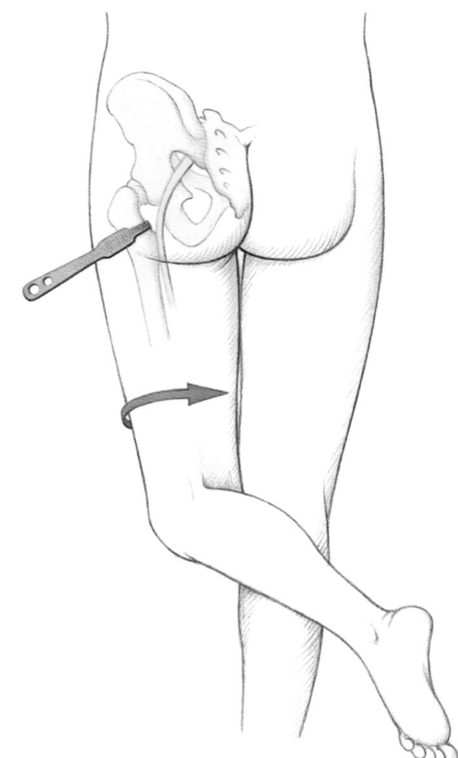

Fig. 9.30 Schematic representation of the position of the posterior Hohmann retractor in relation to the sciatic nerve during external rotation (relatively small distance). The Hohmann retractor comes close to the nerve and endangers it due to pressure between the buttock and the operating table.

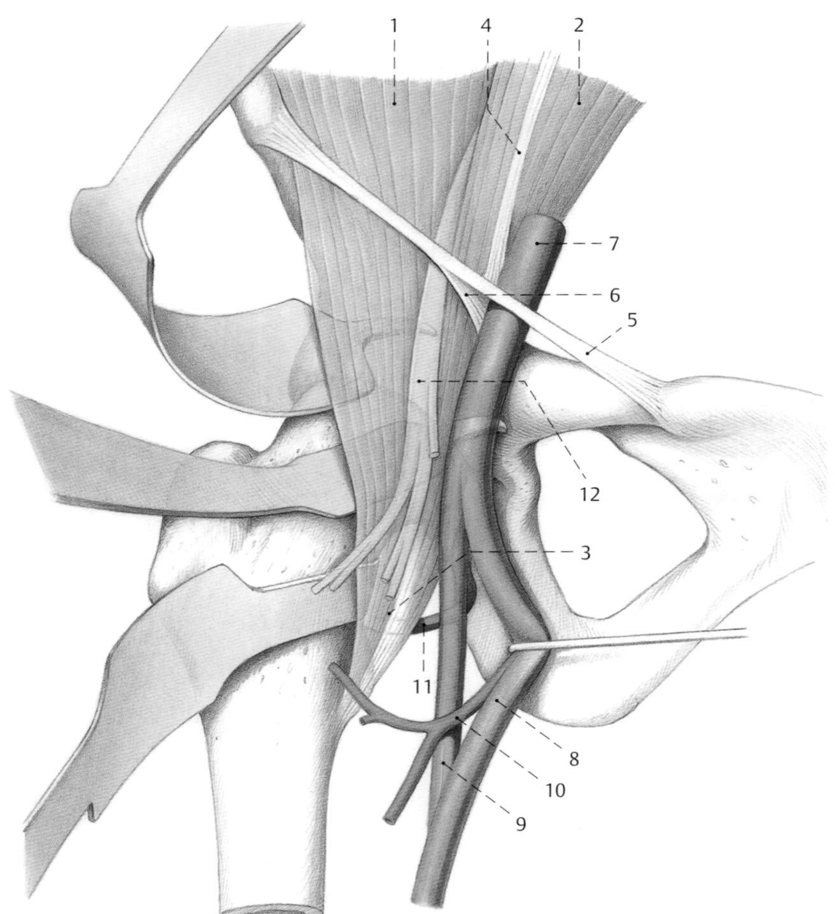

Fig. 9.31 Position of the two anterior and one distal Hohmann retractors in an anterolateral exposure of the hip joint capsule. Caution: there is the possibility of injury to the femoral nerve due to overextension, and to both the femoral artery and the deep femoral artery, which lie directly above the tip of the middle Hohmann retractor. If the distal Hohmann retractor is placed too deeply, the medial circumflex femoral artery may be injured.

1 Iliacus
2 Psoas major
3 Iliopsoas
4 Psoas minor
5 Inguinal ligament
6 Iliopectineal arch
7 External iliac artery
8 Femoral artery
9 Deep femoral artery
10 Lateral circumflex femoral artery
11 Medial circumflex femoral artery
12 Femoral nerve

Exposure of the hip joint capsule by a retractor at the anterior border of the acetabulum medial to rectus femoris is facilitated by division of the reflected head of the origin of rectus femoris (see **Fig. 9.27**).

9.6 Minimally Invasive Anterolateral Approach to the Hip Joint

A. Roth

9.6.1 Principal Indications

- Total joint replacement
- Hemiarthroplasty
- Labrum surgery
- Removal of cam osteophyte
- Femoral neck fractures
- Juvenile slipped femoral epiphysis
- Synovectomy
- Femoral neck osteotomies

9.6.2 Positioning and Incision

The patient is placed in the supine position. With the leg extended, the innominate tubercle is palpated over the greater trochanter. It is usually at the level of the lower border of the acetabulum. The skin incision begins 3 cm anterior and 4–5 cm proximal to the innominate tubercle, and runs at an acute angle of 10–15° from proximal to distal. The incision is between 6 and 10 cm long (**Fig. 9.32**).

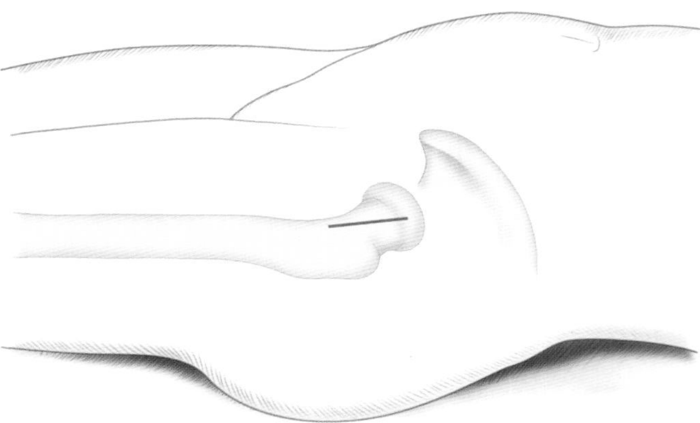

Fig. 9.32 Minimally invasive anterolateral approach. Positioning and incision (left side).

After dividing the subcutaneous tissue parallel to the skin incision, the junction between the iliotibial tract and the tensor of fascia lata comes into view. Roughly 1 cm posterior to this junction, the iliotibial tract is incised parallel to the skin incision. A small vessel is regularly found 1–2 cm proximal to the distal end of the wound, which perforates the iliotibial tract at the junction with the tensor of fascia lata and indicates the correct level of the incision.

9.6.3 Exposure of the Hip Joint Capsule

After transection of the iliotibial tract, a fat pad is seen in front of gluteus medius in the distal part of the approach; this fills the space between gluteus medius and the joint capsule. It is spread with forceps transversely to the direction of the incision. A small vascular bundle is regularly found in about the middle of the approach, which passes through this fat pad from gluteus medius to the tensor of fascia lata and must be coagulated, or ligated and divided (**Fig. 9.33**). The lateral margin of the joint capsule is dissected with a Cobb elevator. The lateral circumflex artery is often visible here. A narrow curved Hohmann retractor is placed at the upper medial boundary of the femoral neck, and a second narrow curved retractor is placed at the upper lateral boundary. The anterior soft tissues are protected by a Langenbeck retractor. Alternatively, a third curved Hohmann retractor can be placed anteriorly at the immediate anterior margin of the acetabulum (**Fig. 9.34**). A Hohmann retractor can optionally be placed at the lower boundary of the femoral neck.

The leg is abducted slightly to allow exposure of the gluteal muscles at the greater trochanter with as little tension as possible. The remaining intact parts of the fat pad described above are then incised as far as the insertion of the gluteal muscles on the greater trochanter.

An L-shaped (right) or reverse L-shaped (left) incision is then made in the capsule. The incision extends from the superior acetabular margin to the lateral border of the femoral neck and then passes distally. The anterior attachment of the capsule is then divided completely from the femur (**Fig. 9.35**).

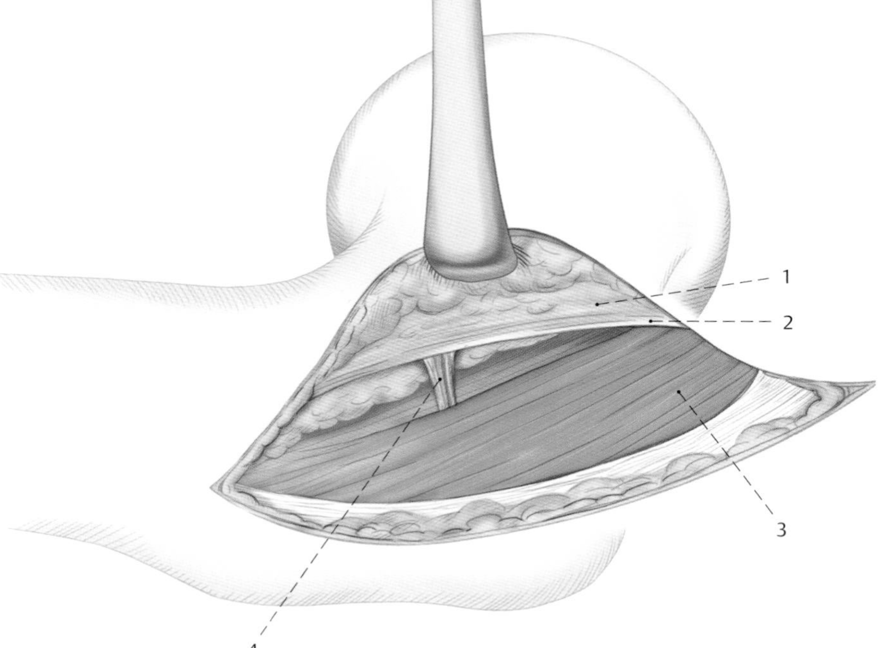

Fig. 9.33 Splitting of fascia lata approximately 1 cm posterior to the tensor of fascia lata, parallel to the line of the muscle.

1 Tensor of fascia lata
2 Fascia lata (iliotibial tract)
3 Gluteus medius
4 Vascular bundle regularly running between the gluteus medius and tensor of fascia lata in the middle of the approach

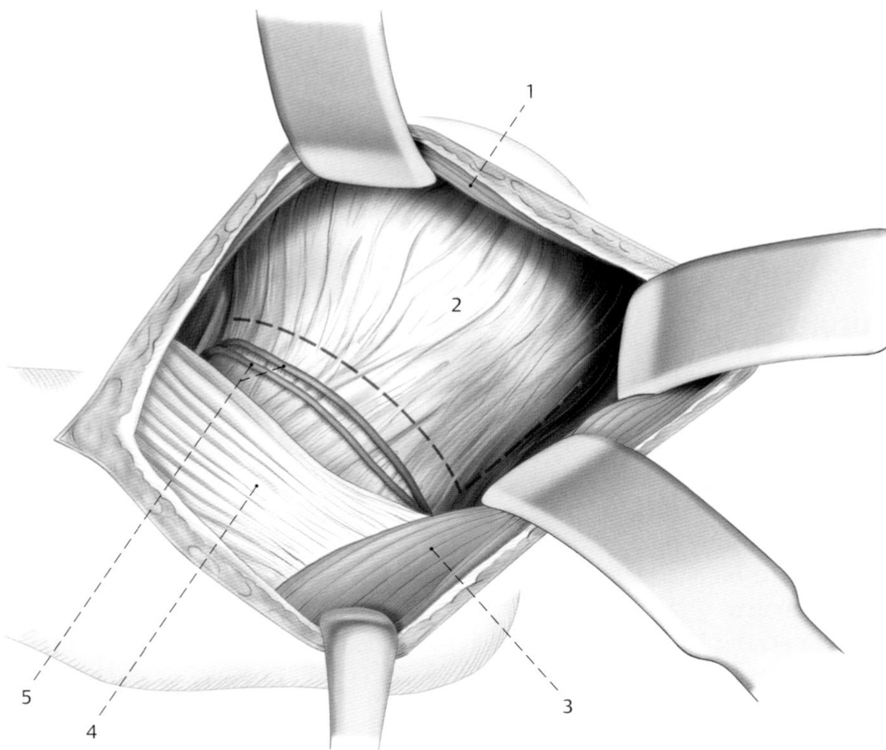

Fig. 9.34 Exposure of the lateral and superior parts of the hip joint capsule. Placement of Hohmann retractors in the anterior and superior positions. This allows cautious retraction of the tensor of fascia lata and gluteus medius. Ligature or electrocoagulation of the small vessels that are regularly found here crossing the Watson-Jones interval is carried out.

1 Tensor of fascia lata
2 Hip joint capsule
3 Gluteus medius
4 Vastus lateralis
5 Lateral circumflex artery and vein

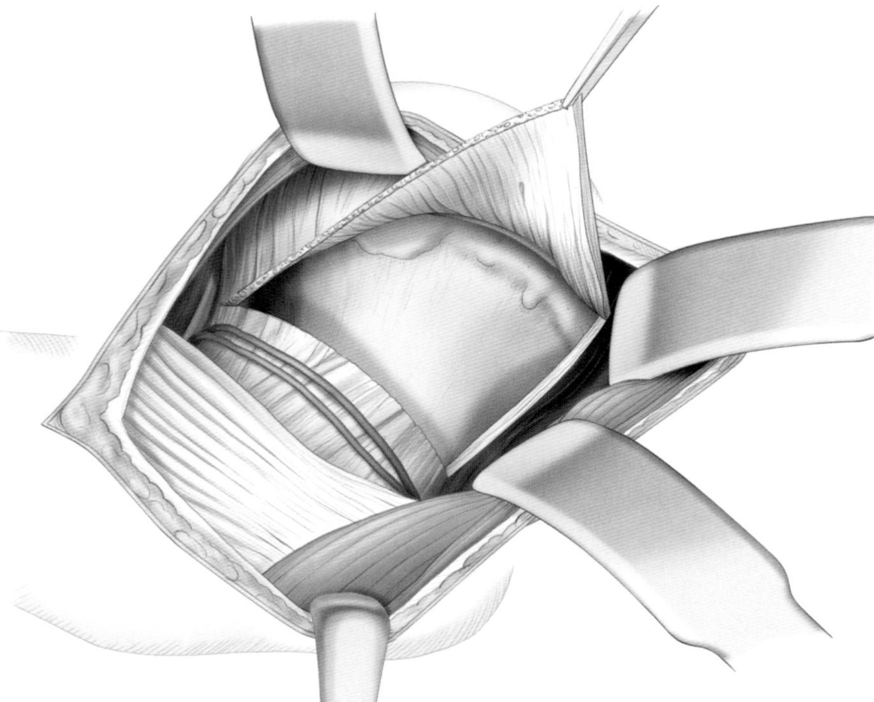

Fig. 9.35 L-shaped incision of the hip joint capsule.

The leg is then flexed by approximately 20°, which relaxes the anterior capsule. The anterior Hohmann retractor is then placed on the anterior margin of the acetabulum below the anterior capsule. By elevating it, any more distal adhesions between the capsule and femoral calcar are exposed.

If required for exposure, the capsule can now be mobilized under vision with a Cobb elevator as far distally as possible toward the lesser trochanter (**Fig. 9.36**).

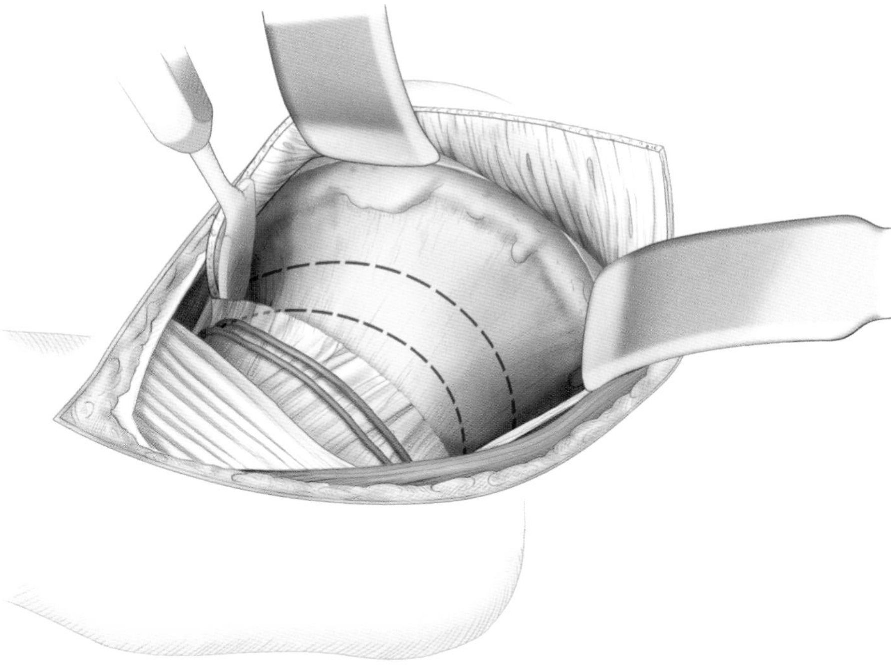

Fig. 9.36 Insertion of a Hohmann retractor on the anterior rim of the acetabulum. The leg is flexed approximately 20°. Subperiosteal dissection of the capsule distally as far as the lesser trochanter with a Cobb elevator. Location of a double osteotomy if removal of the femoral head is planned.

9.6.4 Anatomical Site

With this approach, several small vessels are potentially encountered, which may be protected but may have to be ligated or coagulated. This is essential to reduce the risk of secondary hemorrhage. The following are the involved vessels:

- Branches of the superior gluteal artery and vein: emerge at the anterior border of gluteus medius, cross the Watson-Jones interval, and pass to the tensor of fascia lata.
- Lateral circumflex artery: comes from below and runs anteriorly on the lateral femoral neck.
- Medial circumflex femoral artery: runs over the inferior joint capsule and then turns in a cranial direction, passing posteriorly along the lateral femoral neck. Anastomoses with the lateral circumflex artery cranial to the lateral femoral neck.
- Ascending branch of the lateral circumflex artery: runs in an anterolateral direction in the proximal part of vastus lateralis.
- Deep femoral artery: lies distal to the inferior joint margin.
- Superficial circumflex iliac artery: at the upper border of the acetabulum.
- Inferior branch of the superior gluteal artery: approximately 3 cm above the tip of the greater trochanter in the muscle.

9.6.5 Wound Closure

If the capsule is preserved, the cranial division can be sutured closed. The fascia is closed by interrupted absorbable sutures, sparing the tensor of fascia lata.

9.6.6 Dangers

There may be excessive pressure from the anterior retractor on the tensor of fascia lata with damage to the muscle. The superior gluteal nerve may be damaged by excessive retraction.

Superficial damage of the gluteal muscles may be caused by excessive retraction or the use of Hohmann retractors with relatively sharp edges.

9.6.7 Note

If arthroplasty is planned, the trochanter is positioned approximately 5 cm proximal to the break in the operating table where the distal parts of the table can be lowered with both legs. In cases of dysplasia or coxa vara, an incision starting more distal to the innominate tubercle may be necessary. This distance should be determined on X-ray.

To avoid damage to the gluteal muscles and tensor of fascia lata, especially in a very muscular or large-boned patient, the approach can be extended in the proximal and distal directions. This can also be combined with division of the distal parts of gluteus medius and gluteus minimus, as in the classic anterolateral approach. The capsule can also be resected after an inverted T-shaped incision. When this approach is used for hip arthroplasty, a double osteotomy of the femoral neck is recommended (**Fig. 9.37**). The resulting bone fragment and the rest of the femoral head can be removed successively. Dislocation of the hip is obsolete as the gluteal muscles are overstretched by this.

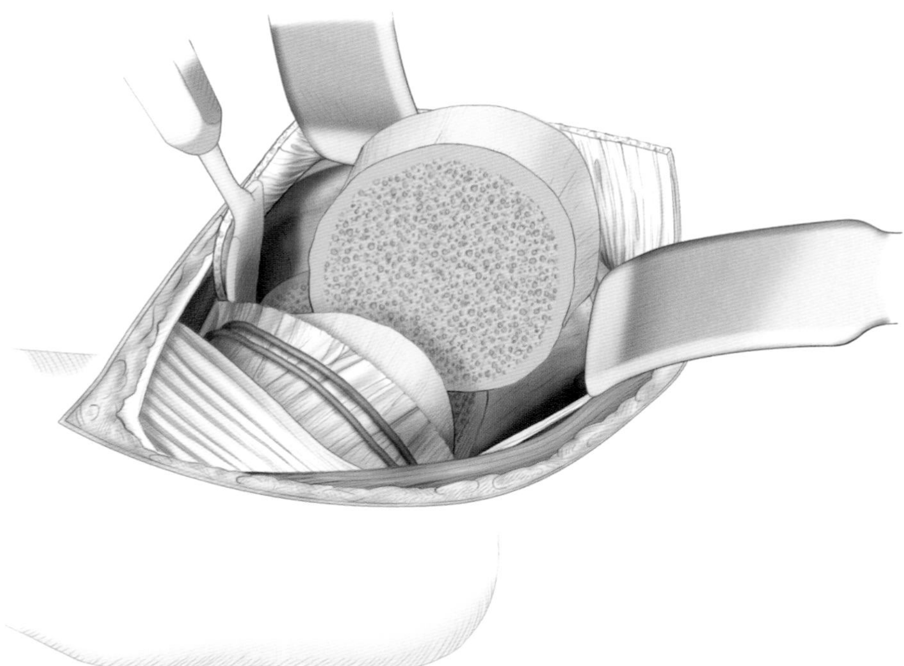

Fig. 9.37 Double osteotomy of the femoral neck and removal of a bone fragment when arthroplasty is planned. The remainder of the femoral head can then be readily extracted.

9.7 Anterior Approach to the Hip Joint

R. Bauer, F. Kerschbaumer, S. Poisel

9.7.1 Principal Indications

- Open reduction of congenital hip joint dislocation
- Pelvic osteotomies
- Total joint replacement
- Iliac fractures
- Tumors
- Osteomyelitis
- Arthrodesis

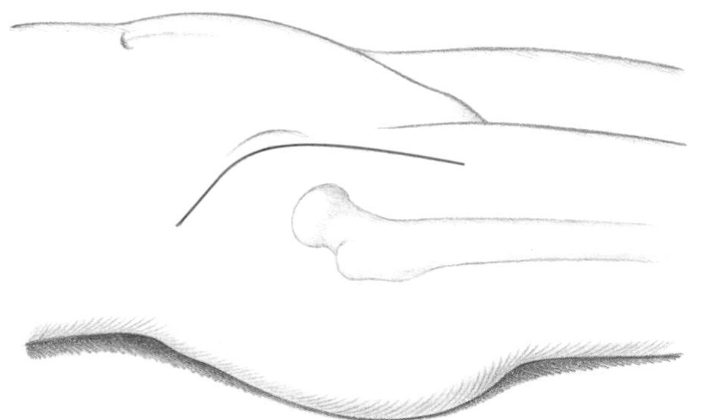

Fig. 9.38 Anterior approach to hip joint. Positioning and incision (right leg).

9.7.2 Positioning and Incision

The patient is placed in the supine position with the leg draped so as to allow free movement. The skin incision begins at the highest point of the iliac crest (iliac tubercle) and continues laterally to it to the anterior superior iliac spine. From here, it runs in a straight line distally for 15 cm (**Fig. 9.38**). It should be noted that the skin incision must be lateral to the iliac crest so that troublesome adhesions between the skin and the iliac crest may be avoided. After division of the skin and subcutaneous tissue, the fascia is incised in a straight line over the tensor of fascia lata (**Fig. 9.39**). This procedure spares the lateral femoral cutaneous nerve, which pierces the fascia between the tensor of fascia lata on one hand, and the sartorius muscle on the other (**Fig. 9.40**). The layer between the tensor of fascia lata and the sartorius is now dissected, both muscles being retracted laterally. Subsequently, the tensor of fascia lata and gluteus minimus and gluteus medius are detached from the ilium in one layer.

9.7.3 Exposure of the Hip Joint Capsule

If possible, the tensor of fascia lata muscle and the gluteal muscles should be detached from the iliac crest subperiosteally. In children, the cartilaginous iliac crest is first split for this purpose. The periosteum adhering to it can easily be stripped off the iliac crest with a raspatory. In adults, this dissection is more difficult and requires careful hemostasis. The gluteal surface may be exposed as far as the greater sciatic foramen. Then a Hohmann elevator is inserted, with which the gluteal muscles can be retracted. A large curved Hohmann elevator may be placed between the anterior portions of the capsule and the origin of rectus femoris (**Fig. 9.41**). A T-shaped opening is made in the hip joint capsule. For wide exposure of

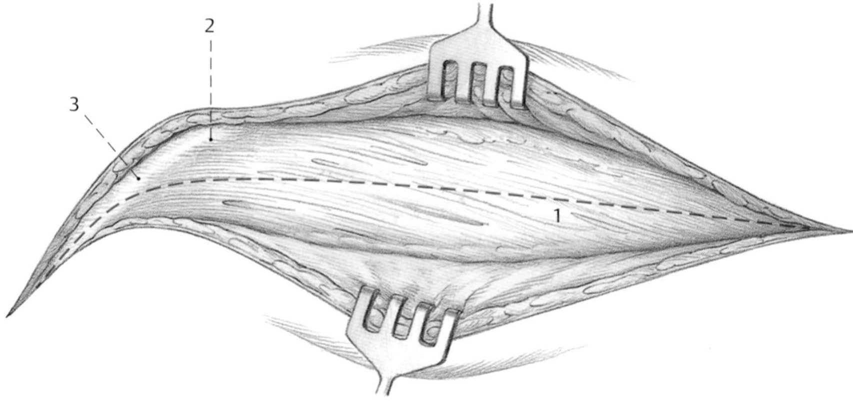

Fig. 9.39 Splitting of fascia parallel to the skin incision over the tensor of fascia lata.

1 Fascia lata
2 Anterior superior iliac spine
3 Iliac crest

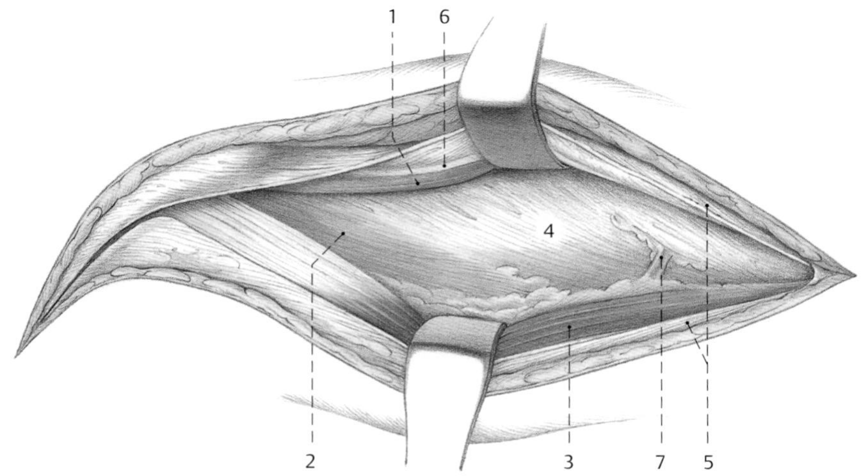

Fig. 9.40 Blunt dissection between sartorius and the tensor of fascia lata as far as the fascia covering rectus femoris. Exposure of branches of the lateral circumflex femoral artery.

1 Sartorius
2 Gluteus minimus
3 Tensor of fascia lata
4 Rectus femoris
5 Fascia lata
6 Lateral femoral cutaneous nerve
7 Lateral circumflex femoral artery, ascending branch

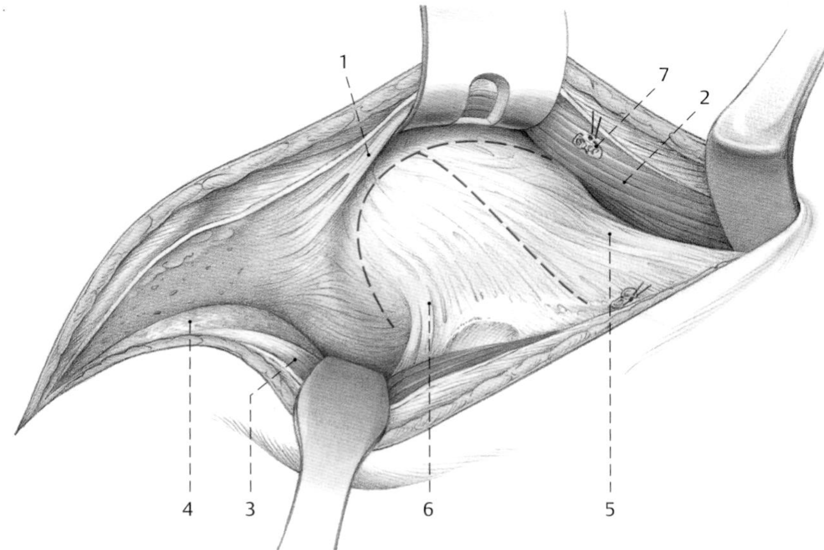

Fig. 9.41 Detachment of the tensor of fascia lata and gluteal muscles from the iliac crest, and subperiosteal dissection, if necessary, as far as the sciatic foramen. Exposure of the hip joint capsule and insertion of Hohmann elevators. A T-shaped incision is made in the hip joint capsule. Ligation and transection of the ascending branch of the lateral circumflex femoral artery.

1 Rectus femoris, reflected head
2 Rectus femoris
3 Tensor of fascia lata
4 Gluteus minimus
5 Iliofemoral ligament, medial portion
6 Iliofemoral ligament, lateral portion
7 Lateral circumflex femoral artery, ascending branch

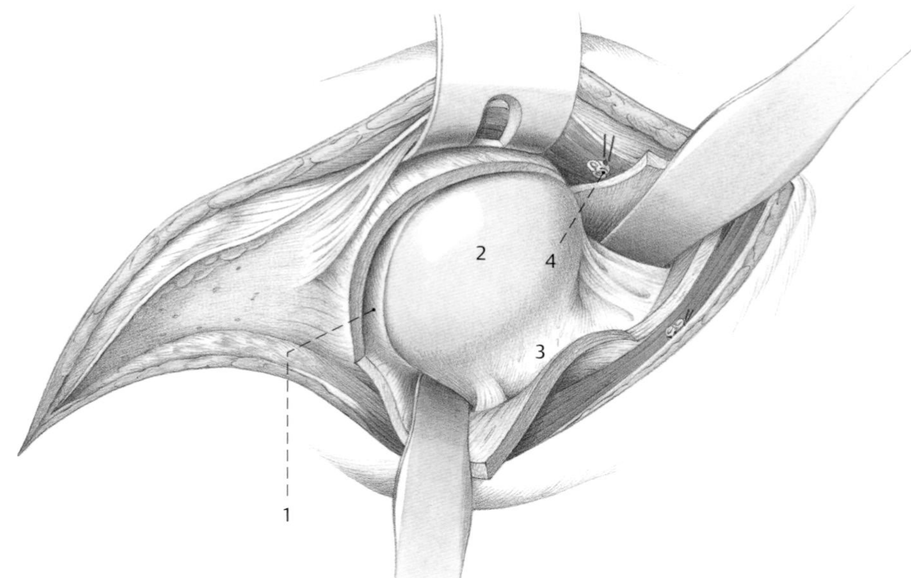

Fig. 9.42 Operative site after opening the hip joint capsule. Hohmann elevators were inserted behind the neck of the femur. The leg was adducted and externally rotated.

1 Acetabular labrum
2 Head of femur
3 Neck of femur
4 Lateral circumflex femoral artery, ascending branch

the hip joint capsule, notably in a distal direction, ligation and transection of the ascending branch of the lateral circumflex femoral artery is required. Following incision of the hip joint capsule, broad Hohmann elevators may be inserted behind the neck of the femur (**Fig. 9.42**). The femoral head can be dislocated by flexion, adduction, and external rotation of the leg.

9.7.4 Wound Closure

Following suture of the hip joint capsule, the gluteal muscles and the tensor of fascia lata are reattached to the iliac crest with interrupted sutures. Then the fascia over the tensor of fascia lata has to be closed.

9.7.5 Note

The anterior approach has been described by Smith-Petersen, Hueter, Callahan, Fahey and others. In certain operations, such as pelvic osteotomy according to Chiari for example, this approach has to be supplemented by detachment of sartorius and iliacus from the anterior superior iliac spine and the iliac fossa, respectively. This is best done by detaching these groups of muscles with a flake of the iliac crest.

Salter used for his osteotomy a skin incision that runs in a nearly straight line from the iliac crest to the groin.

Tönnis recommended an inguinal incision as the approach for the operative treatment of congenital hip joint dislocation.

9.8 Anterior Minimally Invasive Approach

M. C. Michel

9.8.1 Principal Indications

- Total joint replacement
- Hemiarthroplasty
- Femoroacetabular impingement
- Labrum surgery
- Juvenile slipped femoral epiphysis
- Synovectomy
- Femoral neck osteotomy
- Hip revision as a micro-hip approach

9.8.2 Positioning and Incision

The patient is placed in the lateral decubitus position. As the surgeon will stand in front of the patient, the hip comes as close as possible to the edge. The posterior leg plate is removed from the table so that the leg can be hyperextended and externally rotated for better access to the shaft. The pelvis is supported especially on the posterior aspect so that it does not tilt backward (**Fig. 9.43**).

The skin incision begins at the anterior border of the greater trochanter and is directed toward the anterior superior iliac spine (**Fig. 9.44**). The subcutaneous tissue is divided in the same direction down to the fascia of the tensor of fascia lata (**Fig. 9.45**). The junction with the iliotibial tract is exposed. The vessels that always cross the junction can be used as landmarks. In any case, the iliotibial tract is obviously tougher and whiter than the more delicate and reddish fascia of the tensor of fascia lata.

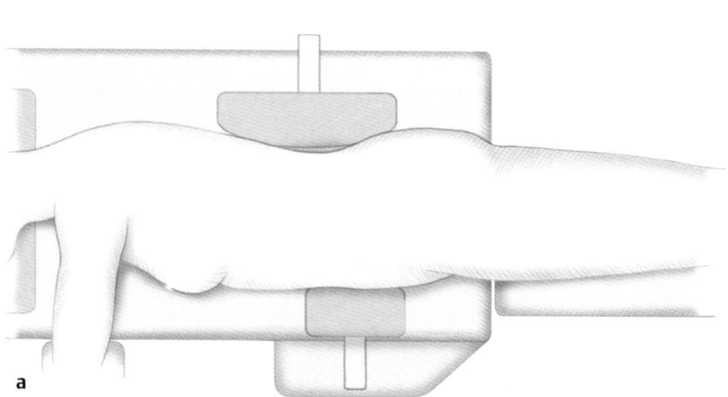

Fig. 9.43 Positioning and incision.

a Lateral position.
b Incision: dashed line = usual incision;
dotted line = micro-hip plus extension.

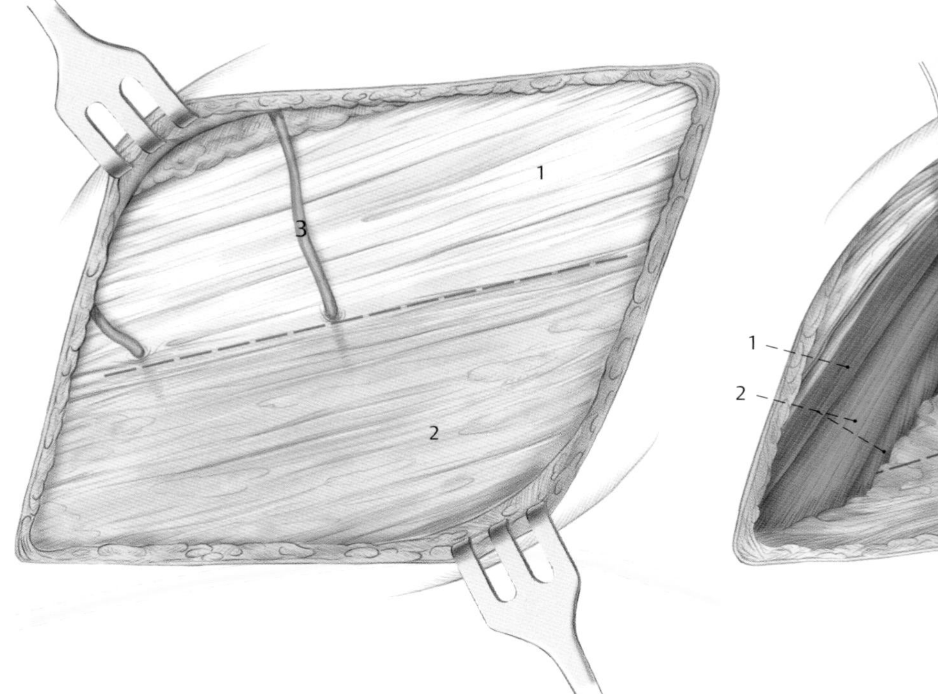

Fig. 9.44 Incision at the junction of the fascia of the tensor of fascia lata and the iliotibial tract.

1 Iliotibial tract
2 Fascia of tensor of fascia lata
3 Vessels crossing the junction

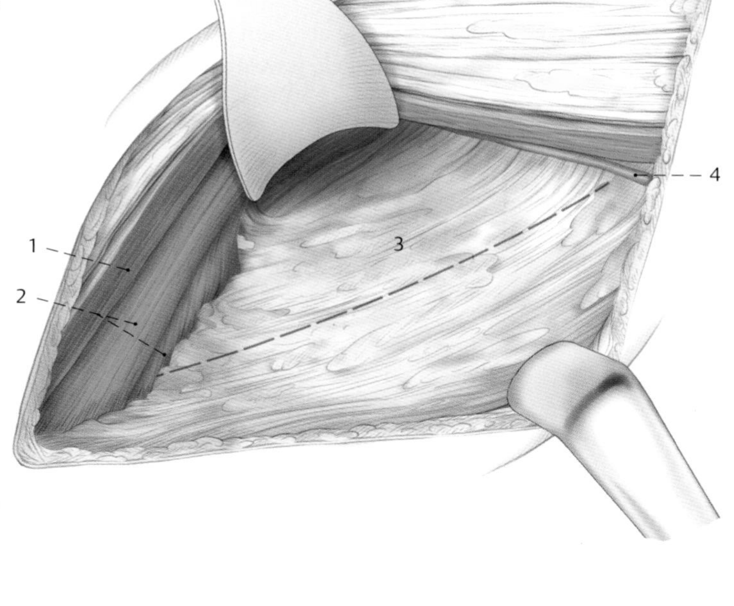

Fig. 9.45 View of the deep anterior fascia.

1 Tensor of fascia lata
2 Gluteus minimus and medius
3 Deep fascia
4 Ascending branch of the lateral circumflex artery

The fascia is split exactly at the junction with the iliotibial tract (but may also be moved 2 mm into the tract to leave a stronger structure for wound closure), and it always runs parallel to the iliotibial tract.

The fascia of the tensor of fascia lata is then lifted with forceps so that the muscle can be dissected and retracted from the inside of the fascia. This technique results in an extremely small risk of injuring the lateral cutaneous nerve of the thigh as this is always outside the fascia.

A blunt Hohmann retractor (capsule retractor) is then advanced over the femoral neck, as close as possible to the greater trochanter. This can be used to elevate the tensor of fascia lata together with gluteus medius and gluteus minimus (**Fig. 9.45**).

At the medial border of the femoral neck, the reflected head of rectus femoris is now palpated.

The fascia is incised laterally, from cranial to caudal. The ascending branch of the lateral circumflex artery is found at the caudal junction. It passes through the fascia to the lower border of the tensor of fascia lata, and can be exposed at this site and ligated.

The reflected head of rectus femoris is then retracted bluntly in a medial direction together with the yellow fat pad, and is held there with a blunt Hohmann retractor (**Fig. 9.46**).

A T-shaped incision is now made in the capsule, lateral to the reflected head of rectus femoris. It runs parallel to the capsule fibers and therefore spares the insertion of the reflected head, but passes through the accessory insertion. Caudally, the capsule is divided in a T-shape from within outward at the intertrochanteric line to spare the main branch of the lateral circumflex artery.

The two blunt Hohmann retractors are then placed in the joint capsule, directly on the femoral neck, providing a clear view of the joint. In addition, the labrum is split cranially, which facilitates dislocation of the head (**Fig. 9.47**).

Accurate exposure of the trochanteric fossa and intertrochanteric line is important as otherwise the osteotomy level cannot be determined.

A good overview should be obtained as this allows cam impingement to be corrected by osteochondroplasty. Even anterior reinsertion of the labrum is readily possible.

Following osteotomy, the femoral neck can be tilted upward. Insertion of a corkscrew allows controlled dislocation, giving a clear view of the acetabulum, including the transverse ligament. In addition, a double-curved Hohmann retractor can be inserted at the lateral insertion, allowing the space to be extended (**Fig. 9.48**).

To expose the femur, the leg is externally rotated, a blunt Hohmann retractor is placed on the outside of the joint capsule at the greater trochanter, and the leg is hyperextended into the free space posterior to the operating table.

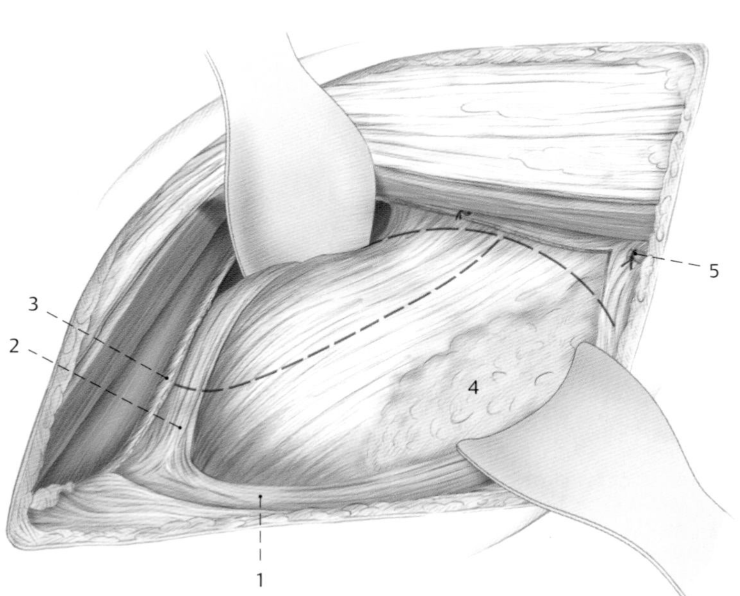

Fig. 9.46 View of the joint capsule after splitting the deep fascia.

1 Reflected head of rectus femoris
2 Accessory fibers of the reflected head of rectus femoris
3 Split superficial fascia
4 Yellow fat pad
5 Ligated ascending branch of the lateral circumflex artery

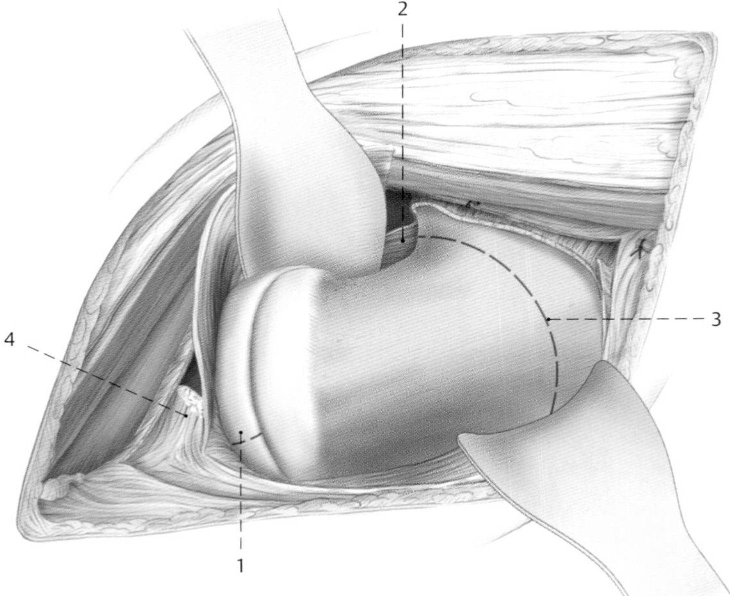

Fig. 9.47 Overview after opening the joint capsule.

1 Split acetabular labrum
2 Trochanteric fossa
3 Osteotomy (depending on implant)
4 Accessory fibers of the reflected head (these are located further caudally = on the right, and are therefore split)

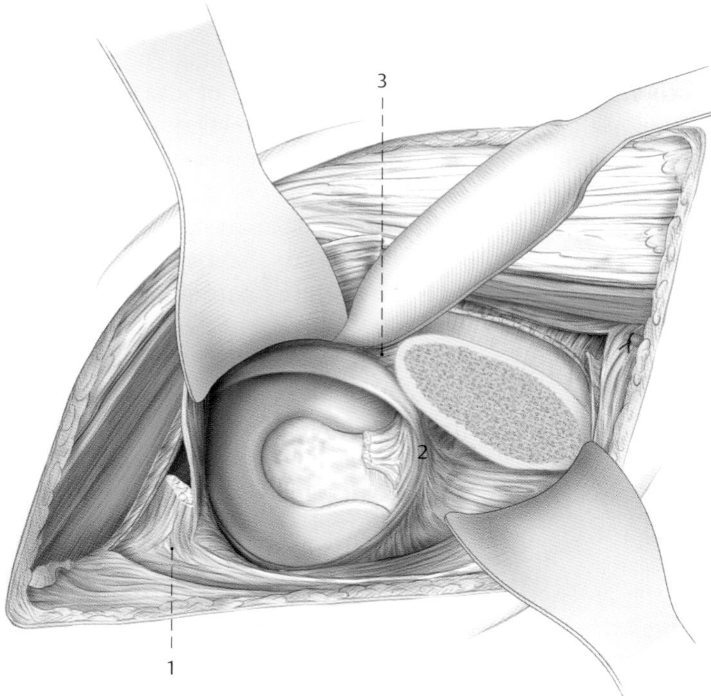

Fig. 9.48 Acetabulum.

1 Reflected head of rectus femoris
2 Transverse acetabular ligament
3 Trochanteric fossa

9.8.3 Wound Closure

Wound closure is limited to closure of the capsule with a few interrupted sutures, and the fascia is closed with a continuous suture.

9.8.4 Dangers

The sensory lateral cutaneous nerve of the thigh runs subcutaneously over the fascia. If dissection is performed inside the fascia, the nerve is not endangered.

Figures 9.45, **9.46**, and **9.47** illustrate the course of the ascending branch of the lateral circumflex artery. This should be ligated or at least coagulated. The lateral circumflex artery runs on the medial border of the intertrochanteric line from posteriorly, and the common trunk may be found further posteriorly. If the medial end of the incision is continued further distally, the medial circumflex femoral artery must be exposed and ligated. Bleeding from these vessels can be fatal.

9.8.5 Note

Although the micro-hip technique is an extremely nontraumatic method, the incision should not be too short, to allow clear visualization at all times. The approach can be readily extended to a micro-hip-plus approach. In this case, the incision is extended longitudinally, and the dangers described above should be noted.

Proximally, the tensor of fascia lata can best be divided completely with a bone squame, allowing even major reconstructions of the acetabulum to be performed. Conversion to an iliofemoral approach is also possible. Distal extension is recommended in revision surgery, identifying and ligating the circumflex artery. This can therefore also be converted to a lateral approach to the femur, which is recommended for extensive femoral fractures. Naturally, the iliotibial tract is then divided not transversely but according to the lateral approach. The extensions for the micro-hip-plus approach are also recommended for revision operations if the surgeon is experienced.

9.9 Arthroscopic Approaches to the Hip Joint

M. Dienst

9.9.1 Principal Indications

- Femoroacetabular impingement
- Early osteoarthritis
- Synovial diseases
- Lesions of the hyaline joint cartilage, acetabular labrum, and ligament of the head of the femur
- Loose bodies in the joint

9.9.2 Positioning and Portals

The patient is placed in the supine position on an extension table. Attaching the extension rails allows switching between stable traction for arthroscopy of the central joint compartment (**Fig. 9.49**) and arthroscopy of the peripheral compartment without traction and with the hip flexed, rotated, and abducted (**Fig. 9.50**). The hip is draped, and a draped image converter is positioned over the operation area with posteroanterior beam path.

The arthroscopic approach to the hip is via anterior, anterolateral, lateral, and posterolateral portals, with at least two portals placed for each compartment. The entry sites, direction, and number of portals vary depending on the indication.

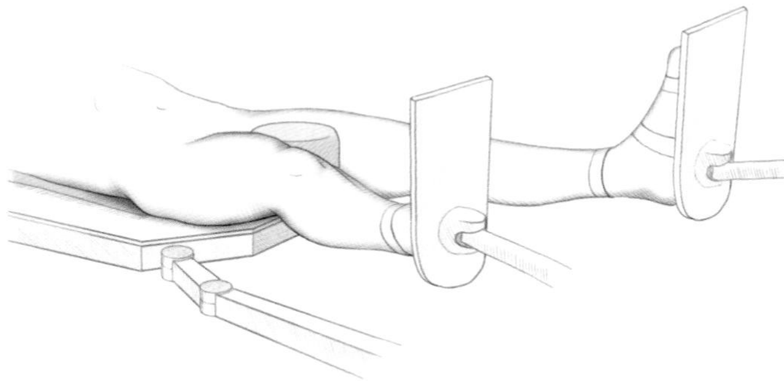

Fig. 9.49 Supine position on an extension table for arthroscopy of the central compartment using traction.

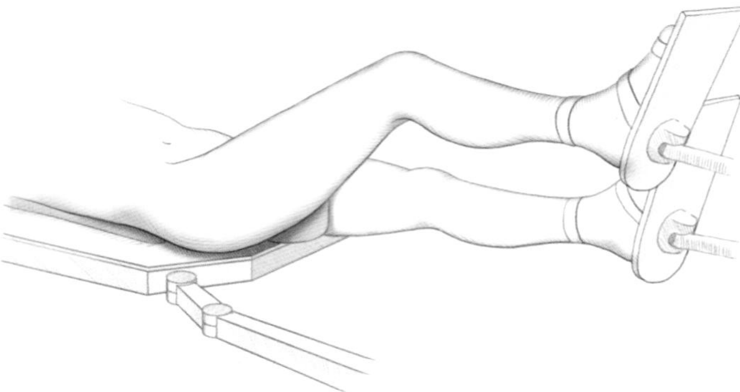

Fig. 9.50 Supine position on an extension table for arthroscopy of the peripheral compartment without traction. By pushing in the table's extension rails, flexing the knee, and opening the locking mechanism on the rail and foot piece, the hip can be flexed, abducted, and rotated.

The portals for the peripheral compartment (**Fig. 9.51**) are placed without traction and with the hip flexed by 10–20°. The proximal anterolateral portal is placed first. The skin incision is on a line joining the anterior superior iliac spine and the tip of the greater trochanter, at the junction of the proximal and middle thirds. The puncture needle is inserted under fluoroscopic control vertical to the axis of the femoral neck and at an angle of approximately 30° in an inferior and approximately 20° in a posterior direction. As it approaches the joint, the needle perforates the posterior part of the tensor of fascia lata and the joint capsule at the anterolateral junction of the femoral head and neck. After distending the joint with approximately 20 mL of fluid, positive backflow confirms a correct intra-articular position. A nitinol wire is advanced as far as the medial capsule. The arthroscope shaft is then inserted through a trocar, and a 70° wide-angle optic is introduced.

For the anterior portal to the peripheral compartment, the arthroscope is adjusted to view the anterior joint capsule above the proximal anterolateral portal, directly cranial to the annular ligament. The skin is incised approximately 4–6 cm distal to the anterior superior iliac spine and 1–2 cm lateral to the vertical line connecting the spine to the upper pole of the patella. The puncture needle is inserted in the sagittal plane almost vertically in posterior direction and inclined approximately 20–30° medially in the horizontal plane. As it passes to the joint, the portal perforates the anterior part of the tensor of fascia lata and the lateral part of rectus femoris before piercing the anterior joint capsule directly cranial to the annular ligament.

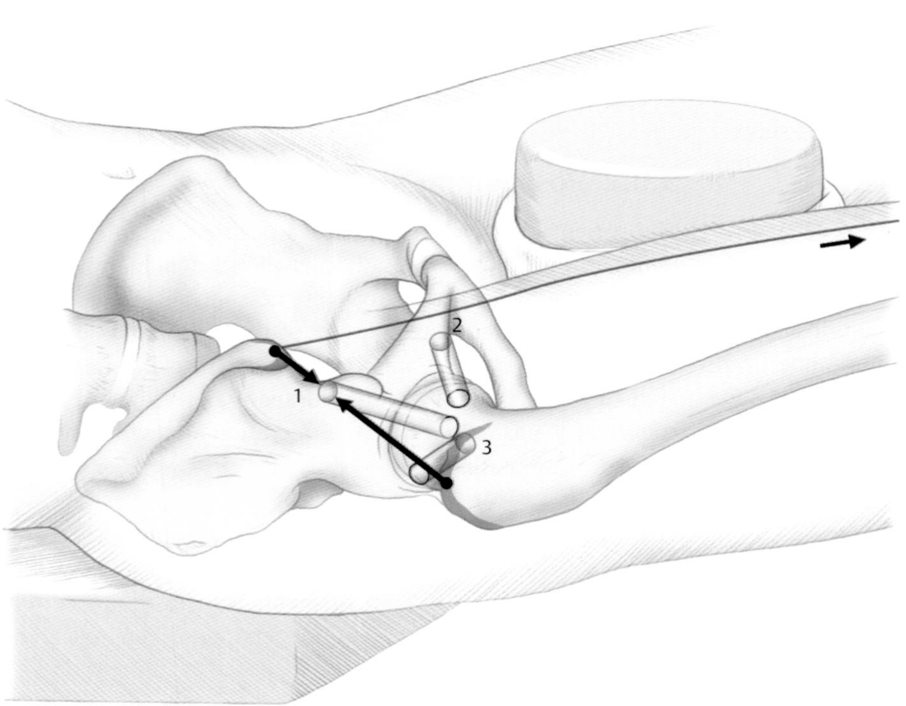

Fig. 9.51 Portals to the peripheral compartment (red circles: skin; black circles: capsule perforation.

1 Proximal anterolateral
2 Anterior
3 Anterolateral

The medial, anterior, and anterolateral peripheral joint cavity can be viewed and instrumented through the proximal anterolateral and anterior portals. For arthroscopy of the posterolateral and posterior parts of the peripheral compartment, an anterolateral portal is created. The skin incision is at the same level as the anterior portal, at the anterior border of the greater trochanter. The metal cannula is directed toward the lateral junction of the femoral head and neck under arthroscopic control with the 70° optic through the proximal anterolateral portal. The capsule is perforated at an approximately 12 o'clock position at the level of the annular ligament.

Placement of the portal for the central compartment is controlled arthroscopically from the periphery to reduce the risk of iatrogenic injury to the acetabular labrum and femoral head cartilage (**Fig. 9.52**). The 70° optic, introduced through the proximal anterolateral portal, is withdrawn as far as possible to the lateral joint capsule, the hip joint is distracted in extension, and the blunt instruments in the anterior and anterolateral portals are advanced between the acetabular labrum and femoral head cartilage into the central compartment. If the joint capsule is tense and the soft tissues are bulky, it may be necessary to create new portals through the existing skin incisions.

To create the anterior portal to the central compartment, the puncture needle is inclined approximately 30° in medial direction and 30° cranially. As it advances toward the joint, the portal perforates the proximal muscle bellies of sartorius and rectus femoris, and parts of the tensor of fascia lata in the case of a lateralized entry site. The capsule is perforated ideally at the often visible junction between the ilium and pubis. To create the anterolateral portal, the puncture needle is inclined approximately 10–20° in a cranial and 20–30° in a posterior direction. En route to the joint, the needle perforates the anterior parts of gluteus medius and also the posterior parts of the tensor of fascia lata if placed more anteriorly. The entry site at the level of the joint capsule is at the 12 o'clock position. The arthroscope shaft introduced through the proximal anterolateral portal is either left anterior to the femoral neck as an outflow cannula or is replaced by a guidewire. The arthroscope is inserted into the central compartment through the anterolateral portal.

The posterolateral and distal anterolateral portals are frequently used accessory approaches. The posteromedial parts of the central compartment, including the caudal parts of the acetabular fossa, are reached through the posterolateral portal, while the distal anterolateral portal is required for therapeutic procedures in the region of the anterolateral acetabular margin. The portal entry site for the posterolateral portal is approximately 3 cm posterior to the posterosuperior angle of the greater trochanter at the same level as the skin incisions for the anterolateral and anterior portals. The puncture needle is directed almost horizontally, angled up to 10° cranially and approximately 30° anteriorly. On the way to the joint, the muscle perforates gluteus maximus, medius, and minimus. The joint capsule is perforated under arthroscopic control through the anterolateral portal between the 9 and 10 o'clock positions, close to the acetabular labrum.

The skin incision for the distal anterolateral portal is 3–4 cm further distally and midway between the anterior and anterolateral portals. Under arthroscopic control through the anterolateral portal, the needle is inclined approximately 15° medially and 45° cranially to perforate the joint capsule between the entry sites of the anterolateral and anterior portals.

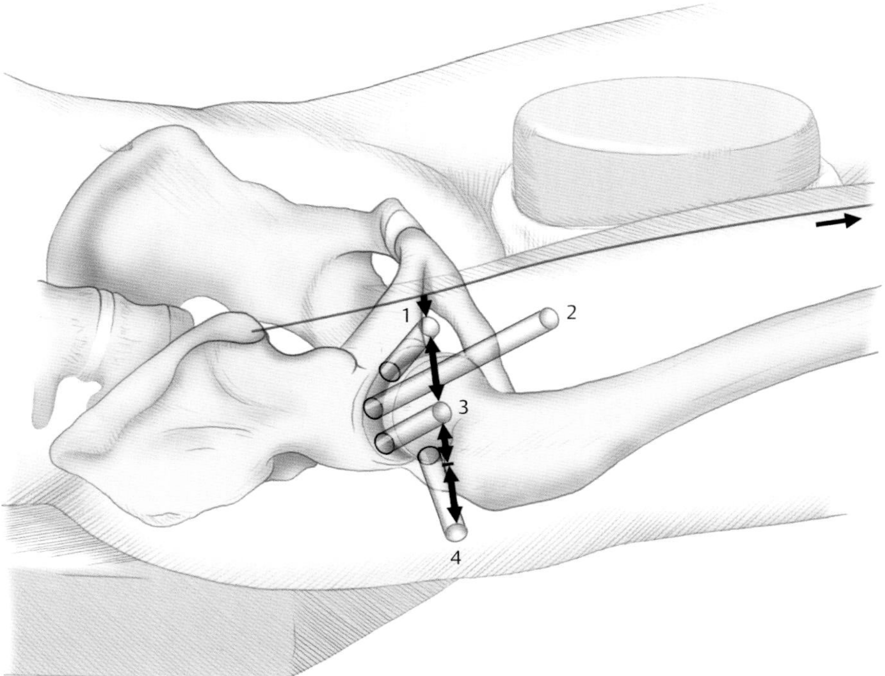

Fig. 9.52 Portals to the central compartment (red circles: skin; black circles: capsule perforation).

1 Anterior
2 Distal anterolateral
3 Anterolateral
4 Posterolateral

9.9.3 Diagnostic Inspection of the Joint Compartments and Arthroscopic Anatomy

Targeted thinning and incision of the joint capsule are essential for complete diagnostic arthroscopy and in preparation for efficient operative therapy. In the peripheral compartment, the annular ligament is thinned from anterior to lateral through the anterior portal using an aggressive shaver and radiofrequency instrument without dividing the longitudinal fibers of the iliofemoral ligament. The longitudinal ligaments in the region of the portal entry sites are notched with a scalpel to allow improved maneuverability of the arthroscope and instruments in the central compartment.

Diagnostic inspection of the peripheral compartment is performed with the 70° optic through the proximal anterolateral portal without traction, with various flexion, rotation, and abduction movements of the hip (**Fig. 9.53**). In the central compartment, the 70° optic is introduced through both the anterolateral and anterior portals and withdrawn from the acetabular fossa as far as the joint capsule, rotating it repeatedly through 180° (**Fig. 9.54**). The integrity of the ligament of the femoral head is checked by internal and external rotation of the hip.

9.9.4 Wound Closure

The wound is closed by approximation of the skin edges with interrupted sutures. Additional closure of the subcutaneous layer is necessary only with longer incisions for the removal of larger loose bodies.

9.9.5 Dangers

The dangers of hip arthroscopy arise mainly from incorrect positioning, excessively prolonged and forceful traction during

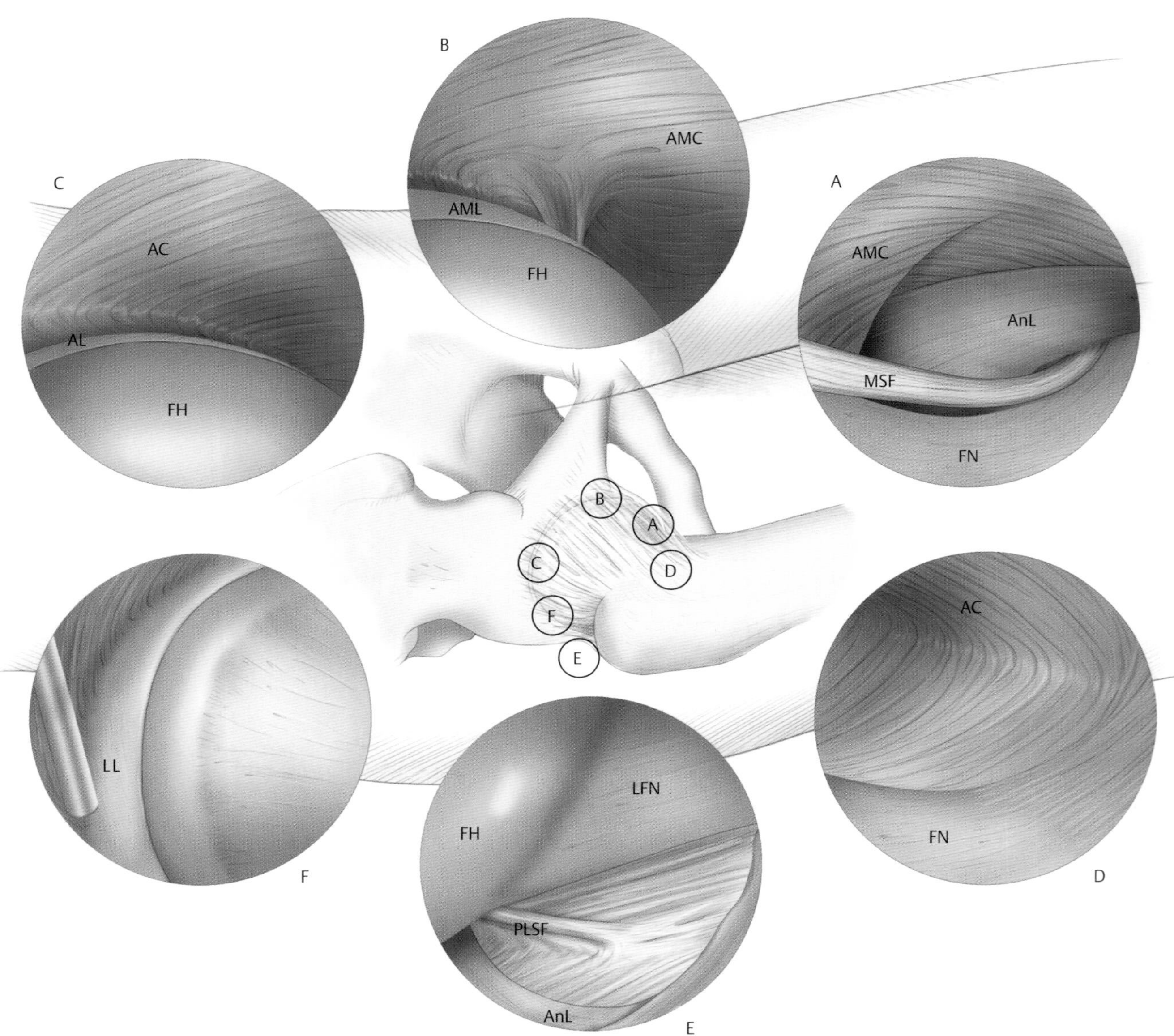

Fig. 9.53 Diagnostic inspection of the peripheral compartment. Anterior (D), medial (A), and posterolateral (E) femoral neck region. Medial (B), anterior (C), and lateral (F) head region. AC, anterior capsule; AL, anterior labrum; AMC, anteromedial capsule; AML, anteromedial labrum; AnL, annular ligament; FH, femoral head; FN, femoral neck; LFN, lateral femoral neck; LL, lateral labrum; MSF, medial synovial fold; PLSF, posterolateral synovial fold.

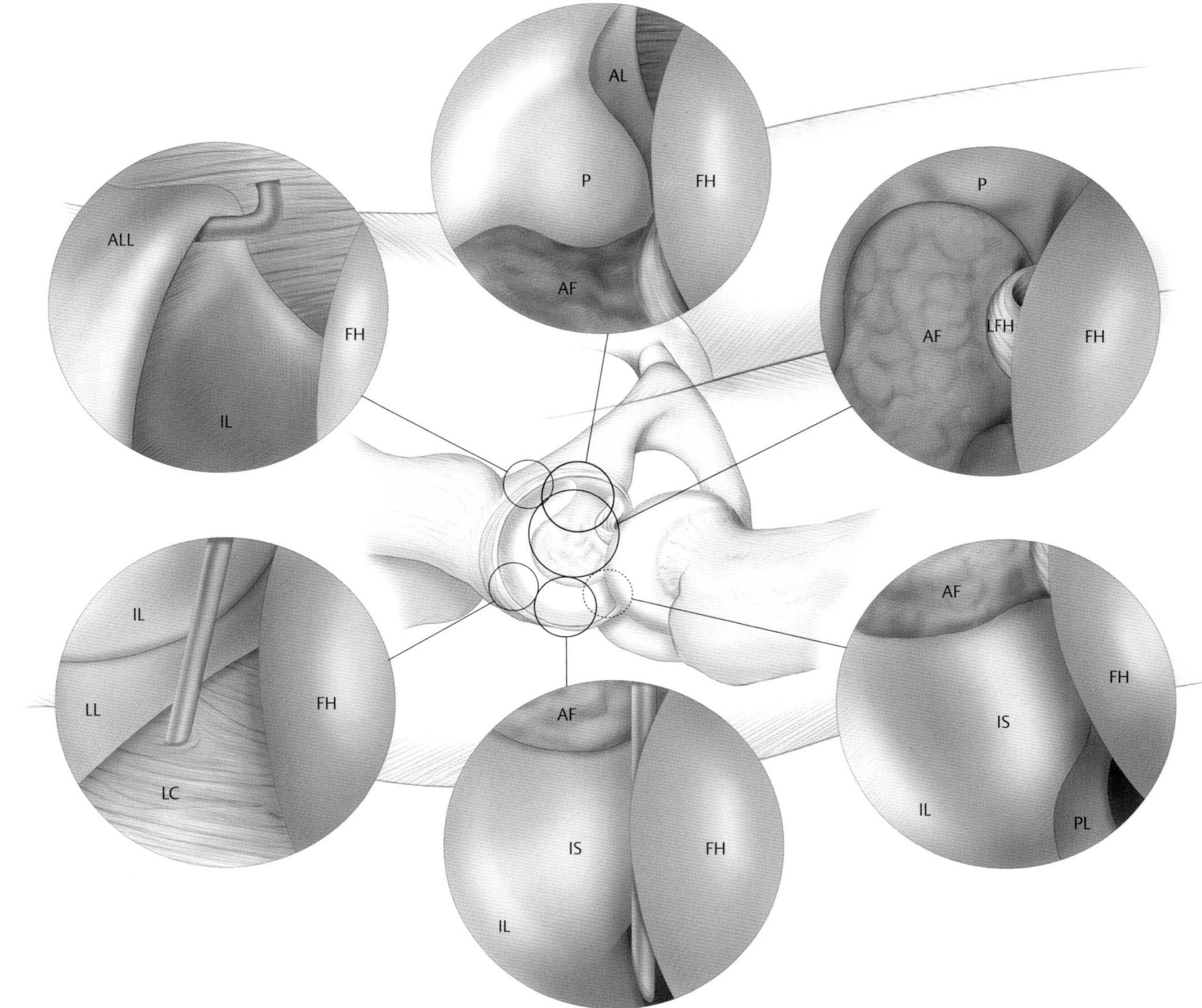

Fig. 9.54 Diagnostic inspection of the central compartment. AF, acetabular fossa; AL, anterior labrum; ALL, anterolateral labrum; FH, femoral head; IL, ilium; IS, ischium; L, labrum; LC, lateral capsule; LFH, ligament of femoral head; LL, lateral labrum; P, pubis; PL, posterior labrum.

arthroscopy of the central compartment, creation of the first portal, and arthroscopy of the central compartment. The pudendal nerve, genital region, and soft tissues and neurovascular structures of the foot and ankle are exposed to the pressure of the countertraction pad and the traction cuff, especially when the operations continue too long with forceful traction. The portal incisions in the skin must be limited to the anterolateral region so as not to injure the branches of the lateral cutaneous nerve of the thigh, which are frequently superficial, especially in thin patients. If the first portal into the central compartment is placed without arthroscopic control from peripherally, there is an increased risk of injury to the acetabular labrum and the femoral head cartilage. Especially when there is little femoroacetabular distraction, the femoral head cartilage is at risk of iatrogenic injury by the arthroscope and instruments. It is important to preserve the terminal branches of the medial circumflex femoral artery at the posterolateral femoral neck, which supply the femoral head.

9.9.6 Note

Other surgeons start with placing the first portal to the central compartment under fluoroscopic control and performing arthroscopy of the peripheral compartment thereafter. The lateral decubitus position is an alternative to supine positioning.

10 Femur

10.1 Anterior Approach

R. Bauer, F. Kerschbaumer, S. Poisel

10.1.1 Principal Indications

- Tumors
- Extensor release procedures for a knee flexion deficit
- Quadriceps necrosis

10.1.2 Positioning and Incision

The patient is placed in the supine position, with the leg draped so as to allow free movement. The incision is straight, following an imaginary line running from the anterior superior iliac spine to the lateral border of the patella. The length of the skin incision depends on individual requirements (**Fig. 10.1**). After the subcutaneous tissue and fascia have been split, the layer between the rectus femoris and vastus lateralis is dissected. The dissection should be made from distal to proximal to avoid injury to the more proximally coursing vessels and nerves (**Fig. 10.2**).

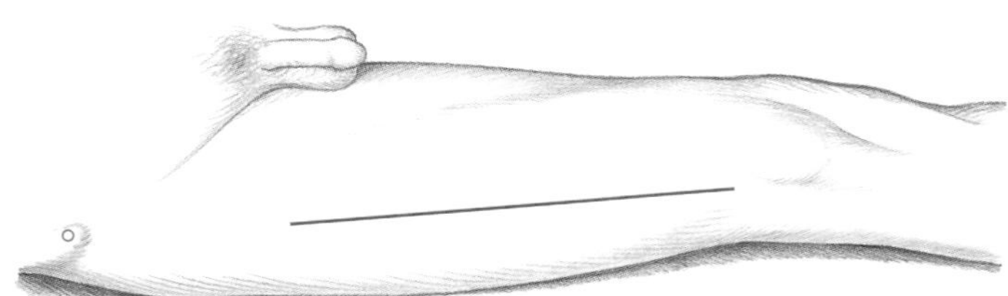

Fig. 10.1 Anterior approach to the femur. Skin incision between the anterior superior iliac spine and the lateral border of the patella (right leg).

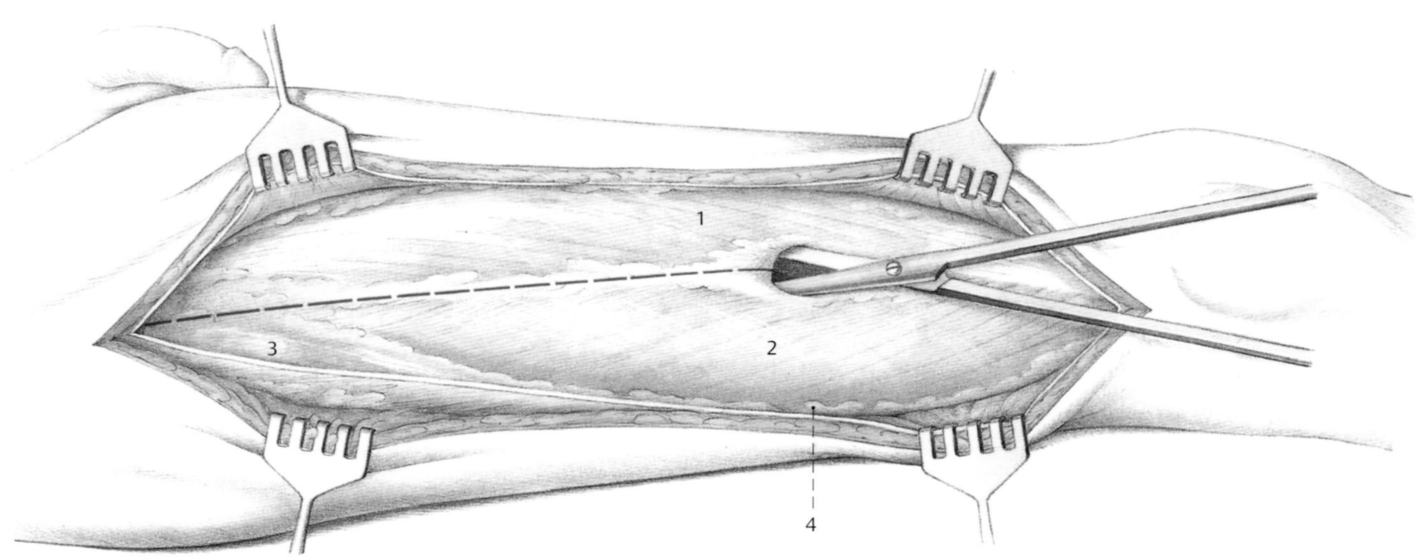

Fig. 10.2 After splitting of the fascia, the rectus femoris and vastus lateralis are separated by scissor dissection.

1 Rectus femoris
2 Vastus lateralis
3 Tensor of fascia lata
4 Fascia lata

10.1.3 Exposure of the Femoral Shaft

Following mobilization of the rectus femoris, this is retracted medially with wound retractors. In the distal region of the wound, the rectus femoris tendon is detached sharply with a scalpel from the vastus lateralis and the subjacent vastus intermedius.

Now the branches of the lateral circumflex femoral artery and vein and the branches of the femoral nerve supplying the vastus lateralis in the middle and upper wound regions are identified and raised (**Fig. 10.3**). More distally, some transversely running vessels need to be transected.

Exposure of the neurovascular bundles, particularly the proximal one, requires transection of the thick fascia covering vastus intermedius. A straight incision is now made in vastus intermedius, extending to the bone. This incision may be made with a diathermy scalpel to minimize bleeding. After medial and lateral retraction of the muscle, Hohmann elevators may be inserted (**Fig. 10.4**). If opening of the knee joint is not intended, vastus intermedius should be incised to at most a handbreadth proximal to the superior border of the patella so that injury to the superior recess of the knee joint capsule (suprapatellar bursa) may be avoided.

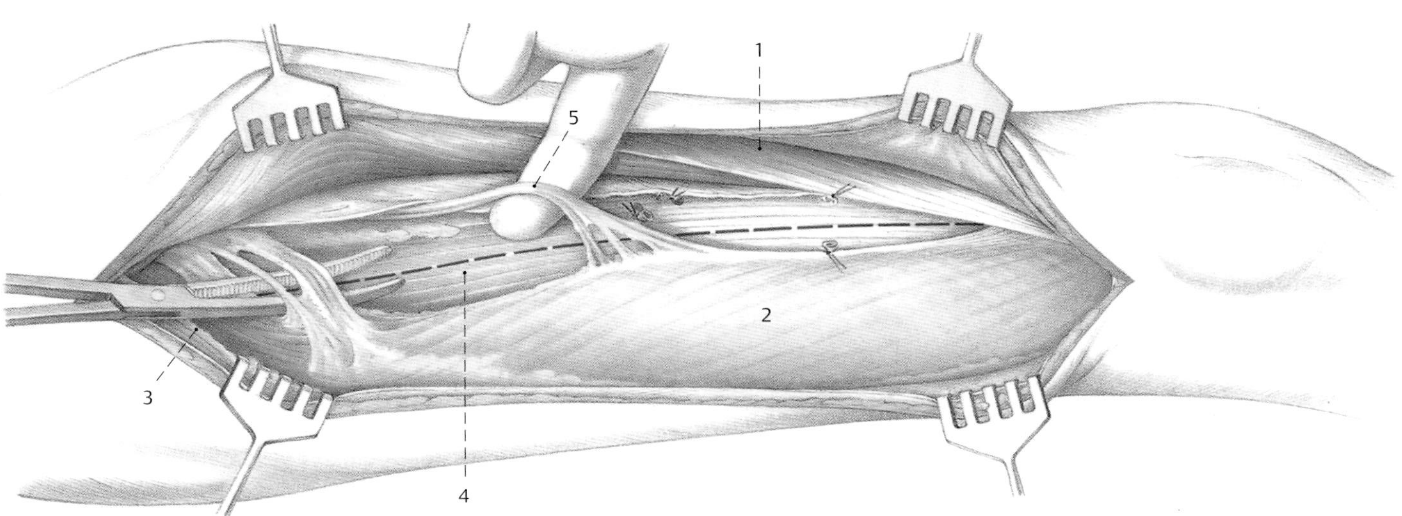

Fig. 10.3 The obliquely coursing vessels and nerves are mobilized and elevated. Subsequently, the vastus intermedius covering the bone is split (dashed line).

1 Rectus femoris
2 Vastus lateralis
3 Tensor of fascia lata
4 Vastus intermedius
5 Muscular branches of the lateral circumflex femoral artery and vein, and femoral nerve

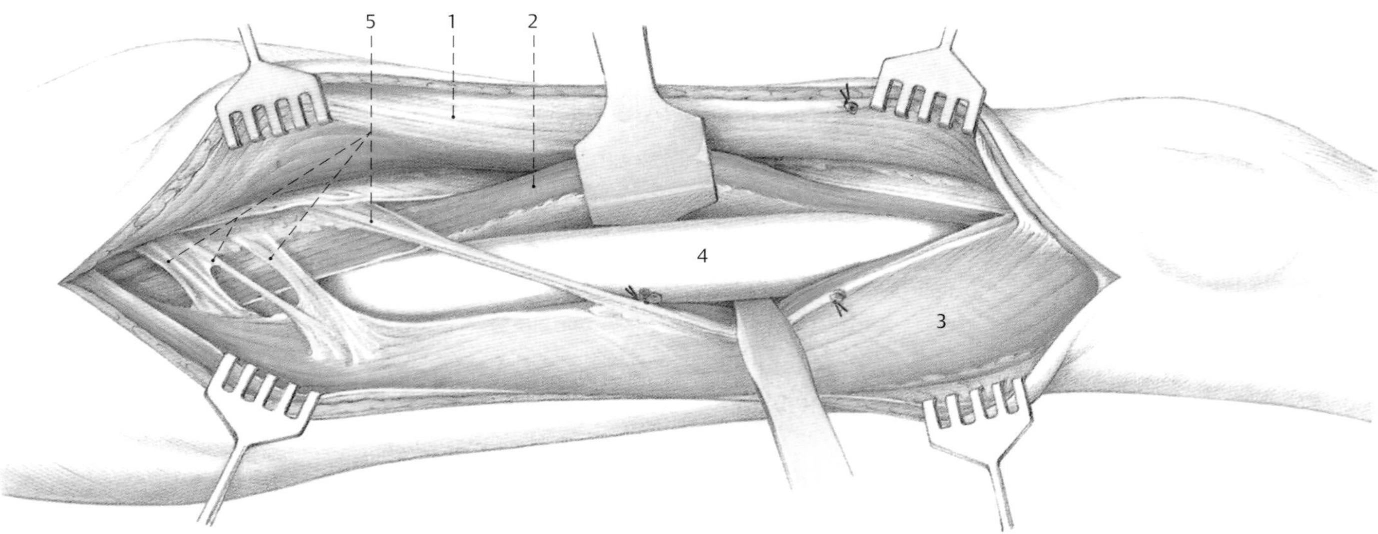

Fig. 10.4 Subperiosteal exposure of femur from the front with inserted Hohmann elevators.

1 Rectus femoris
2 Vastus intermedius
3 Vastus lateralis
4 Body of femur
5 Muscular branches of the lateral circumflex femoral artery and vein, and femoral nerve

10.1.4 Extension of the Approach

The anterior approach to the femur can be extended proximally by lengthening the incision along the iliac crest, as in the anterior, iliofemoral approach to the hip joint. Distal extension of the approach, corresponding to the lateral parapatellar approach to the knee joint, is likewise possible.

10.1.5 Wound Closure

Wound closure is effected by suturing vastus intermedius with interrupted sutures and loose suture of the femoral fascia.

10.1.6 Note

The anterior approach to the femur is employed only in exceptional cases. After using this approach, flexion deficits of the knee joint, probably attributable to iatrogenic damage to the gliding mechanism of the quadriceps, have been observed.

10.2 Lateral Proximal Approach to the Medullary Cavity of the Femur

K. Weise, D. Höntzsch

10.2.1 Principal Indications

- Medullary nailing of the femur
- Fractures
- Pseudarthrosis
- Bone marrow aspiration with a reamer–irrigator–aspirator

10.2.2 Positioning and Incision

Different positions may be used:
- Supine
- Lateral decubitus
- Supine on an extension table
- Lateral decubitus on an extension table

The approach is identical in each case.

It must be ensured that the table is radiolucent as far as the hip. The incision is an extension of the slightly curved long axis of the femur 3–5 cm cranial to the tip of the trochanter (**Fig. 10.5**).

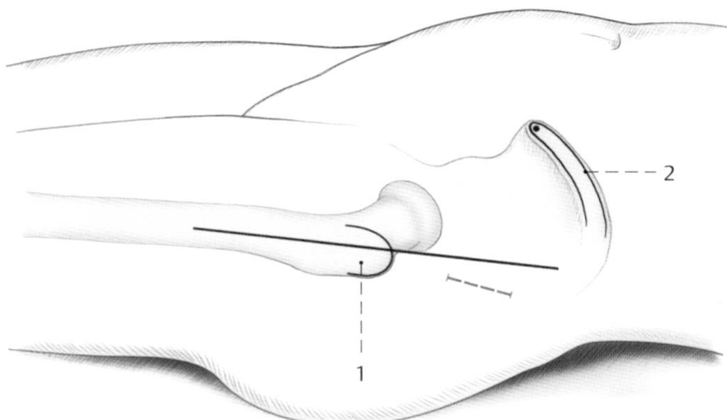

Fig. 10.5 Skin incision continuing the slightly curved axis of the femur 3–5 cm cranial to the tip of the trochanter.

1 Greater trochanter
2 Iliac crest

10.2.3 Exposure of the Proximal Femoral Entry Site

The superficial gluteal fascia is split, followed by the muscle fascia of gluteus medius (**Fig. 10.6**).

The fibers of gluteus medius are divided bluntly and sharply in the line of the fibers. The greater trochanter is palpated deep in the distally directed approach funnel. The desired entry site is found (lateral to the trochanter tip, on the trochanter tip, or in the trochanteric fossa).

After establishing the entry site, the guidewire or opening instrument for nailing is applied and advanced longitudinally in the central axis of the femur (**Fig. 10.7**), here shown with a guidewire.

10.2.4 Wound Closure

The wound is closed in layers.

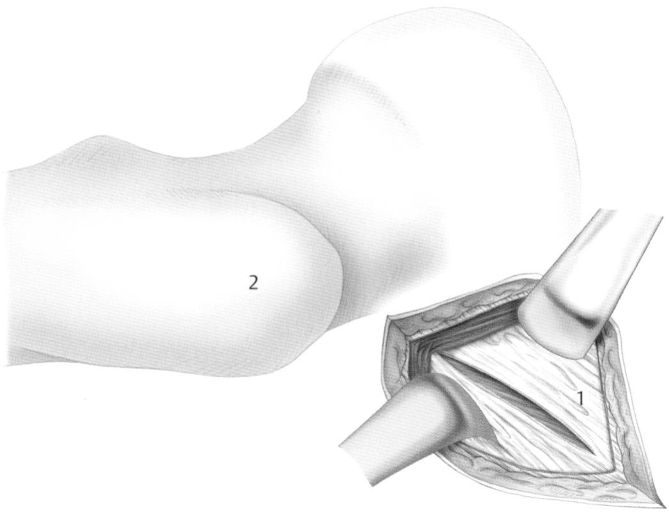

Fig. 10.6 Splitting of the fascia.

1 Fascia
2 Greater trochanter

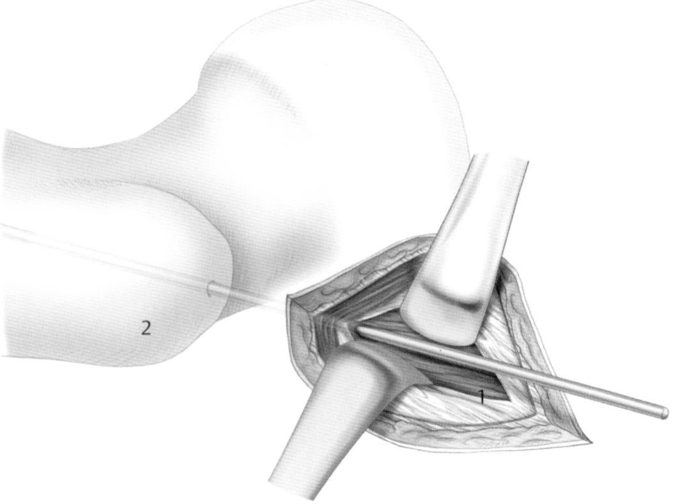

Fig. 10.7 Langenbeck retractors hold the fascia and muscle in an anterior and posterior direction to maintain a funnel-shaped approach to the greater trochanter.

1 Fascia and muscle
2 Greater trochanter

10.3 Lateral Approach to the Femur

R. Bauer, F. Kerschbaumer, S. Poisel

10.3a Lateral Approach—General Points

10.3a.1 Principal Indications

- Osteotomy
- Pseudarthrosis
- Lengthening of the femur
- Fractures

10.3a.2 Positioning and Incision

The patient is placed in the supine position with a pad under the buttocks. The skin incision follows an imaginary line from the greater trochanter to the lateral epicondyle of the femur (**Fig. 10.8**). The length of the incision depends on requirements. After transection of the skin and subcutaneous tissue, the fascia lata is split in line with the skin incision.

10.3a.3 Note

The lateral approach is considered to be the **standard approach to the femur**. This approach generally presents no technical problems and spares the innervation of vastus lateralis. In a broad lateral exposure of the femoral shaft, detachment of the periosteum in the area of the linea aspera should be avoided if possible. A drawback of this approach is transection of the perforating arteries, which adversely affects the blood supply in the region of vastus lateralis.

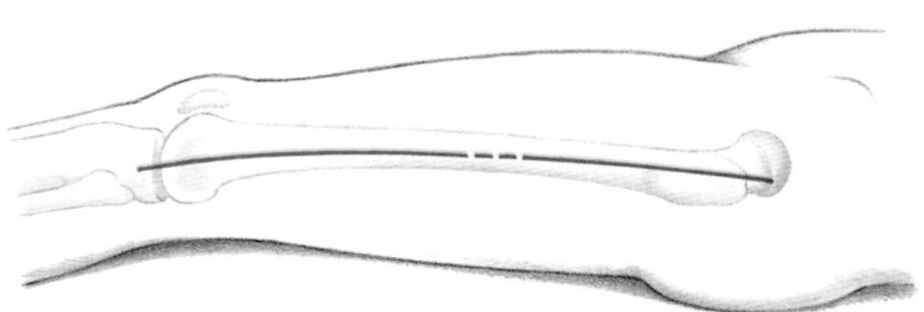

Fig. 10.8 Lateral approach to the femur (left leg). Positioning and incision. The solid line shows the incision for exposure of the proximal and distal femoral segment, respectively. If necessary, the two approaches may be combined (dashed line).

10.3b Lateral Approach—Exposure of the Proximal Femur

For exposure of the proximal portion of the femur, the posterior portion of the fascia lata is first of all detached as far posteriorly as possible from the vastus lateralis.

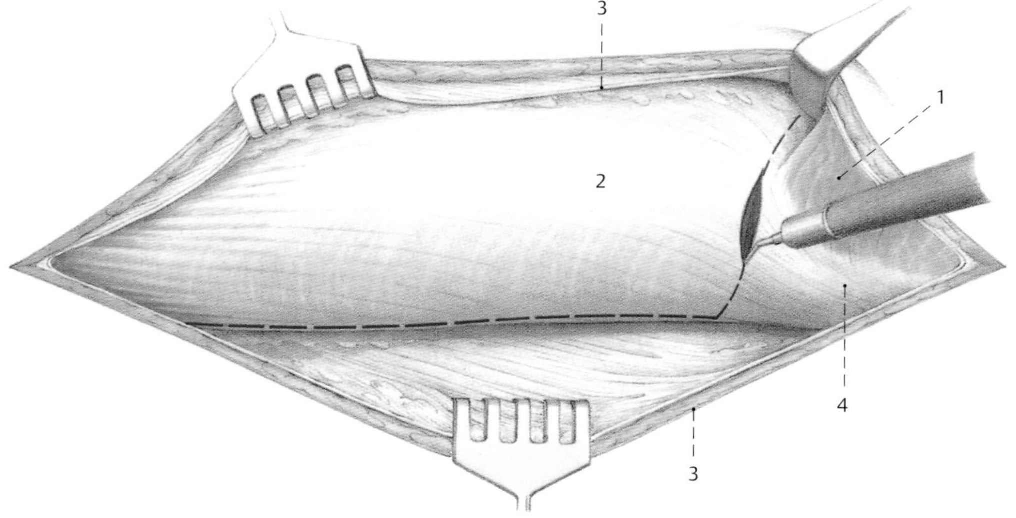

Fig. 10.9 Lateral exposure of the proximal third of the femur. The L-shaped incision in vastus lateralis is made with the aid of diathermy.

1 Gluteus medius
2 Vastus lateralis
3 Fascia lata, cut border
4 Greater trochanter

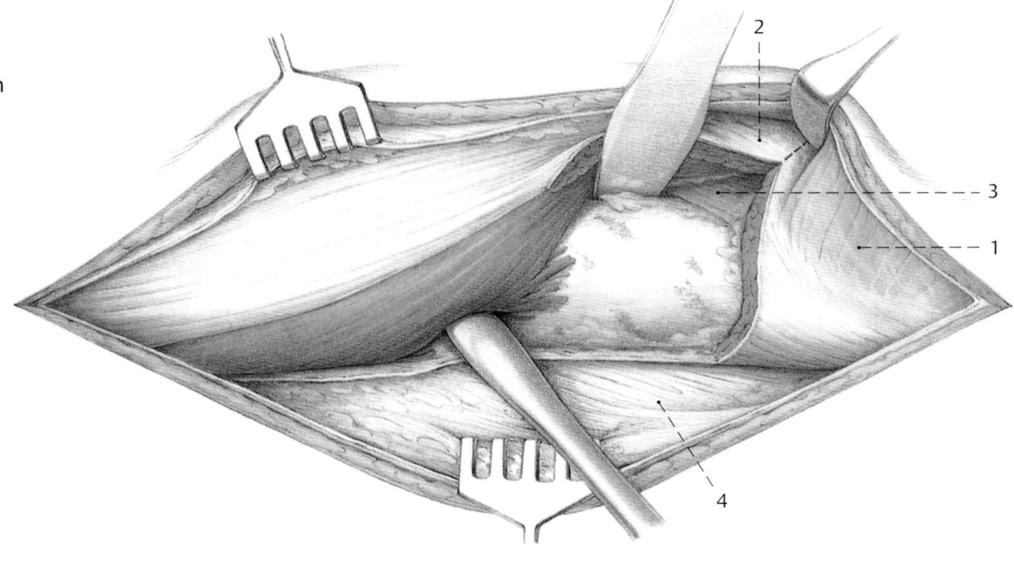

Fig. 10.10 Retraction of vastus lateralis from the lateral femoral intermuscular septum and femur with a raspatory. The dashed line in the upper corner of the wound shows the incisions in vastus lateralis and vastus intermedius for exposure of the intertrochanteric region, should this be required.

1 Gluteus medius
2 Vastus lateralis
3 Vastus intermedius
4 Fascia lata

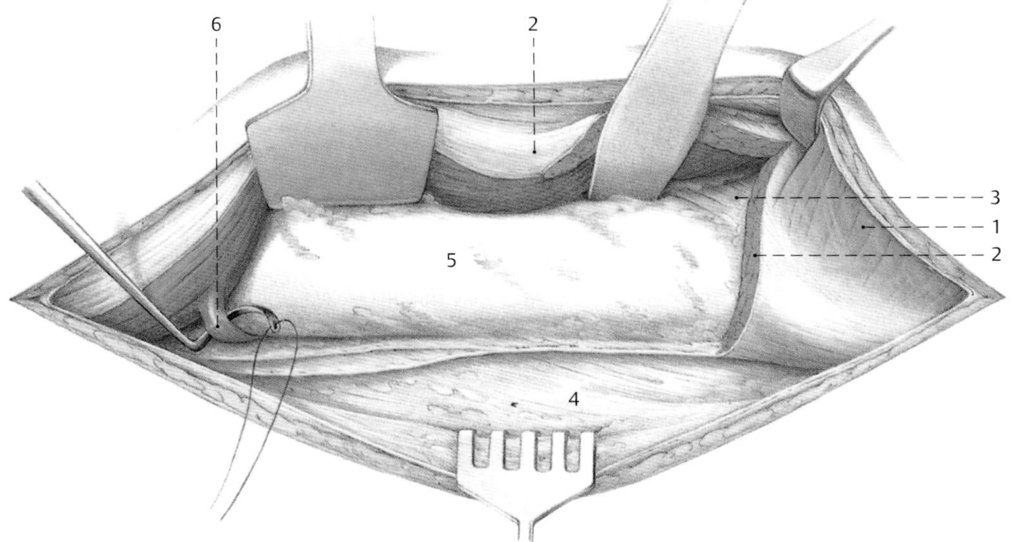

Fig. 10.11 Lateral exposure of the femur. Ligation of the perforating vessels.

1 Gluteus medius
2 Vastus lateralis
3 Vastus intermedius
4 Fascia lata
5 Body of femur
6 Perforating vessels

An L-shaped incision extending to the bone is then made in the vastus lateralis with the diathermy scalpel (**Fig. 10.9**). If an intertrocanteric exposure is desired, proximal retraction of the gluteal muscles with a Langenbeck retractor is advisable. This also allows detachment of the vastus intermedius fibers as far as the neck of the femur. The muscle can now be retracted anteriorly from the lateral femoral intermuscular septum with a raspatory (**Fig. 10.10**). Next Hohmann elevators are inserted for medial retraction of the muscle. In the distal wound area, the first perforating vessels have to be found and ligated (**Fig. 10.11**). For exposure of the intertrochanteric region and distal portions of the hip joint capsule, the gluteal muscles are proximally retracted with a Langenbeck retractor, after which the remaining parts of the vastus intermedius are split. Using the raspatory, the femoral neck can now be exposed from the medial side, and a Hohmann elevator may be inserted at this site (**Fig. 10.12**).

10.3b.1 Anatomical Site

The cross-sectional diagram (**Fig. 10.13**) shows that the vastus lateralis projects posteriorly beyond the femoral shaft. Careful

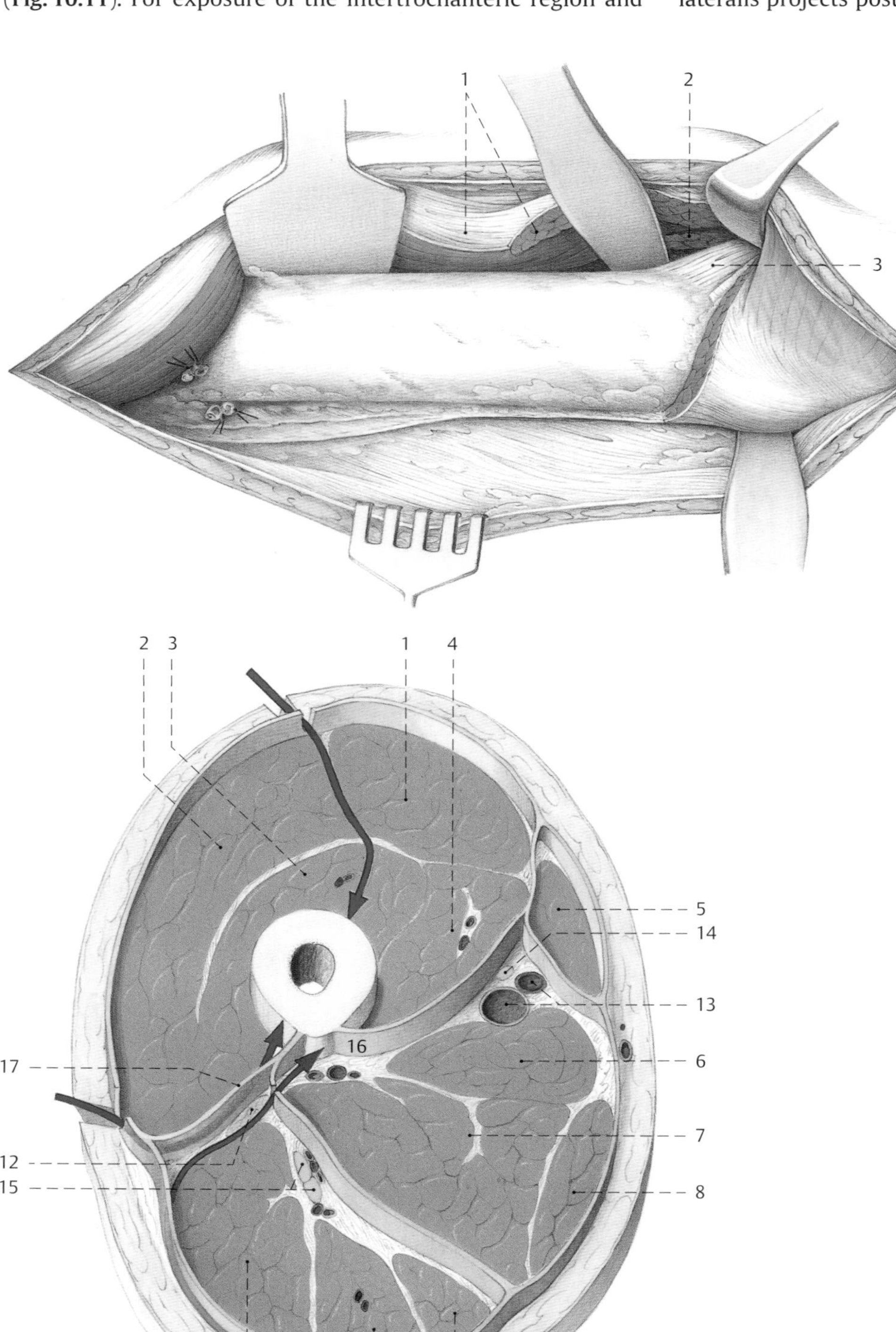

Fig. 10.12 Exposure of the proximal femur and intertrochanteric region, and of the distal portions of the capsule. Insertion of Hohmann retractors.

1 Vastus lateralis
2 Vastus intermedius
3 Iliofemoral ligament, joint capsule

Fig. 10.13 Anatomical site. The schematic cross-section of the proximal third of the femur shows the lateral, anterior, and posterior approaches to the femur (arrows, left leg, view from proximal).

1 Rectus femoris
2 Vastus lateralis
3 Vastus intermedius
4 Vastus medialis
5 Sartorius
6 Adductor longus
7 Adductor magnus
8 Gracilis
9 Semimembranosus
10 Semitendinosus
11 Biceps femoris, long head
12 Biceps femoris, short head
13 Femoral artery and vein
14 Saphenous nerve
15 Tibial and common peroneal nerves
16 Anteromedial intermuscular septum
17 Lateral femoral intermuscular septum

detachment of the vastus lateralis from the lateral femoral intermuscular septum as far as the linea aspera is therefore required.

Dissection behind the lateral femoral intermuscular septum may cause injury to the perforating vessels.

10.3b.2 Wound Closure

The vastus lateralis is reattached both proximally and laterally. The wound is further closed by suture of the fascia lata.

10.3b.3 Dangers

Inadvertent transection of a perforating vessel may lead to mediad retraction of the end of the artery. If this happens, detachment of the periosteum at the linea aspera should be attempted so that the bleeding vessel may be grasped and ligated. If exposure in this manner is not feasible, it may be necessary to identify the deep femoral artery and to ligate it as far distally as possible.

10.3c Lateral Approach—Exposure of the Distal Femur

If exposure of the distal femoral shaft is necessary, the skin incision is extended to a point just proximal to Gerdy's tubercle. The iliotibial band is split along a line paralleling the skin incision (**Fig. 10.14**). If exposure of the lateral femoral condyle is required, the lateral superior genicular artery and vein have to be ligated and transected (**Fig. 10.15**). Subse-

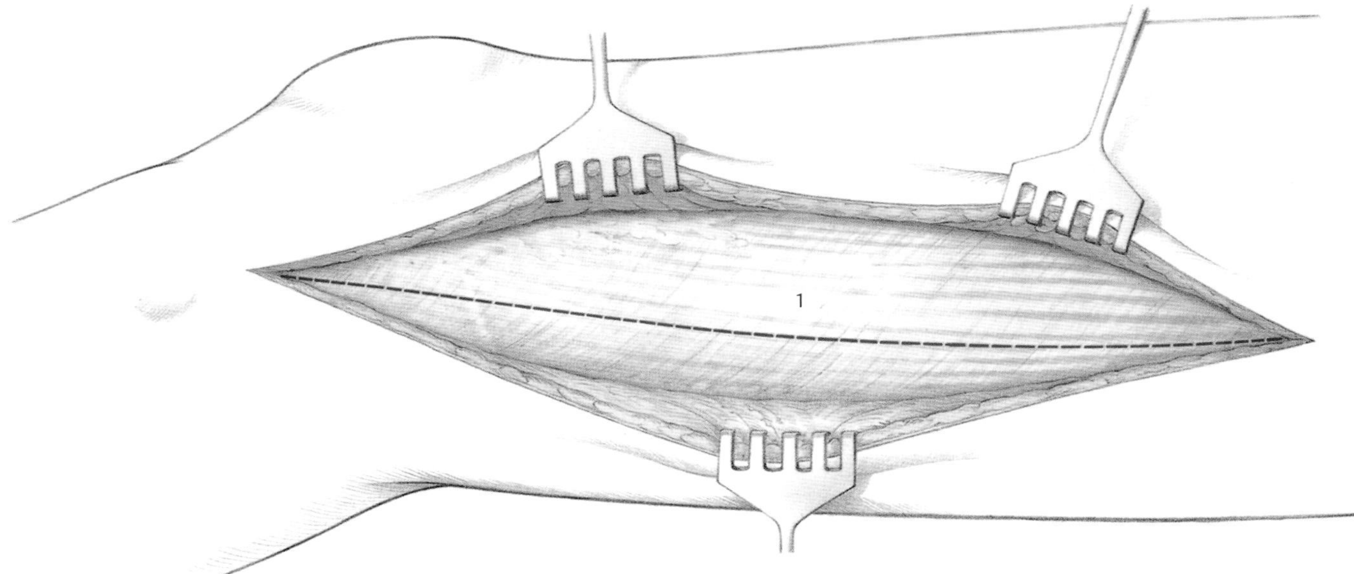

Fig. 10.14 Exposure of the middle and distal thirds of the femur from laterally (left leg). Incision of the iliotibial tract.

1 Iliotibial tract

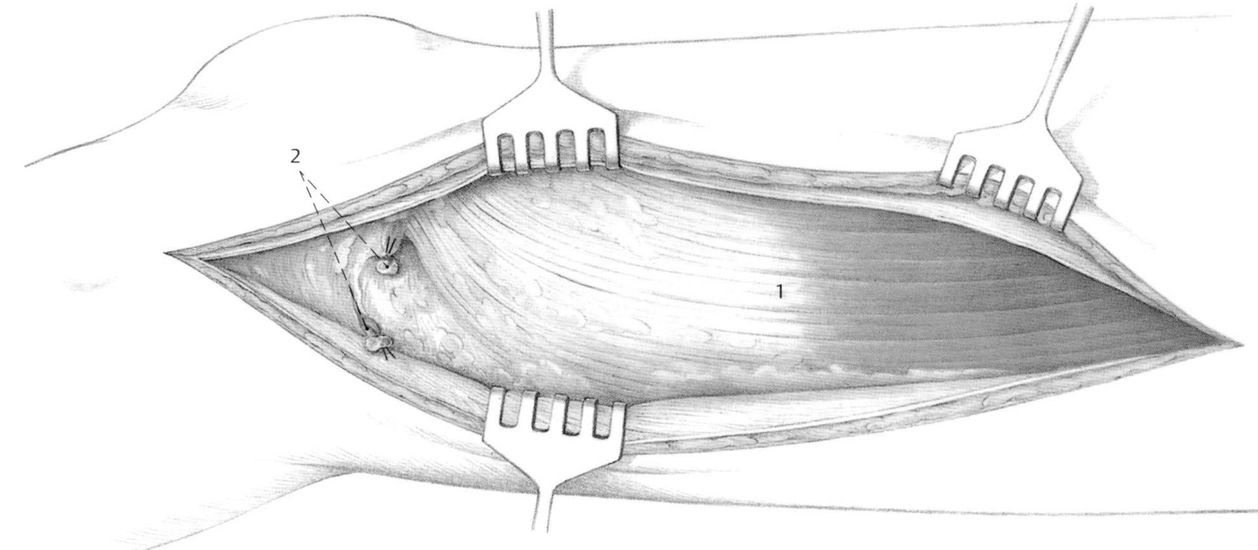

Fig. 10.15 Ligation of the lateral superior genicular artery and vein; mobilization of vastus lateralis.

1 Vastus lateralis
2 Lateral superior genicular artery and vein

quently, the index finger is inserted between vastus lateralis and the femoral periosteum from the distal side, and the muscle is cautiously lifted up. Further dissection of the muscle is carried out in a proximal direction with a raspatory. Perforating vessels need to be ligated and transected (**Fig. 10.16**). Vastus lateralis, thus mobilized, is retracted medially with Hohmann elevators. If necessary, a Hohmann elevator may also be inserted posteriorly. Any subperiosteal exposure of the posterior aspect of the femur or at the linea aspera has to be done very sparingly in order not to compromise the blood supply of the bone (**Fig. 10.17**). The two nutrient arteries that supply the femoral shaft at the boundary between the proximal and the middle thirds and between the middle and distal thirds must be spared.

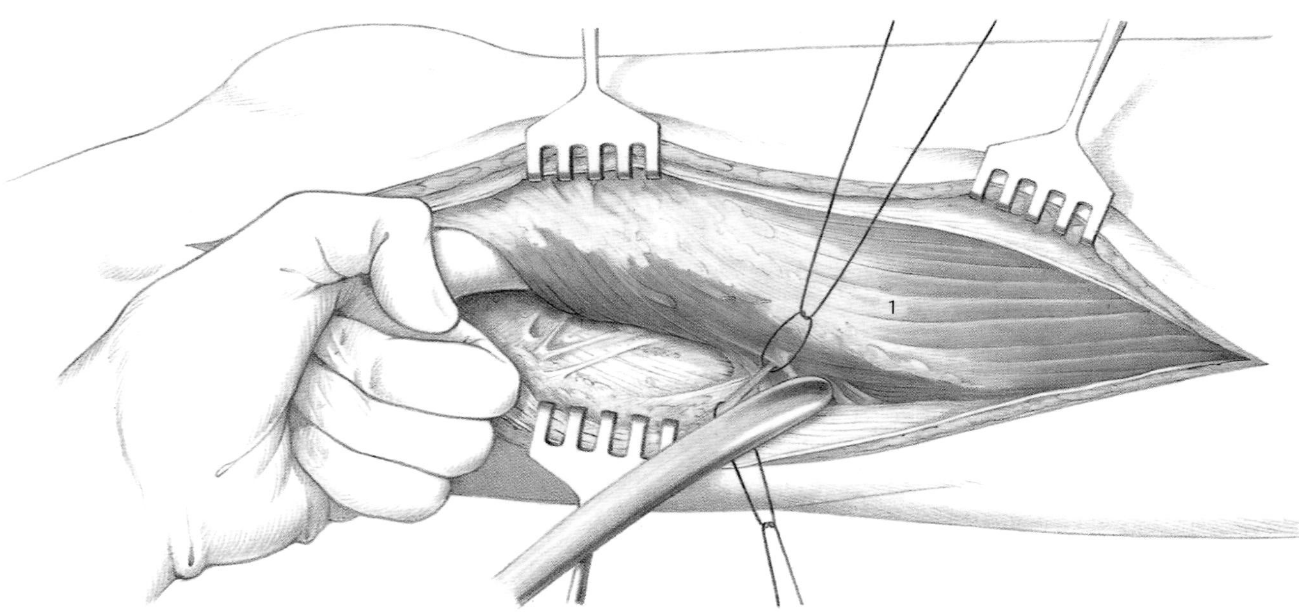

Fig. 10.16 Retraction of vastus lateralis from the lateral intermuscular septum. Ligation of the perforating vessels.

1 Vastus lateralis

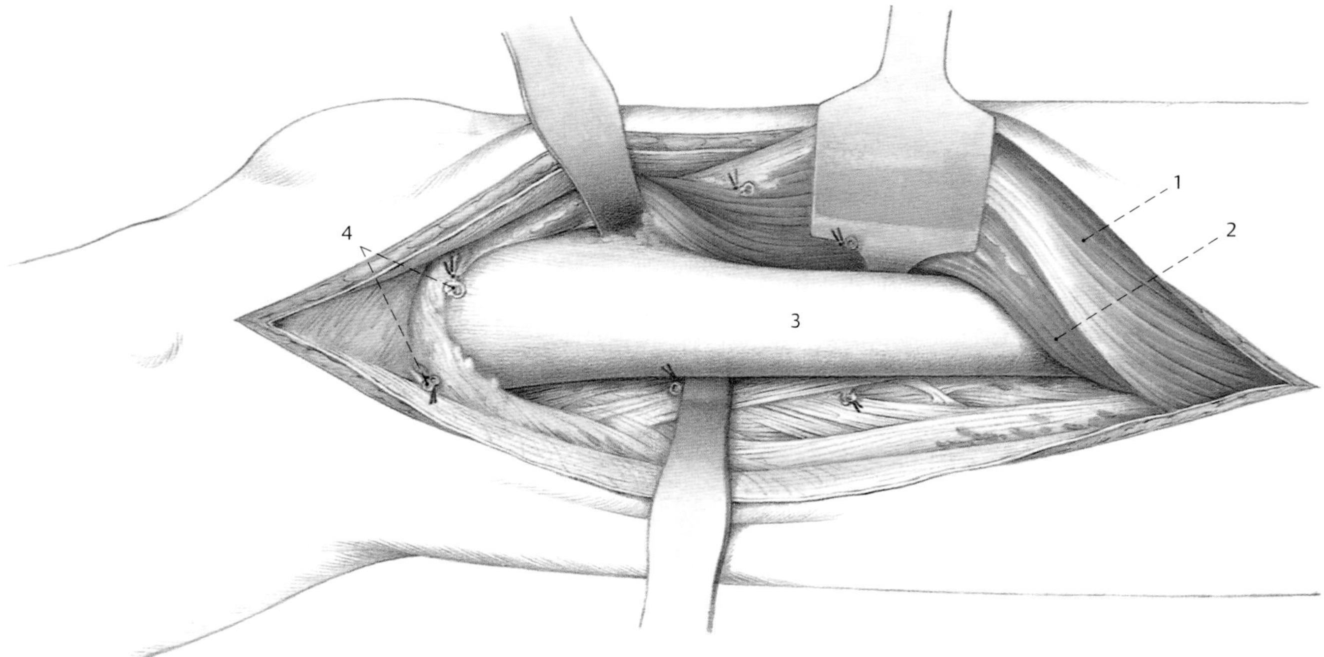

Fig. 10.17 Lateral subperiosteal exposure of the middle and distal thirds of the femur.

1 Vastus lateralis
2 Vastus intermedius
3 Body of femur
4 Lateral superior genicular artery and vein

If possible, the synovial knee joint capsule should not be opened. Properly cautious dissection allows the infrapatellar synovial fold to be recognized both laterally and in the area of the superior recess, and to be lifted off the underlying bone.

10.3c.1 Anatomical Site

The diagrammatic cross-section through the distal third of the femur shows that, in this area, the muscle mass of vastus lateralis is distinctly smaller than it is proximally, and that it barely extends posteriorly beyond the femur (**Fig. 10.18**).

10.3c.2 Wound Closure

The wound is closed by attaching vastus lateralis to the lateral femoral intermuscular septum with loose apposition sutures, and closing the fascia lata by means of interrupted sutures.

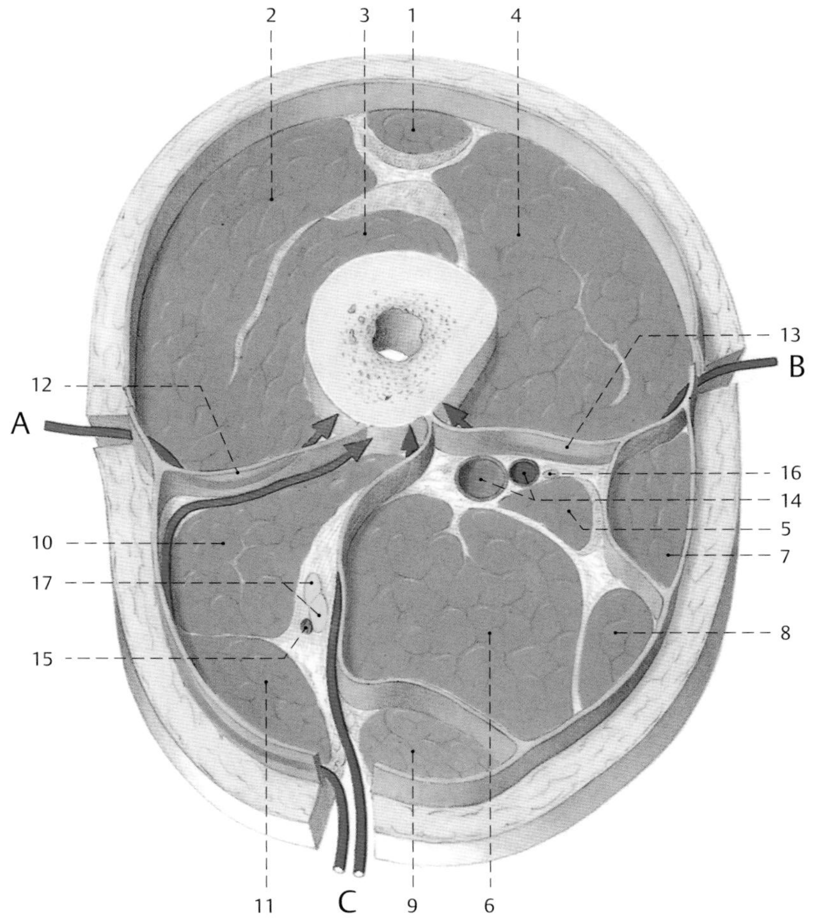

Fig. 10.18 Anatomical site. Cross-section of the distal third of the femur. Representation of the two posterior approaches and the lateral and medial approaches (arrows, left leg, view from proximal).

1 Rectus femoris
2 Vastus lateralis
3 Vastus intermedius
4 Vastus medialis
5 Adductor longus
6 Adductor magnus
7 Sartorius
8 Gracilis
9 Semimembranosus
10 Biceps femoris, short head
11 Biceps femoris, long head
12 Lateral femoral intermuscular septum
13 Medial femoral intermuscular septum
14 Femoral artery and vein
15 Perforating artery I
16 Saphenous nerve
17 Tibial and common peroneal nerves

A Lateral approach
B Medial approach
C Posterior approach

10.4 Minimally Invasive Lateral Approach to the Femur

K. Weise, D. Höntzsch

10.4.1 Principal Indications

- Midshaft fractures and fractures in the proximal and distal thirds
- Periprosthetic fractures with total hip or knee replacement
- Pseudarthrosis
- After segment transport and lengthening

10.4.2 Positioning and Incision

The patient is placed in the supine position. It must be ensured that the table is radiolucent as far as the hip. It can be an advantage to drape the contralateral leg to allow free movement as this allows rotation and length to be determined securely. Lateral radiography is much easier, especially while the fracture has been reduced but is not yet stabilized.

The incision is similar for the following two options:

From proximal to distal: the longitudinal incisions extend 4–10 cm distally from the greater trochanter and 3–5 cm at the anticipated end of the plate, both in the lateral line. Two or more 1–2 cm incisions are made in the lateral line over the introduced plate for reduction maneuvers and screw insertion (**Fig. 10.19**).

Plates inserted from distal to proximal: the entry incision extends 5–10 cm proximally from the knee joint line pointing to the anticipated end of the plate, and the second is 3–5 cm long in the lateral line. Further incisions are carried out as for the first option (**Fig. 10.19**).

10.4.3 Exposure of the Proximal Entry Site

The proximal femur should be reached at the distal third of the greater trochanter and its first 2–4 cm. The fascia lata is split sufficiently to avoid tension. The fascia of vastus lateralis is then split, followed by blunt and sharp division with a finger and scissors of the muscle in the line of its fibers until the periosteum in the target region is reached. From this point, the vastus lateralis is undermined and retracted in its course and at its attachment in the proximal and distal directions, and also anteriorly and posteriorly. Exposure of 2–6 cm longitudinally and half of the circumference is adequate. The operative field can be held open in the anterior and posterior directions, preferably with Langenbeck retractors, but Hohmann elevators may also be used (**Figs. 10.20** and **10.21**).

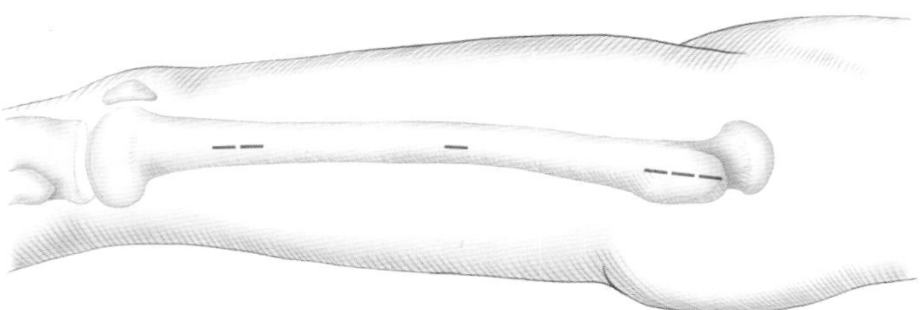

Fig. 10.19 Illustration of the longitudinal incisions over the femur for minimally invasive plate insertion from proximal to distal, and from distal to proximal.

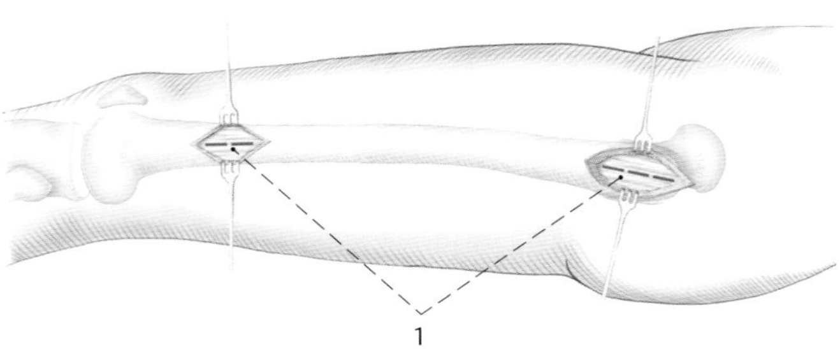

Fig. 10.20 Exposure of the fascia over the greater trochanter and proximal one-fifth of the femur, and at the anticipated end of the selected plate.

1 Fascia lata

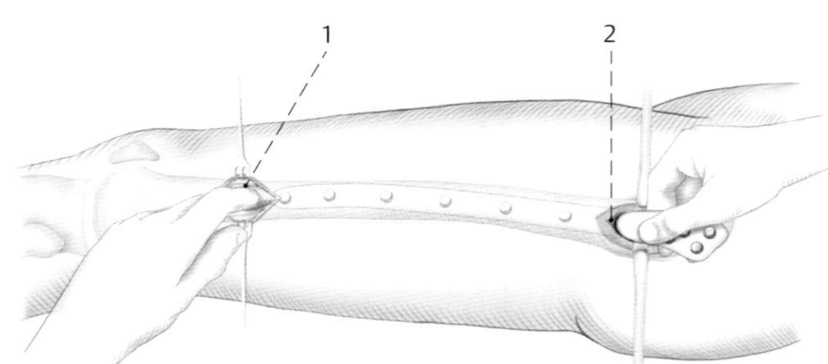

Fig. 10.21 The plate is positioned by pushing it gently back and forth on the periosteum and beneath the muscle and fascia, and the position is checked clinically and radiographically.

1 Fascia lata
2 Vastus lateralis

10.4.4 Minimally Invasive Approaches to the Shaft

A 2–5 cm incision is made in the region of the end of the selected plate (**Fig. 10.22**). The fascia lata and fascia of vastus lateralis are split to the same extent. The muscle is then dissected bluntly and sharply until the periosteum and circumference can be palpated firmly with a finger or instrument (**Fig. 10.22**).

Depending on the technical design of the plate and instruments, the plate is advanced on the femur, on the periosteum and beneath the vastus lateralis muscle, distally toward the finger in the distal incision, crossing the more or less reduced fracture (**Fig. 10.22**).

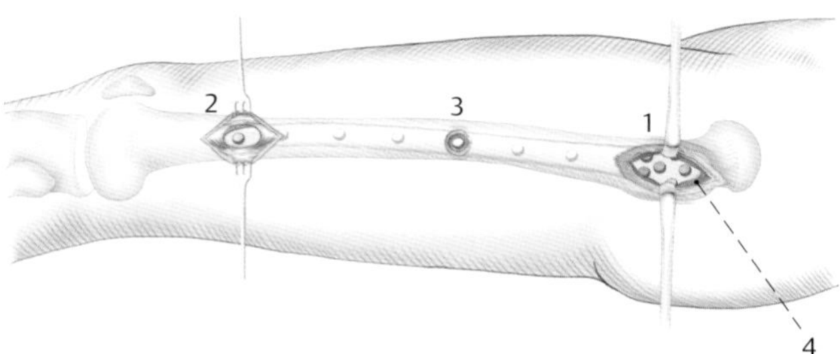

Fig. 10.22 The fascia lata and fascia of vastus lateralis are split. The periosteum of the femur is reached by blunt and sharp dissection in the proximal and distal incisions. The plate is inserted onto the femur from proximal to distal, crossing the fracture, and is advanced toward the palpating finger in the distal incision.

1 Proximal window
2 Distal window
3 Further window for screw placement
4 Vastus lateralis

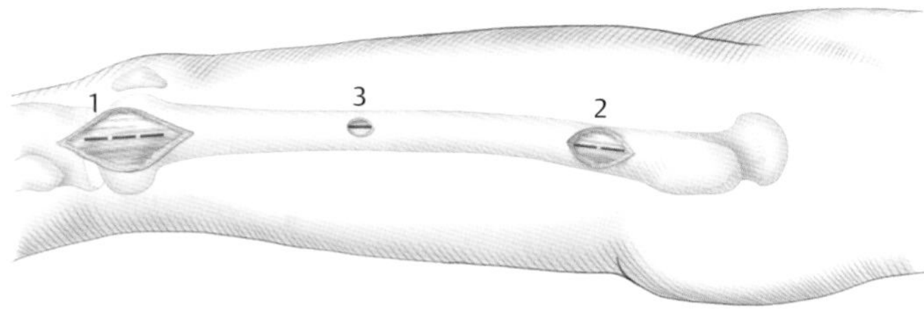

Fig. 10.23 Incision for minimally invasive plate insertion from distal to proximal.

1 Distal window
2 Proximal window
3 Further window for insertion of screws in the plate

A 1–2 cm incision is made for each screw that cannot be inserted through the incisions at the insertion site and end. The fascia lata and vastus lateralis muscle are each split to the same length (so that they are not tensed). The fibers of vastus lateralis are split until the plate can be reached with a finger or instrument for screw insertion without interposed muscle fibers. Screws can be inserted into one or possibly two adjacent plate holes (see **Fig. 10.21**).

10.4.5 Exposure of the Distal Entry Site

The procedure is reversed for positioning the plate from distal to proximal.

The skin is incised for 4–10 cm over the distal femur extending proximally from the knee joint line (**Fig. 10.23**). The distal part of the fascia lata and proximal extensions of the iliotibial tract are split longitudinally (**Fig. 10.24**). The condyle and distal one-fifth of the femur are then dissected bluntly and sharply. The fascia must be mobilized so that the plate will later be inserted beneath and not above this fascia.

The distal part of vastus lateralis is retracted anteriorly with a small incision if necessary. The superior lateral genicular artery and vein must be ligated or coagulated if they cross the operative field.

The rest of the procedure is as described above with an incision over the mid or proximal femur, depending on the location and configuration of the fracture and the selected plate length (**Fig. 10.25**).

10.4.6 Wound Closure

Longer incisions at either end are closed in layers. Full-thickness skin sutures suffice for the stab incisions.

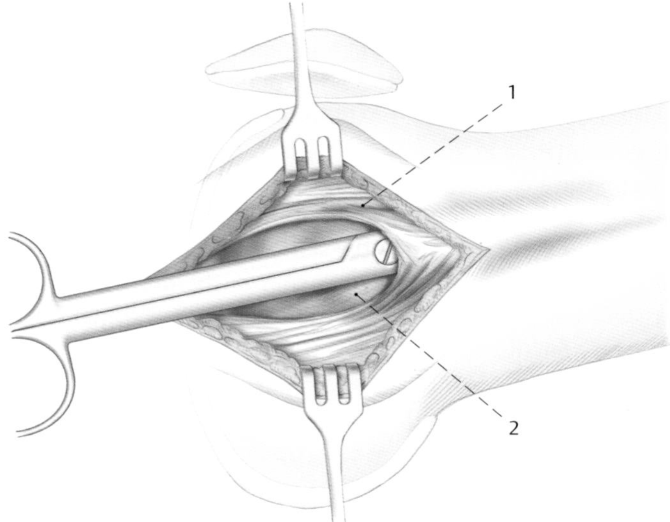

Fig. 10.24 The fascia lata and vastus lateralis muscle are split. The muscle is dissected down to the periosteum of the femur in a funnel shape. Large scissors can be used, but other minimally invasive instruments are also available.

1 Fascia lata
2 Lateral femoral epicondyle

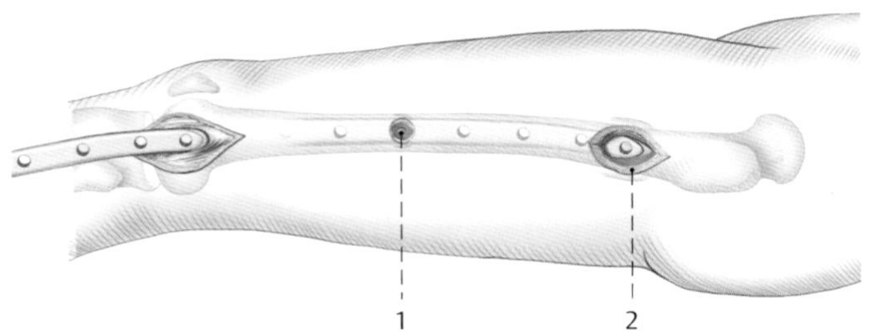

Fig. 10.25 The plate is inserted by pushing it gently back and forth on the periosteum and beneath the muscle. The fracture zone is bridged until the proximal end of the plate has reached the proximal femur. The other plate holes that cannot be reached through the entry window and proximal window are accessed through stab incisions that are dissected down to the plate.

1 Vastus lateralis
2 Fascia lata

10.5 Medial Approach to the Femur

R. Bauer, F. Kerschbaumer, S. Poisel

The medial approach to the femur is especially suitable for exposure of the distal third of the shaft and also, in exceptional cases, for exposure of the middle third.

10.5.1 Principal Indications

- Osteotomy
- Fractures
- Tumors
- Osteomyelitis

10.5.2 Positioning and Incision

The patient is placed supine on the operating table with a pad under the buttocks and the thigh so that the leg to be operated on is slightly higher than the other one (**Fig. 10.26**). The skin incision begins two fingerbreadths distal to the medial femoral epicondyle and continues 15 cm in a proximal direction. For exposure of the middle third of the shaft, an appropriate proximally direction extension of the incision is possible (**Fig. 10.26**). After incision of the skin and subcutaneous tissue, the fascia over vastus medialis is split in the line of the skin incision. Division of the patellar retinacula is normally not necessary for this approach (**Fig. 10.27**).

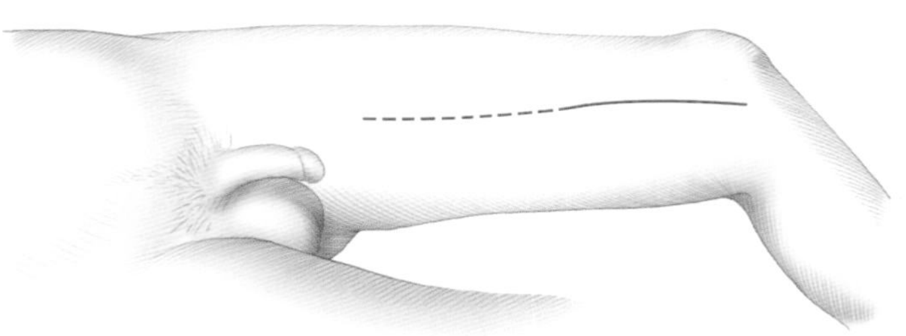

Fig. 10.26 Medial exposure of the distal and middle thirds of the femoral shaft (left leg). Positioning and incision.

10.5.3 Exposure of the Femoral Shaft

Vastus medialis is detached with the index finger from the bone and the medial intermuscular septum, beginning distally. This can be done more easily on the medial than on the lateral side as the vastus medialis does not adhere to the medial femoral intermuscular septum in the distal segment (**Fig. 10.28**). Vastus medialis is supplied by branches of the descending genicular artery, which are transected (**Figs. 10.29** and **10.30**). Subsequently, vastus medialis is laterally retracted from the periosteum, and Hohmann elevators can be inserted. Opening of the superior recess of the knee joint capsule should be avoided. If further exposure of the femur is required in the proximal direction, the vastoadductor membrane has to be split as shown in **Fig. 10.31**. After ligation of several muscular branches of the femoral artery, vastus medialis can now be further dissected proximally. Clear exposure of the middle third of the femoral shaft is thus also possible from the medial side (**Fig. 10.32**).

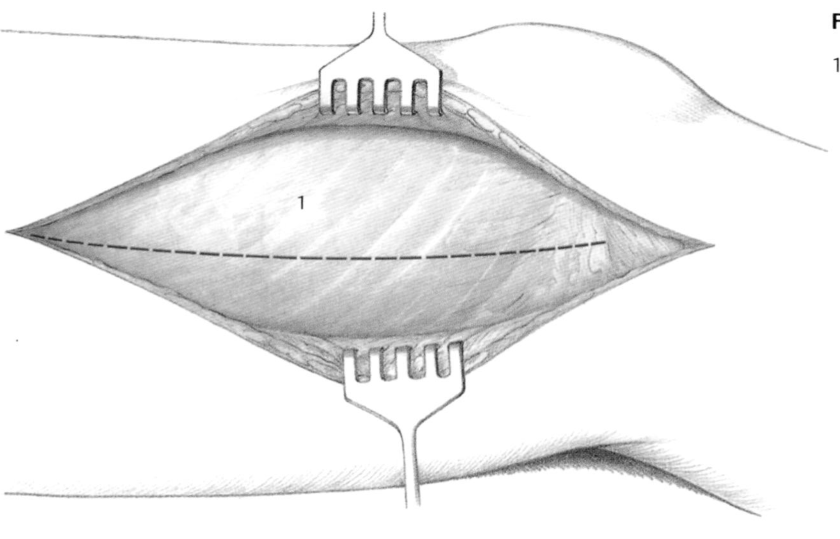

Fig. 10.27 Splitting of the fascia over vastus medialis.

1 Vastus medialis

Fig. 10.28 Detachment of vastus medialis from the medial femoral intermuscular septum.

1 Vastus medialis

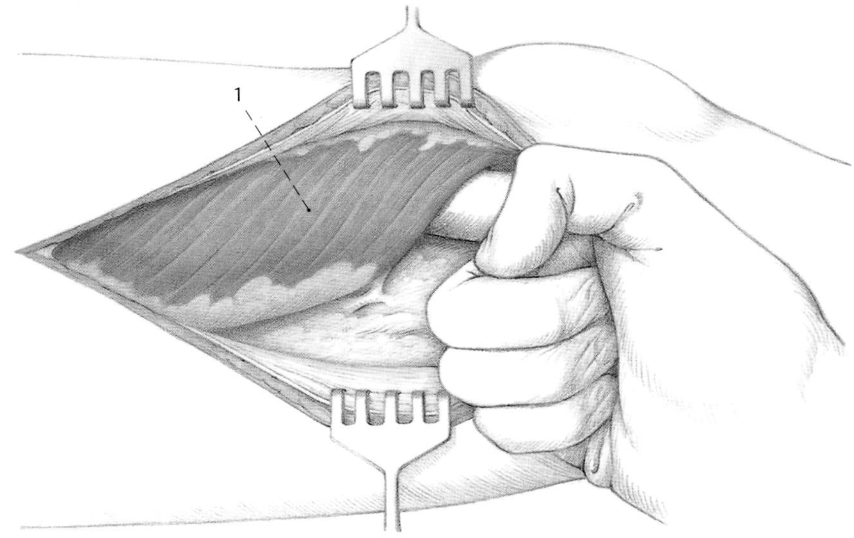

Fig. 10.29 Dissection of vastus medialis from the bone, and placement of a Hohmann elevator.

1 Vastus medialis
2 Tendon of adductor magnus
3 Body of femur
4 Descending genicular artery, muscular branches

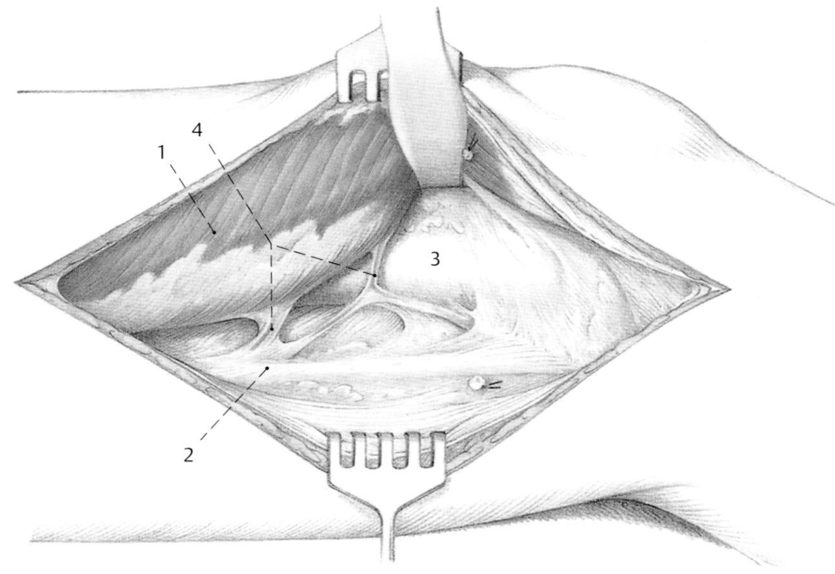

Fig. 10.30 Operative site following ligation of the muscular branches of the descending genicular artery.

1 Vastus medialis
2 Tendon of adductor magnus
3 Body of femur
4 Descending genicular artery, muscular branches

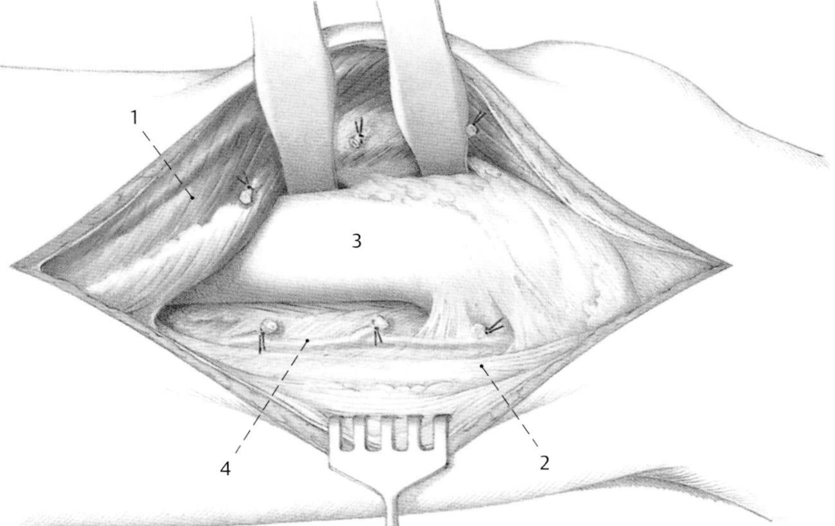

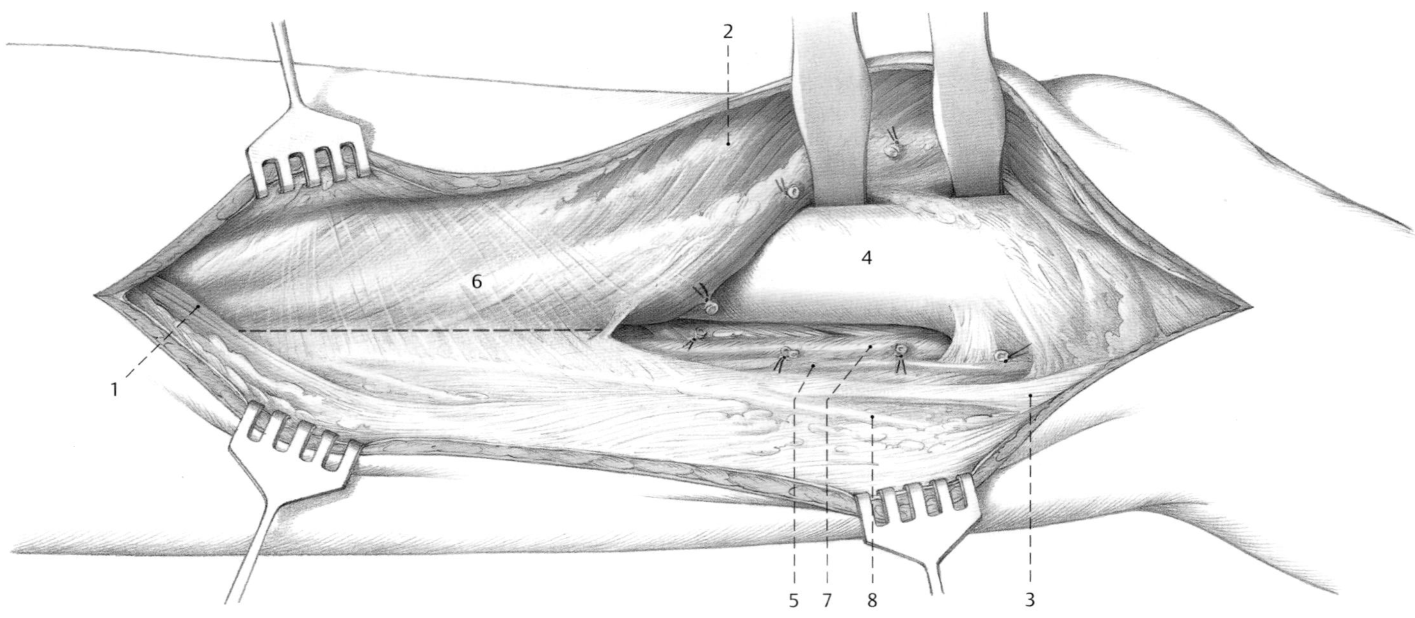

Fig. 10.31 Splitting of the vastoadductor membrane for exposure of the middle third of the shaft.

1 Sartorius
2 Vastus medialis
3 Tendon of adductor magnus
4 Body of femur
5 Descending genicular artery
6 Vastoadductor membrane
7 Femoral vessels
8 Saphenous nerve

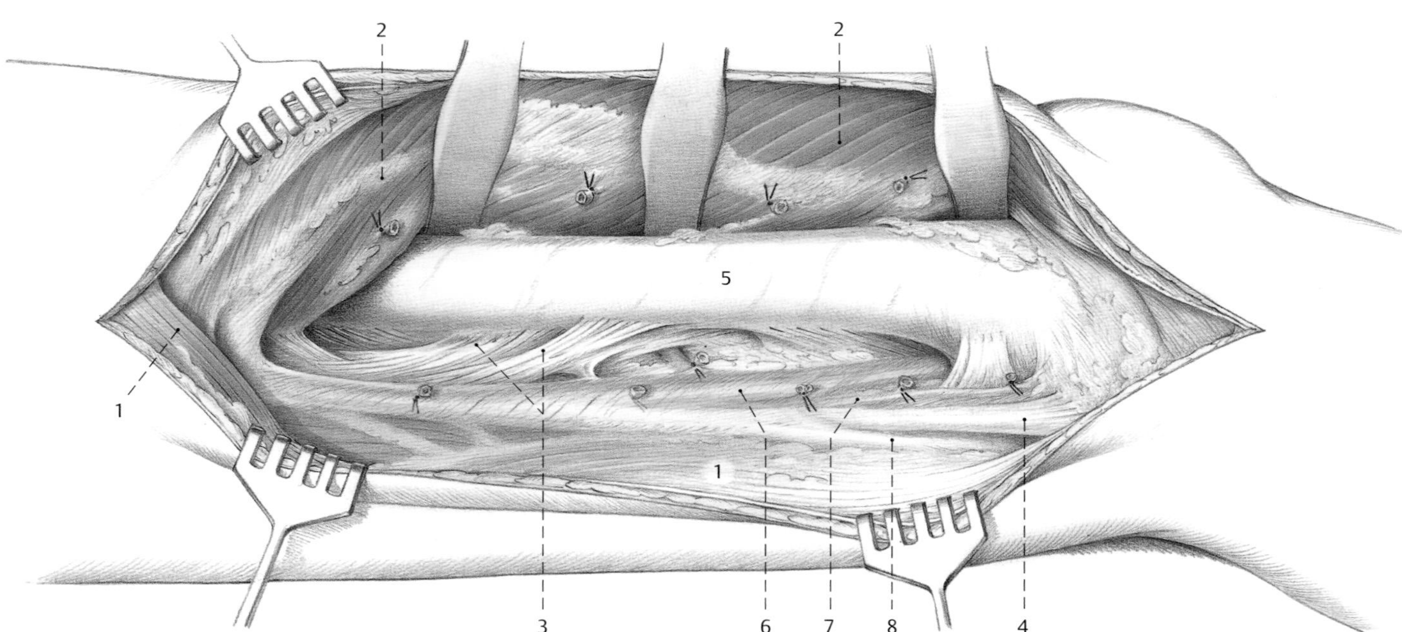

Fig. 10.32 Exposure of the middle and distal thirds of the femoral shaft from medially after ligation and transection of the muscular branches of the femoral artery.

1 Sartorius
2 Vastus medialis
3 Tendon of adductor longus
4 Tendon of adductor magnus
5 Body of femur
6 Femoral vessels
7 Descending genicular artery
8 Saphenous nerve

10.5.4 Extension of the Approach

This approach can be extended distally by lengthening the skin incision analogously to a medial parapatellar incision (**Fig. 11.8**).

Extension of the approach in a proximal direction is not recommended as the branches of the femoral nerve and the deep femoral artery and vein hinder access to the bone. If conditions warrant, sartorius may be stripped off its fascia and reflected upward anteriorly to expose the transition from the middle to the proximal third of the shaft.

10.5.5 Anatomical Site

In **Fig. 10.33**, the tendinous attachment of adductor longus to the femur has been detached to expose the course of the deep femoral artery and vein, and their relation to the femur. Generally, two nutrient arteries that supply the femur at the junction of the proximal and middle thirds and the junction of the middle and distal thirds at the linea aspera arise from the deep femoral artery. The three perforating arteries pass through the lateral femoral intermuscular septum of the femur and supply the vastus lateralis.

To expose the femoral vessels and the saphenous nerve, the vastoadductor membrane and the perivascular sheath have been removed. Note that the saphenous nerve and the descending genicular artery pierce the vastoadductor membrane. In dissecting vastus medialis, attention must be paid to the muscular branch of the femoral nerve that supplies it.

10.5.6 Wound Closure

Muscle sutures are unnecessary in the medial approach to the femur unless parts of the adductor muscles have been detached. Loose closure of the fascia generally suffices.

10.5.7 Dangers

Lack of caution in performing the dissection can cause damage to the saphenous nerve and the femoral or popliteal vessels in the distal wound region.

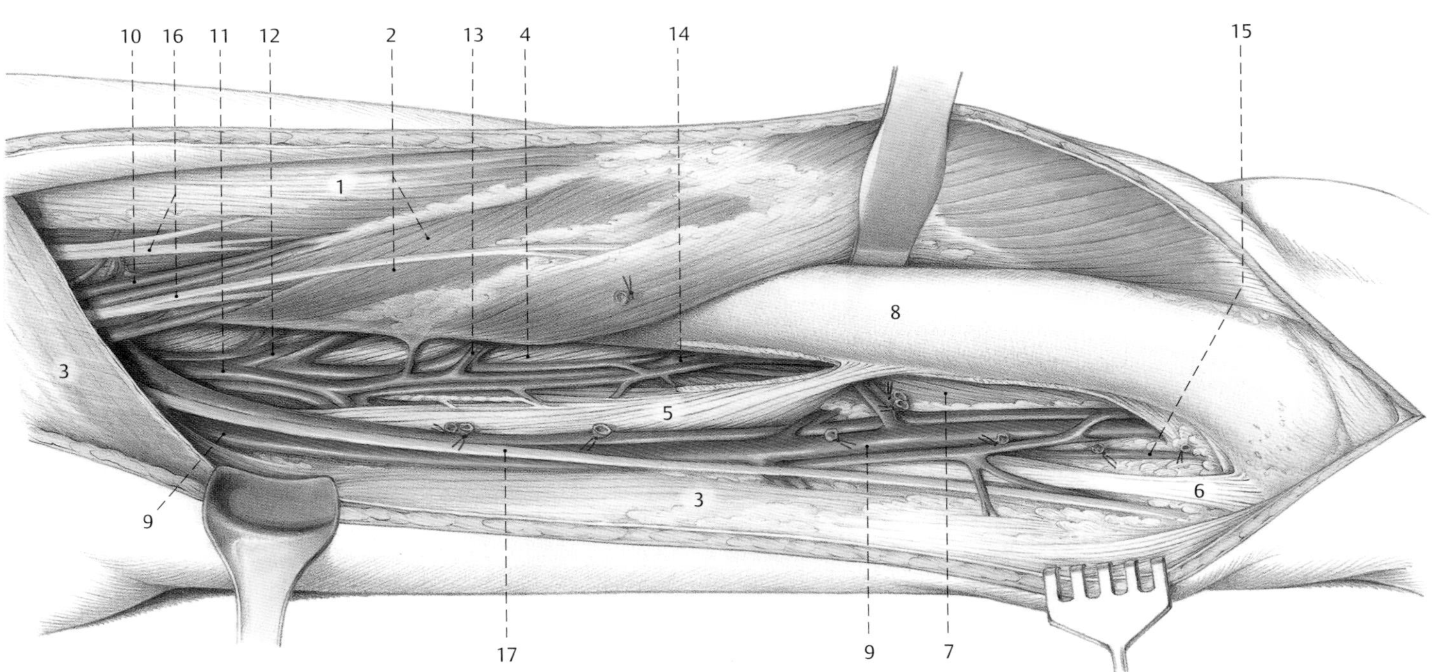

Fig. 10.33 Anatomical site of the left femur, medial view.

1 Rectus femoris
2 Vastus medialis
3 Sartorius
4 Adductor brevis
5 Adductor longus
6 Tendon of adductor magnus
7 Biceps femoris, short head
8 Body of femur
9 Femoral artery
10 Descending branch of the lateral circumflex femoral artery
11 Deep femoral artery
12 Perforating artery I
13 Perforating artery II
14 Perforating artery III
15 Descending genicular artery
16 Muscular branches of femoral nerve
17 Saphenous nerve

10.6 Posterior Approach to Femur

R. Bauer, F. Kerschbaumer, S. Poisel

10.6.1 Principal Indications

- Fractures with injury to the sciatic nerve
- Tumors

10.6.2 Positioning and Incision

The patient is placed in the prone position with the leg draped to allow free movement.

The skin incision is begun two fingerbreadths proximal to the gluteal fold and continued to the middle of the popliteal fossa (**Fig. 10.34**).

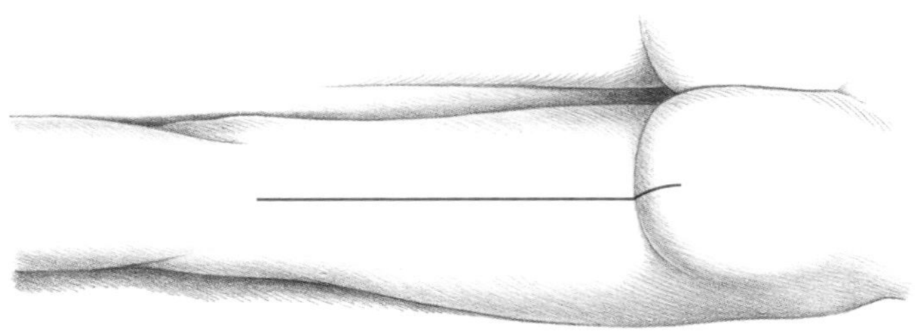

Fig. 10.34 Posterior approach to the femur (right leg). Positioning and incision.

10.6.3 Exposure of the Proximal and Middle Thirds of the Femoral Shaft

Following incision of the skin and subcutaneous tissue, the lateral skin flap is freed to some extent from the fascia. Then the fascia is split laterally to the posterior femoral cutaneous nerve (**Fig. 10.35**). The long head of the biceps is mobilized and retracted medially. Close to the lateral border of the fascia, the short head of the biceps is now also moved away from the more anteriorly situated lateral femoral intermuscular septum (**Fig. 10.36**). The muscular branch of the common peroneal nerve, which supplies the short head of the biceps, should be spared.

Now the periosteum between the lateral femoral intermuscular septum and the origin of the short head of the biceps is incised in the area of the linea aspera. Using a raspatory, the bone is now exposed subperiosteally, dissecting from lateral to medial. In the process, portions of the adductor magnus are also detached from the middle femur. Perforating vessels have to be ligated and transected (**Fig. 10.37**). After insertion of Hohmann elevators, the proximal and middle portions of the femur are exposed posteriorly.

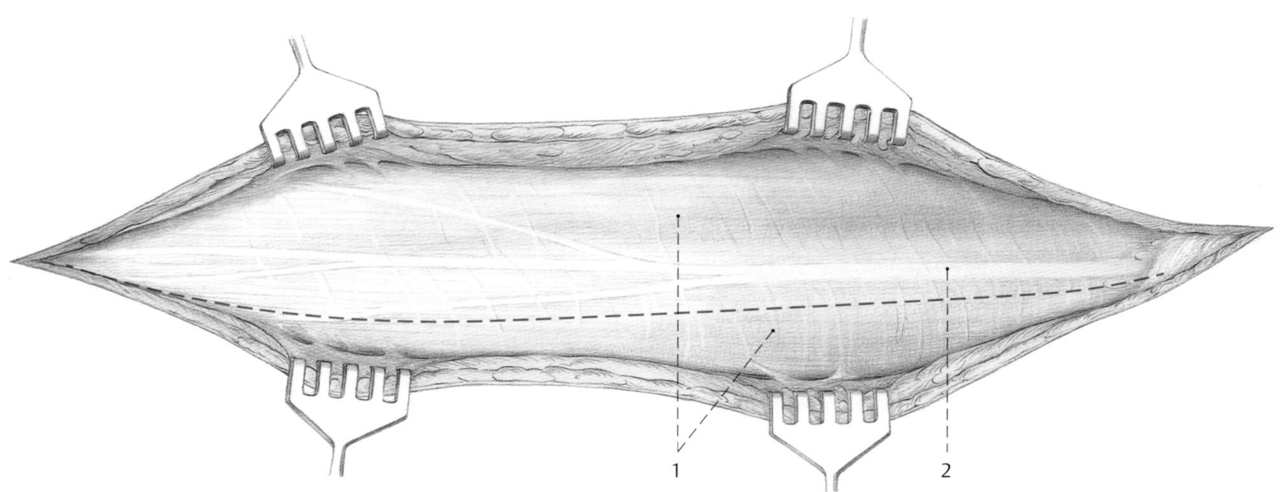

Fig. 10.35 Exposure of the proximal and middle thirds of the shaft. Incision of the fascia lateral to the posterior femoral cutaneous nerve.

1 Fascia lata
2 Posterior femoral cutaneous nerve

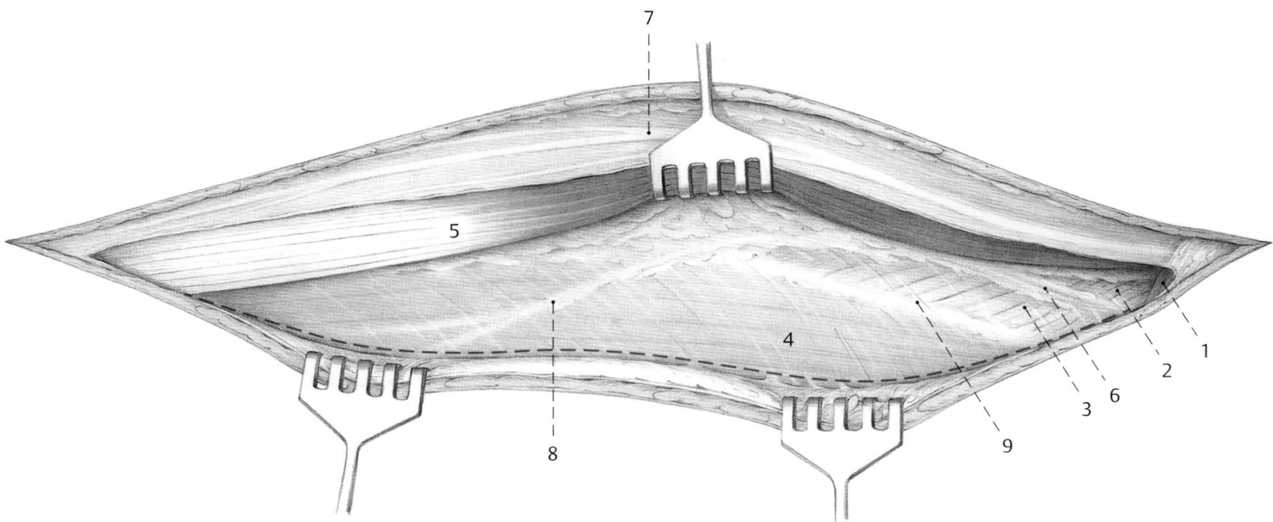

Fig. 10.36 Retraction of the long head of biceps in a medial direction, and detachment of the short head of biceps from the lateral femoral intermuscular septum along the dashed line.

1 Gluteus maximus
2 Adductor minimus
3 Adductor magnus
4 Biceps femoris, short head
5 Biceps femoris, long head
6 Perforating artery and vein I
7 Posterior femoral cutaneous nerve
8 Muscular branch of the common peroneal nerve
9 Linea aspera

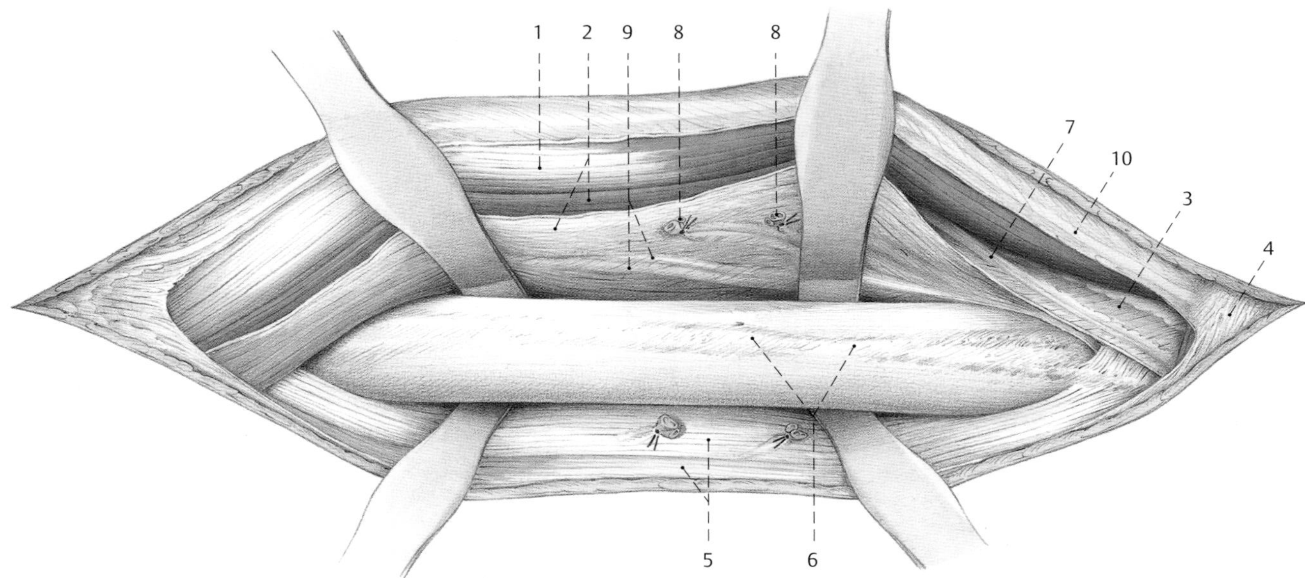

Fig. 10.37 Posterior exposure of the proximal and middle thirds of the femur after detachment of the short head of biceps and the adductor magnus muscle from the linea aspera.

1 Biceps femoris, long head
2 Biceps femoris, short head
3 Adductor minimus
4 Gluteus maximus
5 Vastus lateralis
6 Linea aspera
7 Perforating vessels I
8 Perforating vessels II
9 Perforating vessels III
10 Posterior femoral cutaneous nerve

10.6.4 Anatomical Site

Figure 10.38 shows the course of the deep femoral artery and vein with the perforating vessels. The origin of the short head of the biceps and the attachment of the adductor magnus are freed from the femur at the linea aspera and retracted medially. A nutrient foramen medial to the linea aspera is clearly visible approximately in the middle of the shaft.

To expose the sciatic nerve and the upper portions of the deep artery of the thigh, the gluteus maximus, quadratus femoris, and adductor minimus and pectineus have been split.

10.6.5 Exposure of the Sciatic Nerve

In the event that the sciatic nerve needs to be exposed, or exposure of the distal third of the femur from the posterior side is required, the fascia is split medially to the posterior femoral cutaneous nerve (**Fig. 10.39**). The fascia is then retracted, and the layer between the long head of the biceps laterally and the semitendinosus medially is identified. Both muscle bellies are digitally separated and retracted medially and laterally (**Fig. 10.40**). The sciatic nerve is covered by a fascia-like band that runs between the muscle bellies of semimembranosus and biceps. After splitting of this fascia and retraction of semimembranosus in a medial direction, the sciatic nerve becomes visible. The bifurcation of the nerve is already clearly discernible in the middle and distal areas of the shaft (**Fig. 10.41**).

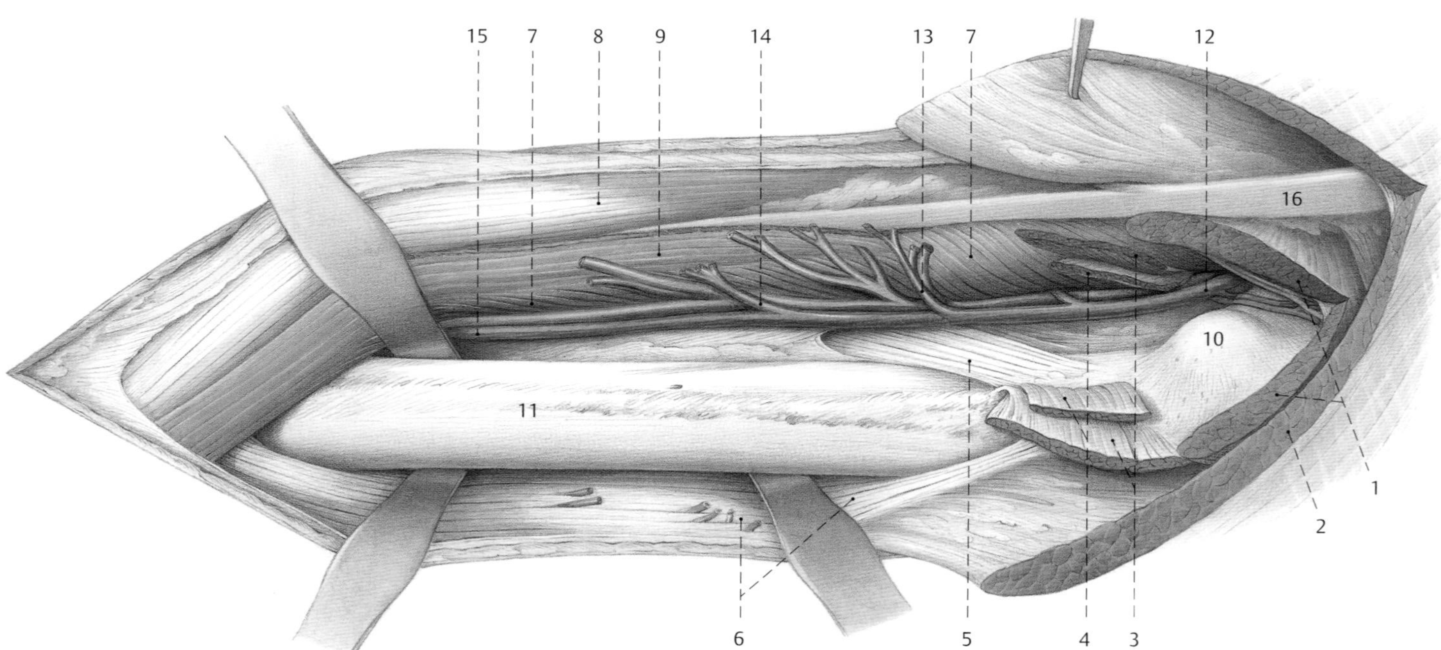

Fig. 10.38 Anatomical site of the proximal and middle thirds of the femur, posterior view. The short head of biceps and the adductor magnus have been stripped off the bone and medially retracted. Gluteus maximus, quadratus femoris, adductor minimus, and pectineus have been split.

1 Quadratus femoris
2 Gluteus maximus
3 Adductor minimus
4 Pectineus
5 Vastus medialis
6 Vastus lateralis
7 Adductor magnus
8 Biceps femoris, long head
9 Biceps femoris, short head
10 Lesser trochanter
11 Body of femur
12 Deep femoral artery
13 Perforating artery I
14 Perforating artery II
15 Perforating artery III
16 Sciatic nerve

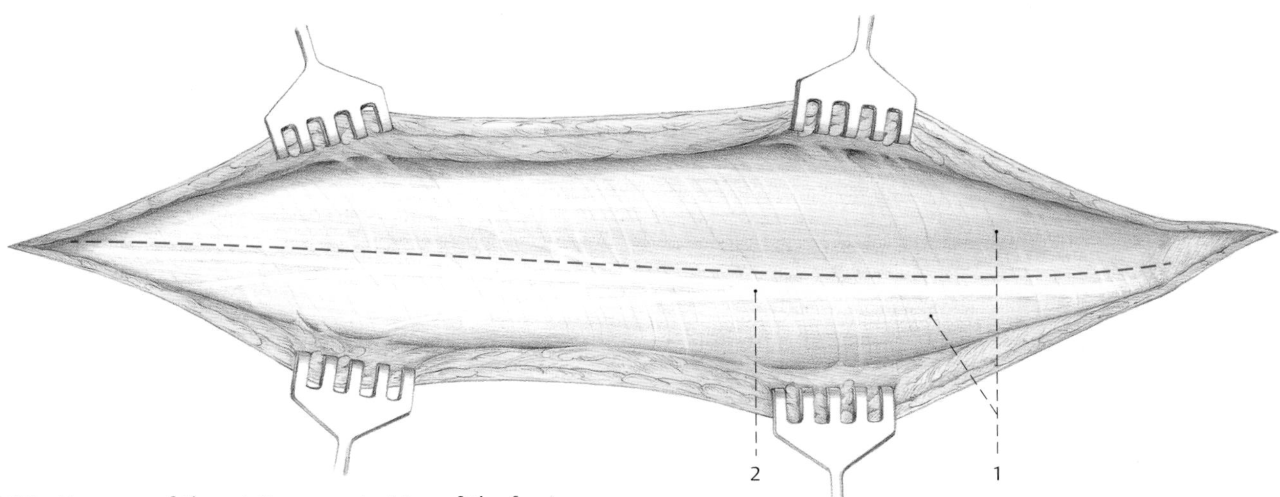

Fig. 10.39 Exposure of the sciatic nerve. Incision of the fascia medial to the posterior femoral cutaneous nerve of the thigh.

1 Fascia lata
2 Posterior femoral cutaneous nerve

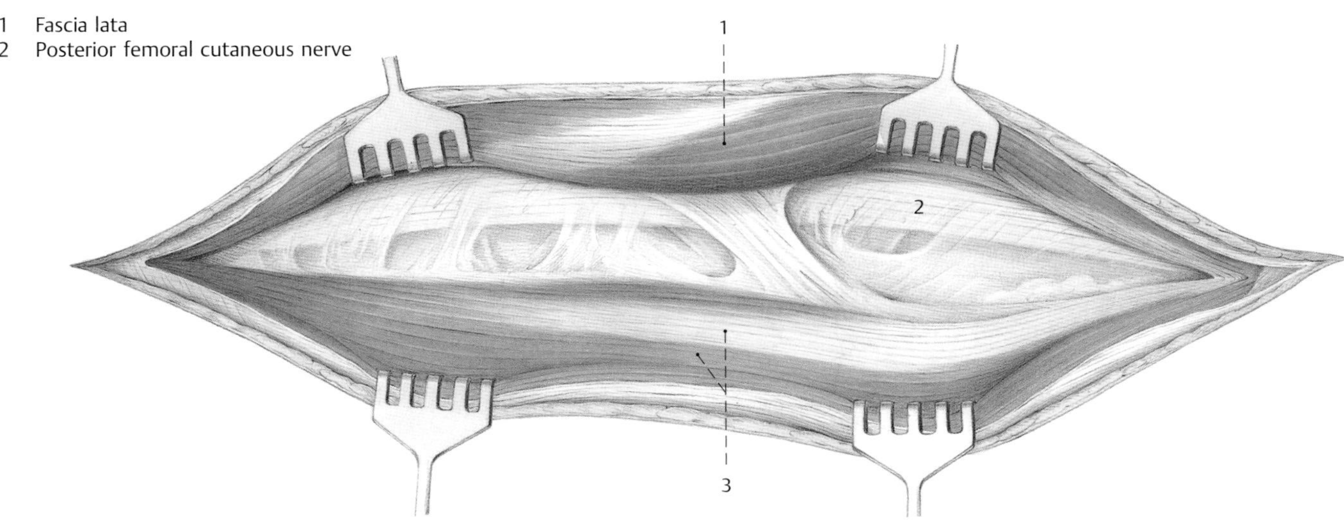

Fig. 10.40 Retraction of semitendinosus in a medial direction, and lateral retraction of the long head of biceps.

1 Semitendinosus
2 Semimembranosus
3 Biceps femoris, long head

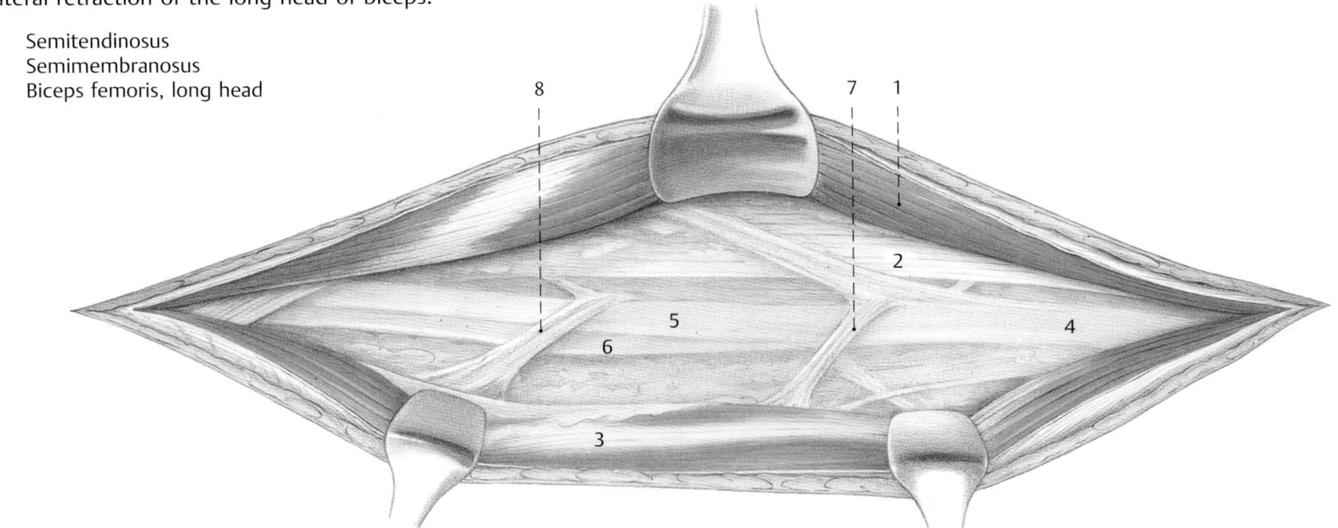

Fig. 10.41 After splitting of the fascia over the sciatic nerve, the semitendinosus and semimembranosus are medially retracted, and the long head of the biceps is retracted laterally.

1 Semitendinosus
2 Semimembranosus
3 Biceps femoris
4 Sciatic nerve
5 Tibial nerve
6 Common peroneal nerve
7 Perforating artery and vein II
8 Perforating artery and vein III

10.6.6 Anatomical Site of the Sciatic Nerve

Figure 10.42 depicts the relation of the sciatic nerve to the ischiocrural muscles, the femur, the femoral vessels, and the adductor magnus. For better exposure of the nerve, the superficial and deep fascia have been removed.

10.6.7 Distal Extension of the Approach

If the distal third of the femur is to be exposed, the sciatic nerve and peroneal nerve are dissected free, snared, and retracted laterally. The periosteum is then incised above the linea aspera between the adductor magnus on one side, and the short head of the biceps on the other. By this means, the distal third of the femoral shaft can be subperiosteally exposed.

10.6.8 Anatomical Site

A schematic cross-section through the distal third of the femur (see **Fig. 10.18**) shows the two possible posterior approaches to the femoral shaft as well as the lateral and medial approaches. For exposure of the proximal third of the femoral shaft from the back, the femoral shaft is accessed between the biceps and the lateral femoral intermuscular septum. For exposure of the distal portions of the femur, on the other hand, the dissection is performed between the two heads of the biceps and the sciatic nerve, as well as between semitendinosus and semimembranosus.

10.6.9 Wound Closure

Wound closure presents no problem; suture of the muscle is not necessary.

10.6.10 Note

A disadvantage of the posterior approach to the femur is the need for subperiosteal exposure of the linea aspera, which requires detachment of the nutrient arteries of the bone. This approach should therefore be used only in exceptional cases.

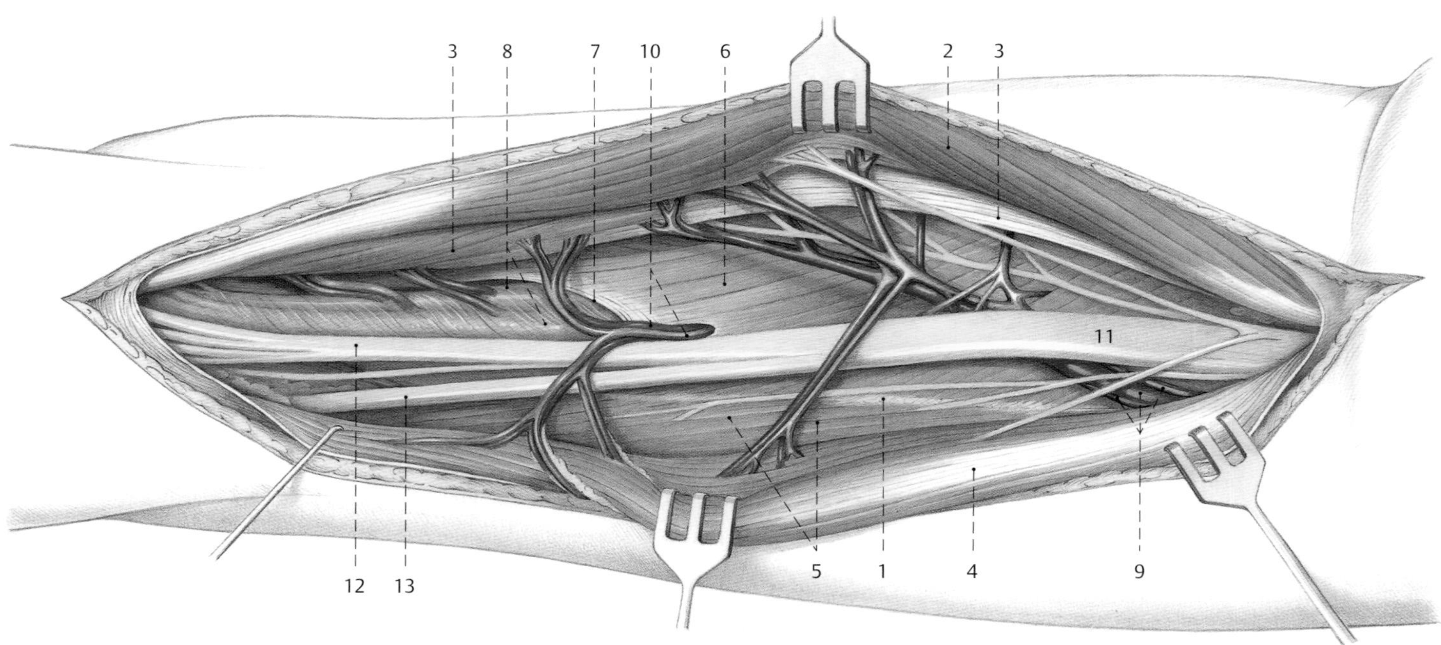

Fig. 10.42 Anatomical site of the posterior femoral region. The superficial and deep fasciae and the perineural tissue have been removed.

1 Linea aspera
2 Semitendinosus
3 Semimembranosus
4 Biceps femoris, long head
5 Biceps femoris, short head
6 Adductor magnus
7 Adductor hiatus
8 Popliteal vessels
9 Perforating artery and vein II
10 Perforating artery and vein III
11 Sciatic nerve
12 Tibial nerve
13 Common peroneal nerve

10.7 Transarticular Medullary Cavity Approach to the Distal Femur

K. Weise, D. Höntzsch

10.7.1 Principal Indications

- Retrograde medullary nailing of the femur
- Fractures
- Pseudarthrosis

10.7.2 Positioning and Incision

The patient is placed in the supine position. The knee must be flexed by 60–80° (no more and no less) by allowing the leg to hang down.

The tip of the patella must not block the entry channel when the knee is flexed, which would be the case with 90° flexion. With flexion of less than 60°, the desired entry point and in particular the desired direction of entry cannot be obtained.

The skin is incised over the center of the patellar tendon (**Fig. 10.43**).

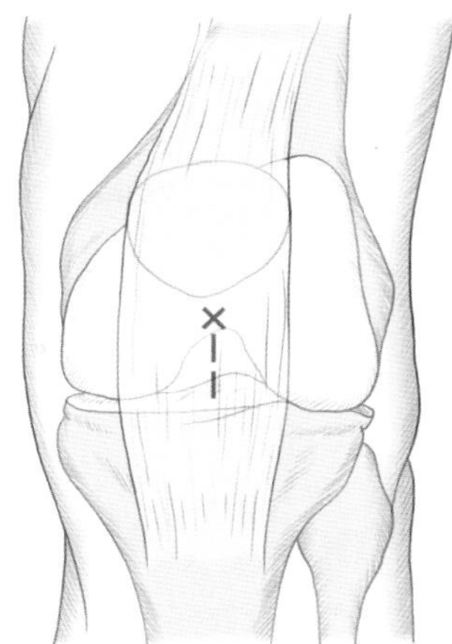

Fig. 10.43 Longitudinal incision over the patellar ligament.

10.7.3 Exposure of the Distal Entry Site to the Femoral Canal

The subcutaneous tissue is split down to the patellar tendon (**Fig. 10.44**).

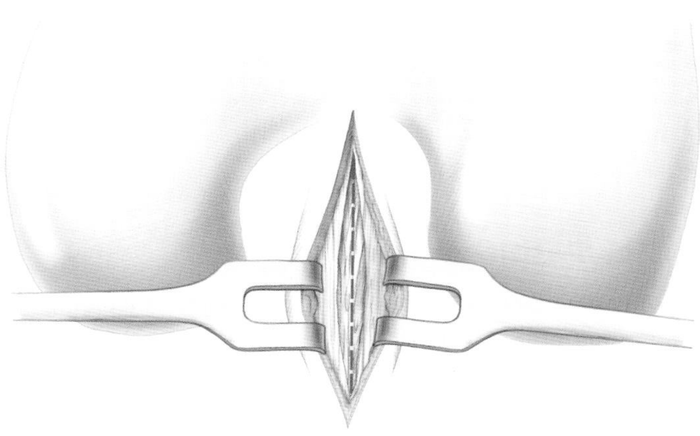

Fig. 10.44 Longitudinal incision of the subcutaneous tissue down to the patellar ligament.

The patellar ligament is then split through all layers over the entire length of the skin incision and a little beyond it from the distal tip of the patella to above its insertion onto the tibial tuberosity. The patellar ligament is retracted with Langenbeck retractors to allow tension-free instrumentation (**Fig. 10.45**). The entry point is usually broached over a guidewire, and this is then inserted centrally in the long axis of the femoral canal. The entry point is exactly in the notch in front of the insertion of the cruciate ligaments and posterior to the margin of the joint surface. The entry point and direction are usually determined and checked with the image converter.

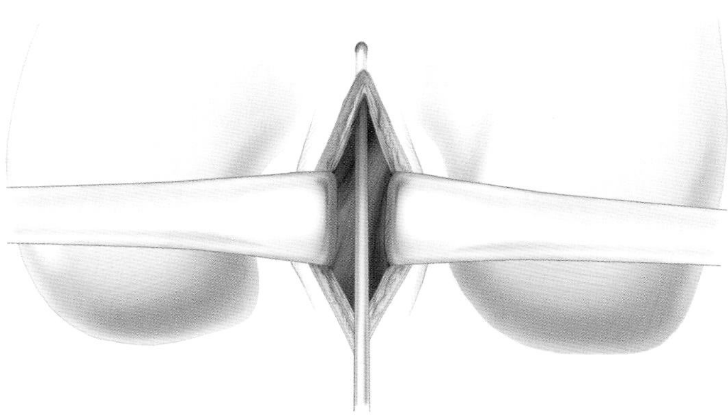

Fig. 10.45 The patellar ligament is split and retracted with Langenbeck retractors as required by the instruments being used. A proximally directed guidewire is inserted at the correct entry point in the central axis of the medullary canal.

10.7.4 Wound Closure

Suture of the patellar ligament through all layers, subcutaneous suture, and skin suture are carried out.

11 Knee

11.1 Anteromedial Minimally Invasive Approaches to the Knee Joint

C. J. Wirth

11.1.1 Principal Indications

- Medial hemiarthroplasty
- Allo-arthroplasty
- Intra-articular fractures
- Partial synovectomy

11.1.2 Positioning and Incision

The patient is placed in the supine position. After optional application of a tourniquet as far proximally on the thigh as possible, the leg is draped to allow free movement. The longitudinal parapatellar incision begins at the tibial tuberosity and runs in a slight curve along the medial border of the patellar ligament to the proximal pole of the patella (**Fig. 11.1**). After flexing the knee to approximately 30°, the subcutaneous tissue is divided. The medial retinaculum and fascia over vastus medialis are exposed parallel to the skin incision (**Fig. 11.2**).

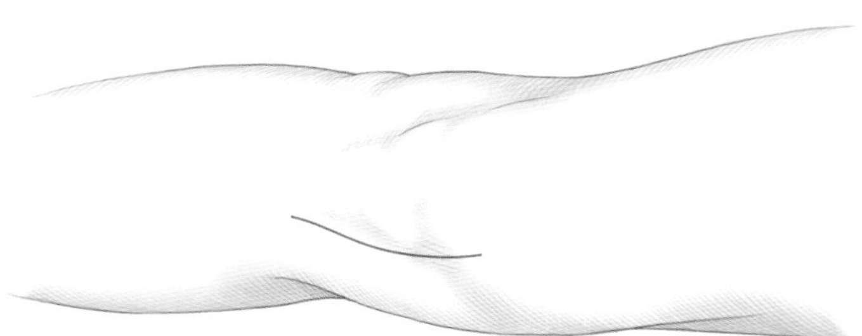

Fig. 11.1 Minimally invasive anteromedial approach to the knee joint. The skin incision is made proximally from the tibial tuberosity to the medial pole of the patella (right knee).

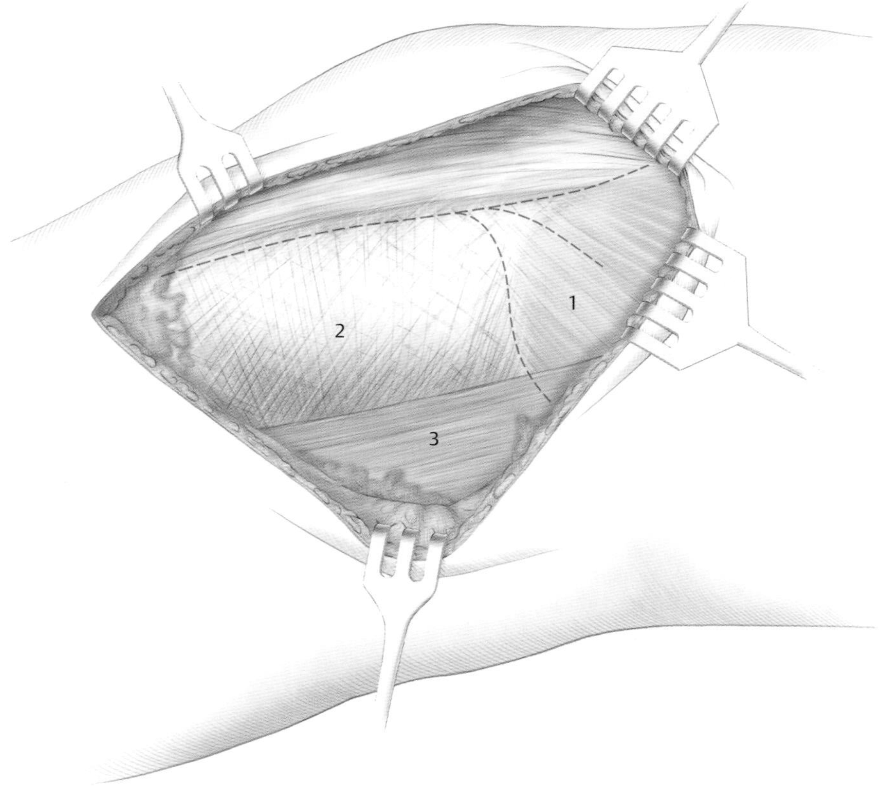

Fig. 11.2 Division of the retinaculum medial to the patella and patellar ligament. In the subvastus approach, the incision in the retinaculum turns in a right angle on the lower border of vastus medialis toward the intermuscular septum. In the midvastus approach, the incision in the retinaculum extends to the middle of the muscle insertion on the proximal medial pole of the patella, and as far as the quadriceps tendon in the case of a quadriceps-sparing approach.

1 Vastus medialis
2 Medial patellar retinaculum
3 Sartorius

In the **mini subvastus approach**, a right-angled incision is made in the medial retinaculum distal to the vastus medialis tendon, with one limb of the incision extending to the medial tibial plateau medial to the patella and patellar tendon, and the other running at the lower border of the vastus medialis toward the intermuscular septum. There, the muscle is dissected bluntly from the septum and the underlying joint capsule (**Fig. 11.3**).

The **mini midvastus approach** involves splitting the vastus medialis where it meets the patella (**Fig. 11.4**). The transverse incision begins at the proximal medial pole of the patella. Fascia and muscle are divided in the line of their fibers over a distance of 2–4 cm to avoid denervation of the distal part of the muscle.

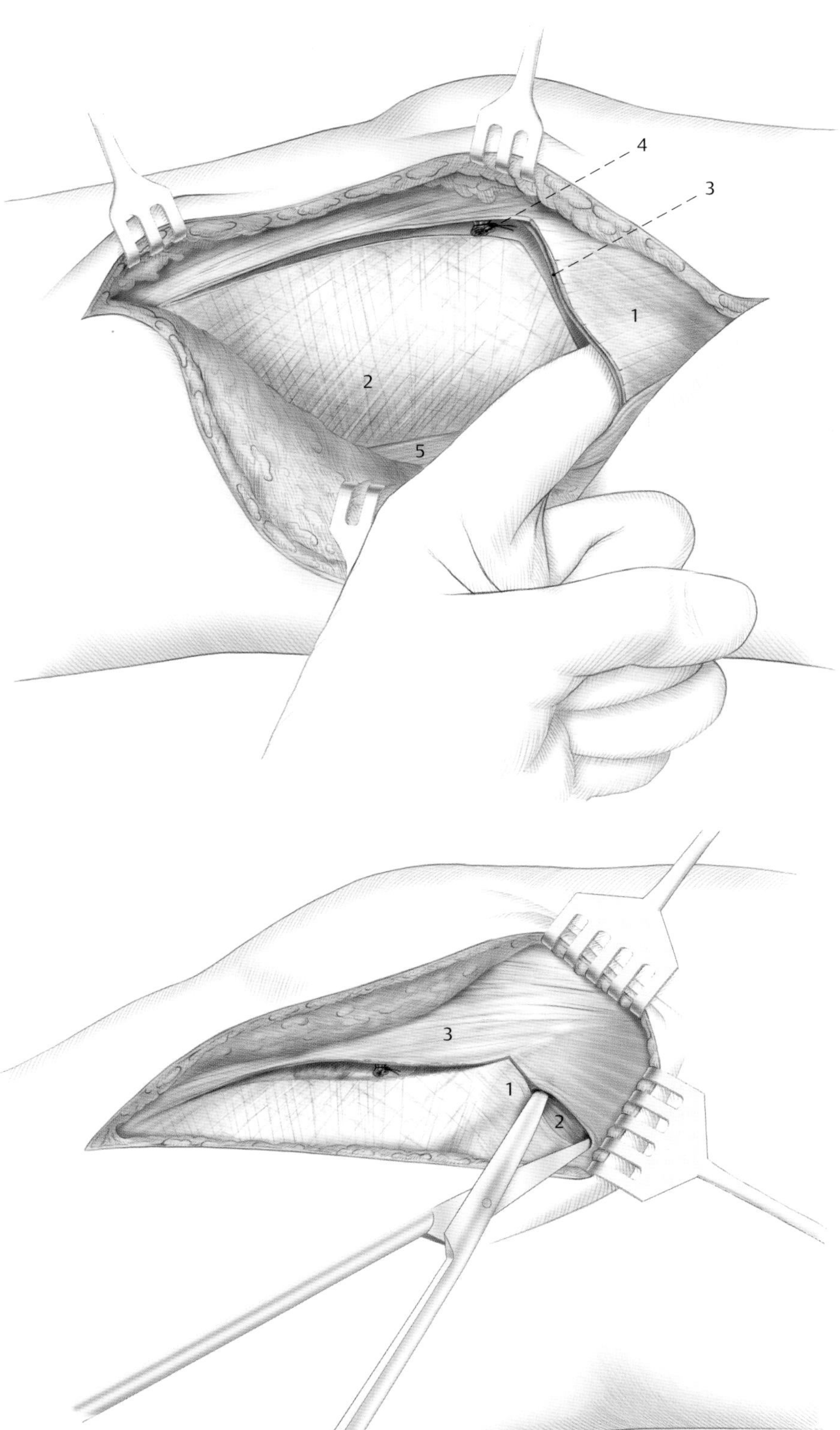

Fig. 11.3 Subvastus approach. The vastus medialis is divided at its lower border and dissected bluntly off the intermuscular septum and joint capsule (beware the femoral artery and vein in the adductor canal). Side branches of the superior medial genicular artery and vein are ligated.

1 Vastus medialis
2 Medial patellar retinaculum
3 Joint capsule
4 Branches of the superior medial genicular artery and vein
5 Sartorius

Fig. 11.4 Midvastus approach. Splitting of the transverse part of the vastus medialis tendon at the level of the proximal medial pole of the patella. Division of the muscle fascia and splitting of the muscle belly in the line of their fibers as far as the joint capsule over a distance of 2–4 cm.

1 Fascia
2 Vastus medialis
3 Longitudinal medial patellar retinaculum

The **quadriceps-sparing approach** is a parapatellar approach that ends at the proximal medial pole of the patella and can be extended as far as the quadriceps tendon if necessary. As in the midvastus approach, the transverse insertion of the vastus medialis muscle is divided from the medial border of the patella as far as its proximal pole (**Fig. 11.5**).

The joint capsule is split in a proximal direction beneath the vastus medialis muscle as far as the suprapatellar recess (**Fig. 11.6**). To expose the joint, the patella can be lateralized (not everted) with the attached vastus medialis.

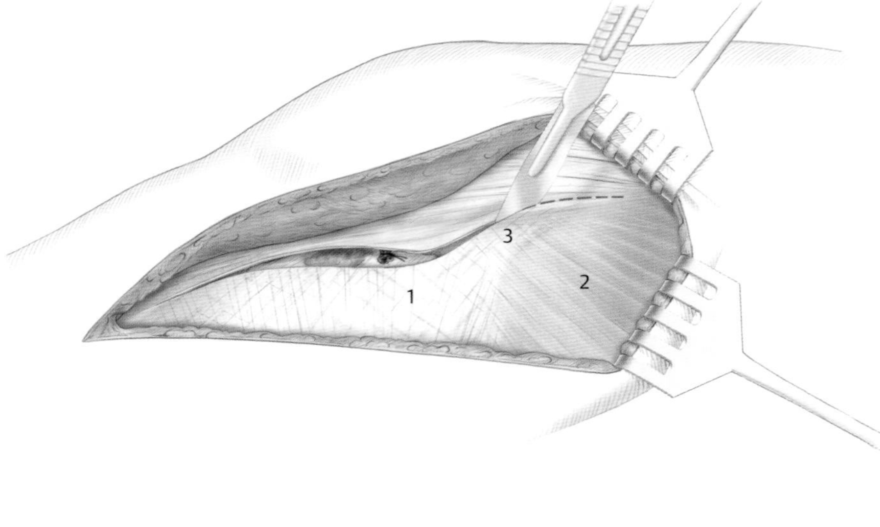

Fig. 11.5 Quadriceps-sparing approach. The incision in the retinaculum runs along the medial border of the patellar tendon and patella to the level of the proximal medial patellar pole. Vastus medialis is not incised.

1 Fascia
2 Vastus medialis
3 Longitudinal medial patellar retinaculum

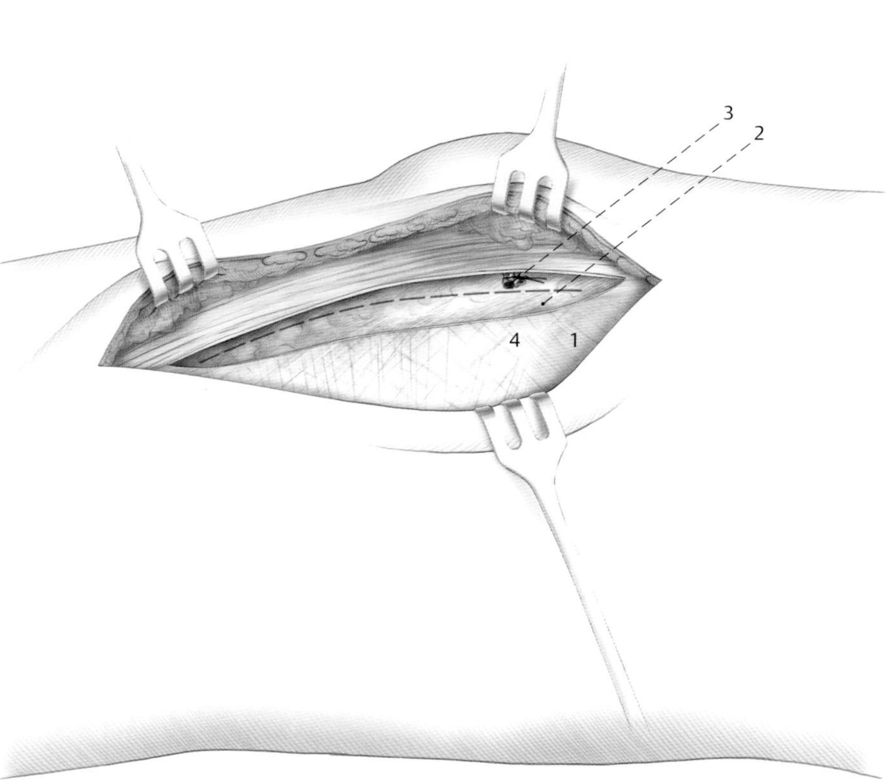

Fig. 11.6 Opening of the knee joint capsule in a longitudinal direction parallel to the split in the retinaculum.

1 Vastus medialis
2 Joint capsule
3 Branches of the superior medial genicular artery and vein
4 Medial patellar retinaculum

11.1.3 Exposure of the Knee Joint

No further dissection is required for exposure of the medial joint compartment. The tibial plateau and femoral condyle are readily accessible by moving the soft tissue window with the knee in various degrees of flexion.

If the entire joint is to be visualized, the tibial plateau is exposed subperiosteally from the medial side, proximal to the tibial tuberosity. Hoffa's infrapatellar fat pad and the deep infrapatellar bursa remain attached to the patellar ligament. This allows the patella to be moved laterally without tension with reduced knee flexion. Two Langenbeck retractors are now inserted laterally, the tips of which are supported on the lateral femoral condyle. They hold the patella in a lateralized position while the knee is flexed cautiously to 70–80° (**Fig. 11.7**). This tenses the vastus medialis increasingly over the distal femur, and vastus medialis can tear if the knee is flexed with excessive force, especially with the midvastus approach.

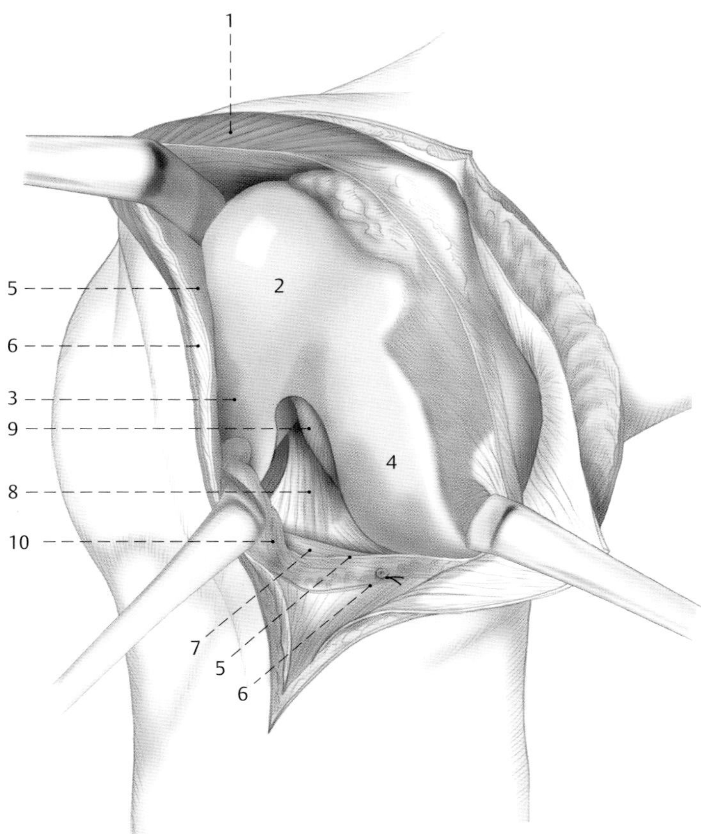

Fig. 11.7 After placing Langenbeck retractors in the suprapatellar recess and behind Hoffa's infrapatellar fat pad, the patella is retracted laterally (not everted) with the knee extended, and the knee is then flexed. To expose the medial femoral condyle, another Langenbeck retractor is placed below the medial collateral ligament.

1 Vastus medialis
2 Patellar surface of the femur
3 Lateral femoral condyle
4 Medial femoral condyle
5 Joint capsule, synovial membrane
6 Joint capsule, fibrous membrane
7 Medial meniscus
8 Anterior cruciate ligament
9 Posterior cruciate ligament
10 Hoffa's infrapatellar fat pad

11.1.4 Wound Closure

Hemostasis is ensured after release of the tourniquet. The joint capsule and divided retinaculum are sutured. In the midvastus approach, the superficial muscle fibers and the muscle fascia are also sutured.

11.1.5 Note

In the minimally invasive approaches, the connection between the quadriceps tendon and vastus medialis is always preserved. This avoids the patella's tendency to postoperative lateralization, and quadriceps function is maintained. During flexion and extension, the joint incision moves proximally or distally like a mobile window, depending on which part of the joint is to be exposed.

In principle, the quadriceps-sparing approach is the least traumatic for the muscles but can be used only in thin patients.

If a bicondylar knee prosthesis is to be inserted via the minimally invasive approach, smaller instruments are required. In the case of contracted knees, greater axial misalignment, muscular or obese patients, or revision surgery, it is advisable to extend the incision to the conventional anteromedial parapatellar approach (**Fig. 11.8**).

11.2 Anteromedial Parapatellar Approach

R. Bauer, F. Kerschbaumer, S. Poisel, C. J. Wirth

11.2.1 Principal Indications

- Allo-arthroplasty
- Synovectomy
- Arthrodesis
- Extension of minimally invasive approaches

11.2.2 Positioning and Incision

The patient is placed in the supine position with the leg extended and draped to allow free movement. The skin incision begins 5 cm proximal to the superior border of the patella, approximately in the center, curves distally 1 cm medial to the medial border of the patella, and then runs to the tibial tuberosity medial to the patellar ligament.

If exposure of the pes anserinus or medial collateral ligament is required, the skin incision may be extended for another 5 cm distally (**Fig. 11.8**). The subcutaneous tissue is now dissected anteriorly and posteriorly, after which the infrapatellar branch of the saphenous nerve is identified (**Fig. 11.9**).

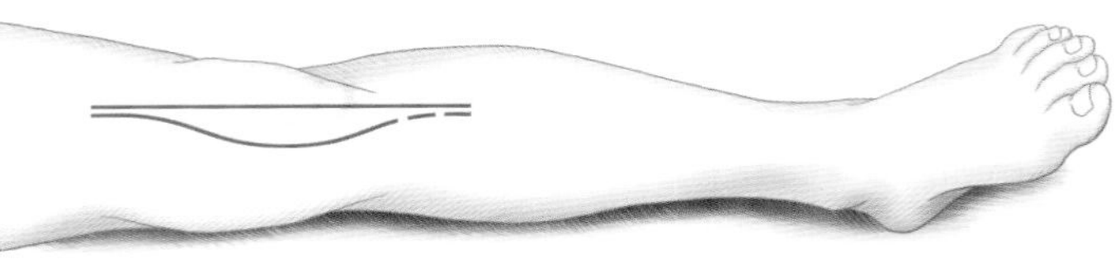

Fig. 11.8 Medial parapatellar approach. The skin incision can curve medial to the patella or run longitudinally over the patella (left knee). It may be extended to expose the pes anserinus and medial capsular and ligamentous apparatus.

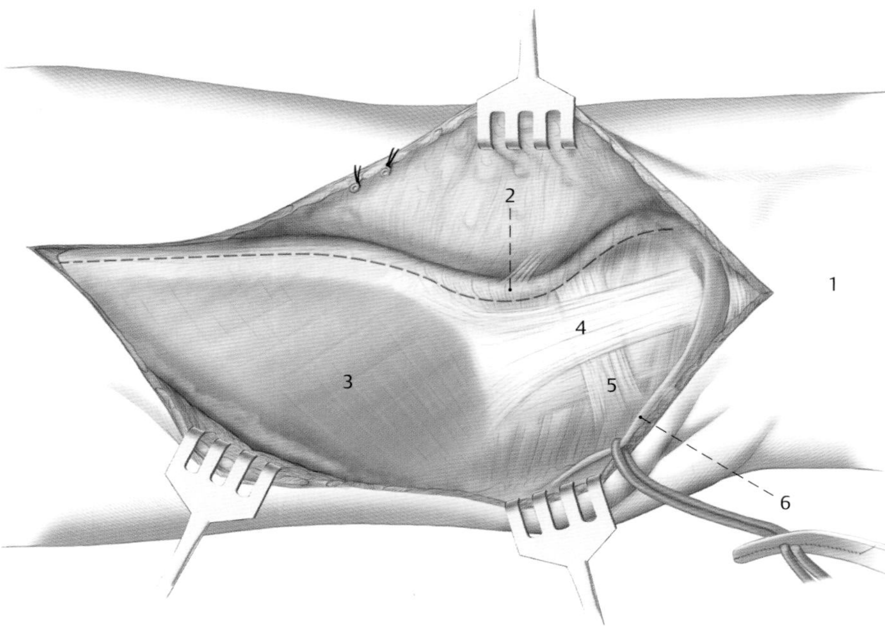

Fig. 11.9 Snaring of the infrapatellar branch of the saphenous nerve. Incision of the medial patellar retinaculum and quadriceps tendon.

1 Tibial tuberosity
2 Patella
3 Vastus medialis
4 Longitudinal medial patellar retinaculum
5 Transverse medial patellar retinaculum
6 Infrapatellar branch of the saphenous nerve

11.2.3 Exposure of the Knee Joint

The medial patellar retinaculum is incised 2 cm medial to the border of the patella. The joint capsule is then bluntly dissected from the retinaculum and the quadriceps tendon with scissors (**Fig. 11.10**). A stay suture is placed in the extensor apparatus of the knee joint at the level of the proximal border of the patella to allow for proper closure of the retinacula. The quadriceps tendon is then split several millimeters lateral to the insertion of vastus medialis. The joint capsule is opened about 2 cm proximal to the medial joint cavity. When dividing the synovial joint capsule distally, account has to be taken of the insertion of the anterior horn of the meniscus (**Fig. 11.11**). The patella can now be retracted laterally and rotated by 180°. If dislocation and rotation of the patella in a lateral direction are not possible, the incision of the quadriceps tendon and the joint capsule should be extended further proximally. In repeat operations, it occasionally proves necessary to detach scar tissue in the area of Hoffa's infrapatellar fat pad and the lateral joint capsule to make complete dislocation and rotation of the patella possible. Then the knee is flexed to 90°, which permits clear exposure of the medial and lateral femoral condyle, the

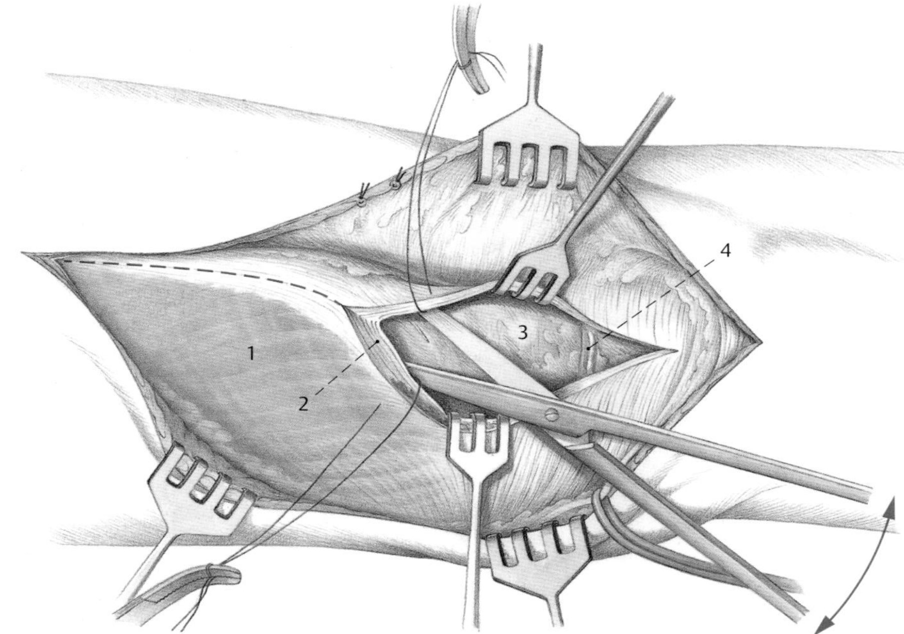

Fig. 11.10 Dissection of the knee joint capsule beneath vastus medialis and the quadriceps tendon. The insertion of vastus medialis is identified by means of stay sutures. Division of the quadriceps tendon is made in a proximal direction.

1 Vastus medialis
2 Tendon of quadriceps
3 Joint capsule, synovial membrane
4 Medial superior genicular artery and vein

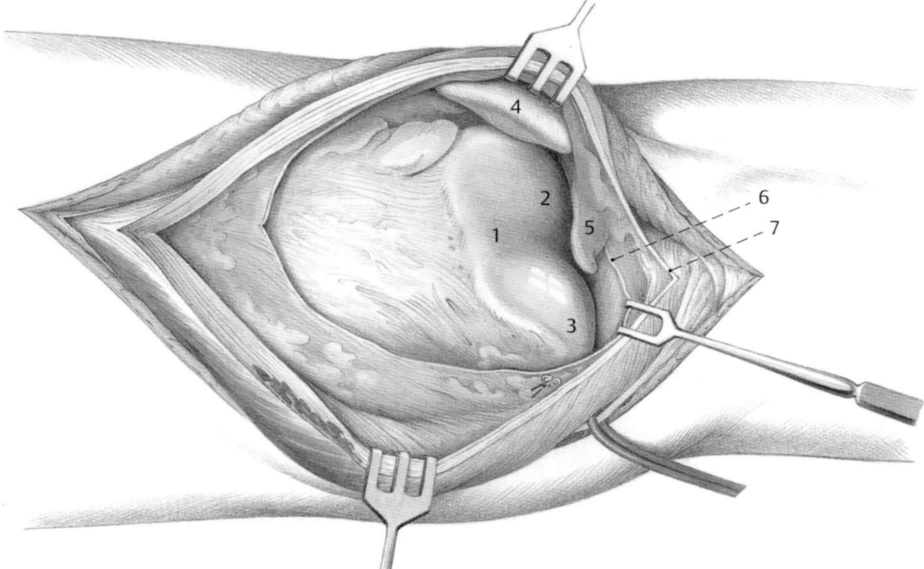

Fig. 11.11 Operative site after opening of the knee joint capsule and lateral displacement of the patella; extended knee joint.

1 Patellar surface of the femur
2 Lateral condyle of the femur
3 Medial condyle of the femur
4 Patella
5 Hoffa's infrapatellar fat pad
6 Joint capsule, synovial membrane
7 Joint capsule, fibrous membrane

intercondylar fossa with both cruciate ligaments, the medial and lateral meniscus, and the tibial plateau (**Fig. 11.12**).

11.2.4 Extension of the Approach

To expose the pes anserinus as well as the medial joint capsule as far as the semimembranosus corner, the incision is extended 5 cm distally from the tibial tuberosity. The skin incision in the proximal region is the same as for the medial parapatellar approach.

After splitting the subcutaneous tissue, the infrapatellar branch of the saphenous nerve is first identified and retracted with a nerve loop. The medial arthrotomy is typically performed via the retinacula 2 cm medial to the internal border of the patella. Subsequently, the layer below the infrapatellar branch is undermined, the nerve is elevated, and beneath it the fascia and the insertion of the superficial part of the pes anserinus are incised. If necessary, the incision may be extended proximally into the quadriceps tendon (**Fig. 11.13**). The knee joint can now be flexed to 90° by hinging down the operating table. In this position, the fascia with the tendons of the superficial part of the pes anserinus can readily be dissected in a posterior direction so that the medial knee joint capsule is clearly exposed. When detaching the superficial part of the pes anserinus from the tibia, care should be taken to spare the underlying attachment of the medial collateral ligament.

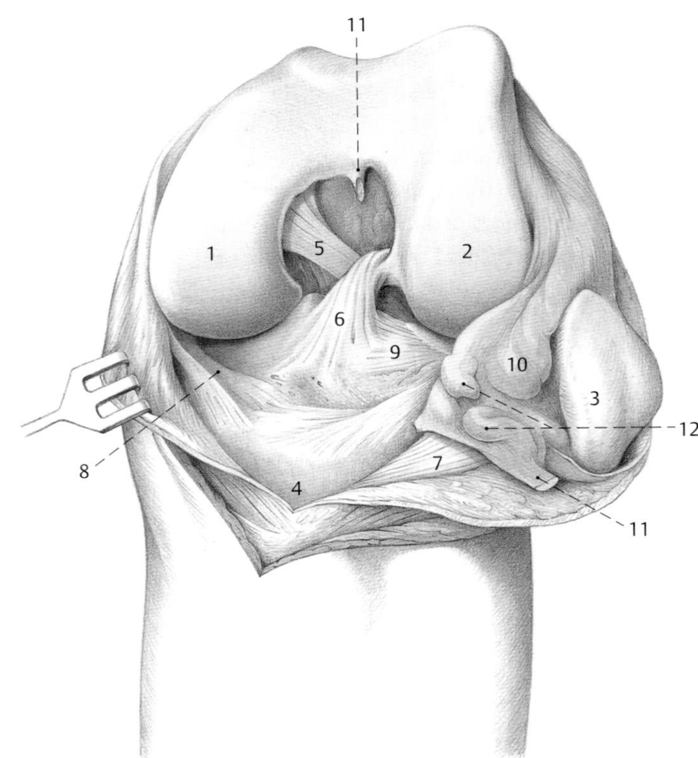

Fig. 11.12 Operative site after 90° flexion of the knee joint, anterior view. The patella has been externally rotated and dislocated.

1 Medial condyle of the femur
2 Lateral condyle of the femur
3 Patella
4 Tibia
5 Posterior cruciate ligament
6 Anterior cruciate ligament
7 Patellar ligament
8 Medial meniscus
9 Lateral meniscus
10 Hoffa's infrapatellar fat pad
11 Infrapatellar synovial fold
12 Alar folds

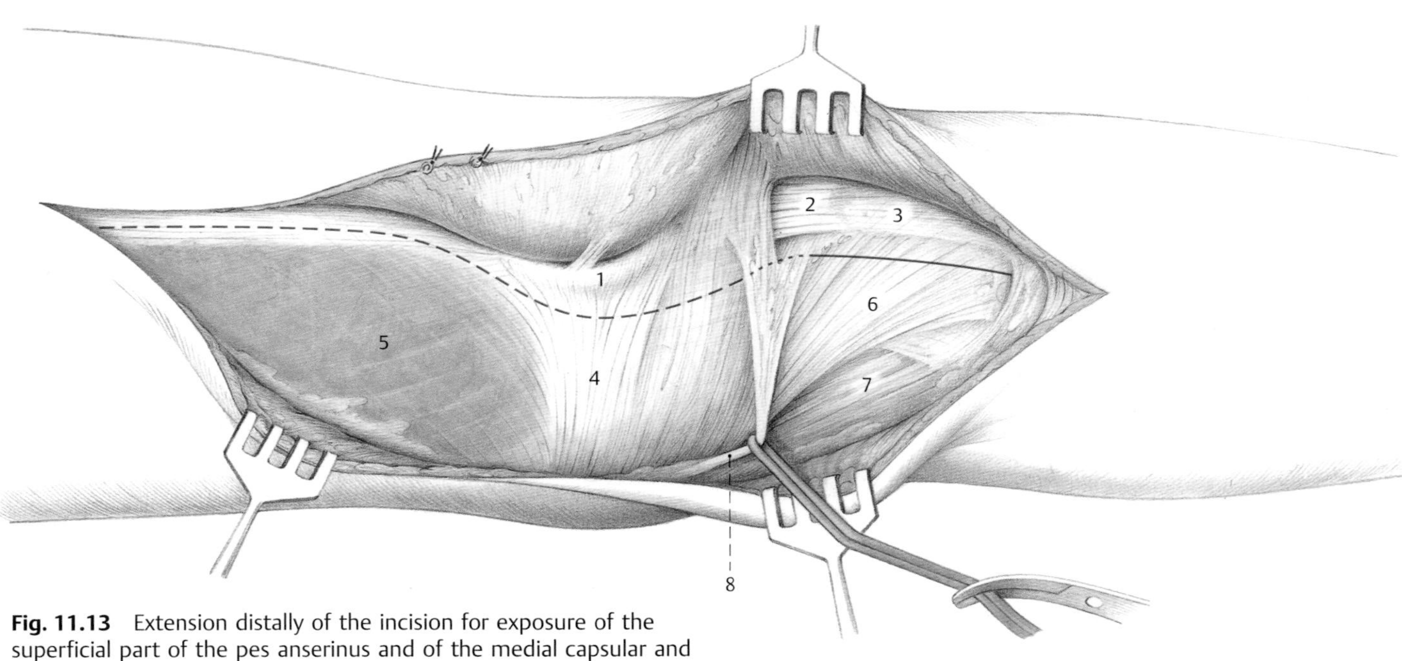

Fig. 11.13 Extension distally of the incision for exposure of the superficial part of the pes anserinus and of the medial capsular and ligamentous apparatus. Incision of the quadriceps tendon, transverse medial patellar retinaculum, and superficial pes anserinus beneath the infrapatellar branch.

1 Patella
2 Patellar ligament
3 Tibial tuberosity
4 Transverse medial patellar retinaculum
5 Vastus medialis
6 Superficial part of pes anserinus
7 Medial head of gastrocnemius
8 Infrapatellar branch of the saphenous nerve

If necessary, the posterior portion of the knee joint can also be inspected from the medial side. The knee joint capsule is opened obliquely behind the posterior medial collateral ligament, and a Langenbeck retractor is inserted (**Fig. 11.14**). This incision generally affords a good overview of the posteromedial corner of the medial meniscus, the posterior joint capsule, and the deep portions of the medial collateral ligament. If exposure of the tibial attachment of the posterior cruciate ligament is required, the incision of the capsule may be extended in a medial direction on the femur, a portion of the medial gastrocnemius head being transected at the same time (**Fig. 11.15**). The tendon of adductor magnus must not be damaged during this incision. The overlying articular nerve of the knee and the branches of the medial superior genicular artery must likewise be spared.

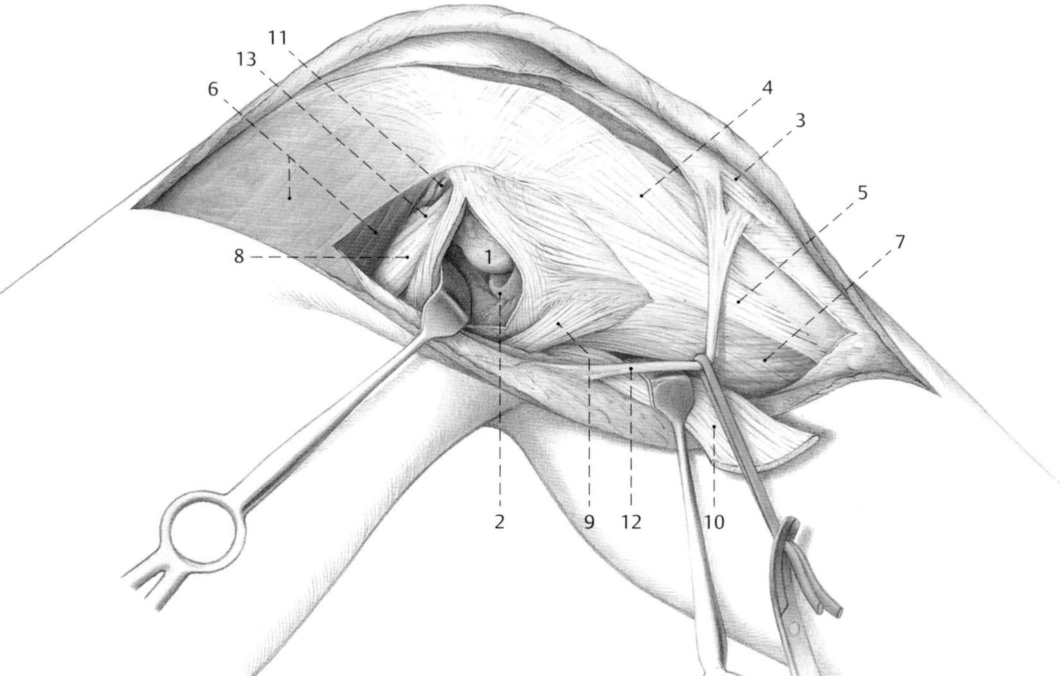

Fig. 11.14 Appearance after detachment of the superficial pes anserinus from the tibia. The posterior portions of the joint capsule have been opened posteriorly to the posterior medial collateral ligament. Care should be taken to spare the medial superior genicular artery and genicular articular nerve.

1 Medial condyle of the femur
2 Medial meniscus
3 Patellar ligament
4 Medial patellar retinaculum
5 Tibial collateral ligament
6 Vastus medialis
7 Popliteus muscle
8 Tendon of adductor magnus
9 Tendon of semimembranosus
10 Superficial part of pes anserinus
11 Medial superior genicular artery and vein
12 Infrapatellar branch of the saphenous nerve
13 Genicular articular nerve

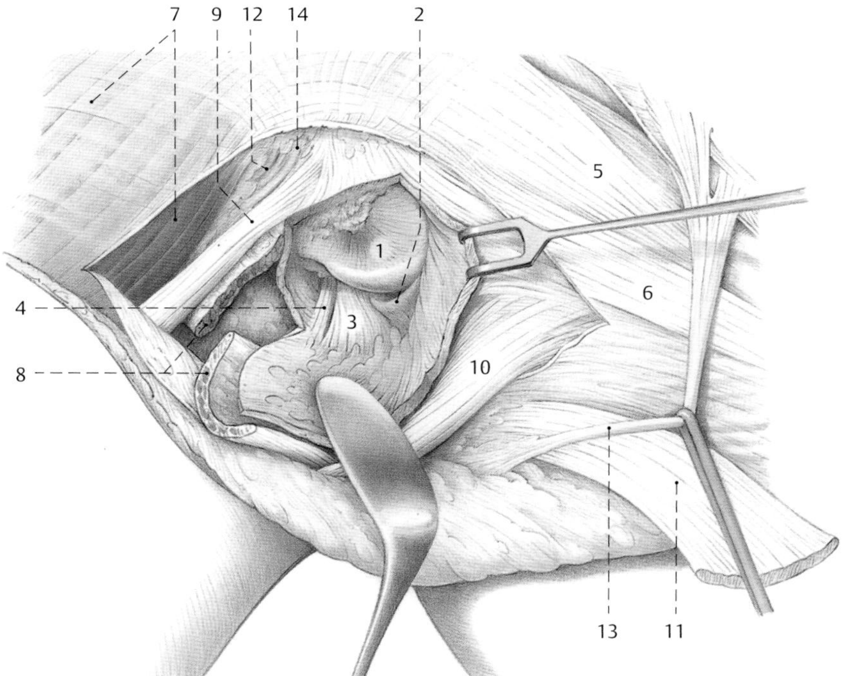

Fig. 11.15 Enlarged opening of the posteromedial portions of the joint capsule by detachment of the medial head of gastrocnemius for exposure of the posterior cruciate ligament.

1 Medial condyle of the femur
2 Medial meniscus
3 Posterior cruciate ligament
4 Posterior meniscofemoral ligament
5 Medial patellar retinaculum
6 Medial collateral ligament
7 Vastus medialis
8 Gastrocnemius muscle, medial head
9 Tendon of adductor magnus
10 Tendon of semimembranosus
11 Superficial part of pes anserinus
12 Medial superior genicular artery and vein
13 Infrapatellar branch of saphenous nerve
14 Genicular articular nerve

11.2.5 Anatomical Site

(**Fig. 11.16**)

The so-called posteromedial joint corner or semimembranosus corner has special significance for the function of the knee joint. The posterior portion of the medial knee joint capsule is dynamically stabilized by the semimembranosus. Semimembranosus has five insertions whose direction is dependent on the flexion of the knee joint. The reflected part runs beneath the medial collateral ligament to the tibia and guards against external rotation on flexion. The direct medial attachment to the tibia causes contraction of the posterior capsule in the extended position. The oblique popliteal ligament is a radiation of the semimembranosus tendon into the posterior joint capsule. Two other fiber tracts radiate into the posterior medial collateral ligament (posterior oblique ligament) on one hand, and into the aponeurosis of the popliteus muscle on the other.

Arthrotomies of the posteromedial portion of the joint may be performed both anterior and posterior to the posterior medial collateral ligament. This femorotibial ligament is closely connected to the posteromedial corner of the medial meniscus. The posterior horn of the meniscus is stabilized by this ligament. Additional dynamic stabilization of this ligament is provided by branches of the semimembranosus tendon.

11.2.6 Wound Closure

The joint capsule, the medial head of gastrocnemius, and the detached pes anserinus are sutured with interrupted sutures. As a rule, tourniquet release and hemostasis are advisable prior to wound closure.

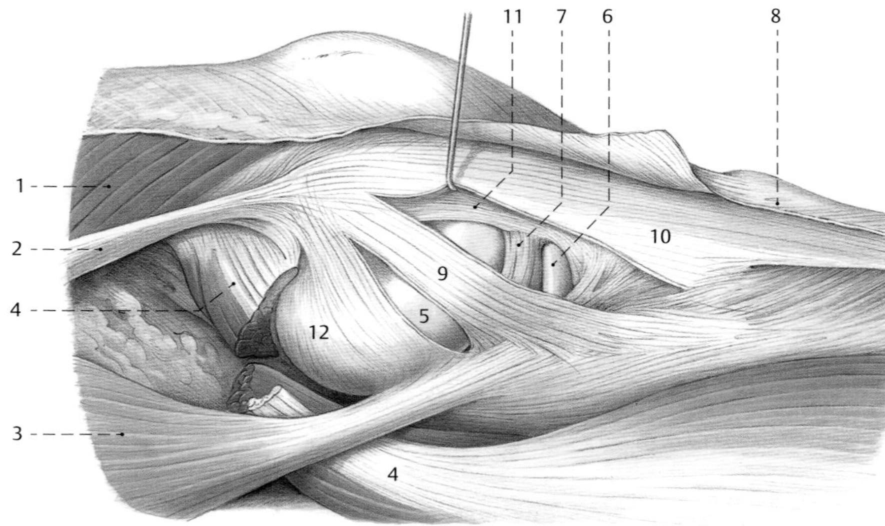

Fig. 11.16 Anatomical site. The medial capsular and ligamentous apparatus of the knee joint.

1 Vastus medialis
2 Tendon of adductor magnus
3 Semimembranosus
4 Gastrocnemius muscle, medial head
5 Medial condyle of the femur
6 Medial condyle of the tibia
7 Medial meniscus
8 Superficial part of pes anserinus
9 Posterior medial collateral ligament
10 Medial collateral ligament
11 Medial capsular ligament
12 Condylar cap

11.2.7 Alternative Skin Incision

Exposure of the knee joint by a medial parapatellar incision of the capsule may be combined with a lateral parapatellar skin incision. Lateral parapatellar incision is preferable for procedures such as synovectomy, arthroplasty, or ligamentous reconstructions since the blood supply and innervation of the skin and subcutaneous tissue on the anterior aspect of the knee are thus impaired to a lesser degree. The prepatellar and infrapatellar innervation of the skin comes mostly from the medial side.

The lateral skin incision may run in a curve or in a straight line from 5 cm proximal to the superior lateral pole of the patella to the tibial tuberosity (**Fig. 11.17**). The following procedure is recommended for atraumatic dissection of the medial skin flap. After splitting the subcutaneous tissue, the underlying fascia is transected in the direction of the incision. The medial skin flap is now subfascially dissected in a medial direction. This procedure can be relied upon to spare the vessels and nerves on the medial side since these run a predominantly extrafascial course (**Fig. 11.18**). Medial arthrotomy is performed in the customary fashion following division of the medial patellar retinaculum and the quadriceps tendon. If necessary, this incision may also be used for a lateral parapatellar arthrotomy, a lateral release, or reconstruction of the lateral ligaments (**Fig. 11.19**).

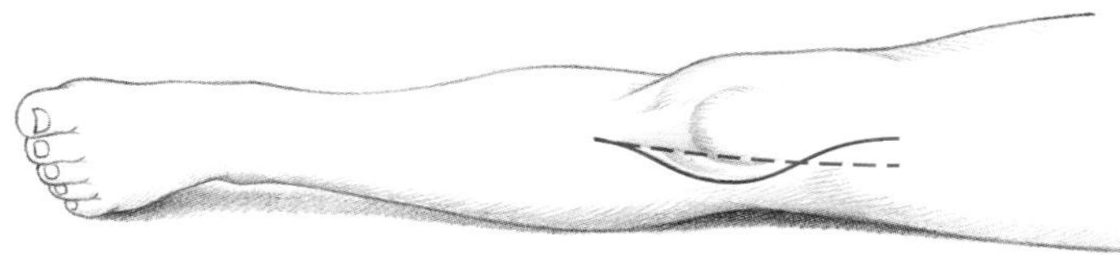

Fig. 11.17 Lateral parapatellar skin incision; this may be straight or curved (left knee joint).

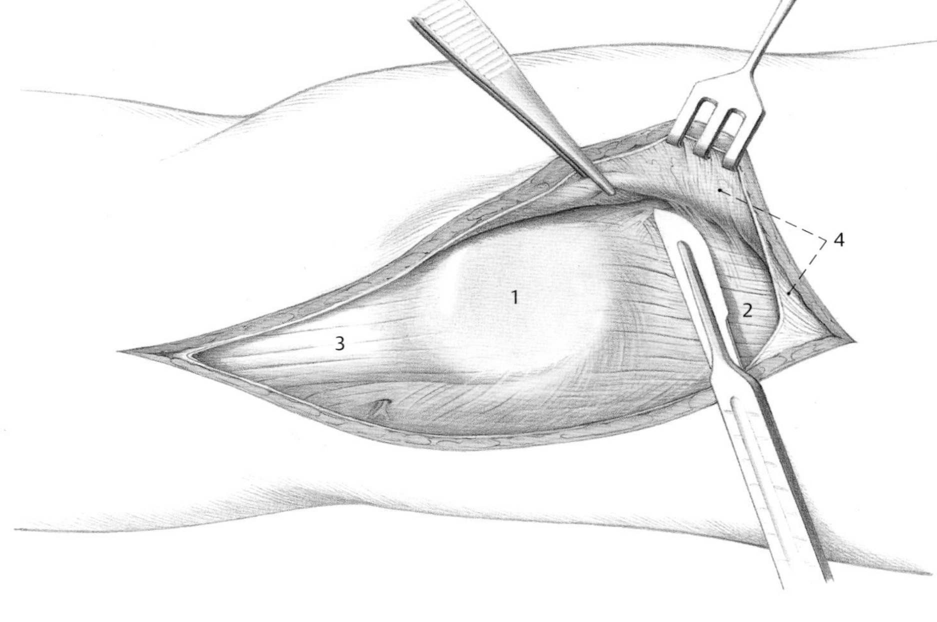

Fig. 11.18 After splitting of the fascia, the medial skin flap is subfascially dissected.

1 Patella
2 Tendon of quadriceps
3 Patellar ligament
4 Fascia

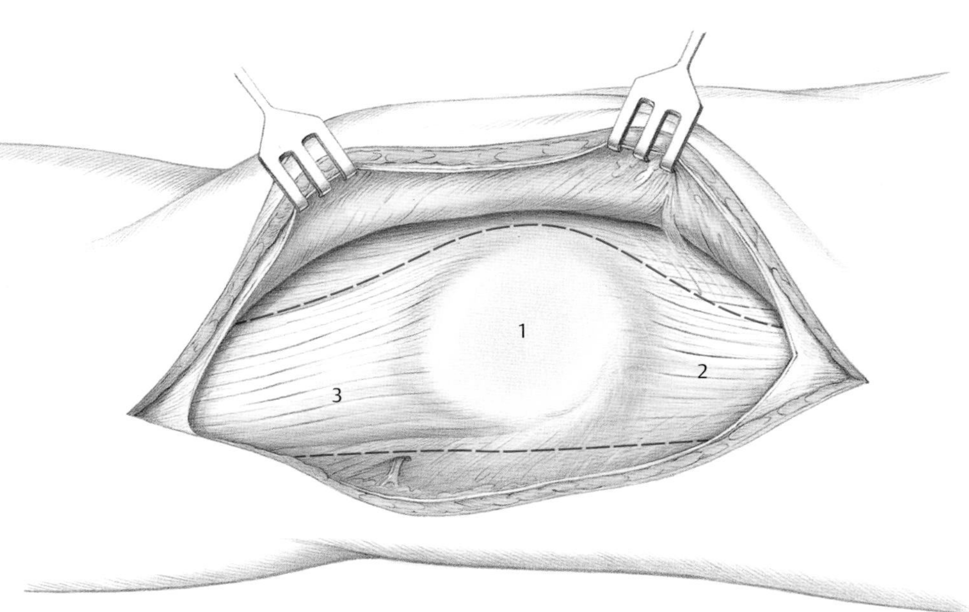

Fig. 11.19 Parapatellar incision of the extensor apparatus (optionally medial or lateral).

1 Patella
2 Tendon of quadriceps
3 Patellar ligament

11.3 Short Medial Approach to the Knee

R. Bauer, F. Kerschbaumer, S. Poisel, C. J. Wirth

11.3.1 Principal Indications

- Medial collateral ligament procedures
- Replacement of the transverse medial patellar retinaculum
- Reattachment of avulsion fractures of the medial patellar border
- Removal of loose articular bodies

11.3.2 Positioning and Incision

The patient is placed in the supine position. Following application of a tourniquet, the knee is draped to allow free movement. The skin incision runs between the medial femoral epicondyle and the medial border of the patella over the joint space (**Fig. 11.20**). After dividing the skin and subcutaneous tissue, the medial retinaculum is exposed. Extending the knee causes the mobile incision window to move to the medial border of the patella (**Fig. 11.21**), and flexion moves it to the medial collateral ligament, medial femoral epicondyle, and proximal border of the pes anserinus (**Fig. 11.22**). The course of the transverse medial patellar retinaculum—from its origin between the bony insertion of the adductor magnus tendon and the medial femoral epicondyle to its insertion onto the upper one-third of the medial patellar border—can be followed by moving the incision window.

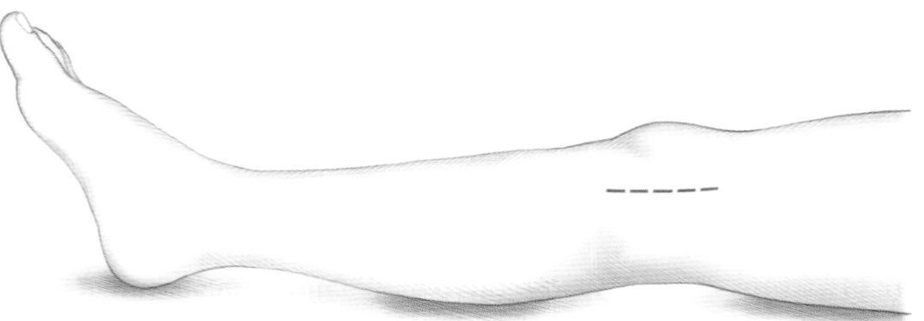

Fig. 11.20 Short medial approach to the knee joint. Skin incision (right knee joint).

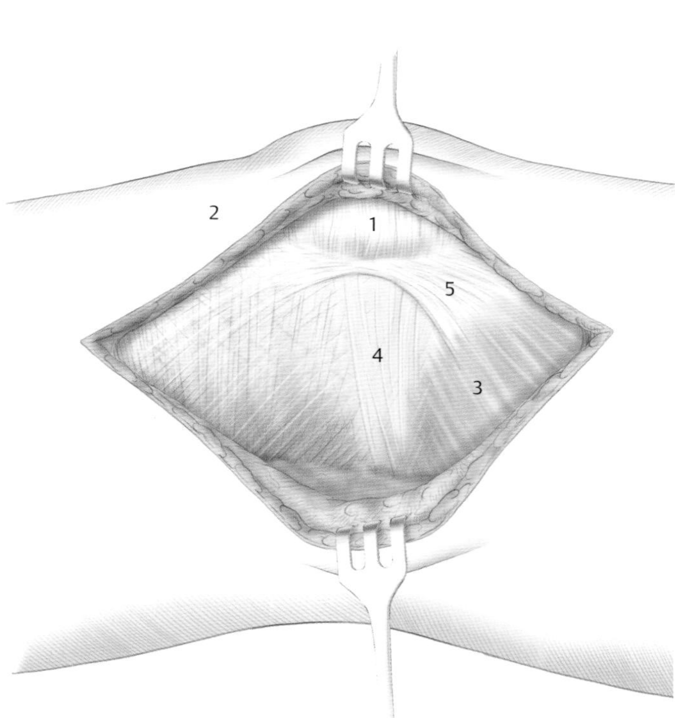

Fig. 11.21 With the knee in extension, the medial border of the patella, parts of the patellar ligament and vastus medialis, and the transverse medial patellar retinaculum are visible through the mobile incision window.

1 Patella
2 Patellar ligament
3 Vastus medialis
4 Transverse medial patellar retinaculum
5 Longitudinal medial patellar retinaculum

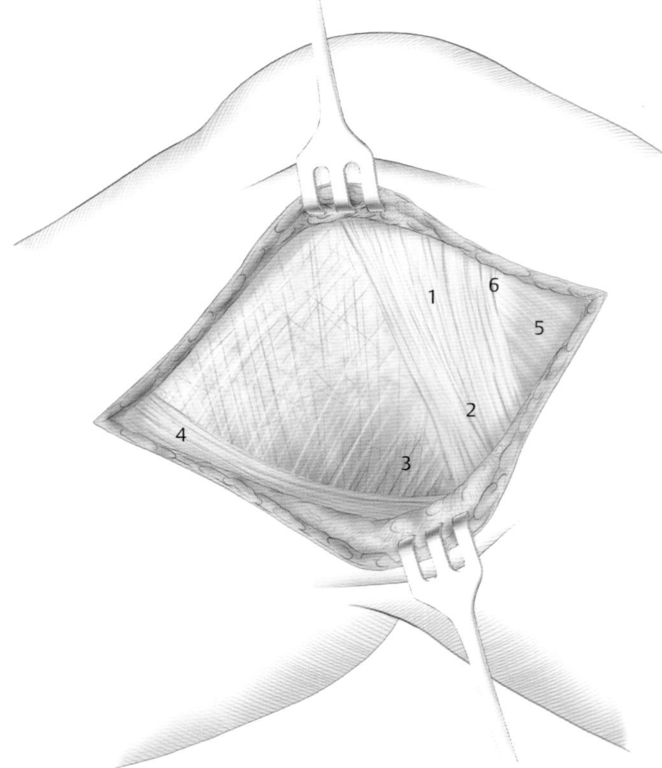

Fig. 11.22 With the knee flexed to 90°, the transverse medial patellar retinaculum can be followed as far as the medial femoral epicondyle and medial collateral ligament. Parts of the pes anserinus and vastus medialis muscle can be seen.

1 Transverse medial patellar retinaculum
2 Medial femoral epicondyle (covered by the transverse medial patellar retinaculum)
3 Tibial collateral ligament
4 Superficial part of pes anserinus
5 Vastus medialis
6 Longitudinal medial patellar retinaculum

11.3.3 Exposure of the Knee Joint

With the knee slightly flexed, the medial retinaculum is divided beside the patella and retracted with wound retractors (see **Fig. 11.23**). The knee joint capsule is incised 2 cm proximally to the medial joint cavity. The incision is then extended to proximal and to distal medial. A Langenbeck retractor is inserted beneath the medial collateral ligament, while a second one laterally retracts Hoffa's infrapatellar fat pad (see **Fig. 11.24**). With the knee flexed to 90°, the medial tibial plateau, the medial femoral condyle, the anterior cruciate ligament, and the anterior horn of the medial meniscus are readily visible.

11.3.4 Wound Closure

After release of the tourniquet and hemostasis, the wound is closed by suture of the capsule and the retinaculum if the joint has been opened, or otherwise by suture of the subcutaneous tissue and skin.

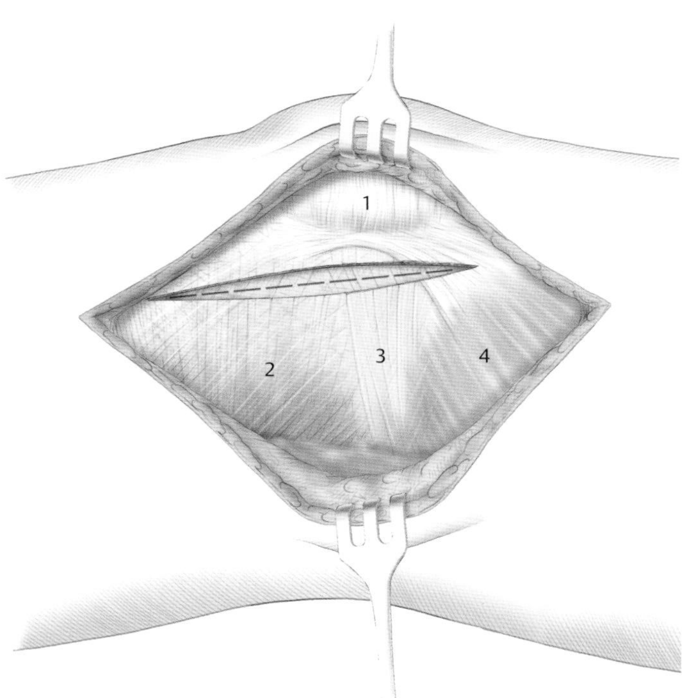

Fig. 11.23 To open the joint, the medial patellar retinaculum and the joint capsule are divided at the parapatellar level.

1 Patella
2 Medial patellar retinaculum
3 Transverse medial patellar retinaculum
4 Vastus medialis

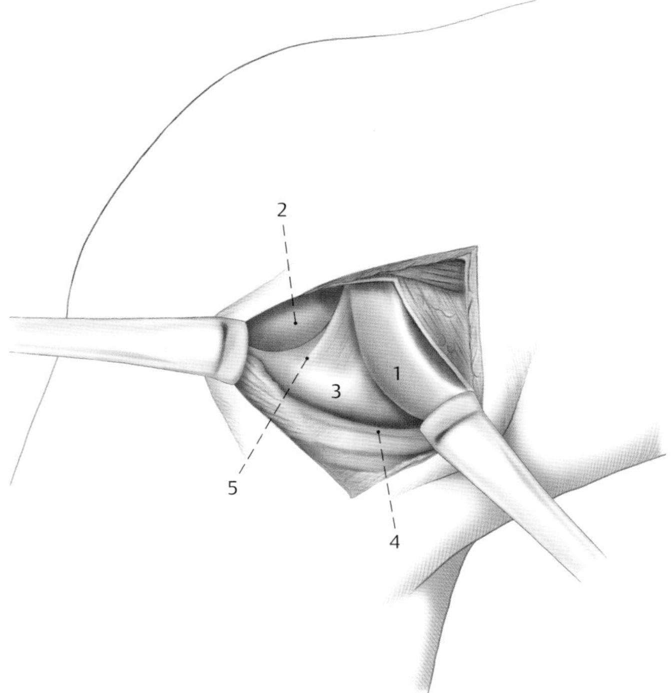

Fig. 11.24 Following the insertion of Langenbeck retractors for retraction of Hoffa's infrapatellar fat pad and the medial collateral ligament, the knee is flexed to a right angle. The anterior horn of the medial meniscus, the medial and part of the lateral femoral condyle, the tibial joint surface, and the anterior cruciate ligament are visible.

1 Medial condyle of the femur
2 Lateral condyle of the femur
3 Superior articular surface of the tibia
4 Medial meniscus
5 Anterior cruciate ligament

11.4 Anterolateral Approach to the Knee Joint

R. Bauer, F. Kerschbaumer, S. Poisel, C. J. Wirth

11.4.1 Principal Indications

- Joint fractures
- Partial synovectomy
- Removal of articular loose bodies

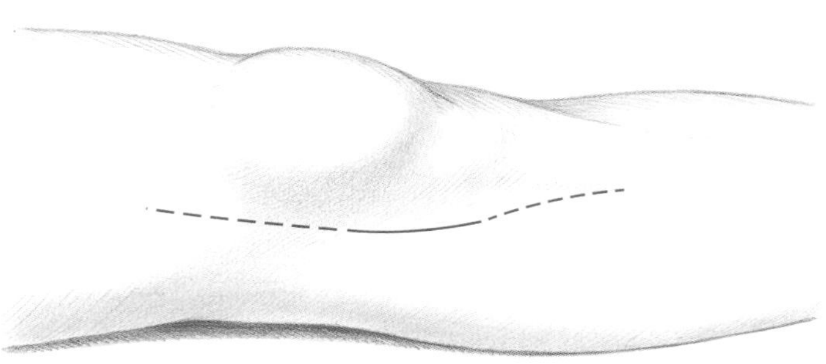

Fig. 11.25 Short anterolateral approach to the knee joint. Skin incision (right knee), with possible extension (dashed line).

11.4.2 Positioning and Incision

The patient is placed in the supine position, and after application of a tourniquet the leg is draped so as to be freely movable. The skin incision is approximately 5 cm long and runs two fingerbreadths laterally to the patella toward Gerdy's tubercle (**Fig. 11.25**).

The skin incision should not be made too obliquely so that it may be extended to a lateral parapatellar incision if necessary or for a repeat operation. After splitting the subcutaneous tissue and inserting retractors, the iliotibial tract is split in the same direction (**Fig. 11.26**).

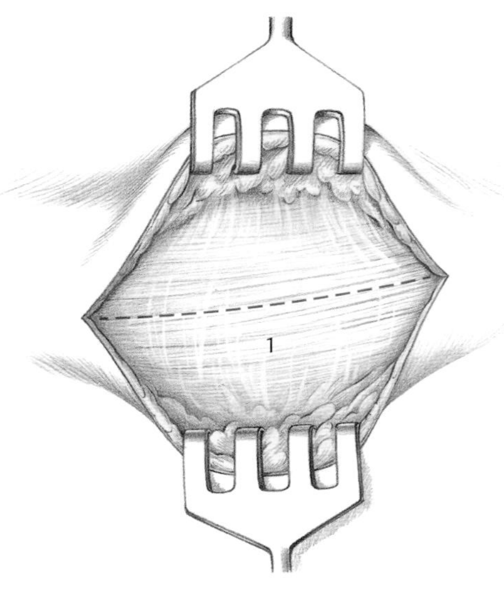

Fig. 11.26 Splitting of the iliotibial tract in the direction of the fibers.

1 Iliotibial tract

11.4.3 Exposure of the Knee Joint

The incision into the lateral knee joint capsule is made obliquely from proximal posterior to distal anterior (**Fig. 11.27**). One Langenbeck retractor is inserted beneath the lateral collateral ligament and one behind Hoffa's infrapatellar fat pad. The knee joint is now flexed. To obtain a complete overview of the lateral meniscus, maximal flexion of the knee joint is recommended. Owing to the oblique course of the lateral collateral ligament, the lateral meniscus can be viewed in this position over its entire circumference. Exposure of the anterior and posterior portions of the meniscus is facilitated by the insertion of a small retractor into the coronary ligament. By slight traction on this retractor, the meniscus can be lateralized to some degree, which facilitates evaluation of its circumference (a completely or partially diskoid meniscus) (**Fig. 11.28**).

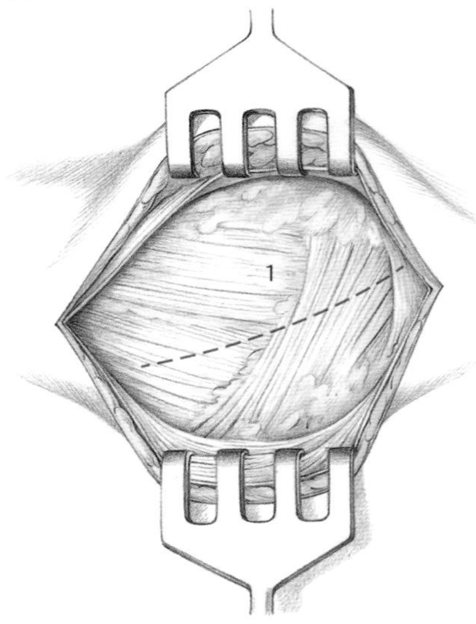

Fig. 11.27 Opening of the knee joint capsule from proximal posterior to distal anterior.

1 Knee joint capsule

11.4.4 Extension of the Approach

If necessary, the short anterolateral incision may be extended to a long parapatellar incision (see **Fig. 11.25** or **Fig. 11.17**). The iliotibial tract is split in line with the skin incision, and the joint capsule is opened as far as the superior recess. The patella can be retracted medially so that an overview of the lateral femoral condyle, the lateral meniscus, and the lateral tibial plateau is obtained. In the presence of intra-articular fractures or in supracondylar osteotomies, the lateral incision can be enlarged in the proximal direction so that the distal femoral metaphysis can be reached by the same approach (see Section 10.3c, **Figs. 10.14, 10.15, 10.16, 10.17**). Distal extension of the approach, for example in the presence of lateral tibial head fractures, is also possible. In this case, the skin incision is obliquely extended in a distal direction as far as the tibial tuberosity.

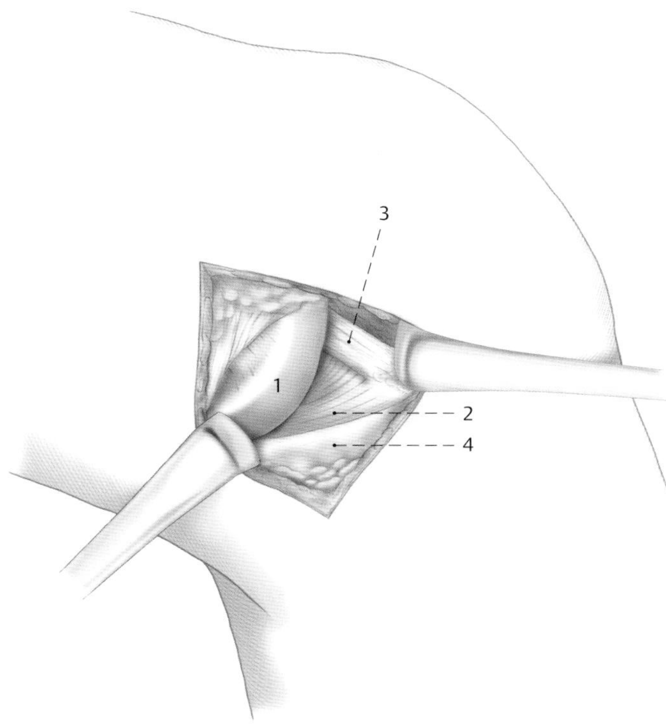

Fig. 11.28 Exposure of the anterolateral segment of the knee joint with the knee flexed. For better exposure of the anterior horn of the meniscus and the anterior cruciate ligament, Hoffa's infrapatellar fat pad and the lateral collateral ligament are each retracted with a Langenbeck retractor.

1 Lateral condyle of the femur
2 Lateral meniscus
3 Anterior cruciate ligament
4 Lateral tibial condyle

11.4.5 Wound Closure

The wound is closed with the knee joint extended by interrupted suture of the knee joint capsule and the iliotibial tract following release of the tourniquet and hemostasis.

11.4.6 Dangers

During resection of the lateral meniscus, the closely subjacent lateral inferior genicular artery may be damaged. After release of the tourniquet, special attention must be paid to this vessel to avert hemorrhage.

11.5 Posterolateral Approach According to Henderson

R. Bauer, F. Kerschbaumer, S. Poisel, C. J. Wirth

11.5.1 Principal Indications

- Iliotibial tractopexy
- Epicondyle transfer
- Removal of articular loose bodies
- Removal of osteochondral plugs

11.5.2 Positioning and Incision

The patient is placed in the supine position. After application of a tourniquet, the leg is draped so as to be freely movable, and the knee joint is slightly flexed by placing a pad under the thigh. The skin incision begins approximately 5 cm proximal to the superior border of the patella on the readily palpable posterior border of the fascia lata, and runs distally to a point approximately one fingerbreadth distal to the head of the fibula (**Fig. 11.29**). After splitting the subcutaneous tissue, the posterior skin flap is dissected free of the fascia, the posterior border of the iliotibial tract is identified, and the fascia at this site is split longitudinally (**Fig. 11.30**).

11.5.3 Exposure of the Knee Joint

It is important to incise the fascia at the right location, that is, behind the lateral intermuscular septum.

After splitting the fascia, its posterior portion together with the biceps muscle is cautiously (common peroneal nerve!) retracted in a posterior direction with a Langenbeck retractor, while the anterior portion of the fascia with the lateral intermuscular septum is retracted anteriorly. The posterior border of the lateral collateral ligament and the lateral head of the

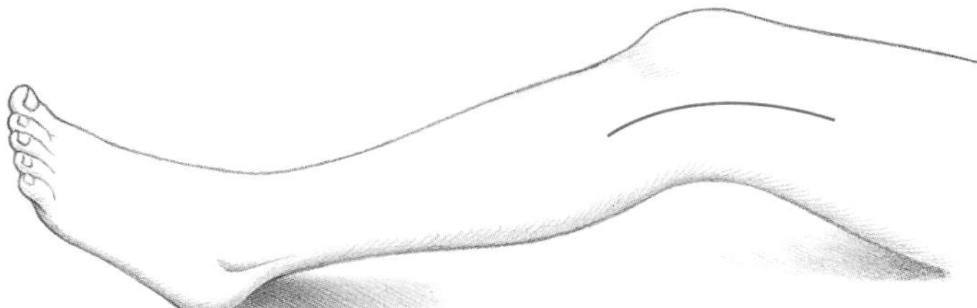

Fig. 11.29 Posterolateral approach to the knee joint. Skin incision (solid line, left knee).

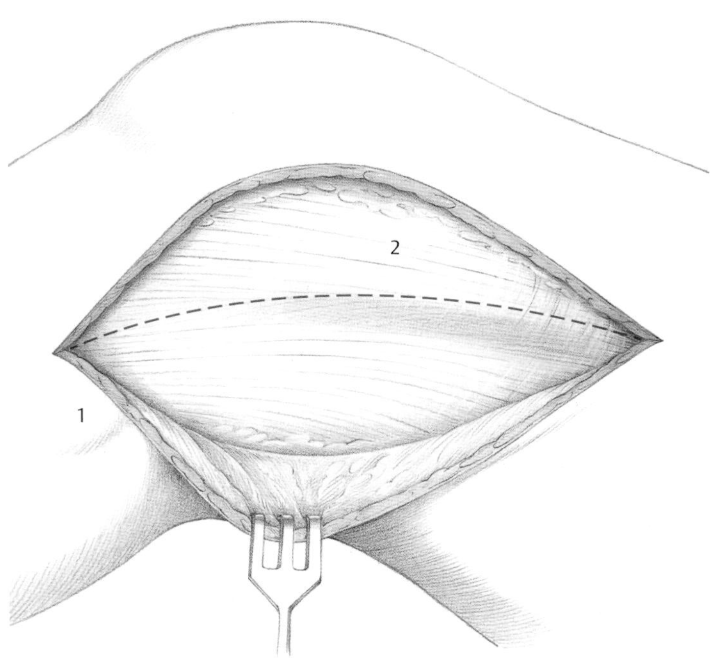

Fig. 11.30 Dissection of the posterior skin flap and splitting of the fascia at the posterior border the of iliotibial tract.

1 Head of the fibula
2 Iliotibial tract

gastrocnemius are dissected free with scissors. An L-shaped incision is made in the capsule behind the lateral collateral ligament, which also transects the lateral gastrocnemius head (**Fig. 11.31**). The lateral collateral ligament and tendon of popliteus can be retracted anteriorly with wound retractors. Insertion of another retractor into the posterior part of the lateral capsule affords a good view of the posterior portion of the lateral femoral condyle, the posterior portion of the lateral meniscus, and the popliteus tendon (**Fig. 11.32**). For better exposure of the lateral femoral condyle, the lateral head of gastrocnemius may be completely detached if necessary.

11.5.4 Extension of the Approach

The approach may be extended proximally to expose the distal end of the femur (see Section 10.3c, **Figs. 10.14**, **10.15**, **10.16**, **10.17**).

11.5.5 Wound Closure

The wound is closed by suture of the capsule and reattachment of the detached lateral head of gastrocnemius.

11.5.6 Dangers

If the knee joint capsule is not opened with sufficient care, the popliteus tendon and the lateral inferior genicular artery may be transected. If the iliotibial band is split anteriorly to the lateral intermuscular septum, further dissection of the capsule becomes extremely difficult.

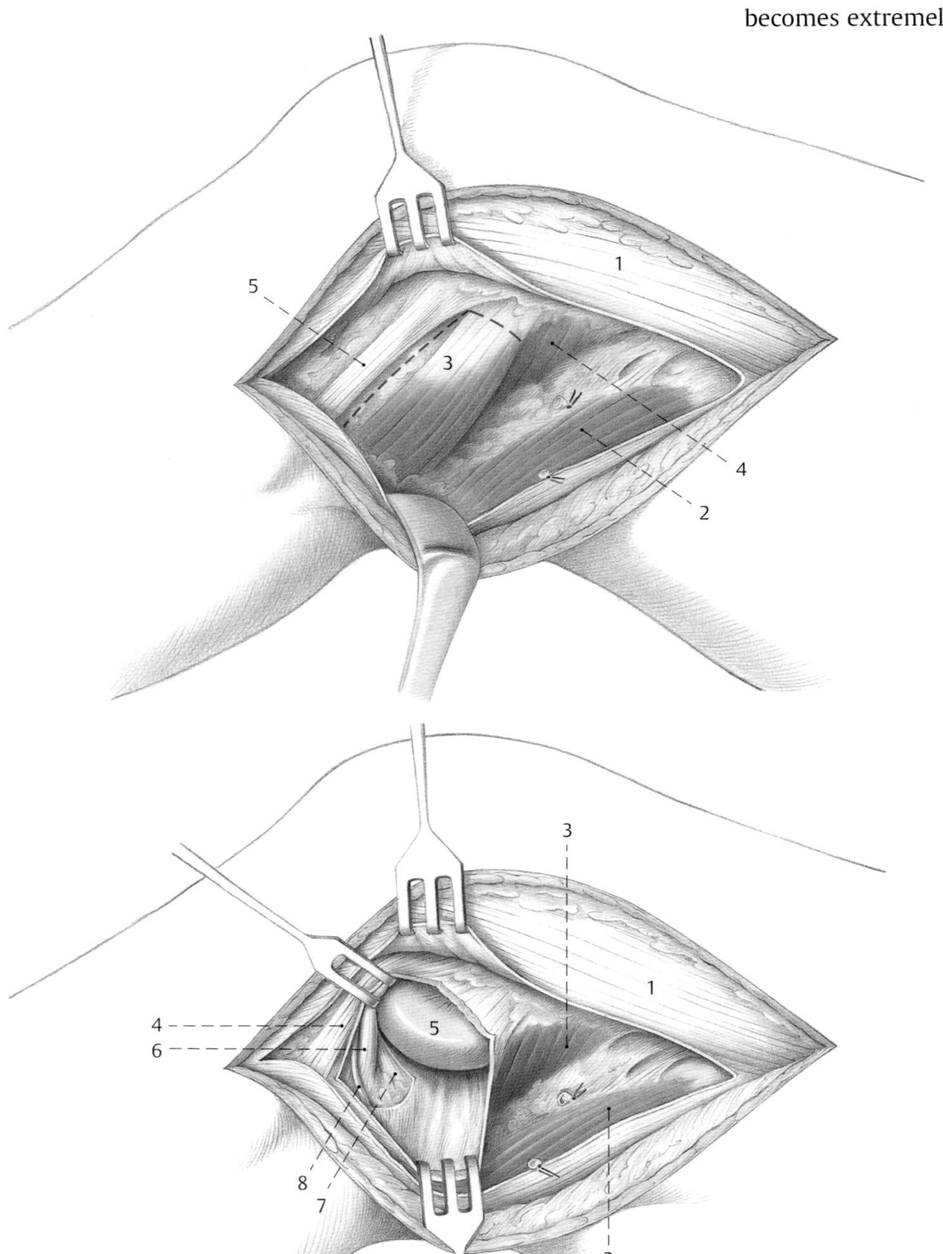

Fig. 11.31 Posterior retraction of the biceps, incision of the capsule behind the lateral collateral ligament, and detachment of the lateral head of gastrocnemius.

1 Iliotibial tract
2 Biceps femoris
3 Gastrocnemius, lateral head
4 Plantaris
5 Fibular collateral ligament

Fig. 11.32 Appearance after opening of the posterolateral portions of the knee joint.

1 Iliotibial tract
2 Biceps femoris
3 Plantaris
4 Fibular collateral ligament
5 Lateral condyle of the femur
6 Tendon of popliteus
7 Lateral meniscus
8 Lateral inferior genicular artery

11.6 Posterior Approach to the Knee Joint According to Trickey

R. Bauer, F. Kerschbaumer, S. Poisel, C. J. Wirth

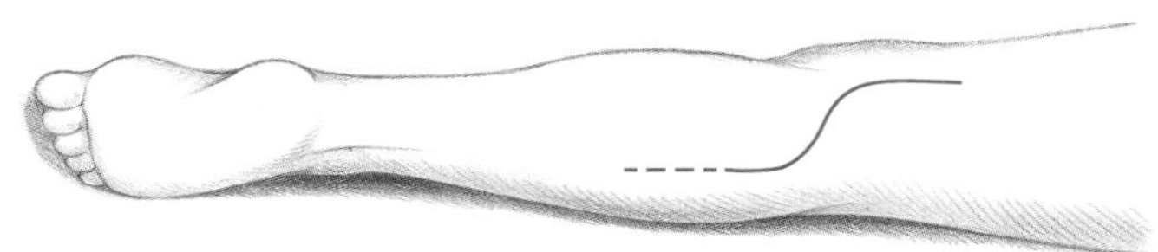

Fig. 11.33 Posterior approach to the knee joint. Skin incision (right knee).

11.6.1 Principal Indications

- Reattachment of the posterior cruciate ligament after an avulsion fracture
- Fractures
- Synovectomy
- Removal of articular loose bodies
- Repair of vessels and nerves in the popliteal fossa
- Popliteal cysts
- Tumors

11.6.2 Positioning and Incision

The patient is placed in the prone position. After application of a tourniquet, the leg is draped to allow free movement. An S-shaped skin incision is made from medial proximal to distal lateral. The central transverse portion of the incision in the popliteal fossa should be at least slightly oblique as closure of the skin is otherwise difficult owing to great tension, notably with flexion contractures (**Fig. 11.33**). For repair of the tibial nerve, the incision may be extended distally (the dashed line in **Fig. 11.33**). After splitting the skin and subcutaneous tissue, the fascia is exposed and incised centrally. The medial sural cutaneous nerve and the accompanying small saphenous vein lie below the fascia in the proximal wound region, and above the fascia in the distal portion of the wound. The fascia should be incised medial to the medial sural cutaneous nerve (**Fig. 11.34**). Extensive splitting of the fascia in the proximal and distal directions is required to expose and retract the vessels and nerves within the popliteal fossa.

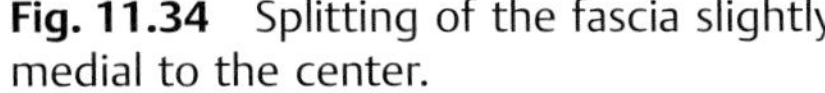

Fig. 11.34 Splitting of the fascia slightly medial to the center.

1 Crural fascia
2 Small saphenous vein
3 Medial sural cutaneous nerve
4 Tendon of semitendinosus

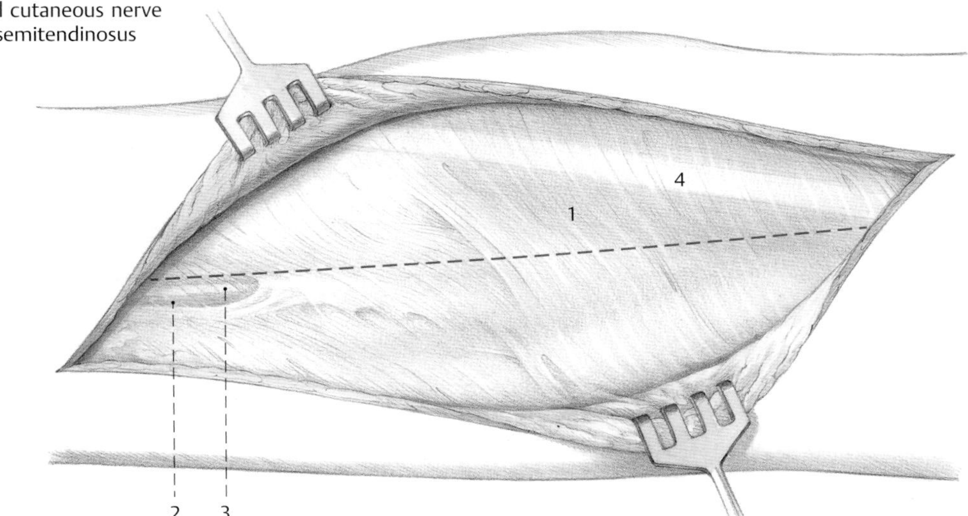

After retraction of the semimembranosus muscle in a medial direction, the tibial nerve is first dissected free and snared. The common peroneal nerve is then dissected free in the same fashion. The branches between the small saphenous and popliteal veins are ligated and transected (**Fig. 11.35**). The popliteal vessels are subsequently exposed and retracted laterally with a blunt retractor or snared. A Langenbeck retractor is then inserted beneath the semimembranosus, being supported by the superior border of the medial femoral condyle (**Fig. 11.36**). The medial head of gastrocnemius is detached approximately one fingerbreadth distal to the tendinous origin.

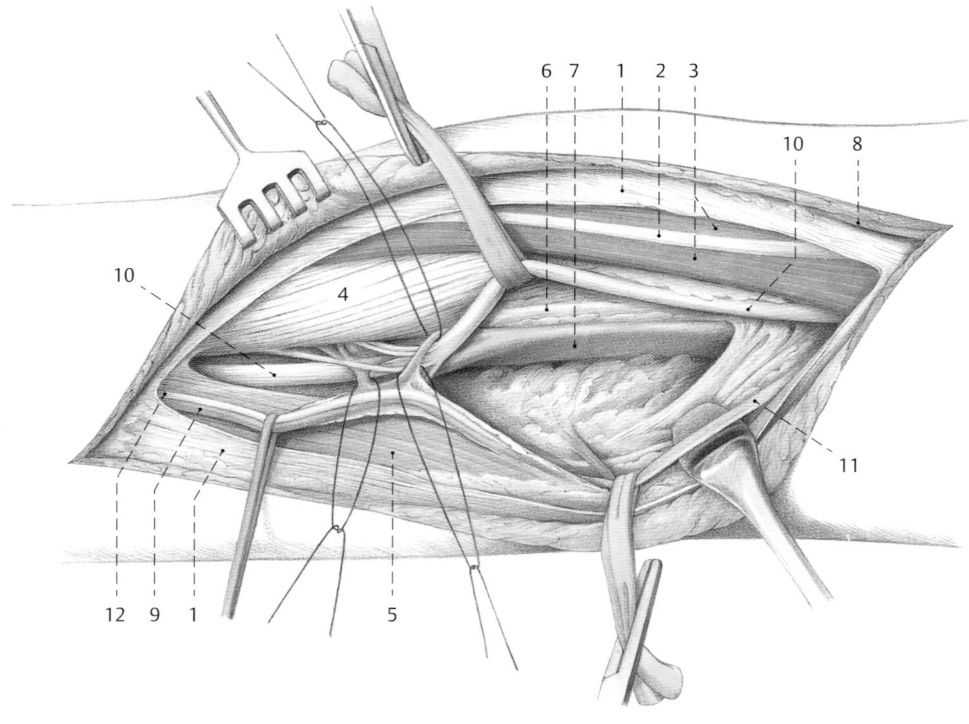

Fig. 11.35 Dissection and snaring of the tibial nerve, common peroneal nerve, medial sural cutaneous nerve, and small saphenous vein. Ligation of the smaller veins between the small saphenous vein and popliteal vein.

1 Crural fascia
2 Semitendinosus
3 Semimembranosus
4 Gastrocnemius, medial head
5 Gastrocnemius, lateral head
6 Popliteal artery
7 Popliteal vein
8 Great saphenous vein
9 Small saphenous vein
10 Tibial nerve
11 Common peroneal nerve
12 Medial sural cutaneous nerve

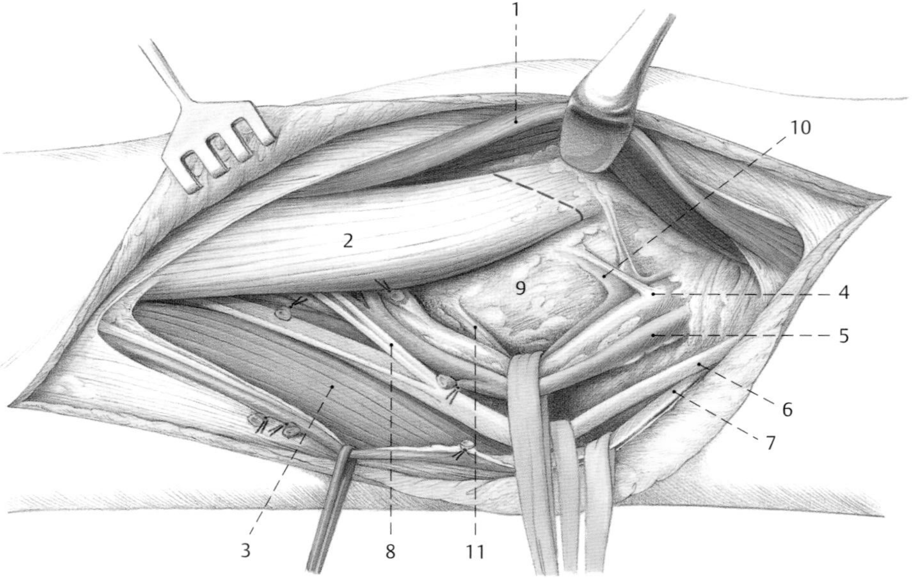

Fig. 11.36 Detachment of the medial head of gastrocnemius one fingerbreadth distal to its origin at the femoral condyle.

1 Semimembranosus
2 Gastrocnemius, medial head
3 Gastrocnemius, lateral head
4 Popliteal artery
5 Popliteal vein
6 Tibial nerve
7 Common peroneal nerve
8 Tibial nerve, muscular branch
9 Joint capsule
10 Medial superior genicular artery and vein
11 Middle genicular artery and vein

11.6.3 Exposure of the Knee Joint Capsule from Posteromedial

The detached head of the gastrocnemius is retracted distally. To avoid overstretching the muscular branches arising from the tibial nerve, excessive tension should be avoided. The joint capsule may be opened with a hinged flap (**Fig. 11.37**). The medial portion of this incision should not be too far medial, to avoid injury to the posterior cruciate ligament and the middle genicular artery. When the flap of the capsule is folded back distally, a good view is obtained of the posterior medial condyle, the course of the posterior cruciate ligament, and the posterior part of the medial meniscus (**Fig. 11.38**).

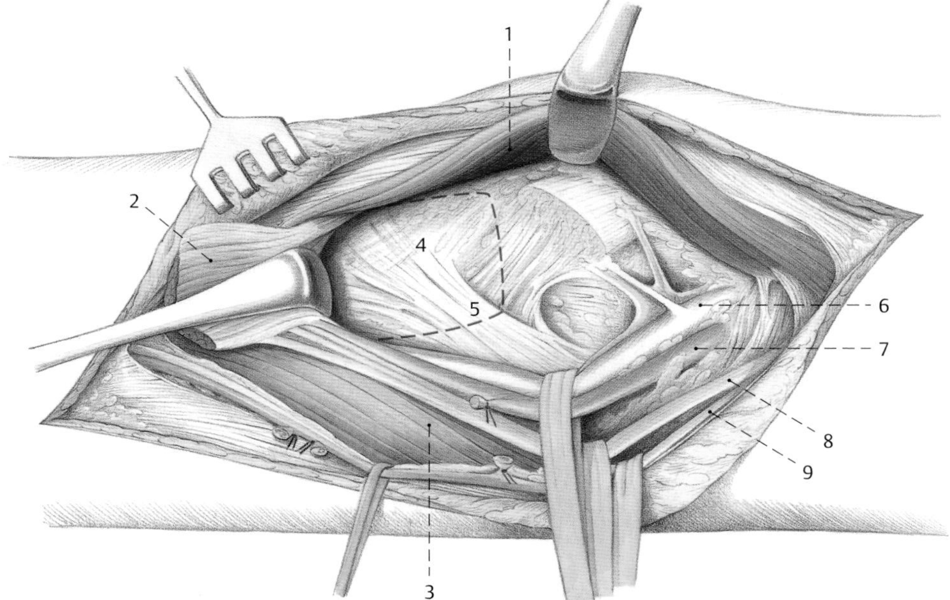

Fig. 11.37 Hinged flap incision of the posterior knee joint capsule after distal retraction of the medial head of gastrocnemius.

1 Semimembranosus
2 Gastrocnemius, medial head
3 Gastrocnemius, lateral head
4 Knee joint capsule
5 Oblique popliteal ligament
6 Popliteal artery
7 Popliteal vein
8 Tibial nerve
9 Common peroneal nerve

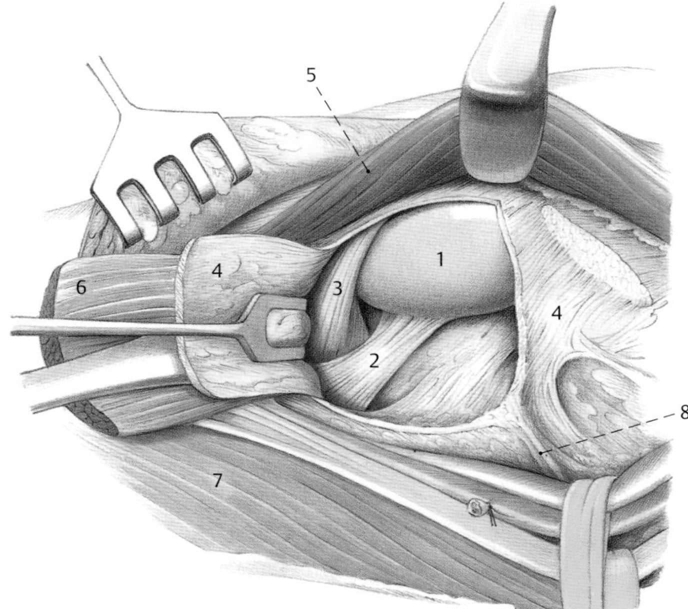

Fig. 11.38 Appearance after opening of the posteromedial portion of the knee joint capsule.

1 Medial condyle of the femur
2 Posterior cruciate ligament
3 Medial meniscus
4 Knee joint capsule
5 Semimembranosus
6 Gastrocnemius, medial head
7 Gastrocnemius, lateral head
8 Middle genicular artery and vein

11.6.4 Exposure of the Knee Joint from Posterolateral

If exposure of the posterolateral portion of the knee joint is necessary, the previously snared popliteal vessels and the tibial nerve are retracted medially. The common peroneal nerve, the biceps femoris, and the medial sural cutaneous nerve are retracted laterally. After ligation of the smaller veins posterior to the knee joint capsule, the lateral head of gastrocnemius, and the origin of the plantaris muscle from the lateral femoral condyle are separated one fingerbreadth distal to their origin (**Fig. 11.39**). Both muscles are then cautiously retracted in distal direction with a Langenbeck retractor, taking account of their vascular and nerve supply (**Fig. 11.40**).

The posterolateral portions of the capsule can now be opened with a hinged flap, similar to the medial portion. Distal reflection of the capsule flap provides a good view of the posterior portions of the lateral condyle, the posterior horn of the lateral meniscus, and the posterior meniscofemoral ligament, as well as the origin of the anterior cruciate ligament on the inner aspect of the lateral femoral condyle (**Fig. 11.41**).

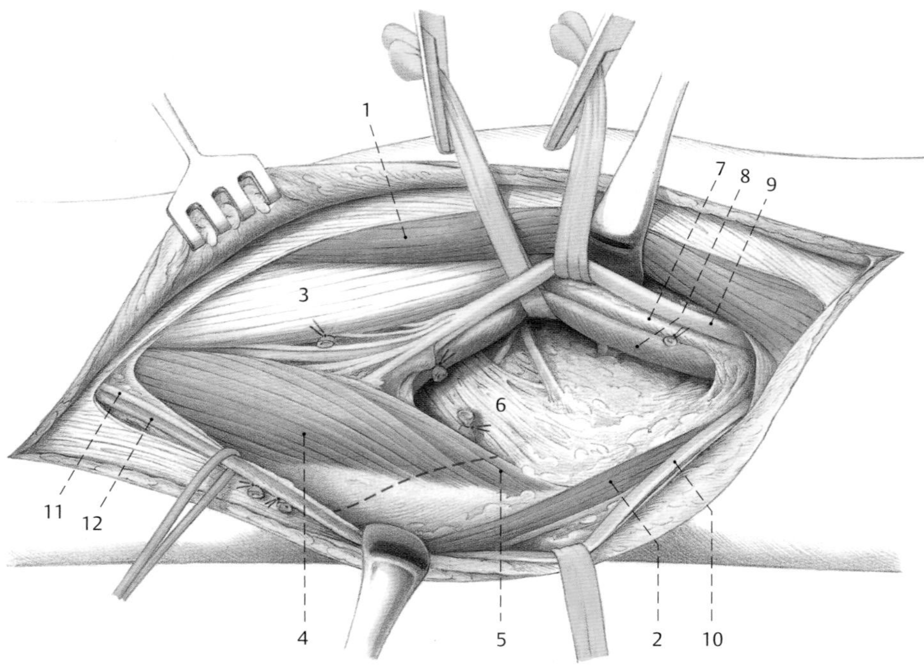

Fig. 11.39 Detachment of the lateral head of gastrocnemius and the origin of plantaris from the lateral condyle of the femur.

1 Semimembranosus
2 Biceps femoris
3 Gastrocnemius, medial head
4 Gastrocnemius, lateral head
5 Plantaris
6 Knee joint capsule
7 Popliteal artery
8 Popliteal vein
9 Tibial nerve
10 Common peroneal nerve
11 Medial sural cutaneous nerve
12 Small saphenous vein

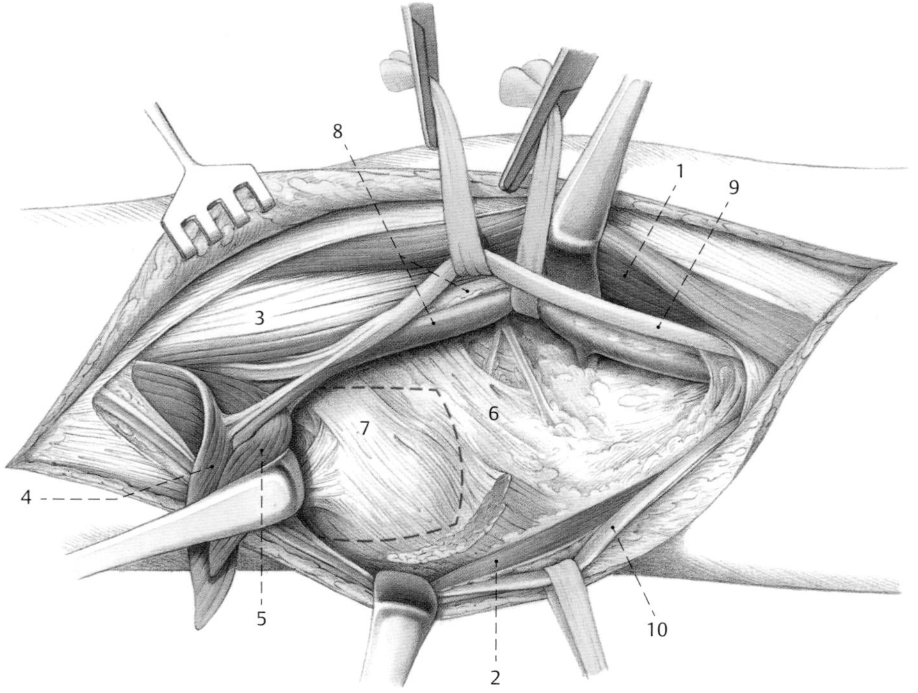

Fig. 11.40 Opening of the posterolateral portions of the knee joint after retraction of the medial head of gastrocnemius.

1 Semimembranosus
2 Biceps femoris
3 Gastrocnemius, medial head
4 Gastrocnemius, lateral head
5 Plantaris
6 Knee joint capsule
7 Oblique popliteal ligament
8 Popliteal vessels
9 Tibial nerve
10 Common peroneal nerve

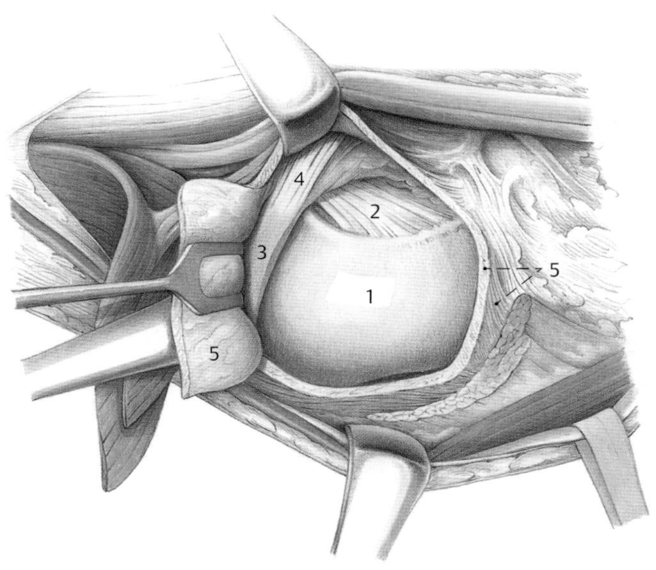

Fig. 11.41 Operative site after opening of the posterolateral portions of the knee joint capsule.

1 Lateral condyle of the femur
2 Anterior cruciate ligament
3 Lateral meniscus
4 Posterior meniscofemoral ligament
5 Knee joint capsule

11.6.5 Anatomical Site

(**Fig. 11.42**)

The medial and lateral heads of gastrocnemius are innervated approximately 7 cm distal to their origin. To prevent denervation of this group of muscles, these muscular branches need to be carefully dissected when exposing the posterior knee joint capsule or in ligament reconstructions involving the medial head of gastrocnemius.

Several centimeters distal to these muscular branches, the tibial nerve and the popliteal vessels enter the plane between the soleus and the popliteus. If repair of the tibial nerve or of the popliteal artery with its branches—the anterior and posterior tibial artery, and the peroneal artery—is necessary, the soleus may be split.

In this case, soleus should be cut medially to the first muscular branch.

11.6.6 Wound Closure

After release of the tourniquet and hemostasis, the capsular incisions are closed by interrupted sutures, and the detached gastrocnemius heads are reattached.

11.6.7 Dangers

Lack of caution during dissection may result in a lesion of the popliteal vessels or their branches. In every case, therefore, the tourniquet is released and hemostasis effected prior to closure of the wound.

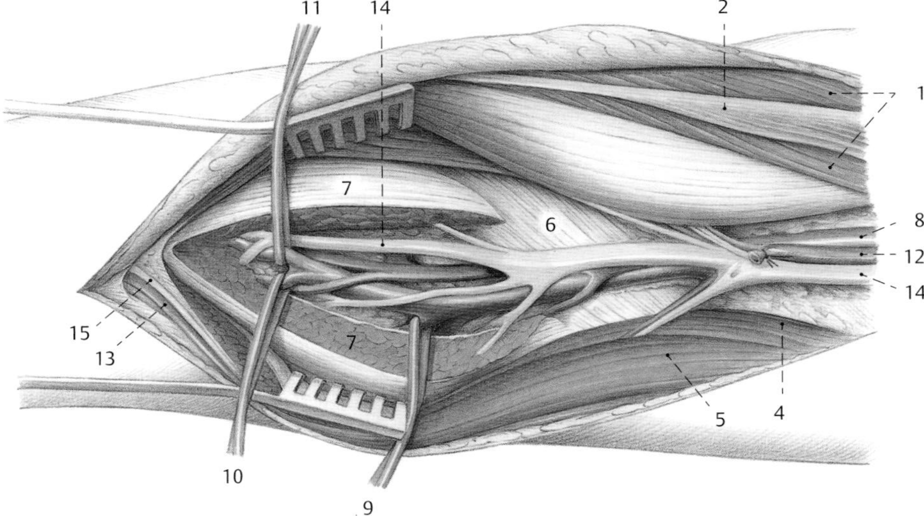

Fig. 11.42 Anatomical site of the popliteal region after partial splitting of gastrocnemius and soleus.

1 Semimembranosus
2 Semitendinosus
3 Gastrocnemius, medial head
4 Plantaris
5 Gastrocnemius, lateral head
6 Popliteus
7 Soleus
8 Popliteal artery
9 Anterior tibial artery
10 Peroneal artery
11 Posterior tibial artery
12 Popliteal vein
13 Small saphenous vein
14 Tibial nerve
15 Sural nerve

11.7 Arthroscopic Approaches

D. Kohn

11.7.1 Principal Indications

- Meniscus lesions
- Cartilage lesions
- Cruciate ligament reconstruction
- Intra-articular fractures

11.7.2 Positioning

All arthroscopic procedures on the knee are performed with the lower leg suspended freely using a thigh holder. The application of a tourniquet inside the thigh holder is recommended. The cuff must not be routinely inflated. Application of a tourniquet makes it more difficult to diagnose bleeding and synovial changes, and it increases the risk of nerve injuries. On the other hand, motorized instruments with a powerful suction action can only be used with application of a tourniquet. The best solution therefore seems to be the routine placement of a cuff that is only inflated if visualization deteriorates if power instruments are used, for particularly firm fixation of the thigh.

Figure 11.43 shows the positioning for knee arthroscopy, with the lower legs suspended freely. To avoid hyperlordosis, the hip on the healthy side is flexed a little.

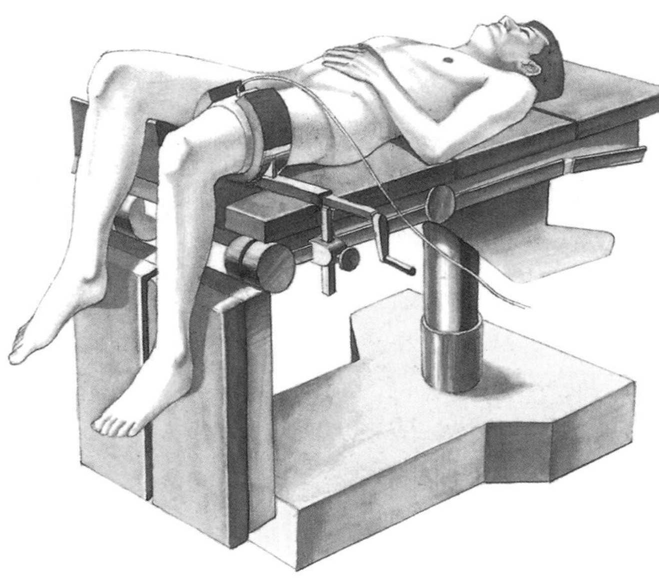

Fig. 11.43 Position for knee arthroscopy. (From: Bauer R, Kerschbaumer F, Poisel S. Becken und untere Extremität. Stuttgart, Thieme; 1995. Orthopädische Operationslehre; Band 2.)

11.7.3 Approaches

The diameter of the arthroscopic approach channels must allow penetration with the arthroscope or auxiliary instruments, but on the other hand these channels must not give rise to a pressure drop due to excessively large leakage. The skin incision length for access of the arthroscope is therefore approximately 7 mm, with an incision length of around 5 mm for instruments. To minimize scarring, all skin incisions should be along Langer's lines. The skin creases in the proximity of joints are horizontal.

The skin is penetrated with a scalpel. The fibrous capsule is penetrated with a scalpel or blunt trocar. The synovial membrane is perforated using a blunt trocar. Penetration of the synovial membrane with a scalpel or sharp trocar is permissible only when the entry portals can be checked intra-articularly with the arthroscope. For less experienced surgeons, probing planned instrument approaches with a size 1 needle is recommended. Working cannulas are usually cumbersome.

Figure 11.44 shows the possible approaches to the knee joint cavity. Some of these approaches are equally suitable for the arthroscope and operating instruments. The central approach is ideal for diagnostic arthroscopy, meniscus operations, removal of loose bodies, biopsy, and plica resection. It allows an assessment of both posterior compartments without shifting the arthroscope. Its position is defined using bony landmarks. The central approach enables the position of the most important instrument approaches to be defined clearly. It allows symmetrical operation on the medial and lateral meniscus. However, the central approach is suitable only for the arthroscope. If performed correctly, trauma to the patellar tendon is negligible and no complaints arise. The fibers of the tendon are pushed aside and never divided.

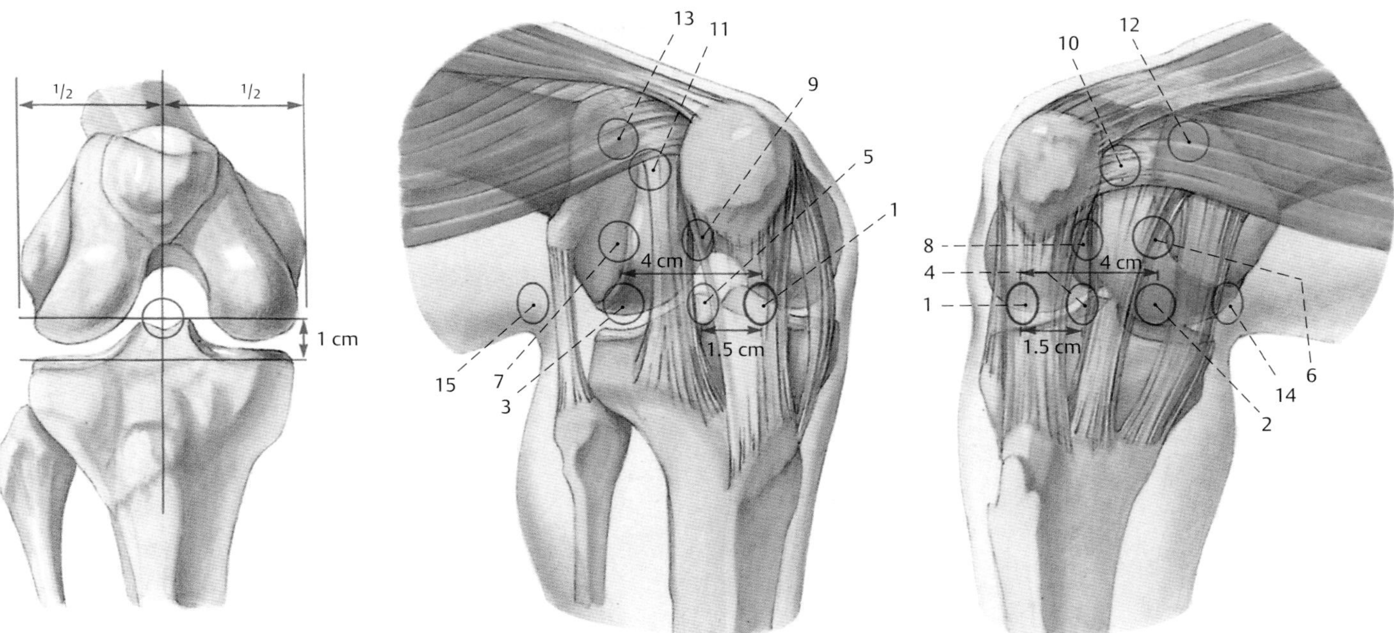

Fig. 11.44 Approaches for knee arthroscopy. (From: Bauer R, Kerschbaumer F, Poisel S. Becken und untere Extremität. Stuttgart, Thieme; 1995. Orthopädische Operationslehre; Band 2.)

1 Central approach, 1 cm above the edge of the medial plateau at the center of the knee
2 Anteromedial approach
3 Anterolateral approach
4 Paracentral medial approach
5 Paracentral lateral approach
6 High anteromedial approach
7 High anterolateral approach
8 High paracentral medial approach
9 High paracentral lateral approach
10 Midpatellar medial approach
11 Midpatellar lateral approach
12 Superomedial approach
13 Superolateral approach
14 Posteromedial approach
15 Posterolateral approach

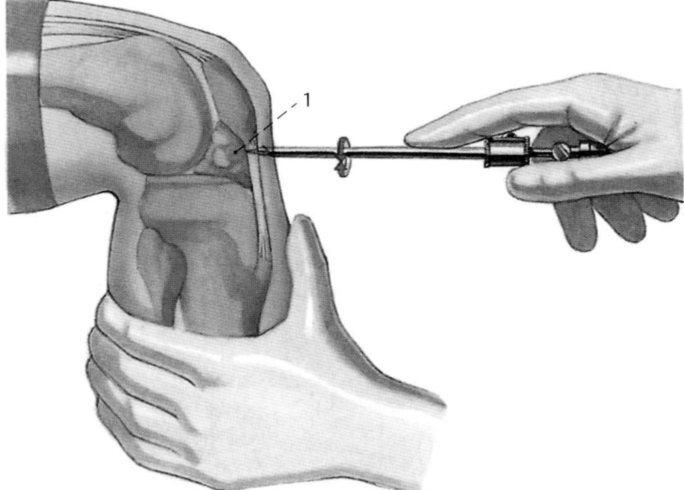

Fig. 11.45 Penetration of the patellar ligament. This is done with the knee flexed to a right angle using controlled pressure and rotating movements of the sharp trocar and sleeve. (From: Bauer R, Kerschbaumer F, Poisel S. Becken und untere Extremität. Stuttgart, Thieme; 1995. Orthopädische Operationslehre; Band 2.)

1 Hoffa's infrapatellar fat pad

11.7.4 Technique

With the knee flexed to 90°, the edge of the medial tibial plateau is palpated and marked. Both epicondyles are palpated, and the distance between them is halved (**Fig. 11.44**). The transverse skin incision is perpendicular to the imaginary knee joint line, 1 cm cranial to the medial edge of the tibial plateau with the knee flexed to 90°. Using cautious rotating movements, the patellar ligament is penetrated with the sharp trocar inside the sleeve (**Fig. 11.45**), the sharp trocar is exchanged for a blunt trocar, and the sleeve with the blunt trocar is advanced into the patellofemoral joint with the knee extended (**Fig. 11.46**).

The blunt trocar is exchanged for the standard optic, which has previously been connected to the camera and fiberoptic cable. After the surgeon has checked on the monitor that the arthroscope is in an intra-articular position, the water supply is connected, and the joint is filled with irrigation fluid through the arthroscope shaft at a pressure of 100 mmHg. When the joint is tense, the superomedial recess is punctured with the outflow cannula. It is connected to an outflow tube with a roller clamp to control the pressure.

As soon as the irrigation system has been started and the surgeon has checked that the outflow is functioning, diagnostic inspection can begin (**Fig. 11.47**).

11.7.5 Wound Closure

The incisions are closed with Steristrips or interrupted sutures.

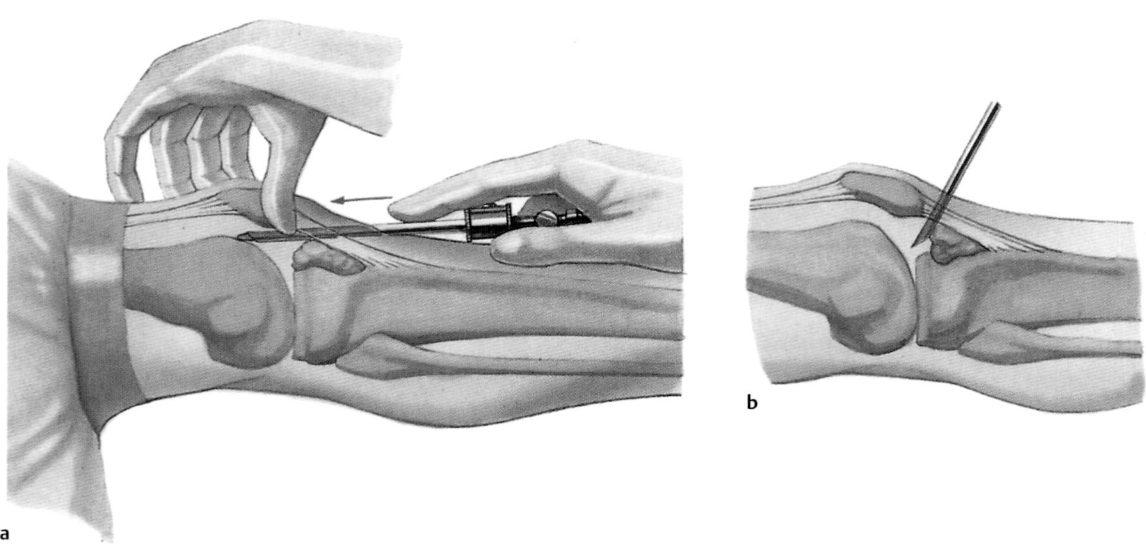

Fig. 11.46 a, b Penetration of the synovial membrane with a blunt trocar/sleeve anterior and superior to Hoffa's infrapatellar fat pad. (From: Bauer R, Kerschbaumer F, Poisel S. Becken und untere Extremität. Stuttgart, Thieme; 1995. Orthopädische Operationslehre; Band 2.)

a The trocar sleeve is first advanced into the patellofemoral joint.
b During subsequent inspection of the femorotibial joint, the fat pad is pushed aside and does not impede visualization.

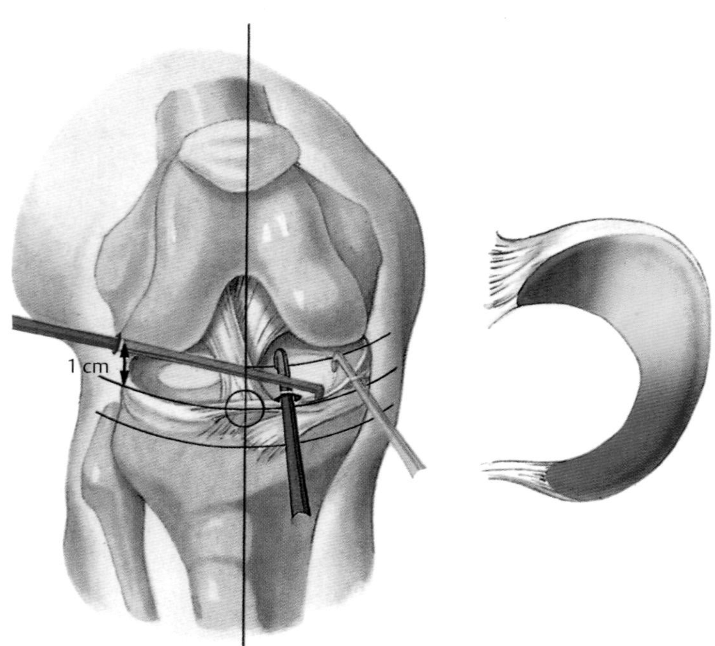

Fig. 11.47 Meniscectomy. Approaches and accessible areas for the medial meniscus depending on the approach (cf. **Fig. 11.44**). (From: Bauer R, Kerschbaumer F, Poisel S. Becken und untere Extremität. Stuttgart, Thieme; 1995. Orthopädische Operationslehre; Band 2.)

Yellow Anteromedial approach
Blue Paracentral medial approach
Red High anterolateral approach

12 Lower Leg

12.1 Proximal Approach to the Medullary Cavity of the Tibia

K. Weise, D. Höntzsch

12.1.1 Principal Indications

- Intramedullary nailing of fractures
- Pseudarthrosis

12.1.2 Positioning and Incision

Various positions are possible:
- Supine with the leg raised
- Supine with the leg hanging down
- On an extension table

The skin incision is centered over the patellar ligament (**Fig. 12.1**). Alternatively, it may be lateral to the patellar ligament, but thereafter the approach is largely identical.

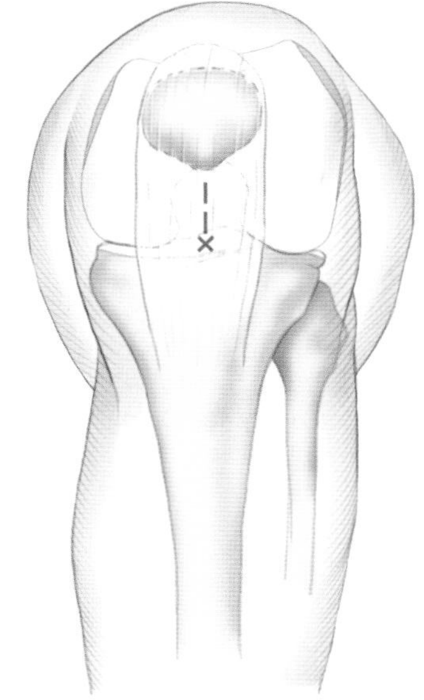

Fig. 12.1 Vertical incision centered over the patellar ligament.

12.1.3 Exposure of the Proximal Approach to the Medullary Cavity of the Tibia

The patellar ligament is split by an incision through all the layers, from the lower pole of the patella and its insertion as far as the tibial tuberosity (**Fig. 12.2**).

The patellar ligament is retracted medially and laterally with Langenbeck retractors (**Fig. 12.3**); alternatively, retaining sutures may be placed.

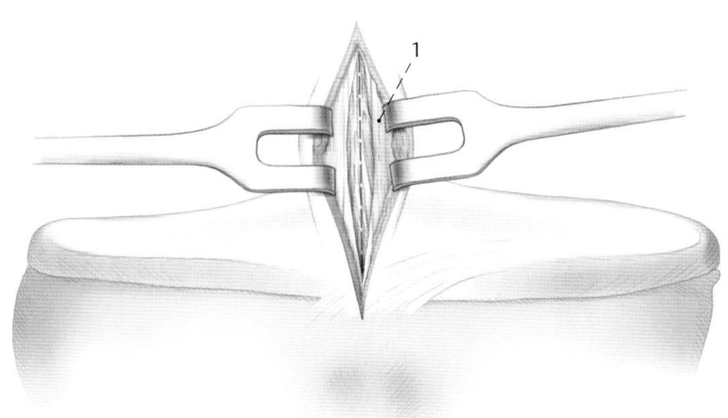

Fig. 12.2 The patellar ligament is split through all layers with a single incision that extends a short distance below the skin.

1 Patellar ligament

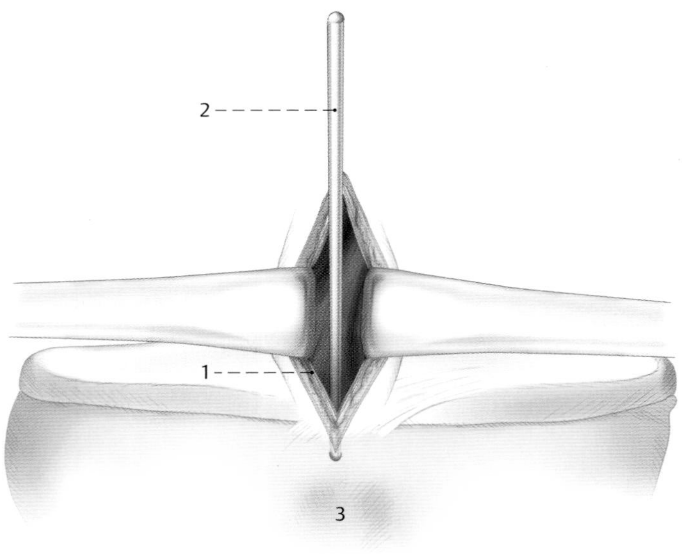

Fig. 12.3 After splitting the patellar ligament, it is held laterally and medially with Langenbeck retractors so that the junction of the joint surface with the tibial tuberosity can be palpated in a distal direction. A guidewire is shown at the desired entry point.

1 Patellar ligament
2 Guidewire
3 Tibial tuberosity

The entry point for the nail is sought by palpation distally and is not shown directly. A guidewire is shown here, but alternative instrumentation may be used.

12.1.4 Wound Closure

The patellar ligament is closed in one layer, followed by subcutaneous suture and skin suture.

12.2 Direct Posterior Approach to the Tibial Plateau

P. Lobenhoffer, O. Yastrebov

12.2.1 Principal Indications

- Posteromedial fracture dislocation of the tibial plateau (medial split fracture)
- Bicondylar fracture dislocation of the tibial plateau
- Tibial bony avulsion of the posterior cruciate ligament

12.2.2 Positioning and Incision

The patient is placed in the prone position. A tourniquet is applied to the operated leg, and the contralateral leg is lowered. The operated leg should be freely mobile. A rolled towel is placed below the thigh or lower leg depending on the direction of reduction.

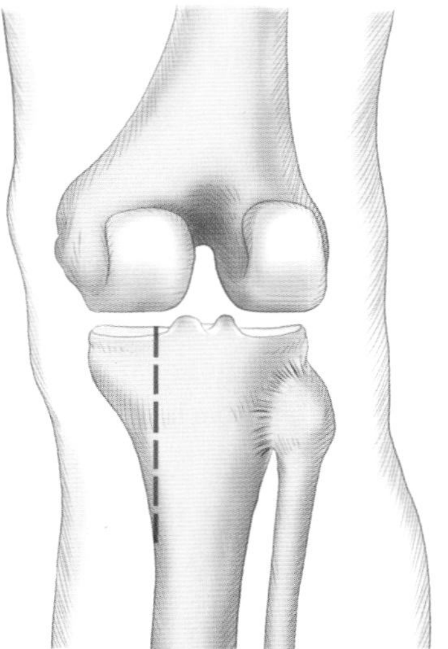

Fig. 12.4 Skin incision extending 7 cm distally from the knee joint line, medial to the popliteal fossa over the medial head of gastrocnemius.

12.2.3 Technique

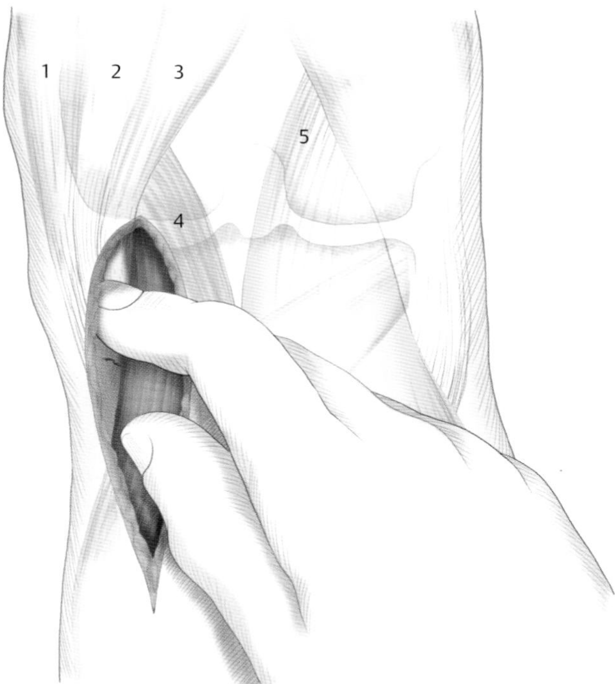

Fig. 12.5 The medial border of the medial head of gastrocnemius is sought following sharp dissection of the subcutaneous tissue and fascia.

1 Gracilis
2 Semitendinosus
3 Semimembranosus
4 Gastrocnemius, medial head
5 Gastrocnemius, lateral head

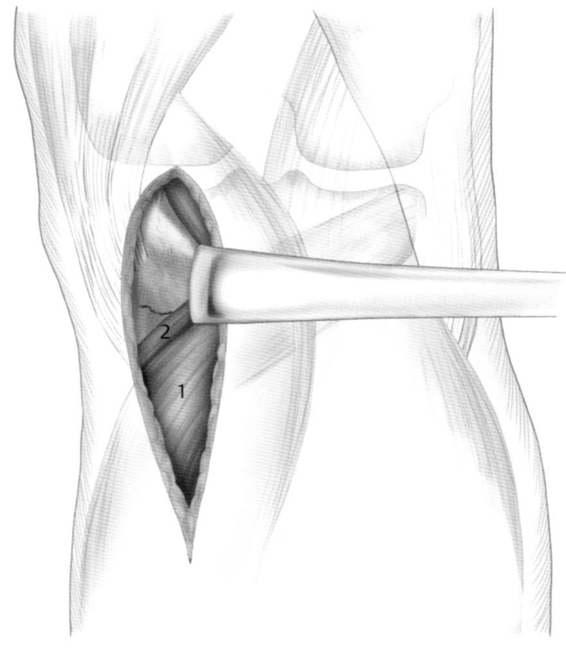

Fig. 12.6 The gastrocnemius is mobilized laterally by blunt dissection and retracted with a vein hook. The popliteus comes into view.

1 Gastrocnemius, medial head
2 Popliteus

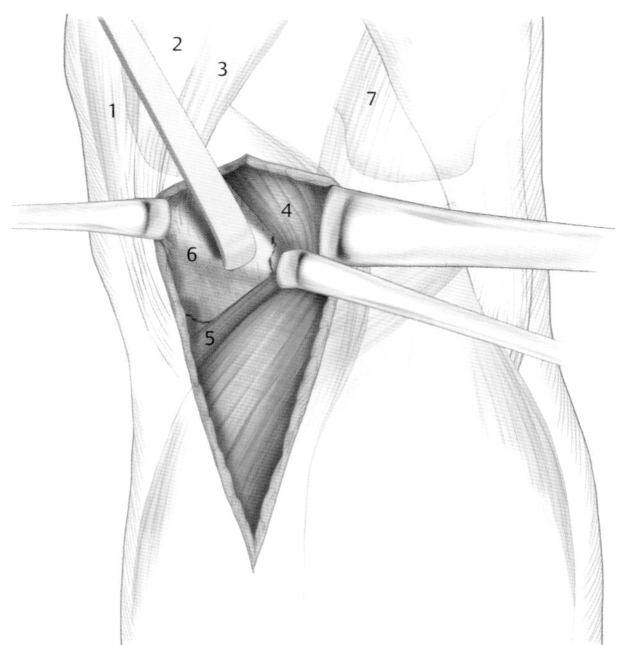

Fig. 12.7 The popliteus is mobilized subperiosteally with a raspatory and retracted distally in a lateral direction. The distal part of the posterior joint capsule is exposed.

1 Gracilis
2 Semitendinosus
3 Semimembranosus
4 Gastrocnemius, medial head
5 Popliteus
6 Medial tibial condyle
7 Gastrocnemius, lateral head

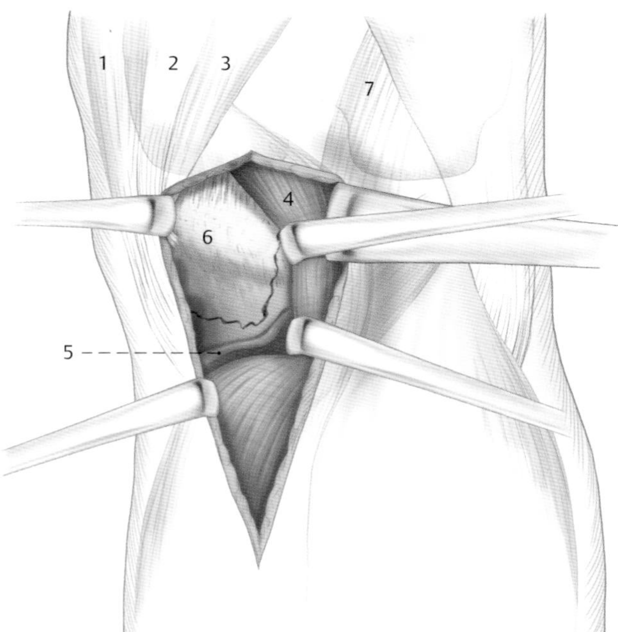

Fig. 12.8 The posterior surface of the medial tibial plateau, the fracture margins, and the caudal fracture tip, which is important for reduction, are exposed. The joint capsule does not have to be opened.

1 Gracilis
2 Semitendinosus
3 Semimembranosus
4 Gastrocnemius, medial head
5 Popliteus
6 Medial tibial condyle
7 Gastrocnemius, lateral head

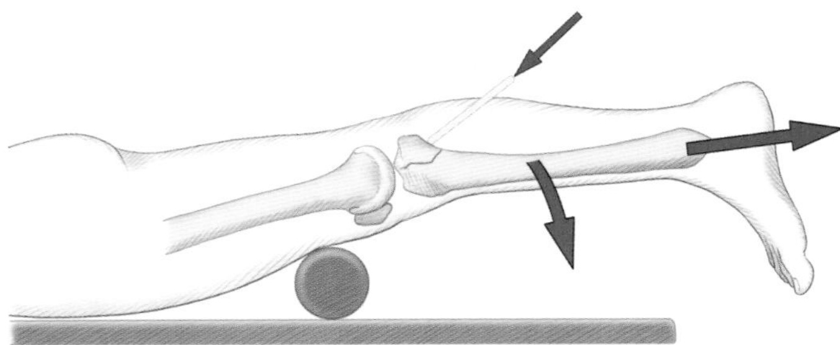

Fig. 12.9 The distal thigh is positioned on a rolled towel. The posteromedial fragment is reduced by extending the knee with simultaneous axial traction on the lower leg. The reduction is supported by a raspatory or oval awl. The fracture is fixed provisionally with Kirschner wires, and final internal fixation is performed after radiographic confirmation of the reduction.

12.2.4 Wound Closure

The soft tissues cover the internal fixation material spontaneously. The popliteus is reapproximated, and the tourniquet is released. Following hemostasis and irrigation, a Redon drain is inserted, the crural fascia is closed, and the wound is closed in layers.

12.2.5 Dangers

- Hematoma
- Deep vein thrombosis
- Infection
- Lower leg compartment syndrome
- Injury to the neurovascular structures

12.3 Posteromedial Approach to the Tibial Plateau

P. Lobenhoffer, O. Yastrebov

12.3.1 Principal Indications

- Posteromedial fracture dislocation of the tibial plateau

12.3.2 Positioning and Incision

The patient is placed supine. A tourniquet is applied to the leg. The side of the thigh is supported. The operated leg is elevated with the knee flexed to 60–70°. The contralateral leg is lowered.

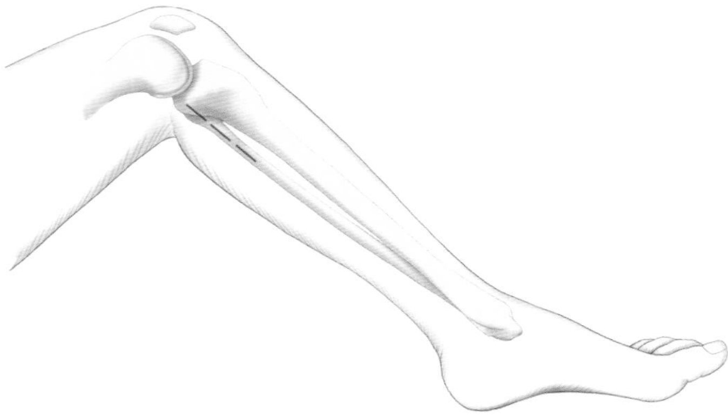

Fig. 12.10 Skin incision approximately 6–7 cm long extending distally from the knee joint line along the posterior tibial border.

12.3.3 Wound Closure

The tourniquet is released. Following hemostasis and irrigation, a Redon drain is inserted if necessary, and the wound is closed in layers.

12.3.4 Dangers

- Hematoma
- Deep vein thrombosis
- Infection
- Lower leg compartment syndrome
- Injury to the neurovascular structures

12.3.5 Technique

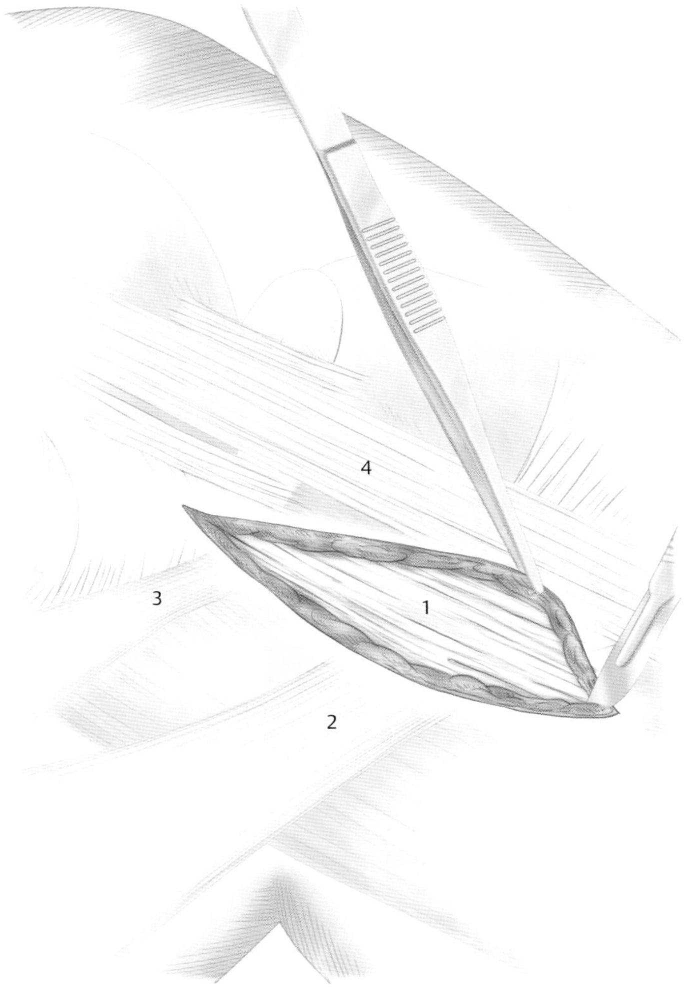

Fig. 12.11 The subcutaneous tissue is divided sharply, and the pes anserinus is identified.

1 Superficial crural fascia
2 Superficial part of the pes anserinus
3 Semimembranosus
4 Tibial collateral ligament

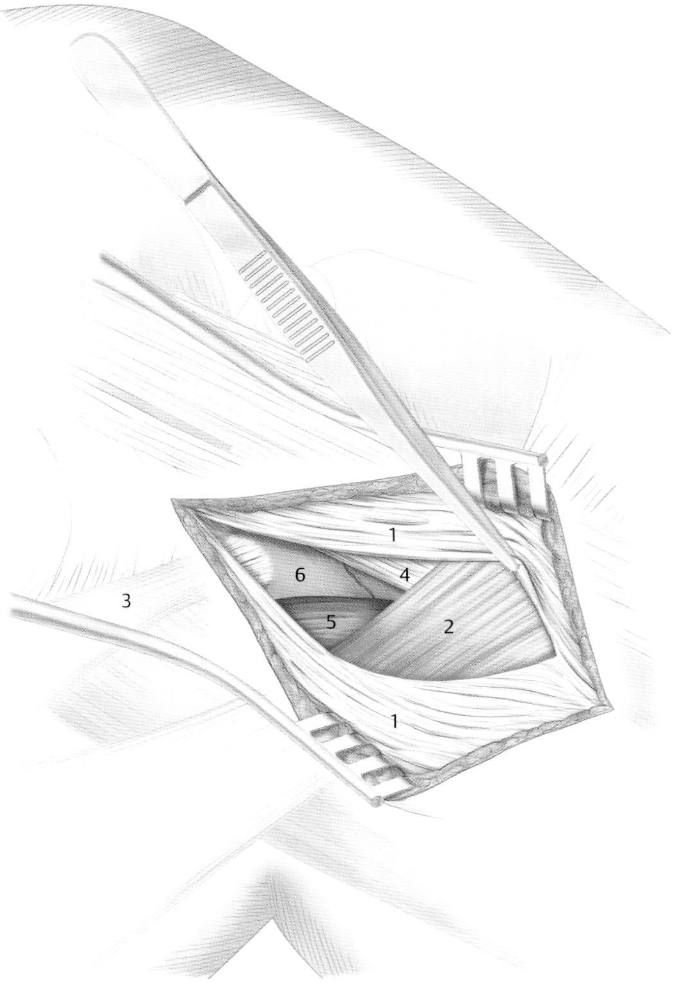

Fig. 12.12 Incision of the crural fascia at the posterior border of the tibial collateral ligament, running from the inferior border of semimembranosus as far as the upper border of the pes anserinus.

1 Superficial crural fascia (incised)
2 Superficial part of the pes anserinus
3 Semimembranosus
4 Tibial collateral ligament
5 Gastrocnemius, medial head
6 Medial tibial condyle

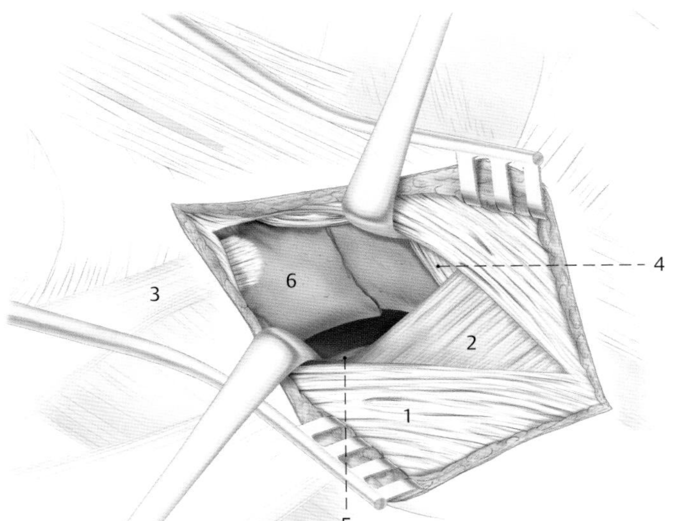

Fig. 12.13 The superficial part of the pes anserinus is retracted caudally, and the medial head of gastrocnemius is retracted posteriorly. The extra-articular fracture components are exposed subperiosteally.

1 Superficial crural fascia (incised)
2 Superficial part of the pes anserinus
3 Semimembranosus
4 Tibial collateral ligament
5 Gastrocnemius, medial head
6 Medial tibial condyle

12.4 Posterolateral Approach to the Tibial Plateau with Osteotomy of the Fibula

P. Lobenhoffer, O. Yastrebov

12.4.1 Principal Indications

- Posterolateral fracture dislocation of the tibial plateau
- Posterolateral depressed fracture of the tibial plateau
- Bicondylar fracture dislocation of the tibial plateau

12.4.2 Positioning and Incision

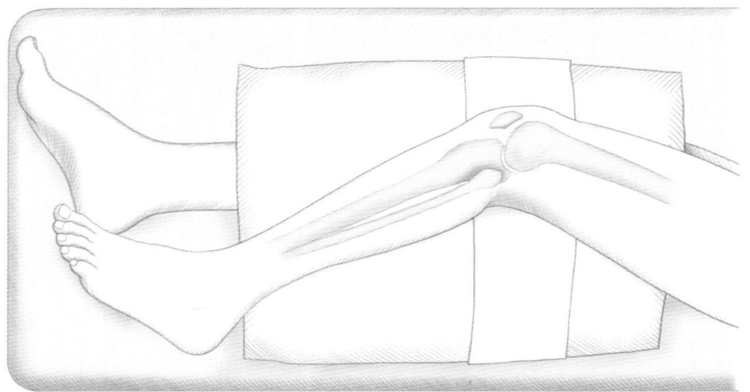

Fig. 12.14 The patient lies supine with the leg raised, or lies on his or her side. Application of a tourniquet. The operated leg is freely mobile.

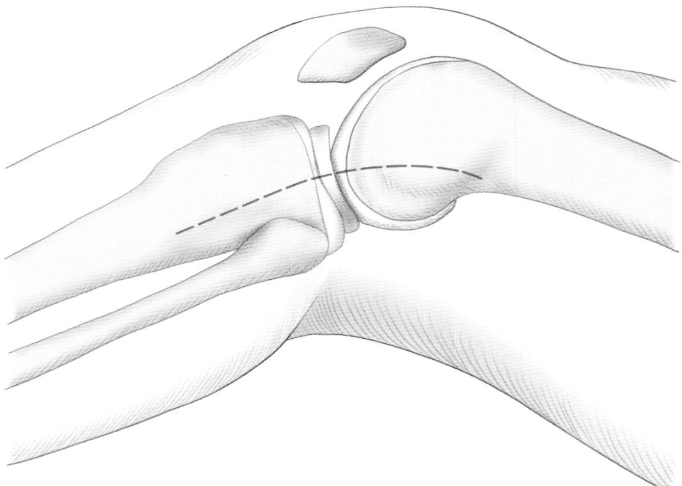

Fig. 12.15 Curved skin incision, approximately 10 cm in length, beginning 3 cm proximal to the joint line and extending distally on the anterolateral surface of the leg.

12.4.3 Technique

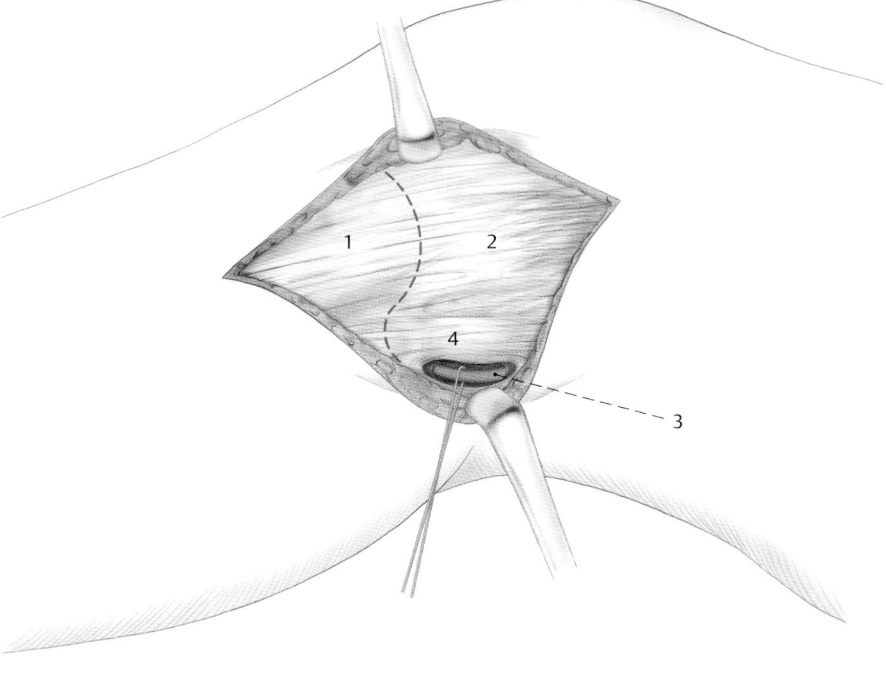

Fig. 12.16 The subcutaneous tissue is divided down to the crural fascia. Subcutaneous dissection continues posteriorly to the head of the fibula. The fascia is split parallel to the fibula, and the common peroneal nerve is exposed and snared. A curved incision is made in the crural fascia along the extensor origin. Note: The superficial peroneal nerve is directly beneath the fascia.

1 Crural fascia
2 Iliotibial tract
3 Common peroneal nerve
4 Head of fibula

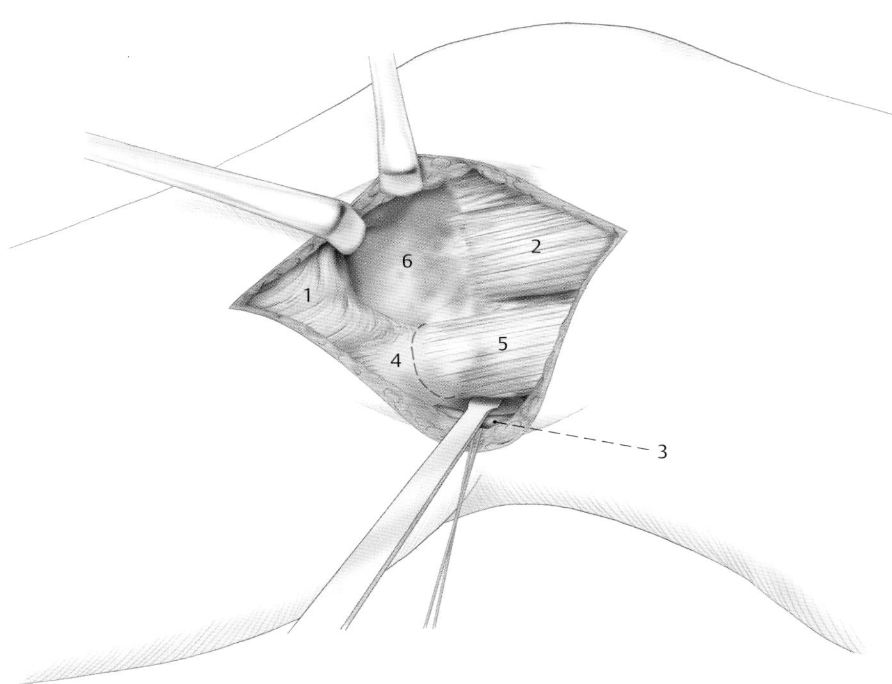

Fig. 12.17 The muscles and fascia are mobilized subperiosteally in a caudal direction. The neck of the fibula is exposed, and an incomplete oblique subcapital osteotomy is performed sparing the common peroneal nerve. The osteotomy is then completed with a chisel, and the head of the fibula is retracted dorsocranially.

1 Origin of the foot extensors (tibialis anterior, extensor digitorum longus)
2 Iliotibial tract
3 Common peroneal nerve
4 Head of the fibula
5 Fibular collateral ligament and tendon of biceps femoris
6 Lateral tibial condyle

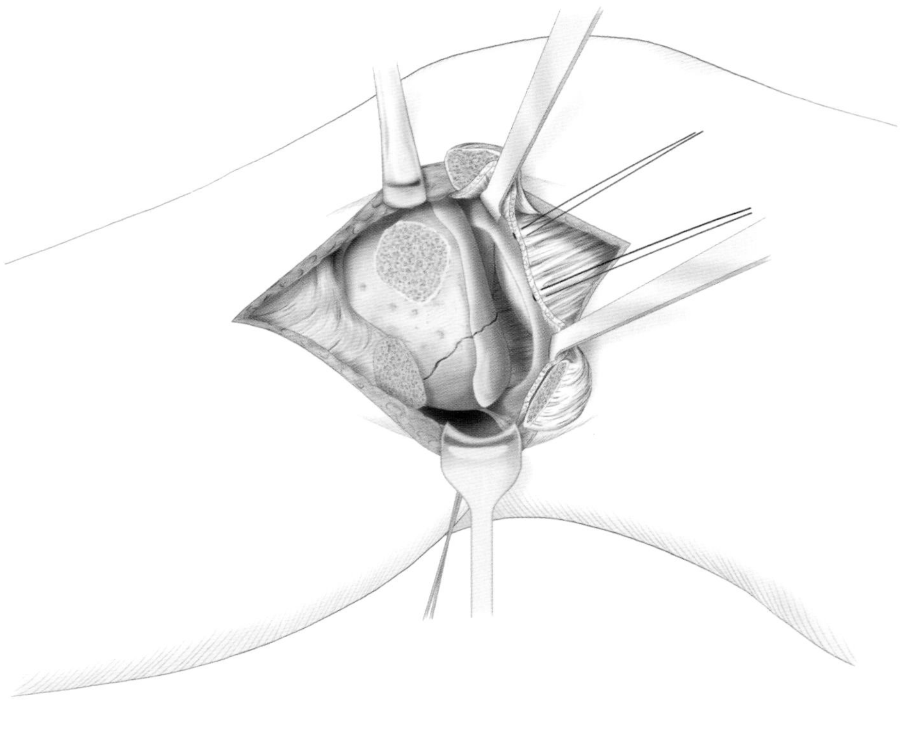

Fig. 12.18 Gerdy's tubercle with the attachment of the iliotibial tract is divided and retracted proximally. The joint capsule is incised and dissected subperiosteally with the meniscotibial ligament. These are held proximally with retaining sutures. The fracture morphology and articular surface of the lateral tibial plateau can be assessed exactly. Exposure of the posterolateral tibial plateau is best achieved with the tibia in varus and internally rotated.

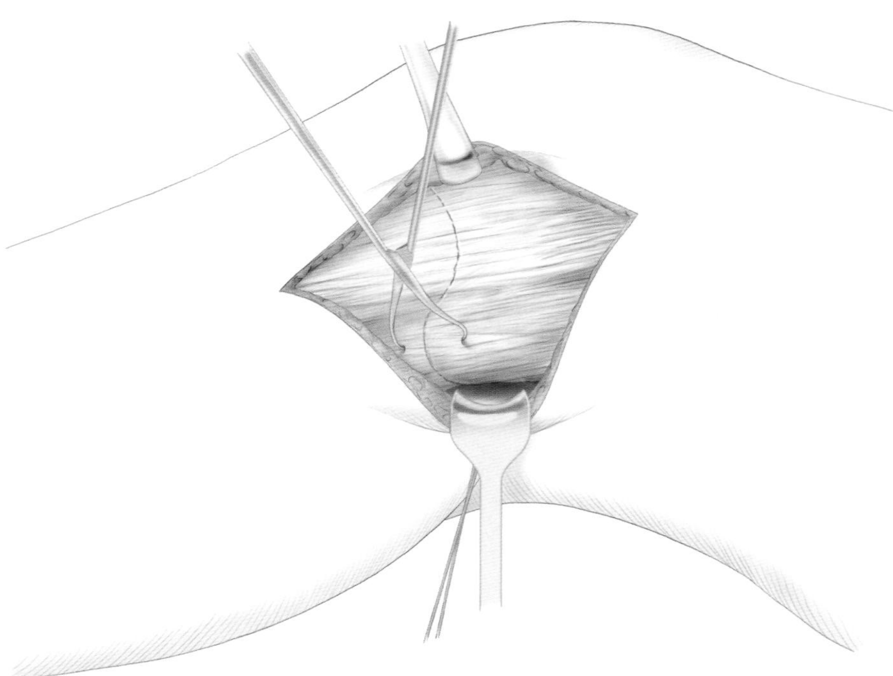

Fig. 12.19 Following internal fixation of the tibial plateau, the fibular head is reduced with pointed reduction forceps, sparing the common peroneal nerve. After predrilling, a small fragment screw is inserted bicortically perpendicular to the osteotomy. Fixation with a wire or tension band is an alternative.

12.4.4 Wound Closure

Closure starts with approximation of the joint capsule and reattachment of Gerdy's tubercle by transosseous suture. The extensors and crural fascia are approximated with a continuous suture. The fascia over the common peroneal nerve is left open. The tourniquet is released. Following hemostasis and irrigation, a Redon drain is inserted if necessary, and the wound is closed in layers.

12.4.5 Dangers

- Hematoma
- Deep vein thrombosis
- Infection
- Lower leg compartment syndrome
- Injury to the neurovascular structures
- Pseudarthrosis of the fibula

12.5 Posterolateral Approach to the Tibia and Fibula

R. Bauer, F. Kerschbaumer, S. Poisel

12.5.1 Principal Indications

- Fractures
- Osteomyelitis
- Infected pseudarthroses

12.5.2 Positioning and Incision

The patient is placed on his or her side. After (optional) application of a tourniquet, the leg is draped so as to allow free movement. The patient may also be placed in a semilateral position, in which case the ipsilateral pelvis has to be well supported. In this position, the lower leg is internally rotated (**Fig. 12.20**). The skin incision begins three fingerbreadths distal to the fibular head and runs toward the external malleolus parallel to the posterior border of the fibula. After dissection of the skin and subcutaneous tissue, the crural fascia is split at the posterior border of the peroneal muscles in line with the skin incision (**Fig. 12.21**).

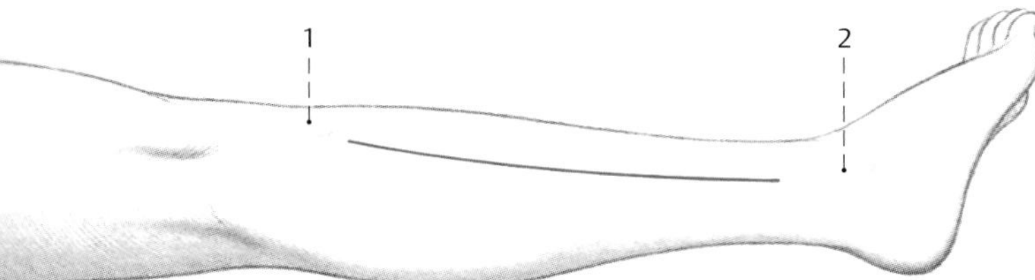

Fig. 12.20 Posterolateral approach to the tibia and fibula. Skin incision (right leg).

1 Head of the fibula
2 Lateral malleolus

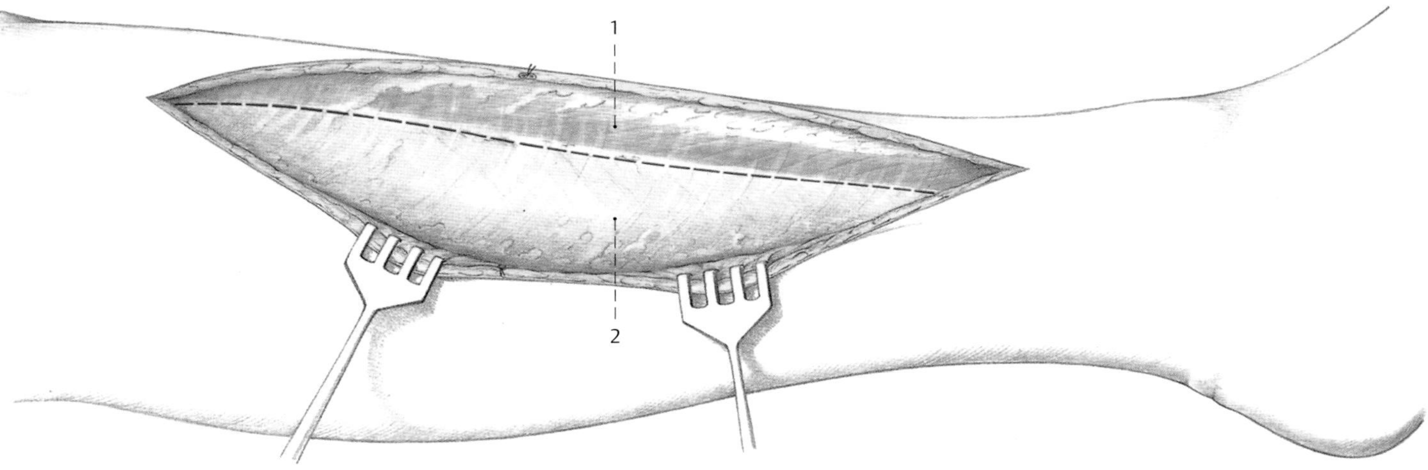

Fig. 12.21 Incision of the crural fascia between peroneus longus and soleus.

1 Crural fascia with peroneus longus
2 Crural fascia with soleus muscle

12.5.3 Posterior Exposure of the Tibia and Fibula

Perforating vessels from the peroneal artery and vein are ligated and transected if necessary. Subsequently, the posterior aspect of the fibula is subperiosteally exposed with a raspatory (**Fig. 12.22**). Note that the direction of dissection with the raspatory must be distal to proximal as this causes less trauma to the muscle. When the posterior surface of the fibula has been uncovered by detachment of the flexor hallucis longus, the tip of the raspatory is used to trace first the interosseous membrane and then the posterior surface of the tibia. Now the tibialis posterior and the flexor digitorum longus muscles are also stripped from the interosseous membrane and the posterior surface of the tibia (**Fig. 12.23**). This should be done as close to the bone as possible to avoid injury to the peroneal vessels. The posterior surface of the tibia should be sparingly exposed for the insertion of Hohmann elevators only (**Fig. 12.24**). In no circumstances should a large portion of the posterior tibial surface be exposed in the medial area of the shaft as the artery that arises from the posterior tibial artery and supplies the posterior tibial surface must be preserved. Maximal internal rotation of the leg can now give a good overview of the posterior surfaces of the tibia and fibula as well as the interosseous membrane, even in the semilateral position.

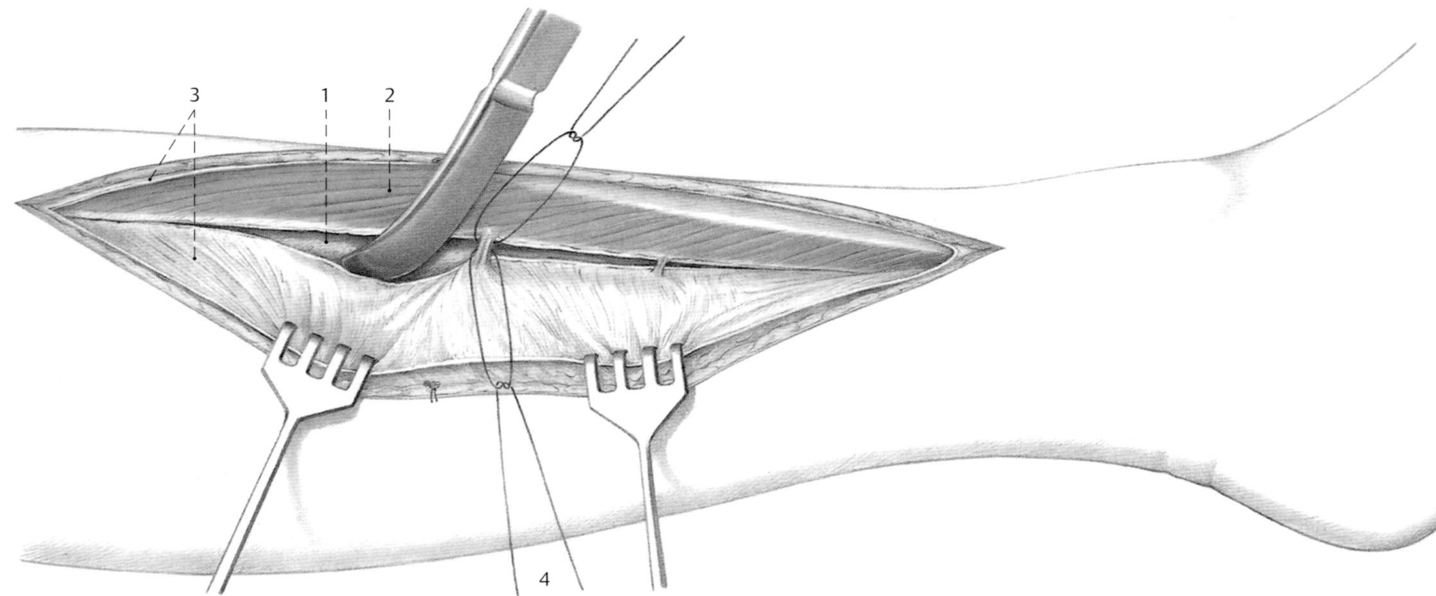

Fig. 12.22 Ligation and transection of the perforating peroneal vessels. Subperiosteal exposure of the fibula with the raspatory anterior to the posterior intermuscular septum of the leg (this should not be done with fractures).

1 Fibula
2 Peroneus longus
3 Crural fascia
4 Muscular branches of the peroneal vessels

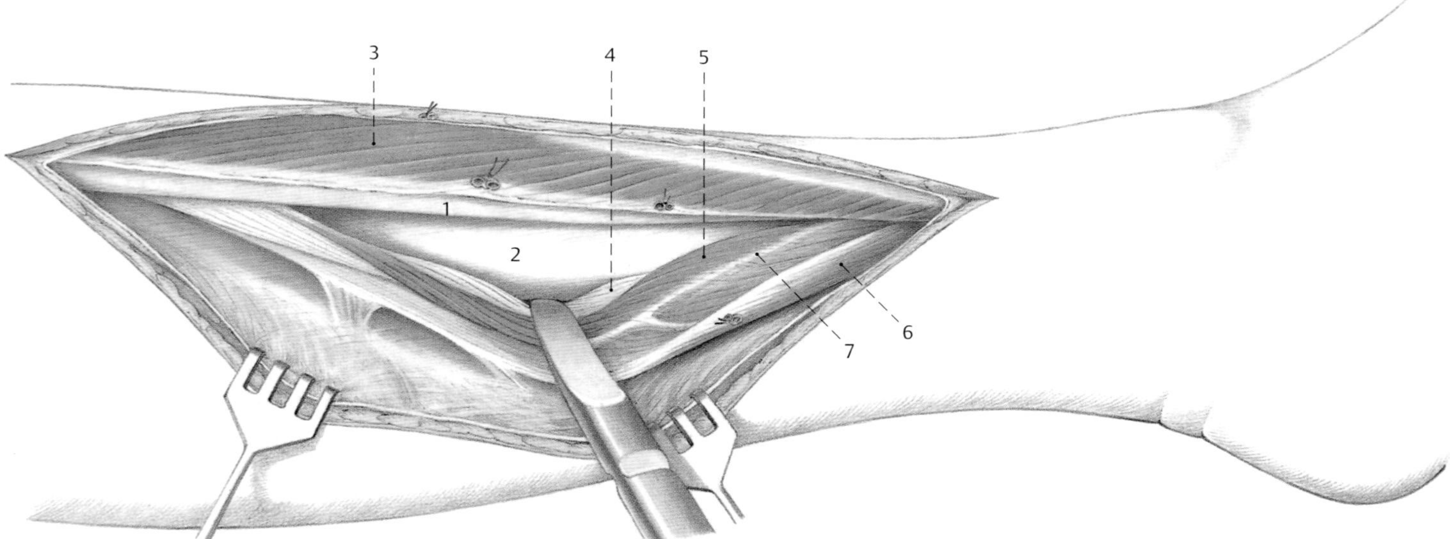

Fig. 12.23 Operative site after detachment of the deep flexor muscles of the leg from the posterior surface of the fibula, interosseous membrane, and posterior aspect of the tibia.

1 Fibula
2 Tibia
3 Peroneus longus
4 Tendons of flexor digitorum longus
5 Tibialis posterior
6 Flexor hallucis longus
7 Peroneal artery and vein

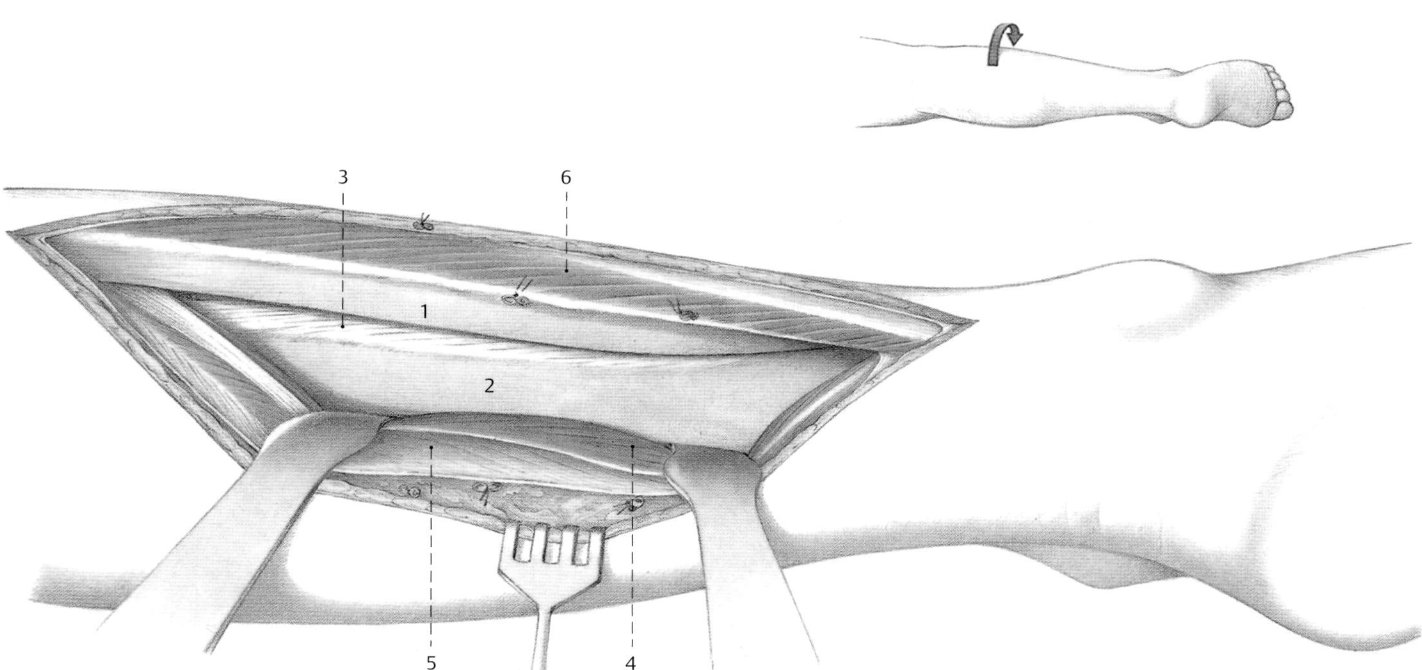

Fig. 12.24 The posterior aspects of the midportions of the fibular and tibial shafts are exposed after internal rotation of the leg and insertion of Hohmann elevators.

1 Fibula
2 Tibia
3 Interosseous membrane
4 Tibialis posterior
5 Flexor hallucis longus
6 Peroneus longus

12.5.4 Anatomical Site

Figure 12.25 presents an anatomical preparation in which, to expose the course of the vessels and nerves in the lower leg, the gastrocnemius (lateral head), soleus, and flexor hallucis longus have been detached from the femur and fibula, respectively, and reflected laterally. The course of the tibial nerve, the popliteal vessels, and their division into the anterior tibial, peroneal, and posterior tibial vessels are shown. Note the direct contact of the peroneal vessels with the fibula. Tibialis posterior has been stripped from the proximal portion of the tibia and the fibula as well as from the interosseous membrane. Proximally, the nutrient artery can be seen arising from the posterior tibial artery. This nutrient artery pierces tibialis posterior to supply the tibia from the posterior side. This vessel and the anterior tibial artery should, if possible, be spared in the posterolateral exposure of the fibula and tibia.

12.5.5 Wound Closure

After release of the tourniquet and hemostasis, the wound is closed by suture of the periosteum over the fibula, as a result of which all the detached muscle groups are brought into apposition again. If the muscles have suffered substantial damage during the operative procedure or if major hemorrhage has occurred, loose suture of the superficial fascia without closure of the deep fascia is advisable in order to avert a deep compartment syndrome after the operation.

12.5.6 Dangers

Extraperiosteal dissection may lead to traumatization of the peroneal vessels, which can give rise to troublesome hemorrhage. Dissection in a proximal direction should not be done at a level higher than four fingerbreadths distal to the fibular head so that injury to the anterior tibial artery and the common peroneal nerve may be avoided.

12.5.7 Note

The approach described above is used mainly for repeat operations on pseudarthrosis of the leg when skin conditions on the anterior side of the leg are unfavorable.

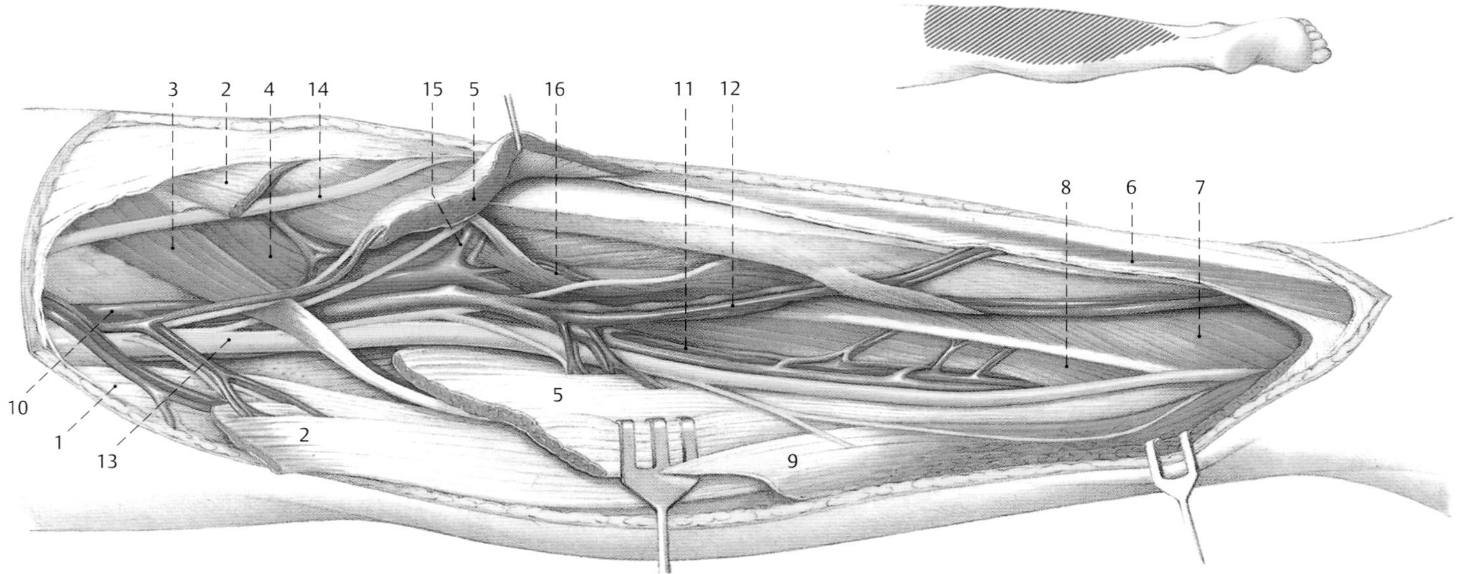

Fig. 12.25 Anatomical site of the deep crural flexor compartment. The lateral head of gastrocnemius, the soleus, and the flexor hallucis longus have been detached from their origins and retracted medially. Distal to the detached origin of soleus, the fibula, the interosseous membrane, and a small portion of the tibia are exposed subperiosteally. Note: The origin of the anterior tibial artery three fingerbreadths distal to the head of the fibula, and the origin of the nutrient artery and course of the peroneal vessels.

1 Gastrocnemius, medial head
2 Gastrocnemius, lateral head
3 Plantaris
4 Popliteus
5 Soleus
6 Peroneus longus
7 Tibialis posterior
8 Flexor digitorum longus
9 Flexor hallucis longus
10 Popliteal artery
11 Posterior tibial artery
12 Peroneal artery
13 Tibial nerve
14 Common peroneal nerve
15 Anterior tibial artery
16 Nutrient artery of the tibia

12.6 Posteromedial Approach to the Tibial Shaft

R. Bauer, F. Kerschbaumer, S. Poisel, K. Weise, D. Höntzsch

12.6.1 Principal Indications

- Fractures
- Leg lengthening

12.6.2 Positioning and Incision

The patient is placed in the supine position. The leg to be operated on is placed over the contralateral leg, and the knee is slightly flexed (**Fig. 12.26**). The skin incision is made two fingerbreadths posterior to the readily palpable medial border of the tibia. It is advisable to split the subcutaneous tissue with caution to spare the saphenous nerve and the great saphenous vein. Transversely running veins must be coagulated or ligated. The fascia is incised behind the saphenous nerve (**Fig. 12.27**).

12.6.3 Exposure of the Tibial Shaft

Insertion of retractors and retraction of the fascia bring into view the medial head of the gastrocnemius, the soleus muscle and, more distally, the origin of flexor digitorum longus, which are covered by the deep layer of the crural fascia (**Fig. 12.28**). The latter and the periosteum are incised at the medial border of the tibia; perforating vessels are coagulated or ligated. The posterior surface of the tibia can be exposed subperiosteally with a raspatory (**Fig. 12.29**). Complete stripping of the periosteum at the interosseous margin of the tibia should be avoided in the middle of the shaft to guard against injury to the nutrient artery.

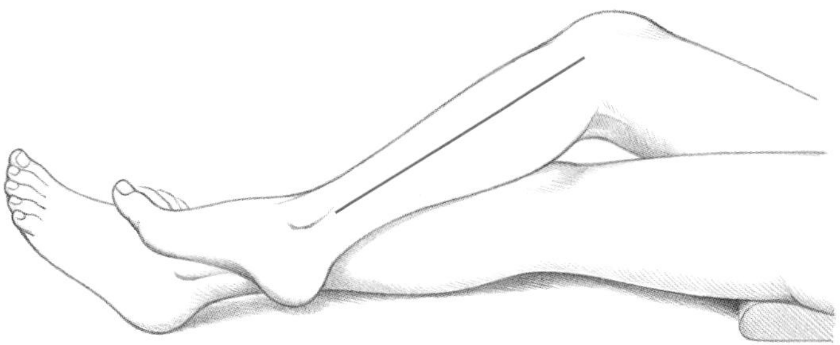

Fig. 12.26 Posteromedial approach to the tibial shaft. Positioning and incision (right leg).

12.6.4 Extension of the Approach

The approach can be extended proximally by continuing the incision as far as the knee joint cavity or by making a curved incision into the popliteal fossa. Distal extension of the approach is likewise possible.

12.6.5 Wound Closure

Following release of the tourniquet and hemostasis, the wound is closed by suture of the superficial crural fascia. To avoid a compartment syndrome, the deep fascial layer should not be sutured. The use of Redon drains is mandatory.

12.6.6 Note

The dorsomedial approach is particularly suitable for exposure of the middle segment of the shaft. The approach described by Banks and Laufmann is better suited for posterior exposure of the proximal shaft.

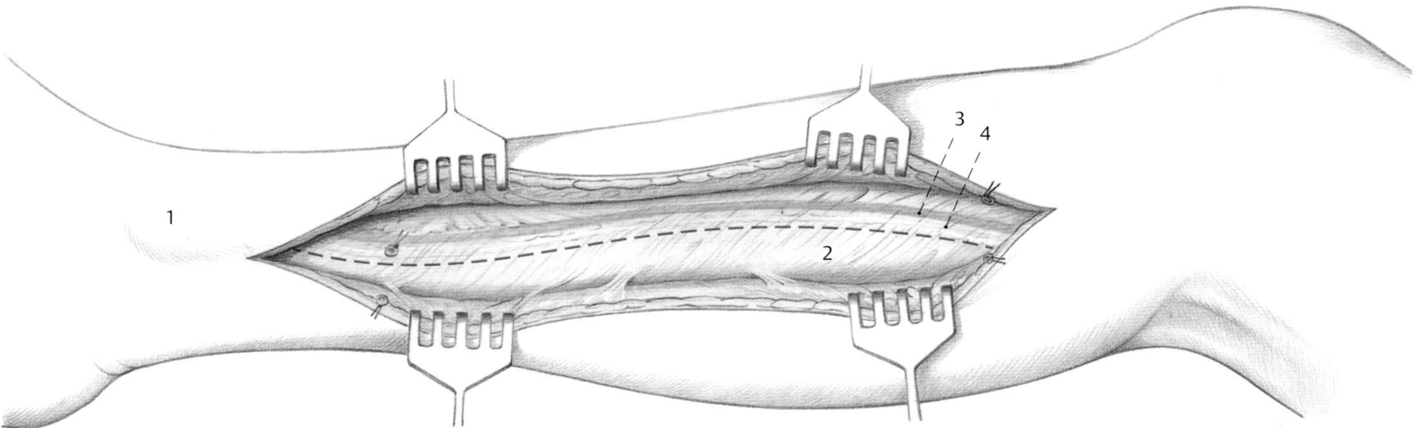

Fig. 12.27 Division of the crural fascia posterior to the saphenous nerve and long saphenous vein.

1 Medial malleolus
2 Crural fascia
3 Great saphenous vein
4 Saphenous nerve

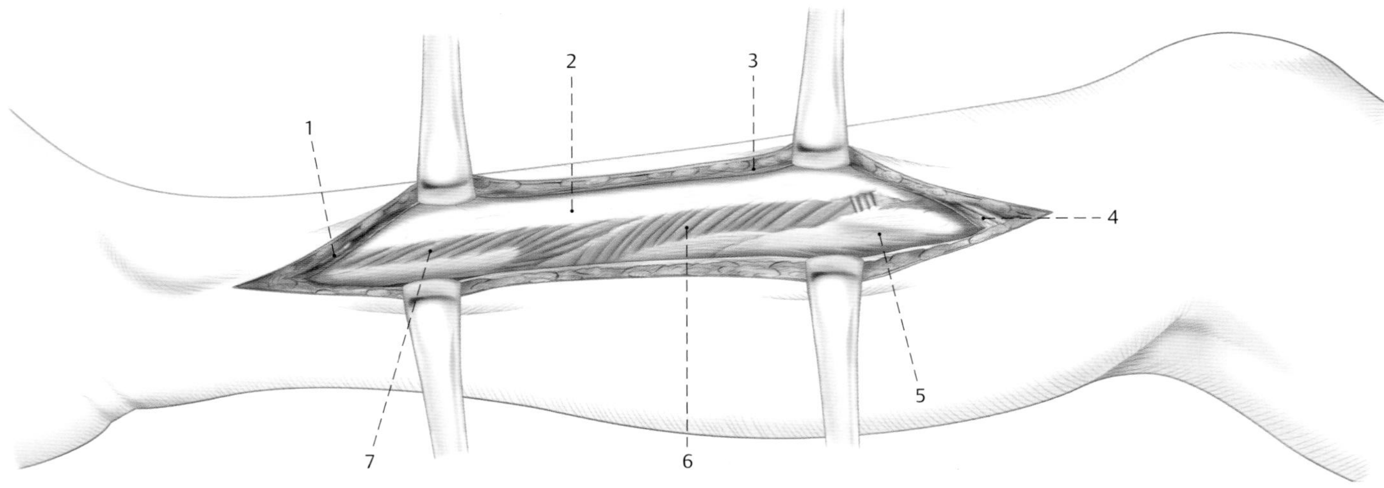

Fig. 12.28 Anterior retraction of the fascia to expose the posterior surface of the tibia.

1 Great saphenous vein
2 Shaft of the tibia
3 Crural fascia
4 Saphenous nerve
5 Gastrocnemius, medial head
6 Soleus
7 Flexor digitorum longus

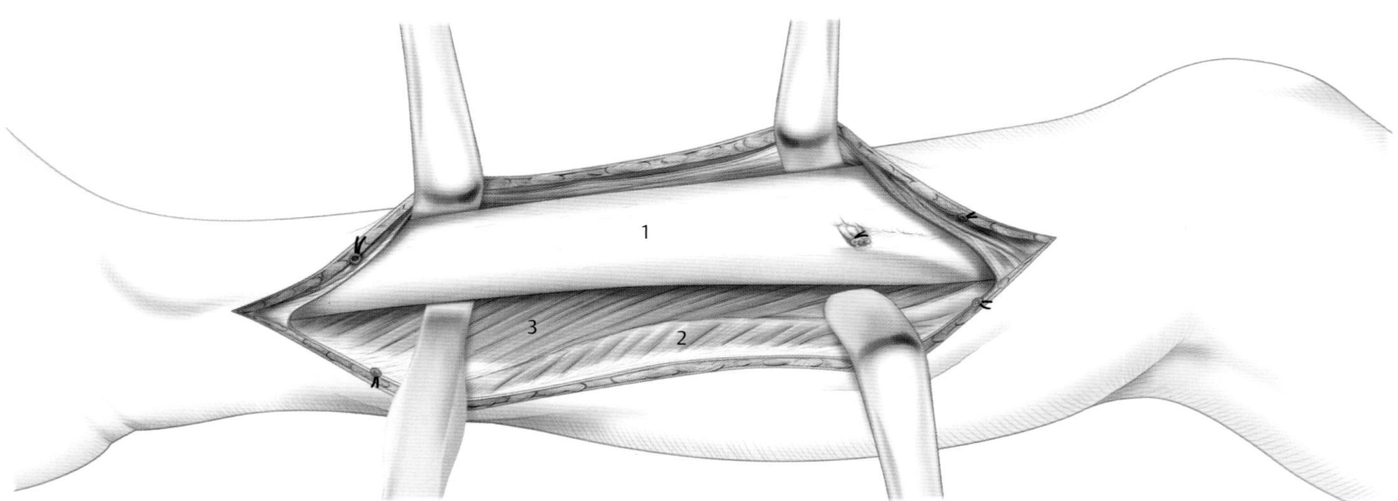

Fig. 12.29 The posterior surface of the tibia is exposed subperiosteally with a raspatory by retraction of the flexor digitorum longus, which must be sharply dissected in the proximal third of the shaft. The medial surface of the tibia is exposed extraperiosteally.

1 Shaft of the tibia
2 Soleus
3 Flexor digitorum longus

12.7 Minimally Invasive Approach to the Medial and Lateral Tibia

K. Weise, D. Höntzsch

12.7.1 Principal Indications

- Fractures from the tibial plateau to the distal tibia
- Pseudarthroses
- Following segment transfer and elongation

12.7.2 Positioning and Incision

The patient is placed supine.

Two incisions are possible:

1. Medial approach to the tibia:
   - From proximal to distal (**Fig. 12.30**):
     The skin incision extends 3–8 cm distally from the medial joint line. A 1–3 cm skin incision is made distally where the end of the selected plate is to be located. Further small incisions are made over the plate holes.
   - From distal to proximal (**Fig. 12.31**):
     The skin incision extends 3–5 cm proximally from the medial malleolus or ankle joint line. A 1–3 cm skin incision is made in the region of the end of the selected plate. Further small incisions are made between these for inserting screws into the shaft.
2. Lateral approach from proximal to distal (**Fig. 12.32**):
   The knee is flexed slightly with a pad under the thigh. A roughly 10 cm skin incision is made slightly obliquely from the lateral femoral epicondyle to about one fingerbreadth posterior to the tibial tuberosity. A further skin incision is made over the expected site of the end of the plate (over the mid shaft or distal shaft, depending on the position of the plate). Small stab incisions for screw insertion are necessary.

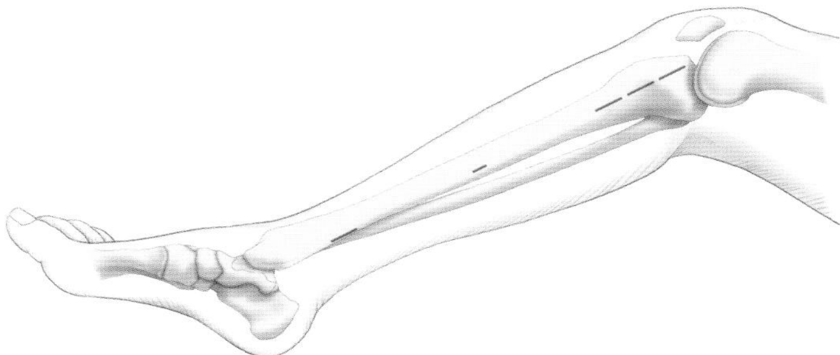

Fig. 12.30 Skin incisions for the minimally invasive approach to the medial tibia, from proximal to distal.

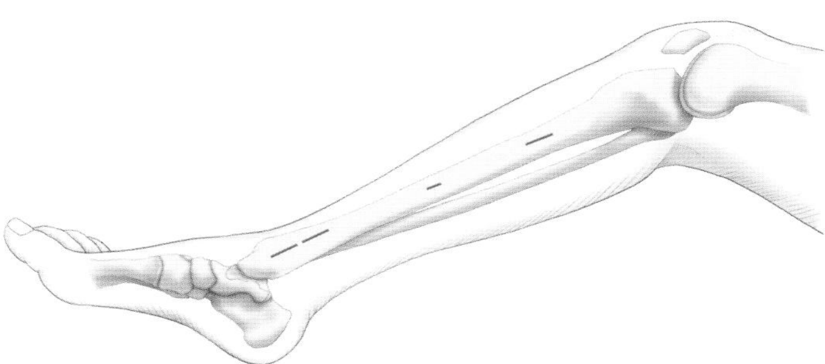

Fig. 12.31 Skin incisions for the minimally invasive approach to the medial tibia, from distal to proximal.

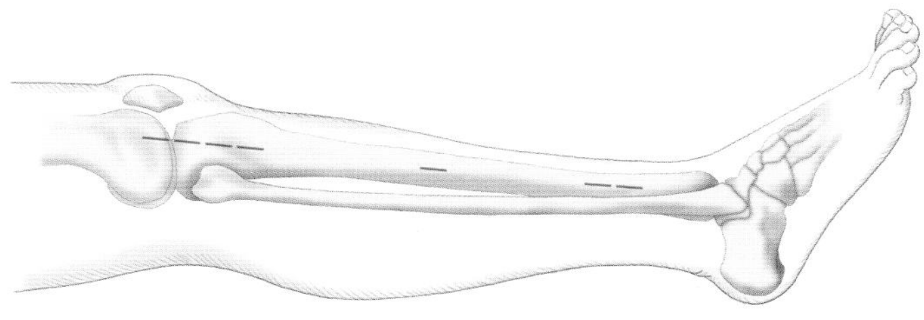

Fig. 12.32 Skin incisions for the minimally invasive approach to the lateral tibia, from proximal to distal.

12.7.3 Exposure of the Medial Approach from Proximal to Distal

For medial minimally invasive insertion from proximal to distal, the subcutaneous fascia is split, and the periosteum of the tibial plateau is exposed. From there, a tunnel is created between the subcutaneous tissue and the tibial periosteum. At the distal end, the fascia is split and the periosteum of the tibia is exposed (**Fig. 12.33**).

The plate, together with auxiliary instruments, can be inserted from proximal to distal, toward a finger in the distal incision. The plate should be positioned centrally over the tibial shaft both proximally and distally (**Fig. 12.34**). This is checked clinically and radiographically.

The screw holes in the shaft are made through stab incisions (**Fig. 12.35**).

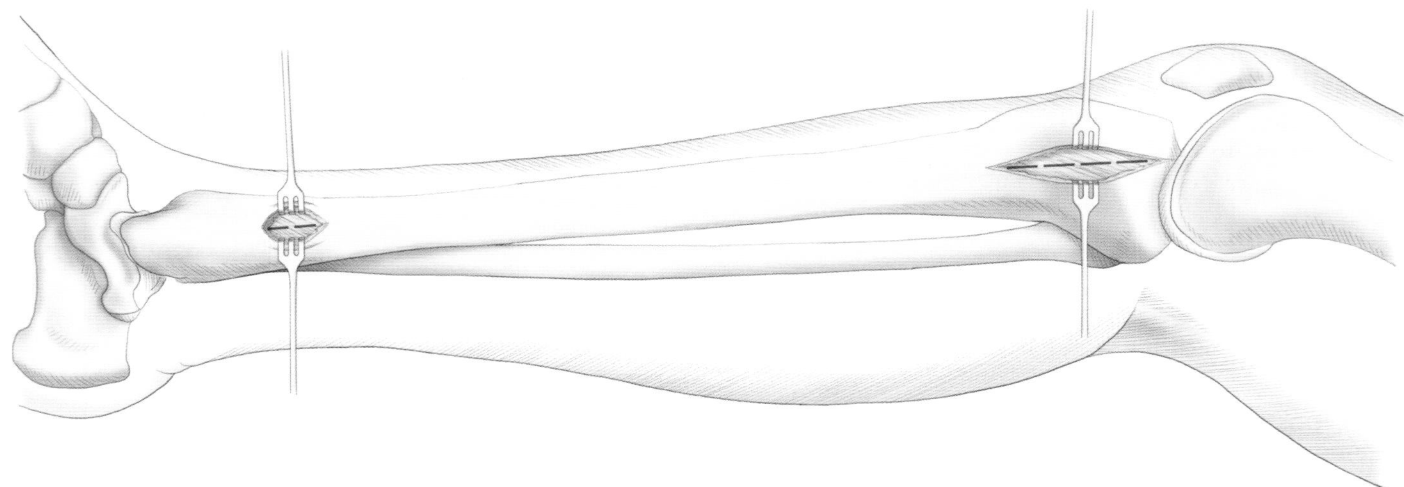

Fig. 12.33 Minimally invasive medial approach to the tibia from proximal to distal. The skin incision is extended so that the periosteum of the tibia is exposed proximally. At the distal end of the selected plate, the skin incision is extended to allow access to the periosteum.

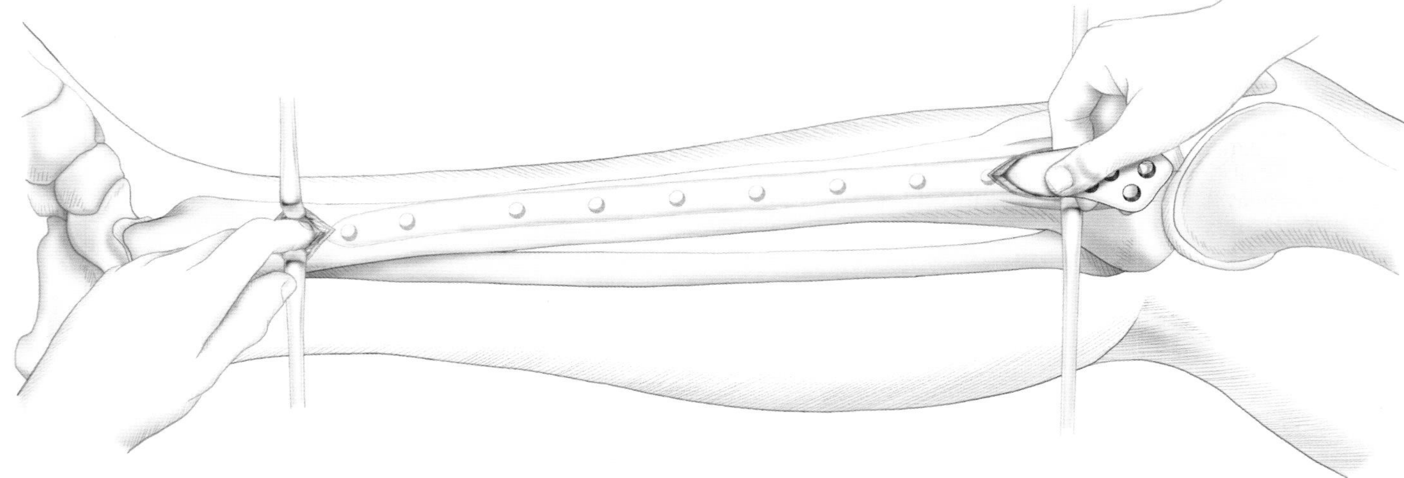

Fig. 12.34 The plate is inserted from proximal to distal toward the distal incision (with a finger), running on the periosteum and bridging the fracture.

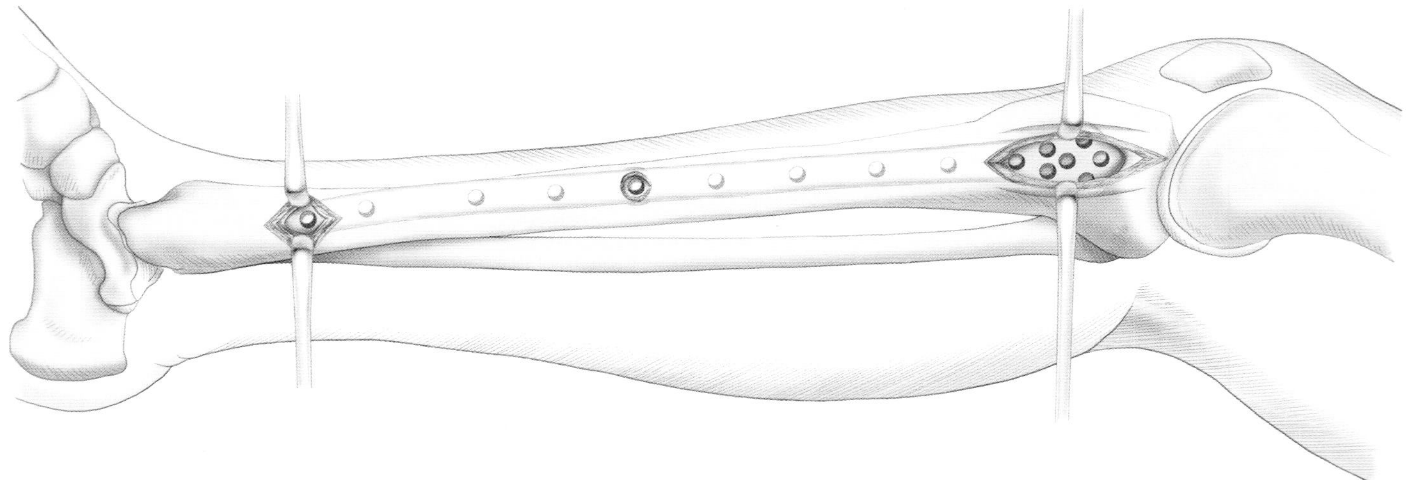

Fig. 12.35 The plate is positioned centrally on the bone both proximally and distally, and its position is checked. Screws are inserted in the shaft through a small stab incision.

12.7.4 Exposure of the Medial Approach from Distal to Proximal

After incising the skin, the crural fascia is split and the tibial periosteum is dissected. A tunnel is created from distal to proximal on the midline of the medial tibial surface. At the site of the end of the chosen plate, the crural fascia is split, and approximately 1–2 cm of the tibial periosteum is exposed (**Fig. 12.36**). The plate is then inserted from distal to proximal toward a finger in the proximal incision (**Fig. 12.37**).

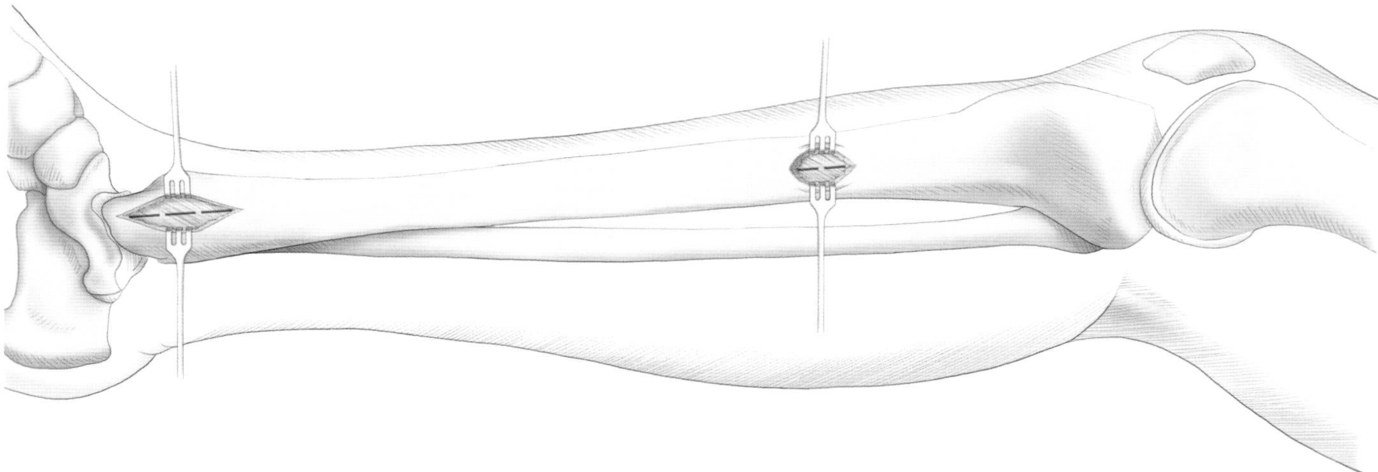

Fig. 12.36 Minimally invasive medial approach to the tibia from distal to proximal. The incision over the medial malleolus and distal leg is extended as far as the tibial periosteum. A funnel-shaped tunnel is then created in a proximal direction. The incision over the end of the plate is deepened down to the periosteum.

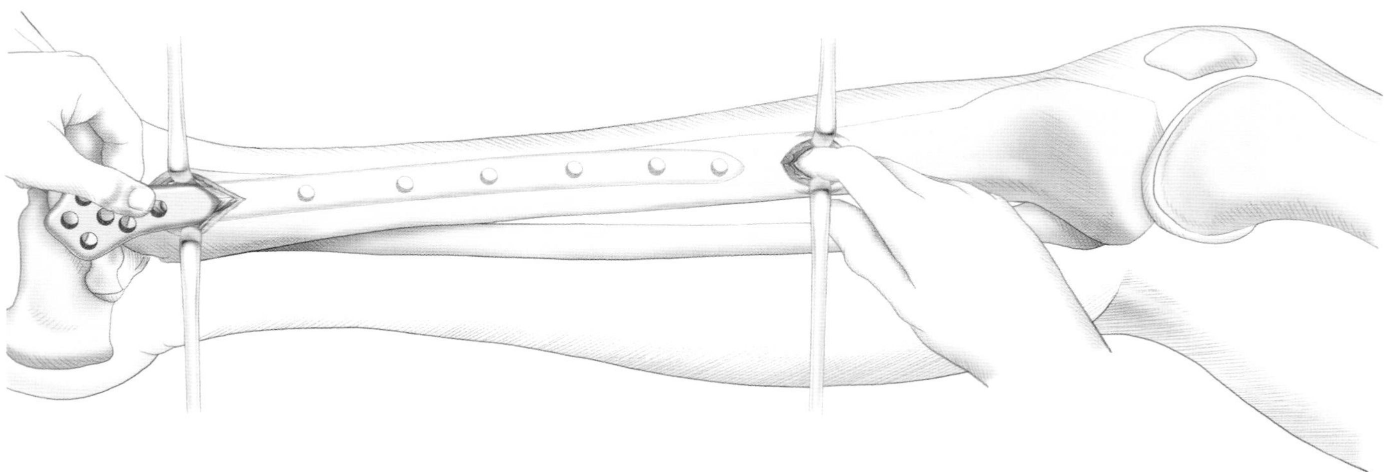

Fig. 12.37 The plate is advanced from distal to proximal across the fracture on the midline of the medial tibial surface toward a finger in the proximal incision.

The plate is then positioned in the distal approach and at its end, and the position is checked clinically and radiographically (**Fig. 12.38**).

Screws are inserted in the shaft through stab incisions (**Fig. 12.38**).

12.7.5 Exposure of the Lateral Approach from Proximal to Distal

Following the skin incision described above, dissection proceeds distally. The fascia of tibialis anterior is split. Tibialis anterior is then peeled out of the fascia and retracted posteriorly, and a tunnel is created in a distal direction (**Fig. 12.39**).

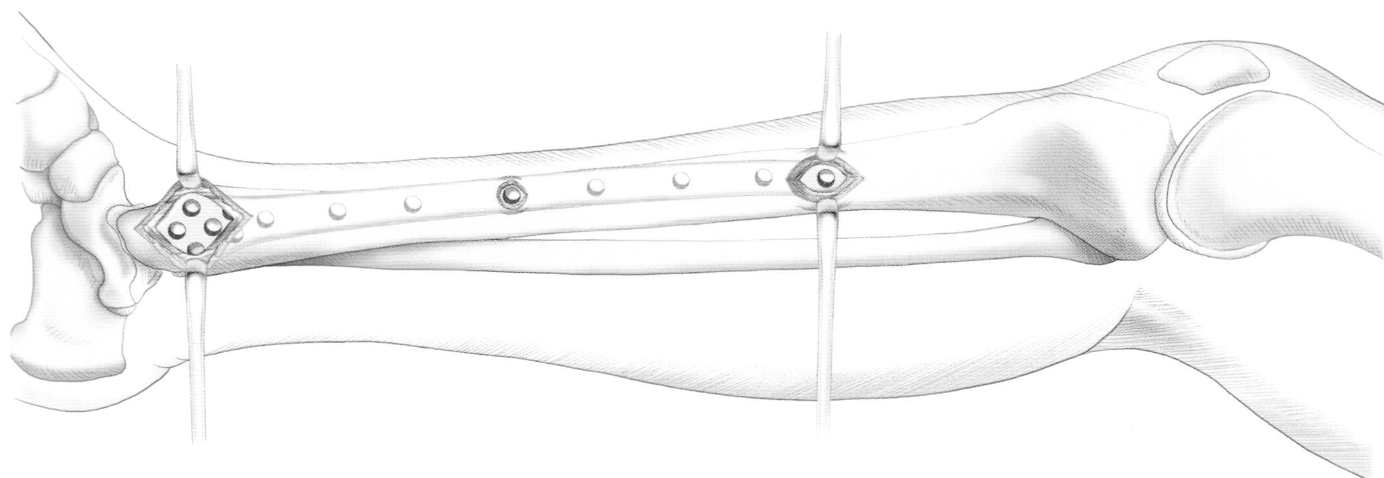

Fig. 12.38 The plate is positioned centrally on the tibia. The position is checked clinically and radiographically. Screws are inserted in the shaft through a stab incision.

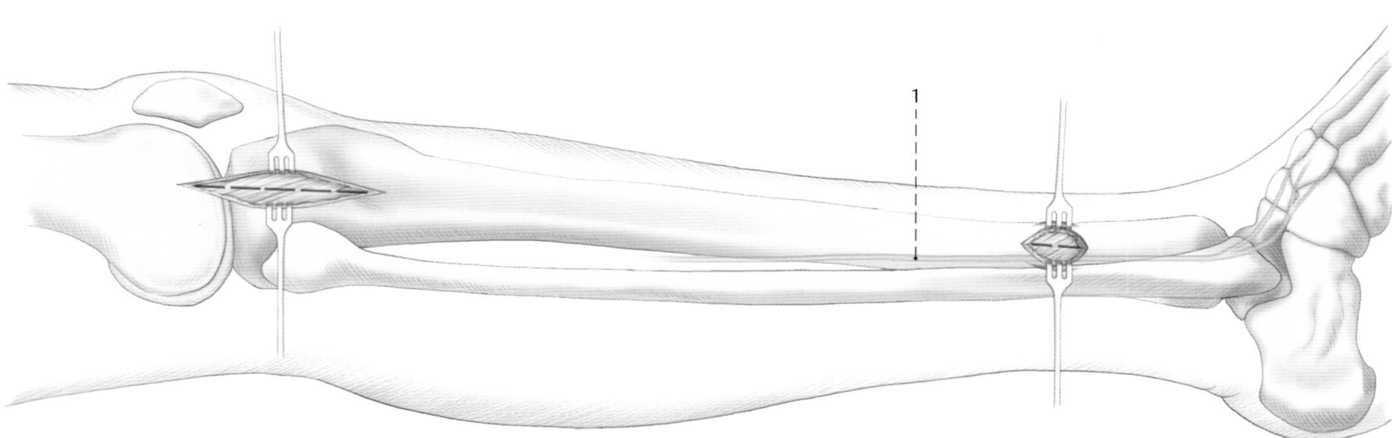

Fig. 12.39 Minimally invasive lateral approach to the tibia, from proximal to distal. The skin incision is deepened distally until the periosteum on the lateral surface of the tibia is reached. Tibialis anterior is then peeled out of its fascia and retracted posteriorly, and a distal tunnel is created centrally on the lateral surface of the tibia. The incision over the end of the chosen plate is deepened. A short incision suffices in the middle of the shaft. In the distal third, the incision must be long enough to allow identification and exposure of the deep peroneal nerve. This is then carefully retracted posteriorly with a Langenbeck retractor.

1 Deep peroneal nerve

In the case of tibial plateau fractures with joint involvement, this approach is extended proximally to the joint line (see Section 11.4).

An incision is made at the site of the end of the plate. This can be short over the middle of the shaft, but has to be 2–4 cm long in the distal third to protect the deep peroneal nerve, which lies in front of the interosseous membrane, where it should be gently exposed (**Fig. 12.40**).

The plate can be advanced along the periosteum in the midline of the lateral surface of the tibia toward the distal incision, facilitated by aiming at a finger toward it in the distal incision. After gentle dissection, the common peroneal nerve must be retracted posteriorly (**Fig. 12.40**).

After insertion of the plate, it is positioned centrally in the proximal funnel and distal incision window; the position is checked clinically and radiographically. When long plates are used, the course of the deep peroneal nerve must be checked in the distal window (**Fig. 12.41**).

Screws are inserted in the shaft through stab incisions.

12.7.6 Wound Closure

In the longer approach region, the wound is closed in layers. Skin closure suffices for short incisions.

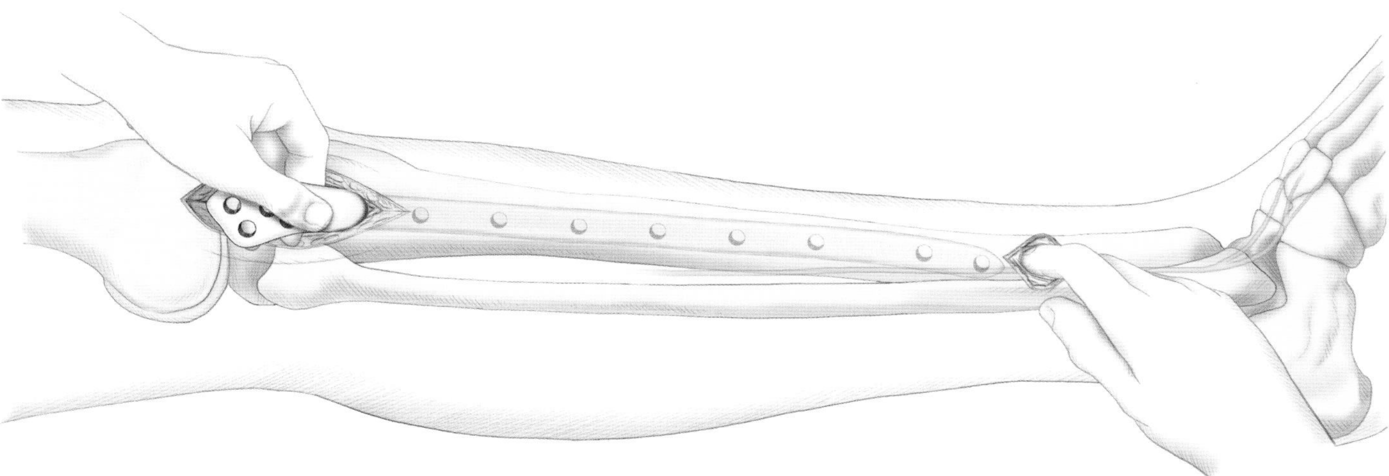

Fig. 12.40 The plate is advanced across the fracture from proximal to distal toward the finger in the distal incision.

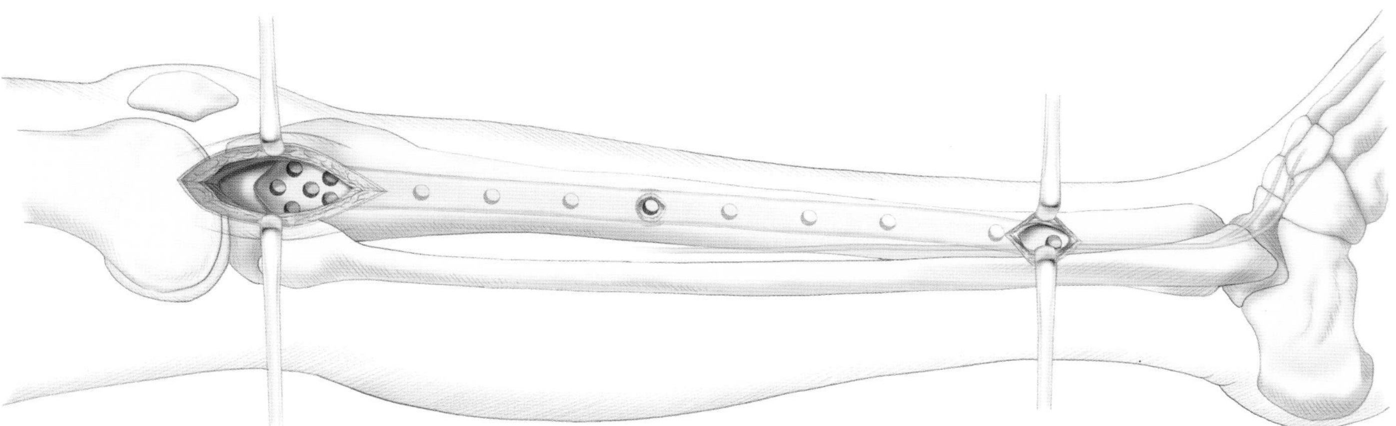

Fig. 12.41 The plate is positioned proximally and distally, and the position is checked clinically and radiographically. The deep peroneal nerve must always be protected distally. It must not be irritated by the plate or indeed lie beneath the plate. It must not be damaged by subsequent screw insertion into the distal holes.

12.8 Lateral Approach to the Fibula

R. Bauer, F. Kerschbaumer, S. Poisel, K. Weise, D. Höntzsch

12.8.1 Principal Indications

- Fractures
- Fibular osteotomy
- Removal of bone grafts from the fibula
- Tumors
- Osteomyelitis

12.8.2 Positioning and Incision

The patient may be placed in a supine, semilateral, or lateral position. After (optional) application of a tourniquet, the leg is draped in a manner allowing free movement. The length of the skin incision depends on the desired extent of fibular exposure. Described below is exposure of the entire fibula according to Henry. The skin incision begins a handbreadth proximal to and 1 cm behind the head of the fibula and extends distally as far as the lateral malleolus (**Fig. 12.42**). The fascia is incised proximally behind the biceps muscle and, to begin with, the common peroneal nerve is identified. After exposure of the nerve, the fascia can be split from proximal to distal (**Fig. 12.43**). Injury to the lateral sural cutaneous nerve should be avoided. The common peroneal nerve is snared with a nerve band and elevated, and the origin of peroneus longus is detached from the neck of the fibula. The periosteum is incised on the posterior border of the fibula between the peroneal muscles and the soleus (**Fig. 12.44**).

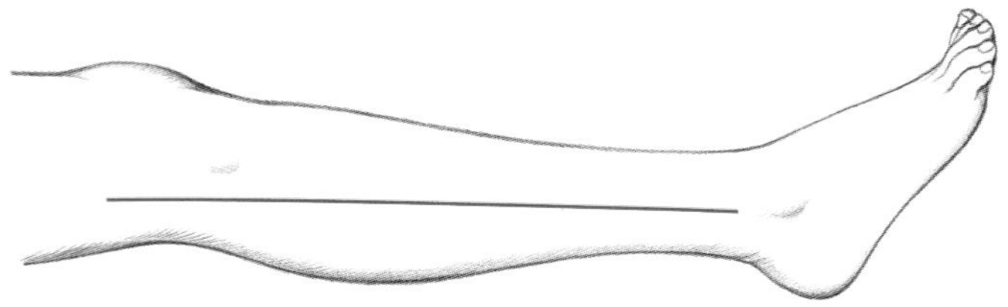

Fig. 12.42 Lateral approach to the fibula according to Henry. Skin incision (right leg).

12.8.3 Exposure of the Fibula

First, the posterior surface of the fibula is exposed subperiosteally, and a Hohmann elevator is inserted. Next the perforating peroneal vessels are ligated and transected. The lateral aspect of the fibula is exposed subperiosteally with a curved raspatory (**Fig. 12.45**) (except for with fractures). Periosteum and muscle should be detached from the fibula from distal to proximal. In this fashion, the peroneal muscles together with the common peroneal nerve can be retracted anteriorly. This permits exposure of the fibula from the head to the distal third of the shaft (**Fig. 12.46**).

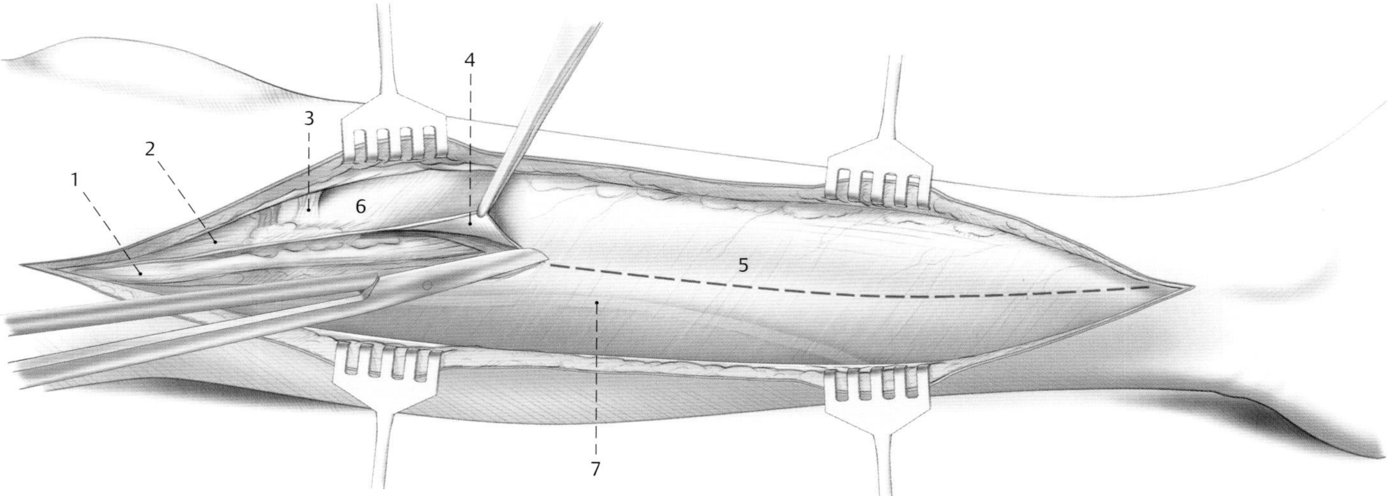

Fig. 12.43 Exposure of the common peroneal nerve in the proximal wound region. Splitting of the crural fascia from proximal to distal.

1 Common peroneal nerve
2 Biceps femoris
3 Anterior ligament of the fibular head
4 Crural fascia
5 Peroneus longus
6 Head of the fibula
7 Lateral sural cutaneous nerve

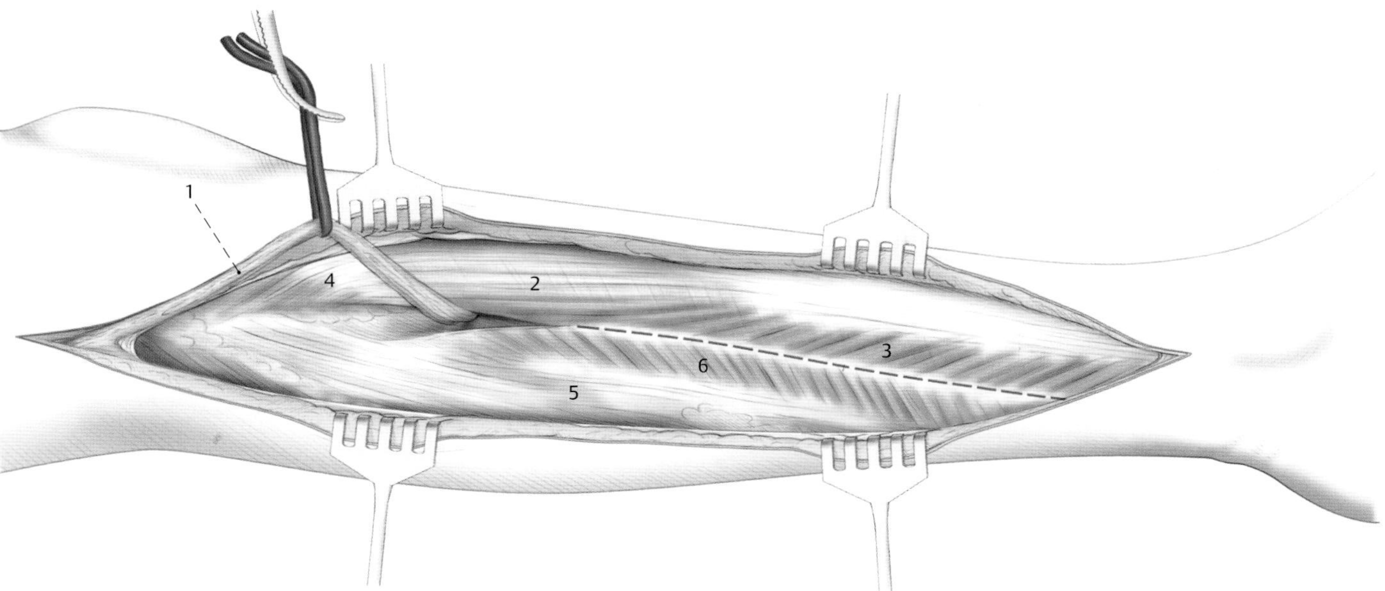

Fig. 12.44 Snaring of the common peroneal nerve. Detachment of peroneus longus from the head of the fibula. Subperiosteal exposure of the fibula between peroneus longus and soleus.

1 Common peroneal nerve
2 Peroneus longus
3 Peroneus brevis
4 Head of the fibula
5 Gastrocnemius muscle, lateral head
6 Soleus

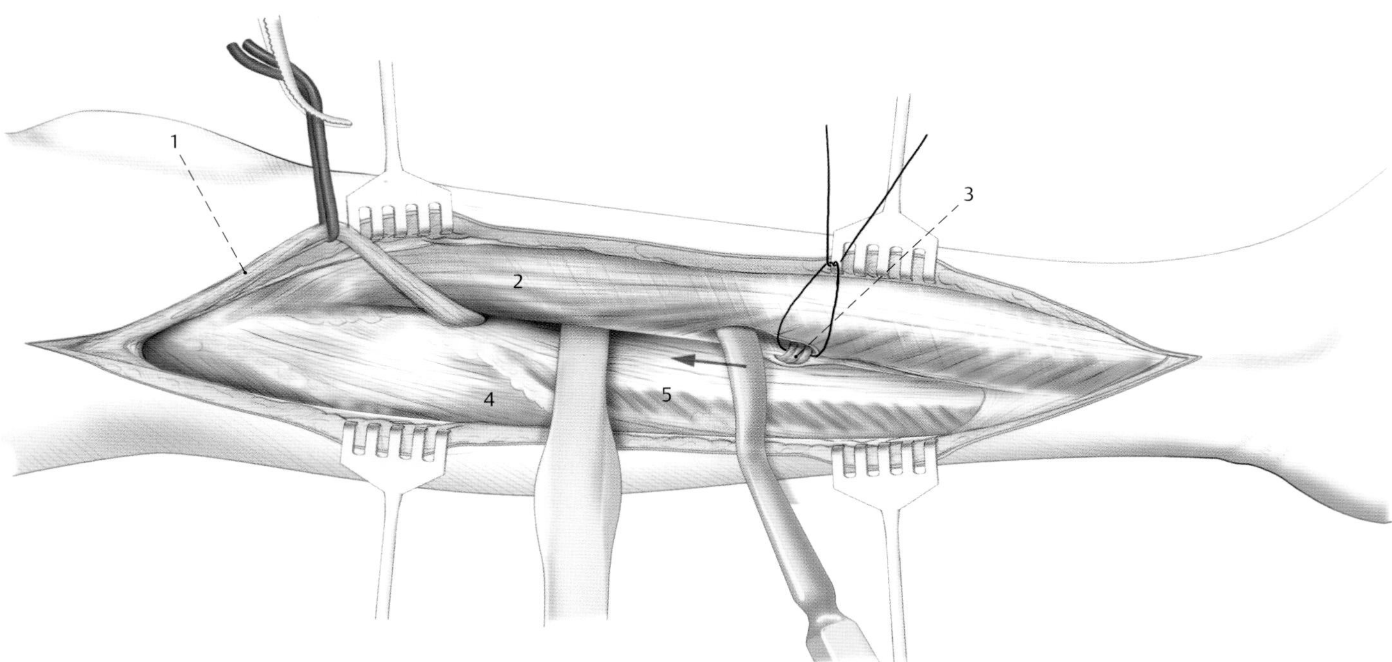

Fig. 12.45 After exposure of the posterior aspect of the fibula, the lateral surface is also subperiosteally revealed. Branches of the peroneal artery are ligated. Note: The direction of exposure is from distal to proximal.

1 Common peroneal nerve
2 Peroneus longus
3 Muscular branches of the peroneal artery and vein
4 Gastrocnemius muscle, lateral head
5 Soleus

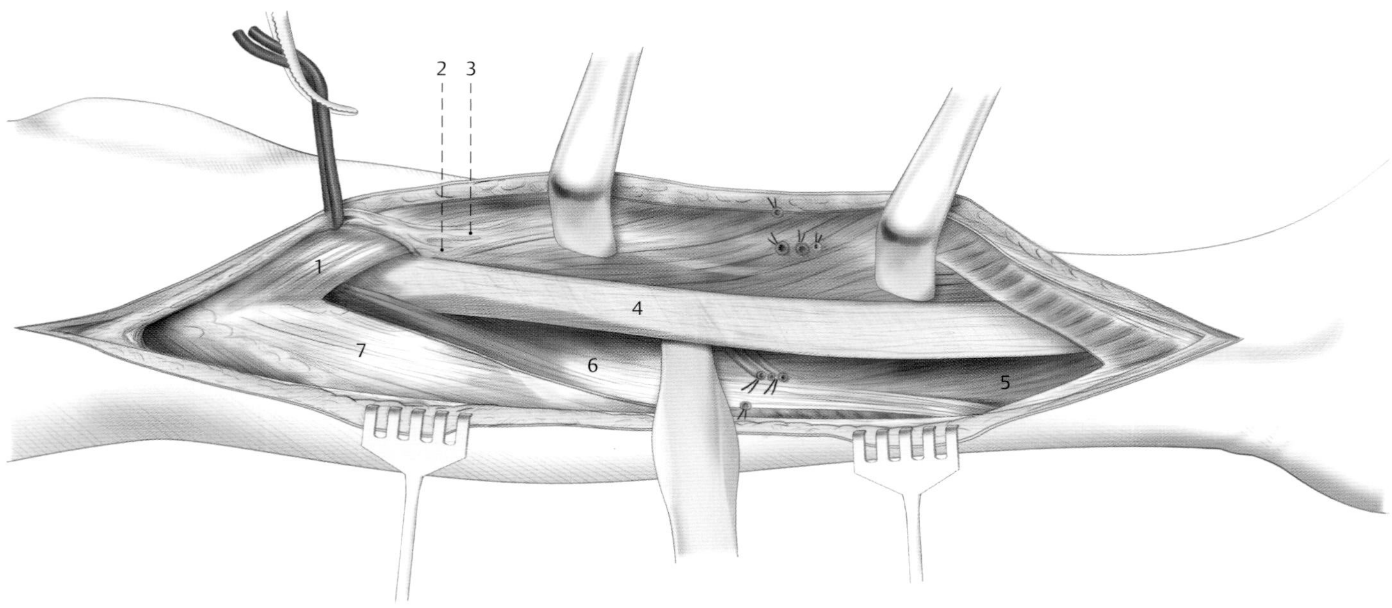

Fig. 12.46 Appearance after exposure of the proximal two-thirds of the fibula.

1 Peroneus longus
2 Deep peroneal nerve
3 Superficial peroneal nerve
4 Shaft of the fibula
5 Flexor hallucis longus
6 Soleus
7 Gastrocnemius muscle, lateral head

12.8.4 Exposure of the Distal Third of the Fibular Shaft

If exposure of the distal portion of the fibula is required, incision of the fascia anterior to the peroneal tendons is recommended. The fibula is exposed with the superficial peroneal nerve preserved. At this site, careful subperiosteal dissection of the fibula is necessary since the peroneal vessels are directly adjacent to the posterior side of the bone.

12.8.5 Anatomical Site

(**Fig. 12.47**)

The cross-section through the distal portion of the lower leg shows the following differences from the proximal cross-section: a posterior position of the fibula relative to the tibia, anterior displacement of the anterior tibial vessels and the deep peroneal branch, and direct contact of the peroneal vessels with the fibula. The possible approaches to the fibula anteriorly and posteriorly to the peroneal muscles, as well as the posterolateral and posteromedial approaches to the tibia, are presented in **Fig. 12.47**.

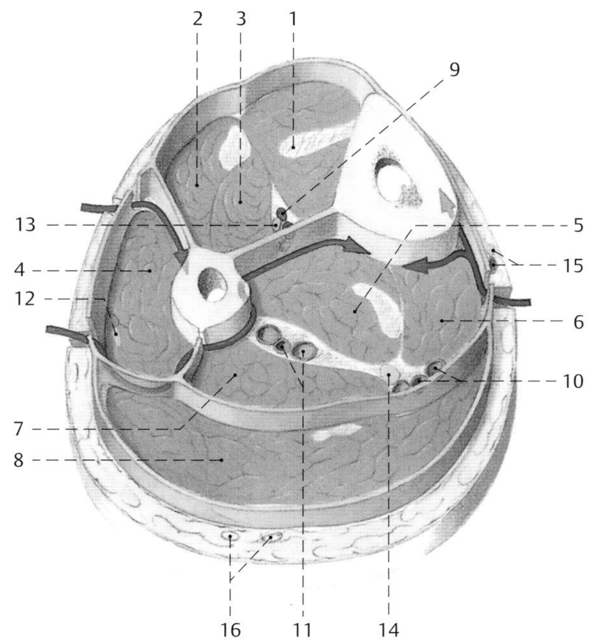

Fig. 12.47 Anatomical site. Schematic cross-section through the distal lower leg. Note: The posterior position of the fibula relative to the tibia, enlargement of the deep flexor compartment, and approaches to the tibia and fibula (left leg, view from proximal).

1 Tibialis anterior
2 Extensor digitorum longus
3 Extensor hallucis longus
4 Peroneal muscles
5 Tibialis posterior
6 Flexor digitorum longus
7 Flexor hallucis longus
8 Triceps surae
9 Anterior tibial vessels
10 Posterior tibial vessels
11 Peroneal vessels
12 Superficial peroneal nerve
13 Deep peroneal nerve
14 Tibial nerve
15 Saphenous nerve and great saphenous vein
16 Sural nerve and small saphenous vein

12.8.6 Wound Closure

Wound closure is effected after release of the tourniquet and hemostasis, by suture of the periosteum and the crural fascia.

12.8.7 Note

The complete exposure of the fibula described above is necessary only in exceptional cases. For fibular osteotomy, short skin incisions in the middle of the shaft or at the level of the proximal half of the shaft are sufficient. Also, in exposure of a short segment of the fibula, dissection is performed on the anterior border of the posterior intermuscular septum of the leg.

13 Foot

13.1 Anterior Approach to the Ankle Joint

R. Bauer, F. Kerschbaumer, S. Poisel

13.1.1 Principal Indications

- Fractures
- Arthrodesis
- Arthroplasty
- Synovectomy

13.1.2 Positioning and Incision

The patient is placed in the supine position. After (optional) application of a tourniquet, the leg is draped in a manner allowing free movement. A pad is placed under the lower leg. The skin incision, approximately 10 cm in length, is straight and passes in the midline over the ankle joint (**Fig. 13.1**). When transecting the subcutaneous tissue, one should watch for the superficial peroneal nerve, which runs an extrafascial course.

The picture of the anatomical site (**Fig. 13.2**) shows the oblique course of this nerve, which crosses the operative field in its distal portion. Lying between the tendons of extensor digitorum longus and extensor hallucis longus are the dorsal artery and vein of the foot and the deep peroneal nerve, the sensory terminal branch of which supplies the skin in the first web space.

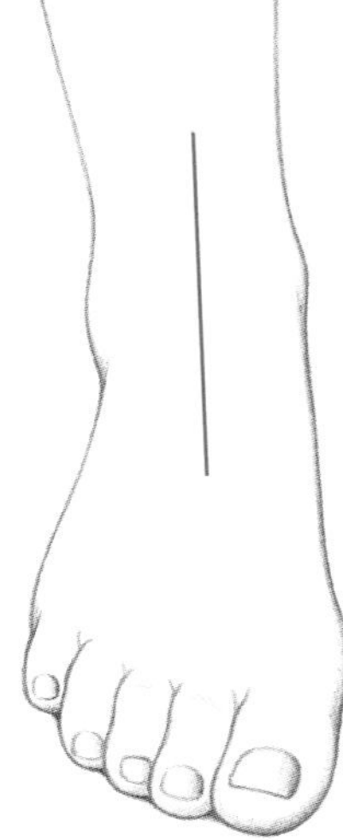

Fig. 13.1 Anterior approach to the ankle joint. Skin incision (right leg).

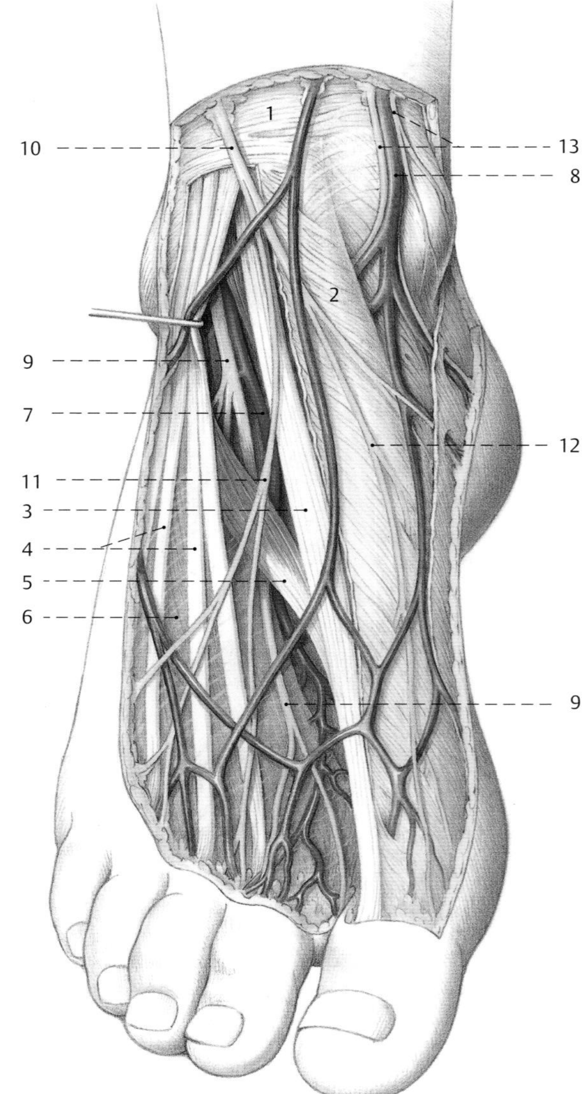

Fig. 13.2 Anatomical site of the dorsum of the foot (right leg).

1 Superior extensor retinaculum
2 Inferior extensor retinaculum
3 Tendon of extensor hallucis longus
4 Tendons of extensor digitorum longus
5 Extensor hallucis brevis
6 Extensor digitorum brevis
7 Dorsal artery of the foot
8 Great saphenous vein
9 Deep peroneal nerve
10 Superficial peroneal nerve
11 Intermediate dorsal cutaneous nerve
12 Medial dorsal cutaneous nerve
13 Saphenous nerve

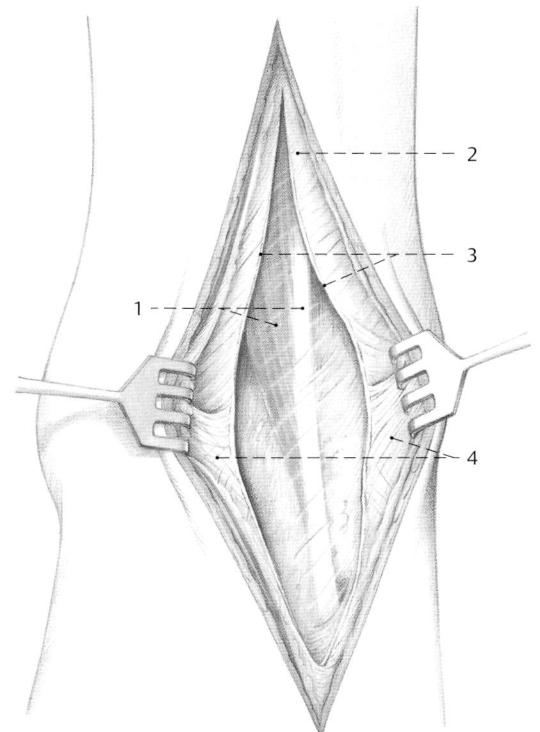

Fig. 13.3 Division of the fascia and exposure of extensor hallucis longus.

1 Extensor hallucis longus
2 Crural fascia
3 Superior extensor retinaculum
4 Inferior extensor retinaculum

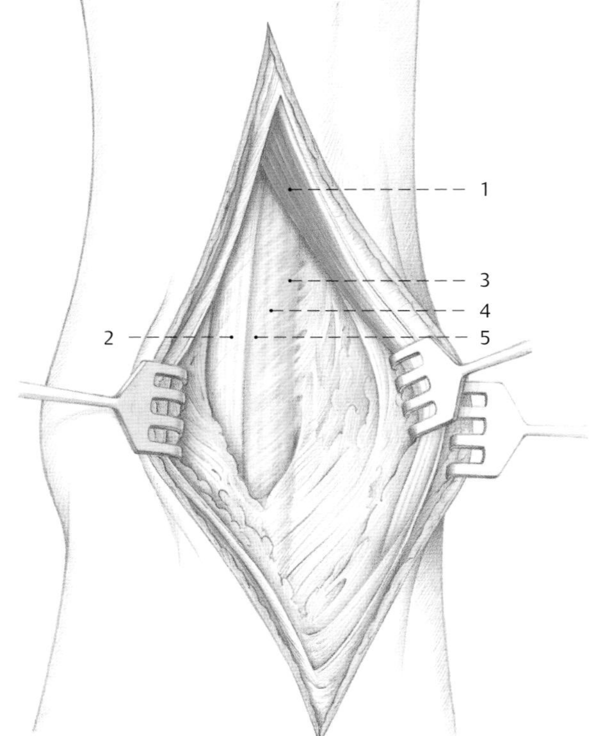

Fig. 13.4 Dissection between extensor hallucis longus and extensor digitorum longus for exposure of the neurovascular bundle.

1 Extensor hallucis longus
2 Tendons of extensor digitorum longus
3 Anterior tibial vein
4 Anterior tibial artery
5 Deep peroneal nerve

After exposure of the fascia and its reinforcing bands (superior and inferior extensor retinacula), these are split in line with the skin incision (**Fig. 13.3**). Medial retraction of extensor hallucis longus and lateral retraction of extensor digitorum longus reveal the neurovascular bundle lying deeply (**Fig. 13.4**).

13.1.3 Exposure of the Ankle Joint

The entire neurovascular bundle with its connective tissue sheath is dissected free and mobilized laterally. Ligation and transection of the medial anterior malleolar artery and vein are recommended if adequate lateral mobilization is to be achieved (**Fig. 13.5**). The capsule of the ankle joint behind the neurovascular bundle is split longitudinally. Incision of the capsule is extended proximally into the periosteum of the tibia so that the ankle joint capsule and the periosteum on the lateral surface of the tibia can be medially and laterally mobilized in one layer with a raspatory. This permits anterior opening of the ankle joint. Now Langenbeck retractors may be inserted medially and laterally, uncovering the distal tibia, the anterior portion of the inner malleolus, and the trochlea and neck of the talus (**Fig. 13.6**).

13.1.4 Wound Closure

After release of the tourniquet and hemostasis, the wound is closed by suture of the capsule and the extensor retinacula.

13.1.5 Note

With this approach, impairment of wound healing is not uncommon. Careful hemostasis and the use of Redon drains are especially important in this procedure.

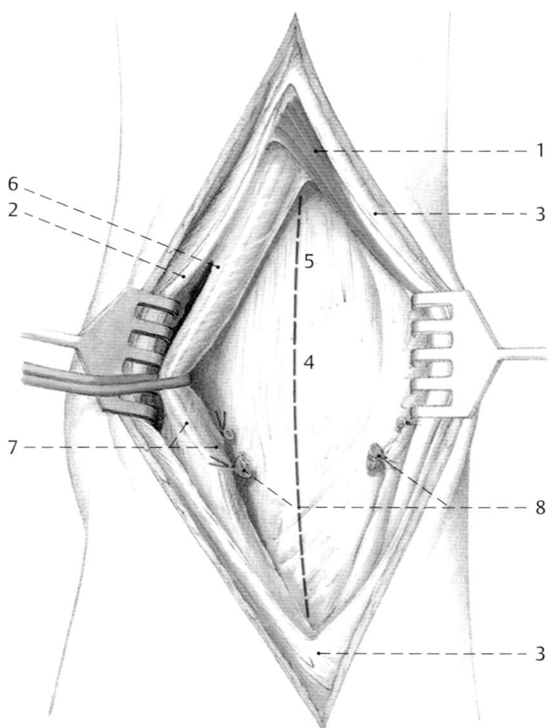

Fig. 13.5 Exposure of the ankle joint capsule following retraction of the neurovascular bundle. The incision made in the capsule may be straight (dashed line) or T-shaped.

1 Extensor hallucis longus
2 Tendons of extensor digitorum longus
3 Crural fascia
4 Talocrural joint capsule
5 Tibia
6 Deep peroneal nerve
7 Anterior tibial artery and vein
8 Medial anterior malleolar artery and vein

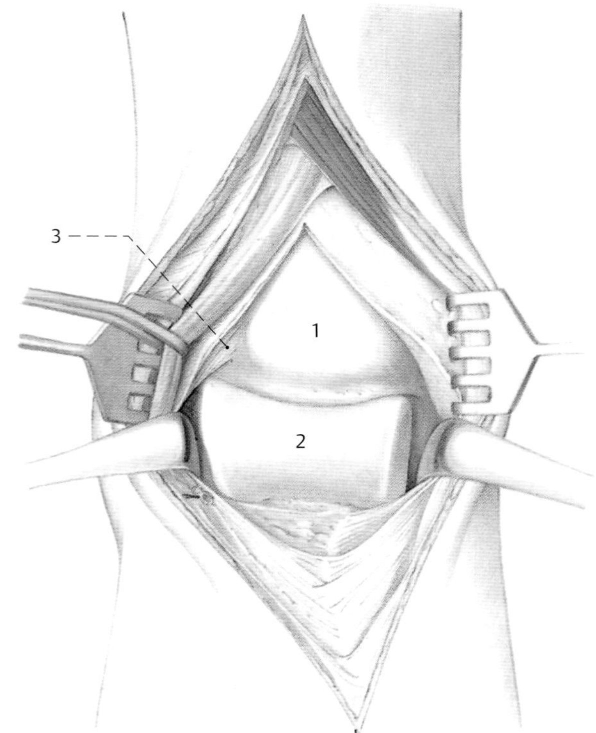

Fig. 13.6 Exposure of the distal end of the tibia and trochlea of the talus after opening of the capsule.

1 Tibia
2 Trochlea of talus
3 Anterior tibiofibular ligament

13.2 Anterolateral Approach to the Ankle Joint and Talocalcaneonavicular Joint

R. Bauer, F. Kerschbaumer, S. Poisel

13.2.1 Principal Indications

- Fractures
- Arthrodesis
- Synovectomy
- Arthroplasty

13.2.2 Positioning and Incision

The patient is placed in the supine position. After (optional) application of a tourniquet, the leg is draped so as to allow free movement. A pad is placed under the lower leg, and this is slightly rotated internally. A skin incision approximately 10 cm long is made laterally to the generally readily palpable extensor digitorum longus anterior to the tibiofibular syndesmosis. If necessary, the incision can be extended distally in the direction of the fourth metatarsal bone (**Fig. 13.7**). After splitting the skin and subcutaneous tissue, the crural fascia is divided with a straight incision, and the inferior extensor retinaculum with an H-shaped incision (**Fig. 13.8**). Care should be taken not to damage the branches of the superficial peroneal nerve lying medial to this incision. The extensor digitorum longus and peroneus tertius muscles can be medially retracted (**Fig. 13.9**).

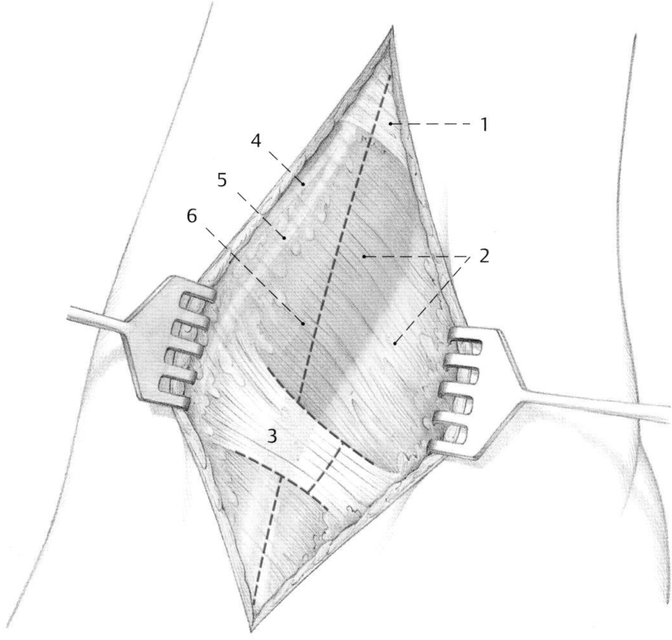

Fig. 13.8 Splitting of the fascia and inferior extensor retinaculum.

1 Superior extensor retinaculum
2 Dorsal fascia of the foot
3 Inferior extensor retinaculum
4 Medial dorsal cutaneous nerve
5 Intermediate dorsal cutaneous nerve
6 Extensor digitorum longus

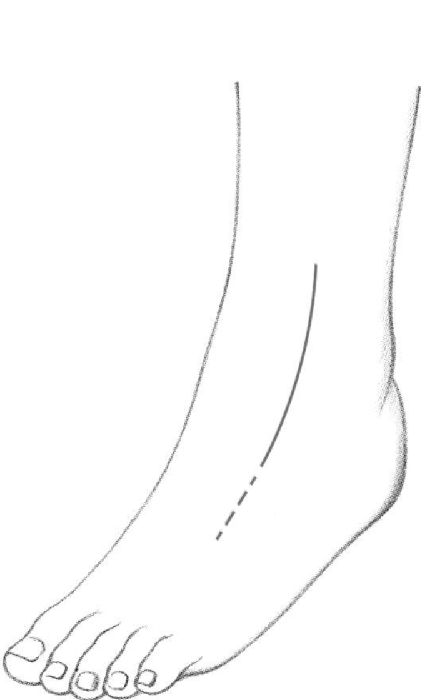

Fig. 13.7 Anterolateral approach to the ankle joint and talocalcaneonavicular joint. Skin incision (left leg).

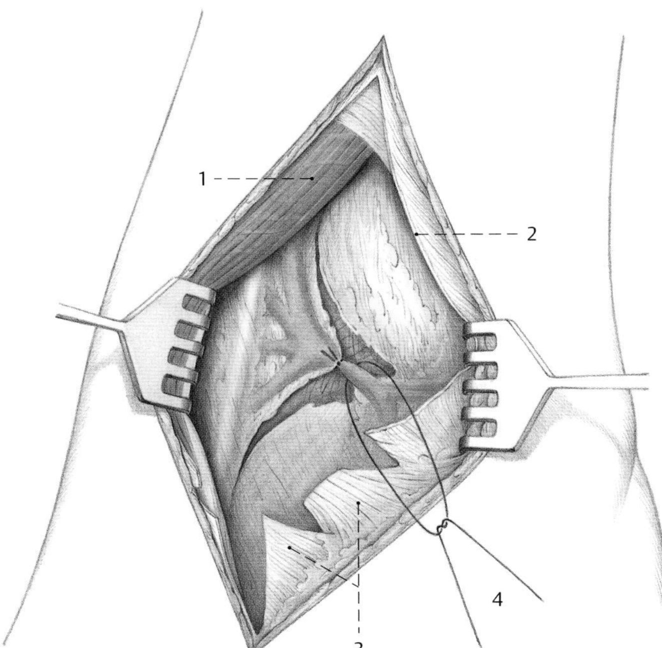

Fig. 13.9 Retraction in a medial direction of extensor digitorum longus and ligation of the transversely coursing veins.

1 Extensor digitorum longus
2 Crural fascia
3 Inferior extensor retinaculum
4 Anterior tibial veins

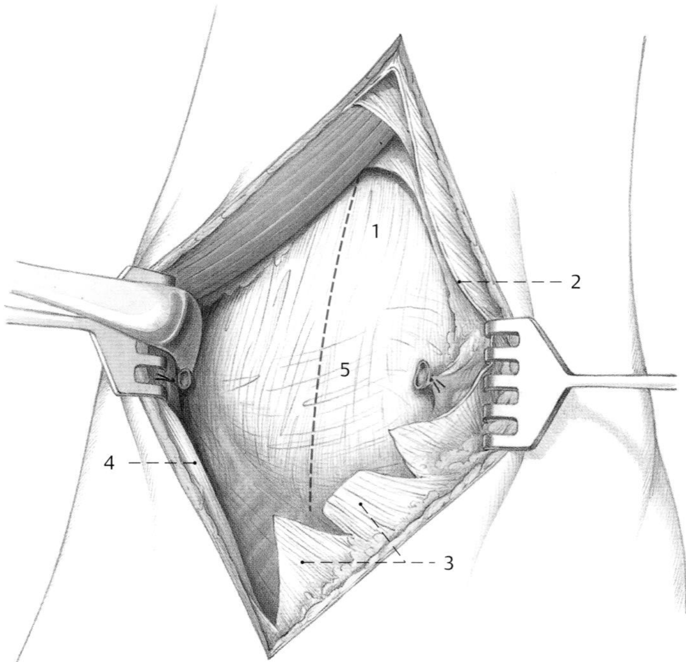

Fig. 13.10 Longitudinal (dashed line) or T-shaped incision of the capsule of the ankle joint.

1 Tibia
2 Crural fascia
3 Inferior extensor retinaculum
4 Tendon of peroneus tertius
5 Talocrural joint capsule

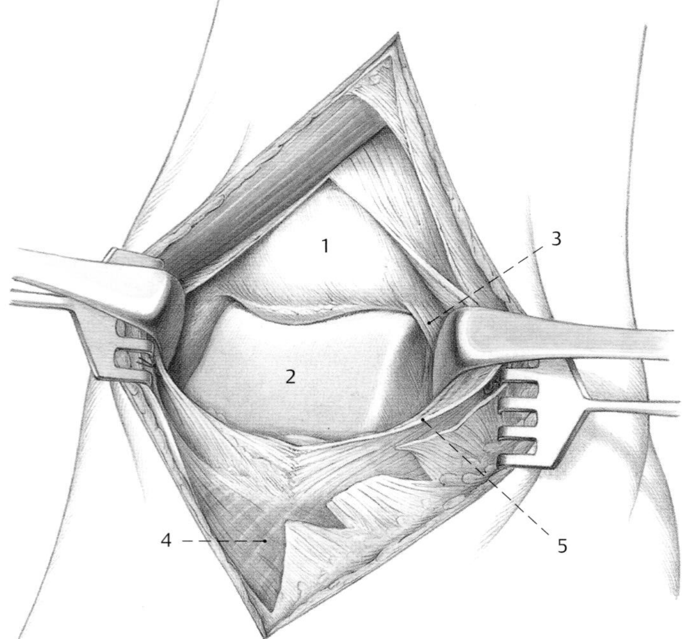

Fig. 13.11 Exposure of the distal tibia and trochlea of the talus after opening of the joint capsule.

1 Tibia
2 Trochlea of the talus
3 Anterior tibiofibular ligament
4 Extensor digitorum brevis
5 Talocrural joint capsule

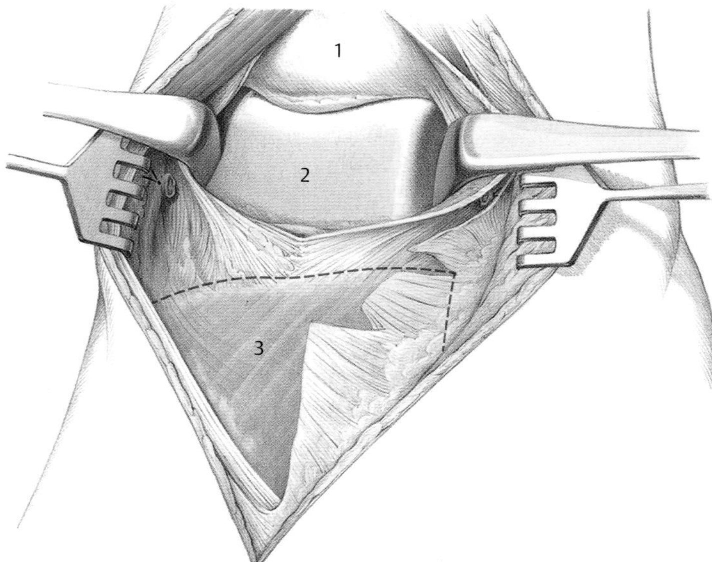

Fig. 13.12 Following distal extension of the skin incision, the short extensor muscle of the toes is detached along the dashed line.

1 Tibia
2 Trochlea of the talus
3 Extensor digitorum brevis

13.2.3 Exposure of the Ankle Joint

The transverse venous branches of the lateral anterior malleolar artery are ligated and transected. With the aid of a raspatory, the neurovascular bundle can be cautiously retracted in a medial direction from the anterior aspect of the ankle joint capsule. Subsequently, a Langenbeck retractor is inserted in the same plane (**Fig. 13.10**). The capsule of the ankle joint is split longitudinally. For liberal exposure of the ankle joint, the periosteum of the tibia proximal to the capsule also has to be split. It is retracted with a raspatory in the same plane as the capsule. Then Langenbeck retractors are inserted into the joint (**Fig. 13.11**).

13.2.4 Distal Extension of the Approach

If exposure of the talocalcaneonavicular joint is required, the skin incision is extended distally. After the fascia has been split, extensor digitorum longus and extensor hallucis brevis are detached from their origins (**Fig. 13.12**). This necessitates transection of the lateral tarsal artery and vein, which course in part beneath these muscles. The muscle flap is retracted distally, and then the medial and lateral Chopart joint is opened with a T-shaped incision (**Fig. 13.13**). Following transection of the bifurcate ligament, the joint surfaces are well exposed if the forefoot is pushed in a plantar direction (**Fig. 13.14**). If necessary, the subtalar joint can also be exposed

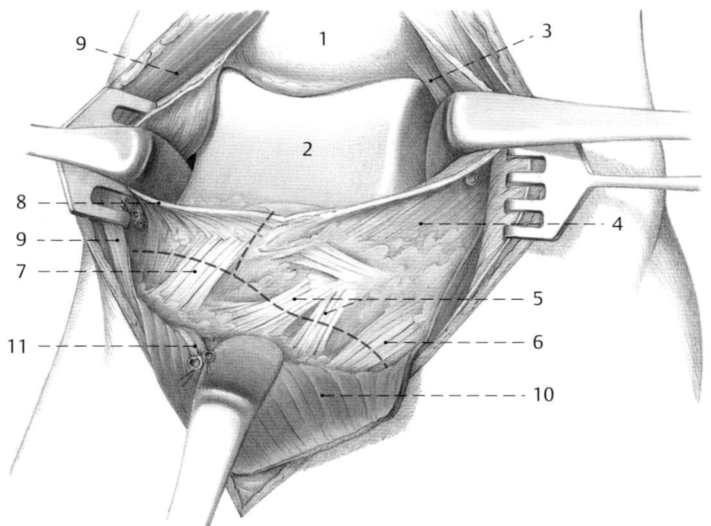

Fig. 13.13 Following dissection of the extensor digitorum brevis, a T-shaped incision is made in the capsules of the medial and lateral Chopart joint line.

1 Tibia
2 Trochlea of the talus
3 Anterior tibiofibular ligament
4 Anterior talofibular ligament
5 Bifurcate ligament
6 Dorsal calcaneocuboid ligament
7 Talonavicular ligament
8 Tibionavicular part of medial ligament
9 Extensor digitorum longus
10 Extensor digitorum brevis
11 Tarsal artery and vein

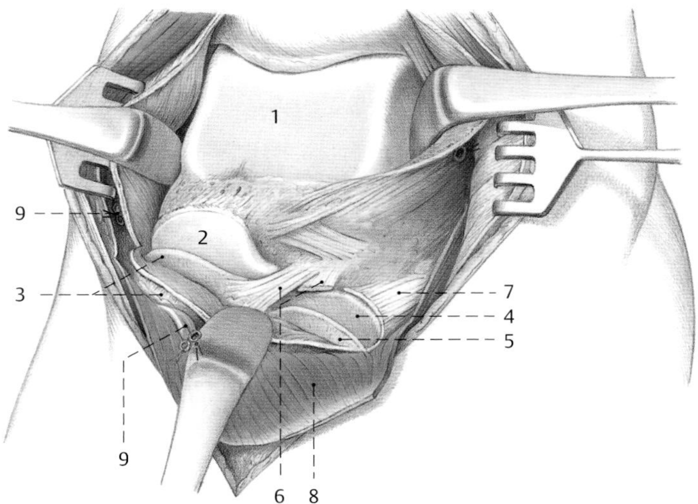

Fig. 13.14 Appearance after opening of the ankle joint and the medial and lateral Chopart joint. Incision of the subtalar joint is along the dashed lines in **Fig. 13.13**.

1 Trochlea of the talus
2 Head of the talus
3 Navicular bone
4 Calcaneus
5 Cuboid bone
6 Bifurcate ligament
7 Dorsal calcaneocuboid ligament
8 Extensor digitorum brevis
9 Lateral tarsal artery and vein

with this approach once the tarsal sinus has been cleared (see Section 13.13, **Fig. 13.65**ff.).

13.2.5 Wound Closure

Wound closure is effected by suture of the ankle joint capsule as well as of the fascia and the retinaculum of the inferior extensor muscles.

13.2.6 Note

This approach is especially suitable for arthrodesis of the talocalcaneonavicular and talocrural joints. Impaired wound healing occurs less frequently in this case than with the anterior approach to the ankle joint.

13.3 Cincinnati Approach

O. Eberhardt, T. Wirth

13.3.1 Principal Indications

- Correction of talipes equinovarus
- Correction of congenital vertical talus
- Posterior, posteromedial, and posterolateral capsulotomies

13.3.2 Positioning and Incision

The patient is usually placed prone. The extent of the incision depends on the planned operation. If only Achilles tendon elongation and posterior arthrolysis are planned, the incision is posterior, above the transverse skin crease over the heel (**Fig. 13.15a**). If posteromedial arthrolysis is to be performed, the incision is extended medially to in front of the medial malleolus (**Fig. 13.15b**). If complete peritalar arthrolysis is necessary, the incision is continued laterally over the lateral malleolus as far as the calcaneocuboid joint (**Fig. 13.15c**).

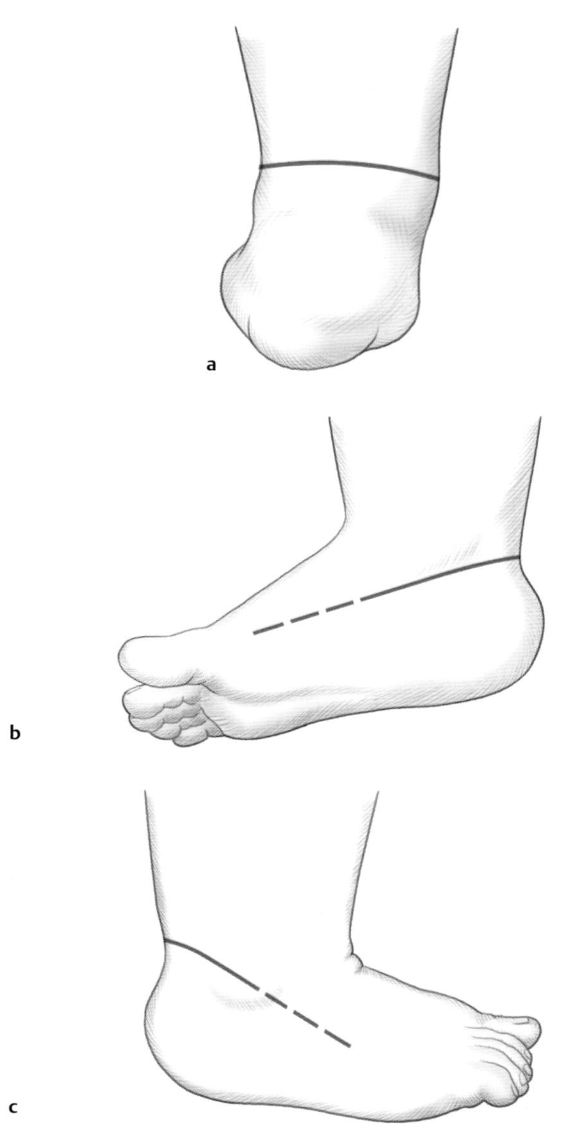

Fig. 13.15 a–c Cincinnati approach incisions.

a The incision is made approximately 0.5–1 cm above the posterior heel skin crease and continues medially to in front of the medial malleolus.
b The incision can be extended medially and laterally as required.
c The approach can be extended laterally over the tip of the fibula as far as the calcaneocuboid joint.

13.3.3 Achilles Tendon Lengthening and Exposure of the Posterior Joint Capsule with Posterior Arthrolysis

For posterior arthrolysis, the Achilles tendon, the lateral neurovascular bundle (sural nerve and accompanying vessels), and the medial neurovascular bundle (tibial nerve, posterior tibial artery and vein) are exposed (**Fig. 13.16**). To lengthen it, the Achilles tendon can be incised in both the frontal and sagittal planes. We prefer elongation in the frontal plane. To expose the posterior joint capsule, the lateral neurovascular bundle and the peroneal tendons (after opening the tendon sheaths), and the flexor hallucis longus and medial neurovascular bundle are retracted.

The flexor hallucis longus points to the talocalcaneonavicular joint. The posterior capsule of the ankle and talocalcaneonavicular joints is exposed together with the posterior fibulotalar ligament (**Fig. 13.16**).

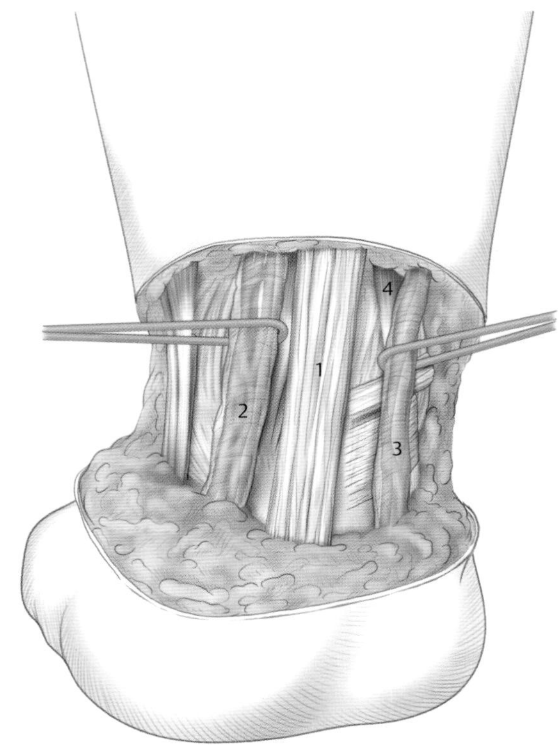

Fig. 13.16 Posterior dissection showing the Achilles tendon, medial and lateral neurovascular bundles, and peroneal tendons. The peroneal tendon sheaths must not be opened completely behind the fibula as this predisposes to dislocation of the peroneal tendons.

1 Calcaneal tendon
2 Medial neurovascular bundle (tibial nerve, posterior tibial artery and vein)
3 Lateral neurovascular bundle (sural nerve, small saphenous vein)
4 Peroneal tendons

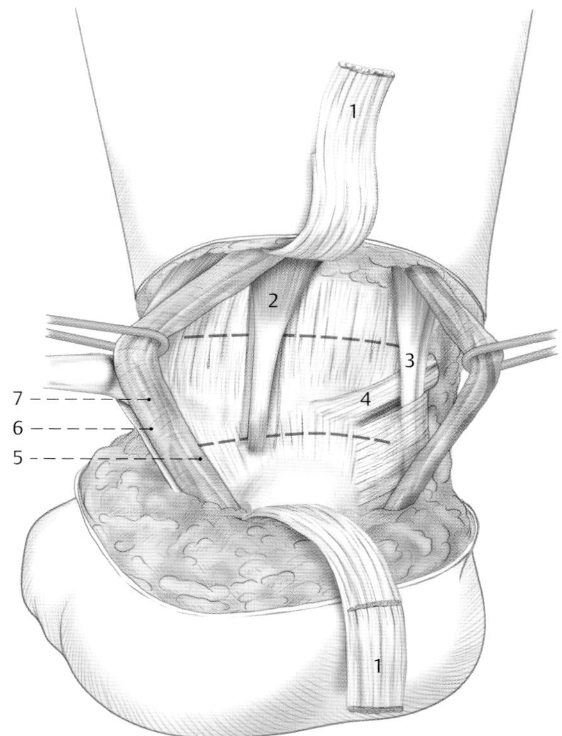

Fig. 13.17 Exposure of the posterior joint capsule structures of the ankle and talocalcaneonavicular joint. The dashed lines show the incisions for arthrolysis in these joints. Flexor hallucis longus passes into the talocalcaneonavicular joint so it acts as a guide.

1 Calcaneal tendon (incised in the frontal plane)
2 Flexor hallucis longus
3 Peroneal tendons
4 Posterior talofibular ligament
5 Tibial nerve
6 Posterior tibial veins
7 Posterior tibial artery

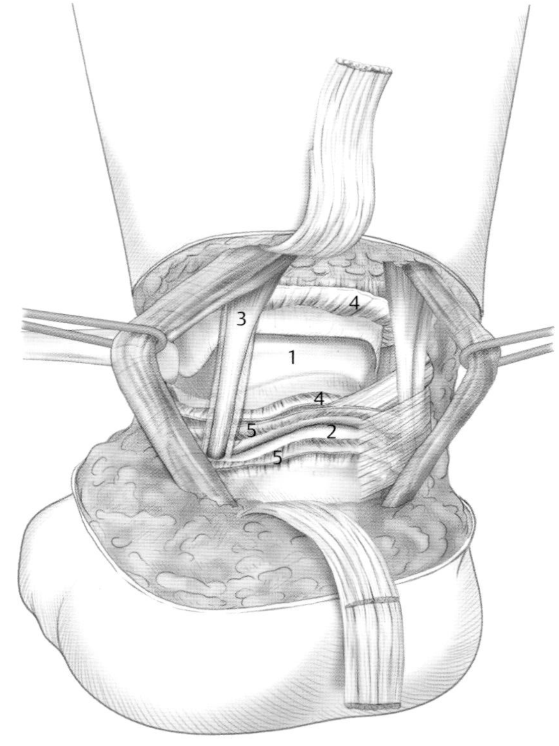

Fig. 13.18 Complete posterior arthrolysis with the ankle and talocalcaneonavicular joints opened. If contracture of flexor hallucis longus is present, its tendon can optionally be lengthened.

1 Talus
2 Calcaneus
3 Flexor hallucis longus
4 Ankle joint capsule
5 Talocalcaneonavicular joint capsule

The capsule is incised transversely, sparing the flexor hallucis longus and posterior fibulotalar ligament (**Figs. 13.17** and **13.18**). If the flexor hallucis longus tendon is shortened, it can be elongated in a Z-shape through the posterior approach.

13.3.4 Medial Arthrolysis, Elongation of Tibialis Posterior and Flexor Digitorum Longus

To expose the medial series of joints, tibialis posterior, and flexor digitorum longus, the fascia of abductor hallucis is first incised. The medial neurovascular bundle is retracted. Behind the medial malleolus, the tendon sheaths of flexor digitorum longus and tibialis posterior are incised, and the tendons are exposed.

The capsule of the talonavicular joint and the anterior part of the subtalar joint can now be exposed (**Fig. 13.19**). The flexor digitorum longus tendon can be dissected as far as the plantar flexor chiasm.

A Z-shaped incision is made in the tendon of tibialis posterior. The distal cut tendon end acts as a guide to the talonavicular joint. Arthrolysis of the talonavicular joint and subtalar joint can be performed from the medial side. The extent of the arthrolysis is determined by the severity of the deformity. The talocalcaneal ligament must on no account be divided as this predisposes to pes valgus. If the flexor tendons are contracted, the tendon of flexor digitorum longus can be lengthened by a Z-shaped incision via the medial approach (**Figs. 13.20** and **13.21**).

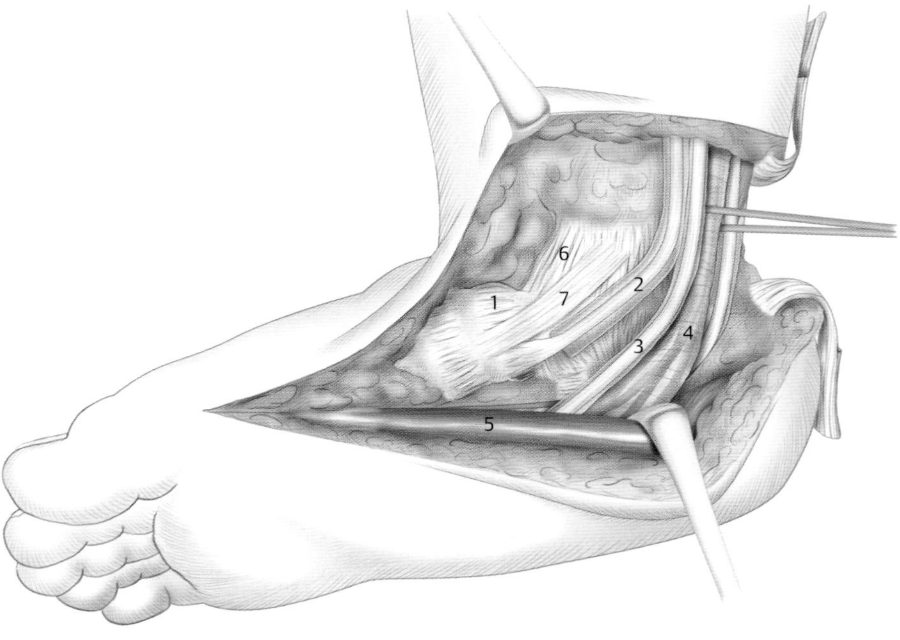

Fig. 13.19 Medial site after division of the abductor hallucis fascia. The talonavicular joint and medial ankle joint can be seen. The tendons of tibialis posterior and flexor digitorum longus are behind the medial malleolus. The tendon sheaths have been opened, and the tendons are intact.

1 Dorsal talonavicular ligament
2 Tibialis posterior
3 Flexor digitorum longus
4 Medial neurovascular bundle
5 Abductor hallucis
6 Deltoid ligament, anterior tibiotalar part
7 Deltoid ligament, tibionavicular part

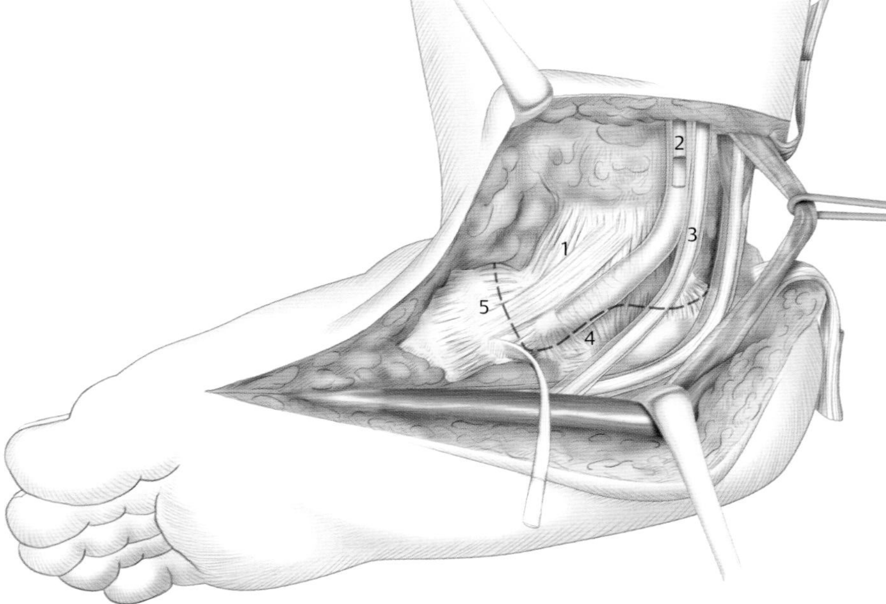

Fig. 13.20 The tendon of tibialis posterior is lengthened using a Z-shaped incision. The dashed line marks the incision for medial arthrolysis that includes the talonavicular joint and subtalar joint. The tibiotalar ligament must not be incised.

1 Deltoid ligament
2 Tibialis posterior
3 Flexor digitorum longus
4 Subtalar joint
5 Talonavicular joint

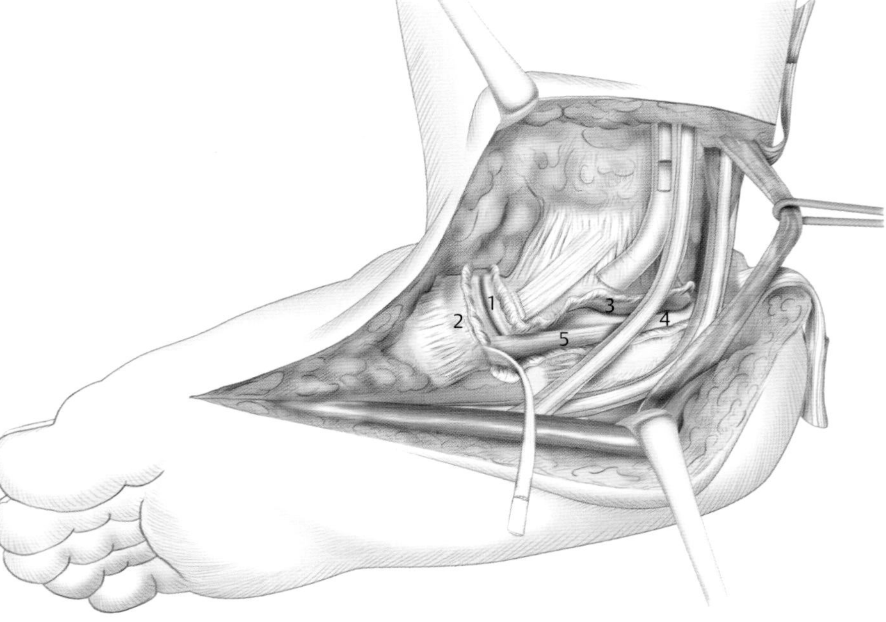

Fig. 13.21 The opened talonavicular joint, through which the head of the talus can be visualized and reduced. The subtalar joint is opened from the medial side, sparing the medial neurovascular bundle, which is snared.

1 Head of the talus
2 Navicular bone
3 Talus
4 Calcaneus
5 Plantar calcaneonavicular ligament

13.3.5 Lateral Arthrolysis, Lengthening of the Peroneal Tendons

The fibula with its ligaments, the peroneal tendons, the calcaneus, and the cuboid bone can be exposed through the lateral part of the approach (**Fig. 13.22**). Lateral arthrolysis is usually performed in the case of very severe deformities. Depending on the severity of the deformity, the arthrolysis can extend from the calcaneocuboid joint via the subtalar joint to the entire gap between the talus, calcaneus, and navicular and cuboid bones (**Figs. 13.23** and **13.24**). The fibulocalcaneal ligament can be divided from the lateral aspect. If the peroneal tendons are contracted, they can be lengthened through the lateral part of the approach. The sural nerve is exposed posteriorly and must also be dissected laterally and spared.

13.3.6 Wound Closure

The tendons are sutured in a neutral position. Both the Achilles tendon and the tibialis posterior tendon must be sutured with adequate tension. Excessive lengthening results in overcorrection with the development of talipes calcaneus or pes valgus. Wound closure can be continuous with an absorbable intracutaneous suture, but interrupted sutures are preferable for critical wounds. After wound closure, a long-leg case is applied. A short-leg cast is preferable in children over 3 years of age.

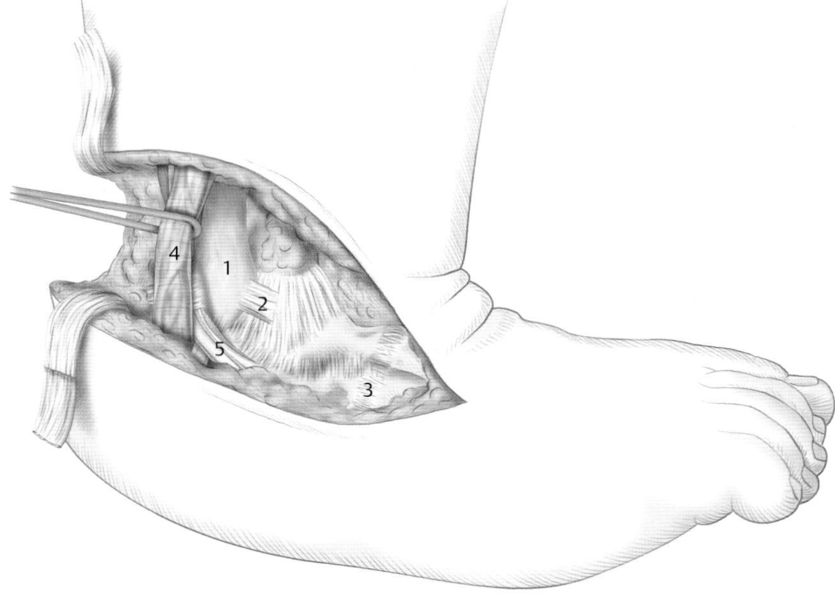

Fig. 13.22 Lateral site after division of the subcutaneous tissue. The lateral neurovascular bundle is snared.

1 Fibula
2 Anterior talofibular ligament
3 Calcaneocuboid joint
4 Lateral neurovascular bundle (posterior tibial artery, posterior tibial veins, tibial nerve)
5 Peroneal tendons

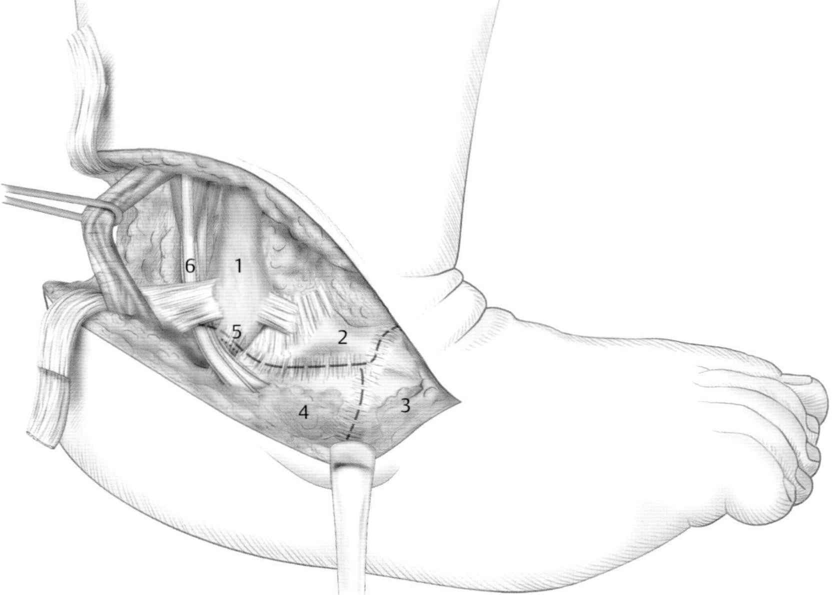

Fig. 13.23 Lateral view with snared neurovascular bundle and visible peroneal tendons. The dashed lines show the optional lateral arthrolyses.

1 Fibula
2 Talus
3 Cuboid
4 Calcaneus
5 Calcaneofibular ligament
6 Peroneal tendons

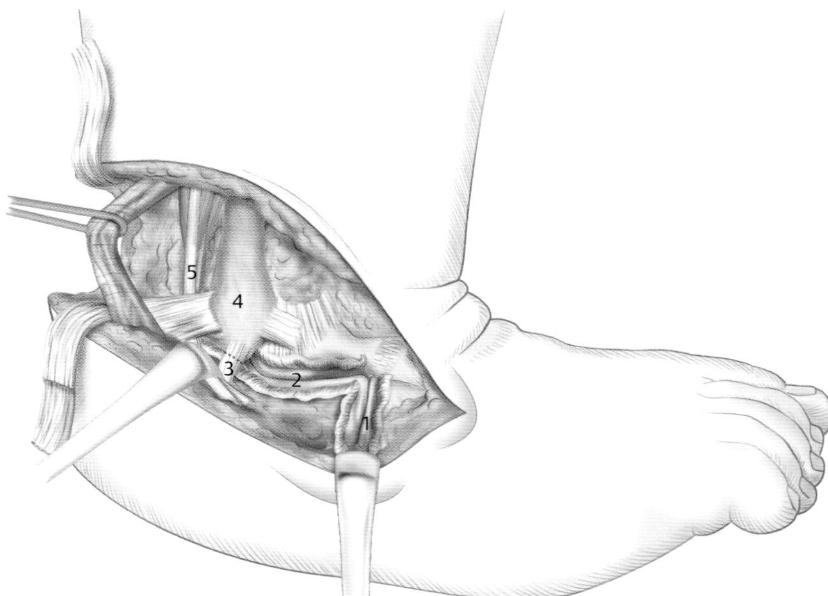

Fig. 13.24 Lateral site with the subtalar joint and calcaneocuboid joint opened, and the talonavicular joint not yet opened. The stippled line shows the division of the calcaneofibular ligament, which is transected with the arthrolysis.

1 Calcaneocuboid joint
2 Subtalar joint
3 Calcaneofibular ligament
4 Fibula
5 Peroneal tendons

13.3.7 Dangers

Since correction is performed during infancy and the site is very small, the neurovascular bundles require special care. Wound closure can be a problem with severe equinovarus deformity. The first postoperative cast is applied with the foot in the equinus position. The equinus is corrected by successive casts that stretch the posterior soft tissues.

13.3.8 Note

Arthrolysis to correct foot deformities in infancy and early childhood must be adjusted to the severity of the deformity. The deformity is corrected “a la carte.” Overextensive arthrolysis leads to overcorrection with the development of even more severe pes valgus.

13.4 Posteromedial Approach to the Ankle Joint and the Medial Side of the Talocalcaneonavicular Joint

R. Bauer, F. Kerschbaumer, S. Poisel

13.4.1 Principal Indications

- Capsulotomy
- Correction of talipes deformities

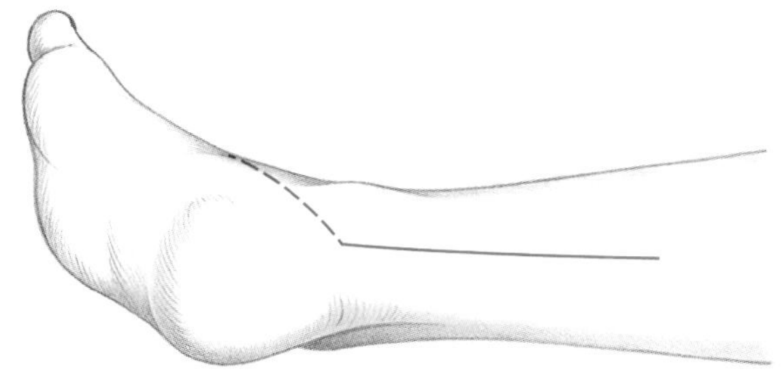

Fig. 13.25 Posteromedial approach to the ankle joint and talocalcaneonavicular joint. Skin incision (right leg).

13.4.2 Positioning and Incision

How the patient is positioned depends on the intended operation. If a purely posterior capsulotomy of the ankle joint with elongation of the Achilles tendon is planned, the patient is placed in the prone position. However, if medial capsulotomy of the talocalcaneonavicular joint is required as well, the supine position with the leg externally rotated is preferable.

The longitudinal incision is made along the medial border of the Achilles tendon and extends to the calcaneal tuberosity. If necessary, the incision may be lengthened anteriorly as far as the insertion of the tibialis anterior tendon (**Fig. 13.25**). After splitting the fascia over the Achilles tendon, this is dissected free of the underlying fat from below. Depending on the nature of the foot deformity, the Achilles tendon may be transected sagittally or frontally. Sagittal tenotomy with section of the medial half of the Achilles tendon at its attachment is particularly necessary for talipes. In cases of talipes equinus alone, the Achilles tendon is tenotomized frontally (**Fig. 13.26**). The transection may be either posterior and distal or posterior and proximal. The type of transection performed depends on the length of the muscular portion of the soleus. If the muscular portion of the soleus extends far distally, frontal lengthening is recommended, the proximal transverse incision being made in a posterior direction, and the distal one in an anterior

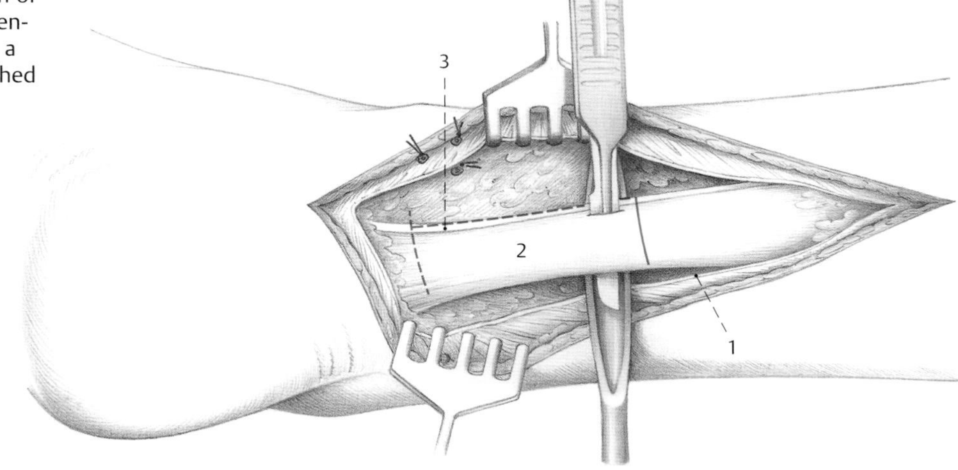

Fig. 13.26 After division of the fascia, the Achilles tendon is undermined, and a Z-shaped tenotomy (dashed lines) is performed.

1 Crural fascia
2 Calcaneal tendon
3 Plantaris tendon

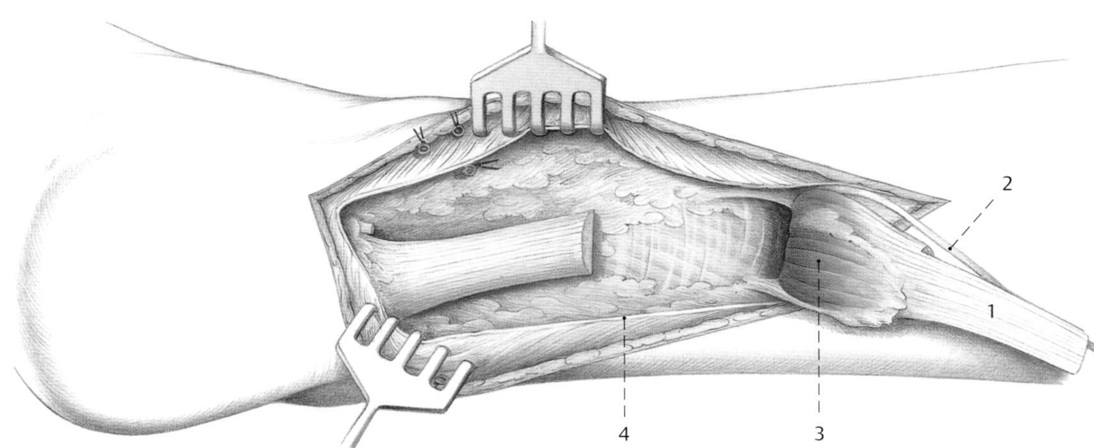

Fig. 13.27 Reflection of the tendon ends from the wound.

1 Calcaneal tendon
2 Plantaris tendon
3 Triceps surae
4 Crural fascia

direction. The tenotomized tendon ends are reflected upward from the wound so that the underlying deep crural fascia is revealed (**Fig. 13.27**). The tendon ends are then covered with moist swabs, and the foot, which is usually in the equinus position, can now be manually set in the neutral position. The deep layer of the crural fascia is incised over the belly of flexor hallucis longus (**Fig. 13.28**).

13.4.3 Exposure of the Joint Capsule

Flexor hallucis longus is recognizable by its typical muscle belly, which extends far distally and covers the posterior surface of the tibia. The tibial nerve and the posterior tibial artery lie medial to flexor hallucis longus.

For posterior exposure of the distal tibia and the capsule of the ankle joint, flexor hallucis longus has to be proximally detached—sharply in part—from its origin, avoiding damage to the peroneal artery. Distally, the tendon sheath of this muscle is split. At this site, branches of the posterior tibial artery have to be transected (**Fig. 13.29**). Posterior capsulotomy of the talocrural and talocalcaneonavicular joints can be effected by means of two transverse incisions or by complete detachment of the capsule as shown in **Fig. 13.29**. For this purpose, the posterior talofibular and calcaneofibular ligaments need to be transected. When transecting the calcaneofibular ligament, the peroneal tendons have to be protected. Medially, the posterior part of the deltoid ligament is transected directly at its attachment to the calcaneus (**Fig. 13.30**).

13.4.4 Extension of the Approach with Medial Release

If exposure of the medial portions of the talocalcaneonavicular joint should subsequently prove necessary, the skin incision may be extended anteriorly and distally. The skin is incised approximately as far as the insertion of tibialis anterior on the inner aspect of the first metatarsal joint. Then the crural fascia over the neurovascular bundle is split from proximal to distal, the superficial layer of the flexor retinaculum being opened distally. It is now possible to pass under the neurovascular bundle and retract it laterally with a rubber band (**Fig. 13.31**). Subsequently, the anterior portion of the flexor retinaculum is split by a curved incision, and now the tendi-

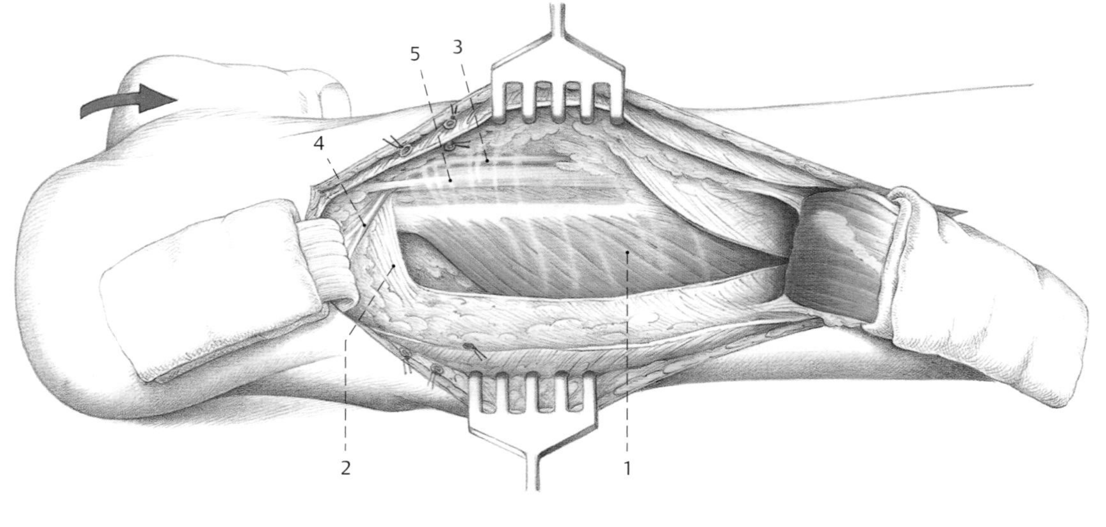

Fig. 13.28 Incision of the deep crural fascia.

1 Flexor hallucis longus
2 Retinaculum of the flexor muscles, superficial layer
3 Posterior tibial artery
4 Calcaneal branch
5 Tibial nerve

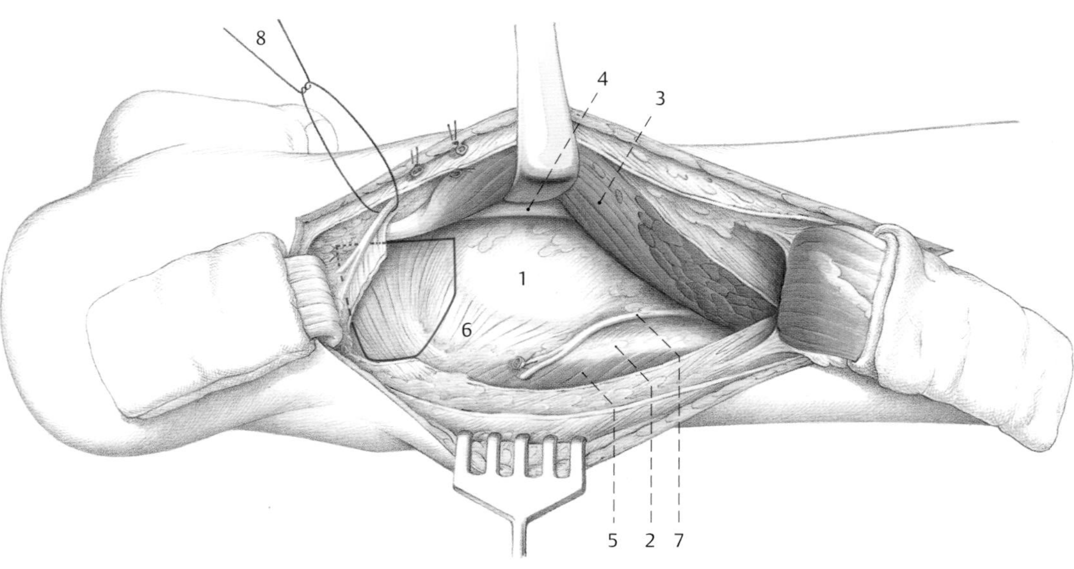

Fig. 13.29 Mediad retraction of flexor hallucis longus and fenestration of the posterior portion of the capsule of the ankle joint and talocalcaneonavicular joint. Note: In its proximal portion, flexor hallucis longus has been partly detached from its origin on the fibula.

1 Tibia
2 Fibula
3 Flexor hallucis longus
4 Tendon of tibialis posterior
5 Short peroneal muscle
6 Posterior tibiofibular ligament
7 Peroneal artery
8 Posterior tibial artery, calcaneal branch

nous compartments of the flexor digitorum longus and tibialis posterior have to be incised (**Fig. 13.32**). If necessary, the tendons of flexor digitorum longus and tibialis posterior are subjected to a Z-shaped tenotomy and pulled out of the wound (**Fig. 13.33**). Through manual lateral displacement of the forefoot, the cavities of the subtalar and talonavicular joints can be located with a needle. Complete splitting of the tendon sheath of flexor hallucis longus is necessary to expose the subtalar articulation. Manual eversion of the foot provides a good overview of the talonavicular and talocalcaneal joints (**Fig. 13.34**).

13.4.5 Wound Closure

Closure of the joint capsule is generally unnecessary after medial and posterior capsulotomy. If conditions warrant, the transected tendons are lengthened by a Z-shaped incision and sutured with interrupted sutures. This incision may entail impaired wound healing owing to skin tension.

13.4.6 Dangers

Transection of the calcaneofibular ligament endangers the peroneal tendons, and transection of the posterior portion of the deltoid ligament endangers the posterior tibial artery and the tibial nerve.

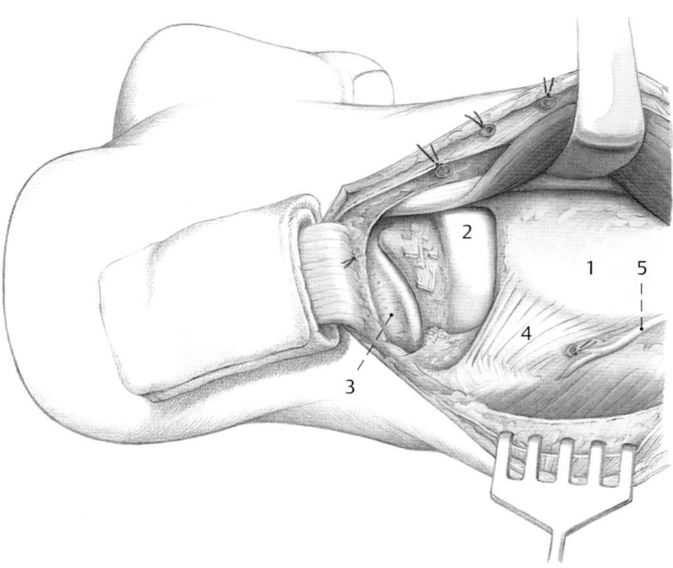

Fig. 13.30 Operative site after resection of the joint capsule; posterior exposure of the talocrural and subtalar joints.

1 Tibia
2 Trochlea of the talus
3 Calcaneus
4 Posterior tibiofibular ligament
5 Peroneal artery

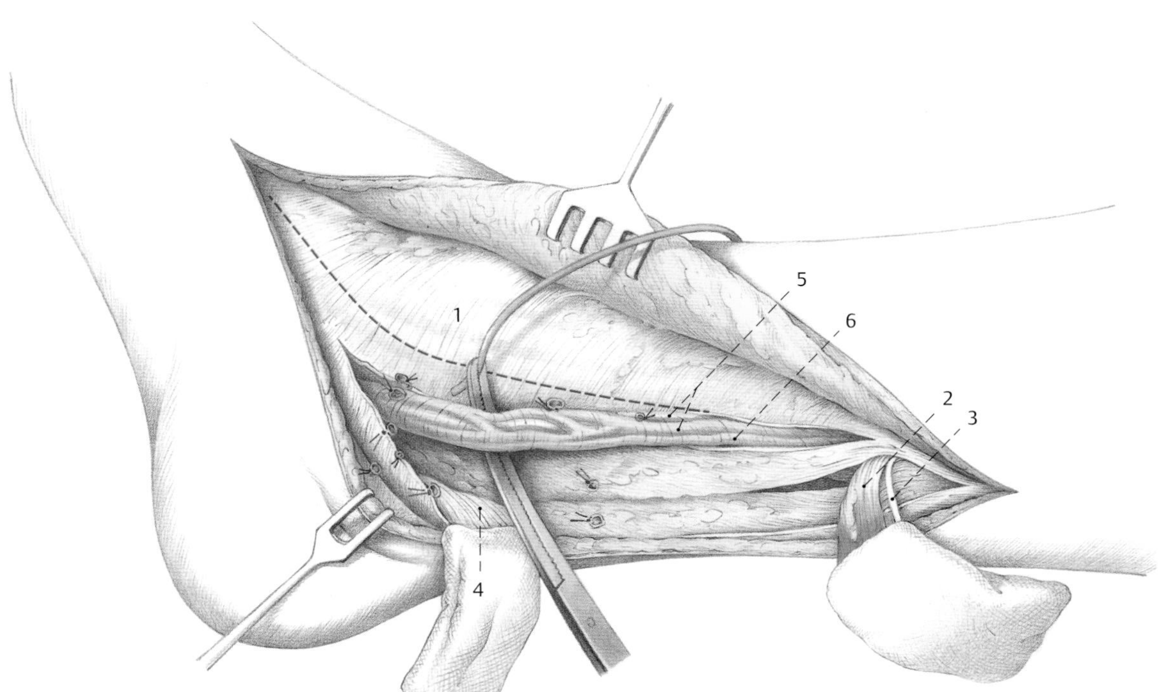

Fig. 13.31 Appearance after extension of the skin incision in a distal and medial direction.

1 Flexor retinaculum
2 Triceps surae
3 Plantaris tendon
4 Calcaneal tendon
5 Posterior tibial artery and accompanying veins
6 Tibial nerve

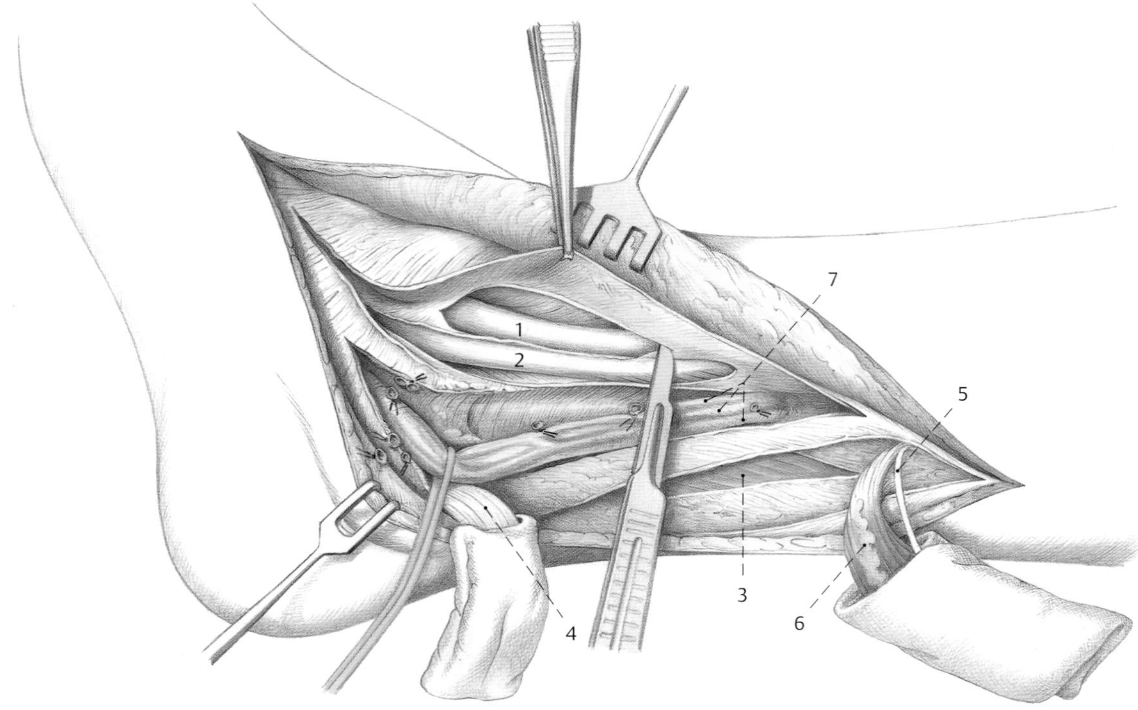

Fig. 13.32 Operative site after incision of the tendon sheaths of flexor digitorum longus and tibialis posterior.

1 Tendon of tibialis posterior
2 Tendon of flexor digitorum longus
3 Flexor hallucis longus
4 Calcaneal tendon
5 Plantaris
6 Triceps surae
7 Posterior tibial vessels and tibial nerve

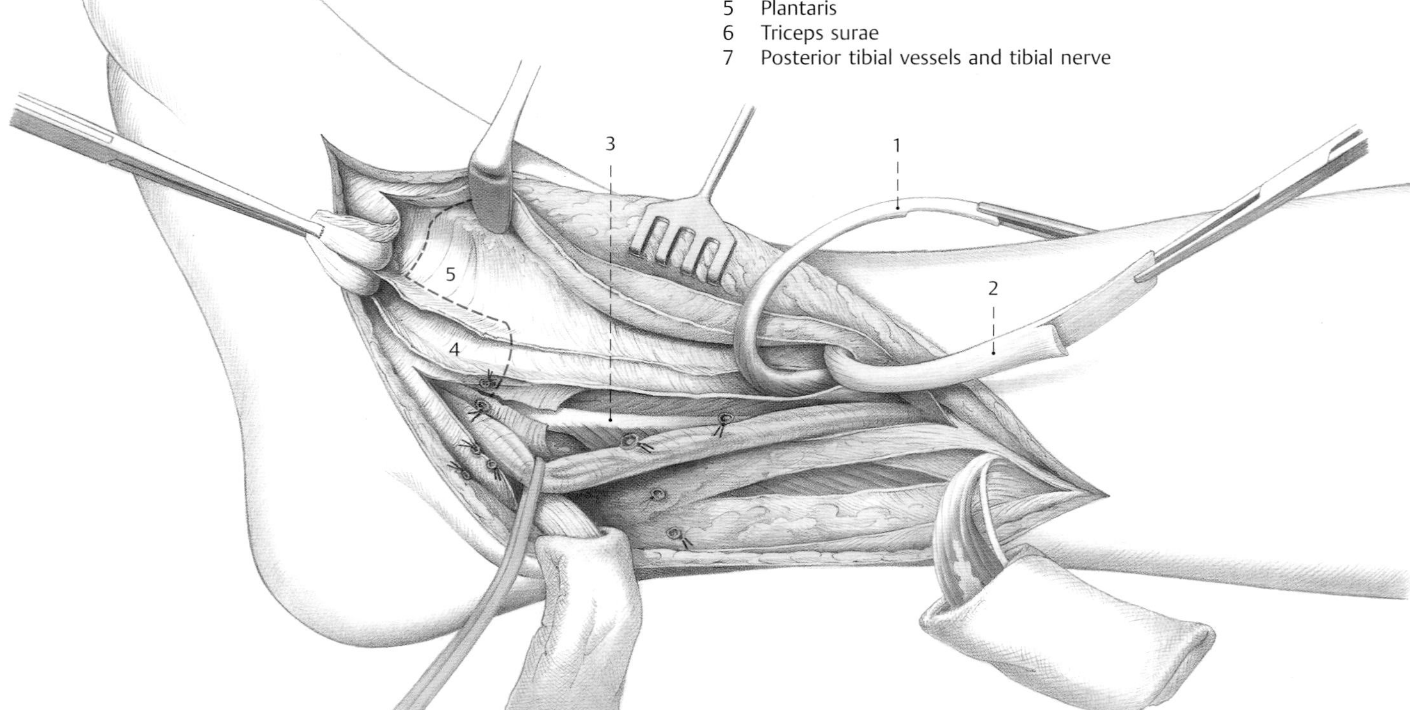

Fig. 13.33 Operative site after Z-shaped tenotomy of flexor digitorum longus and tibialis posterior. The dashed line shows the stepped incision of the talocalcaneonavicular and subtalar joints. The tendon sheath of flexor hallucis longus had previously been split over a long distance in a distal direction.

1 Tendon of flexor digitorum longus
2 Tendon of tibialis posterior
3 Tendon of flexor hallucis longus
4 Tendon sheath of flexor digitorum longus
5 Tendon sheath of tibialis posterior

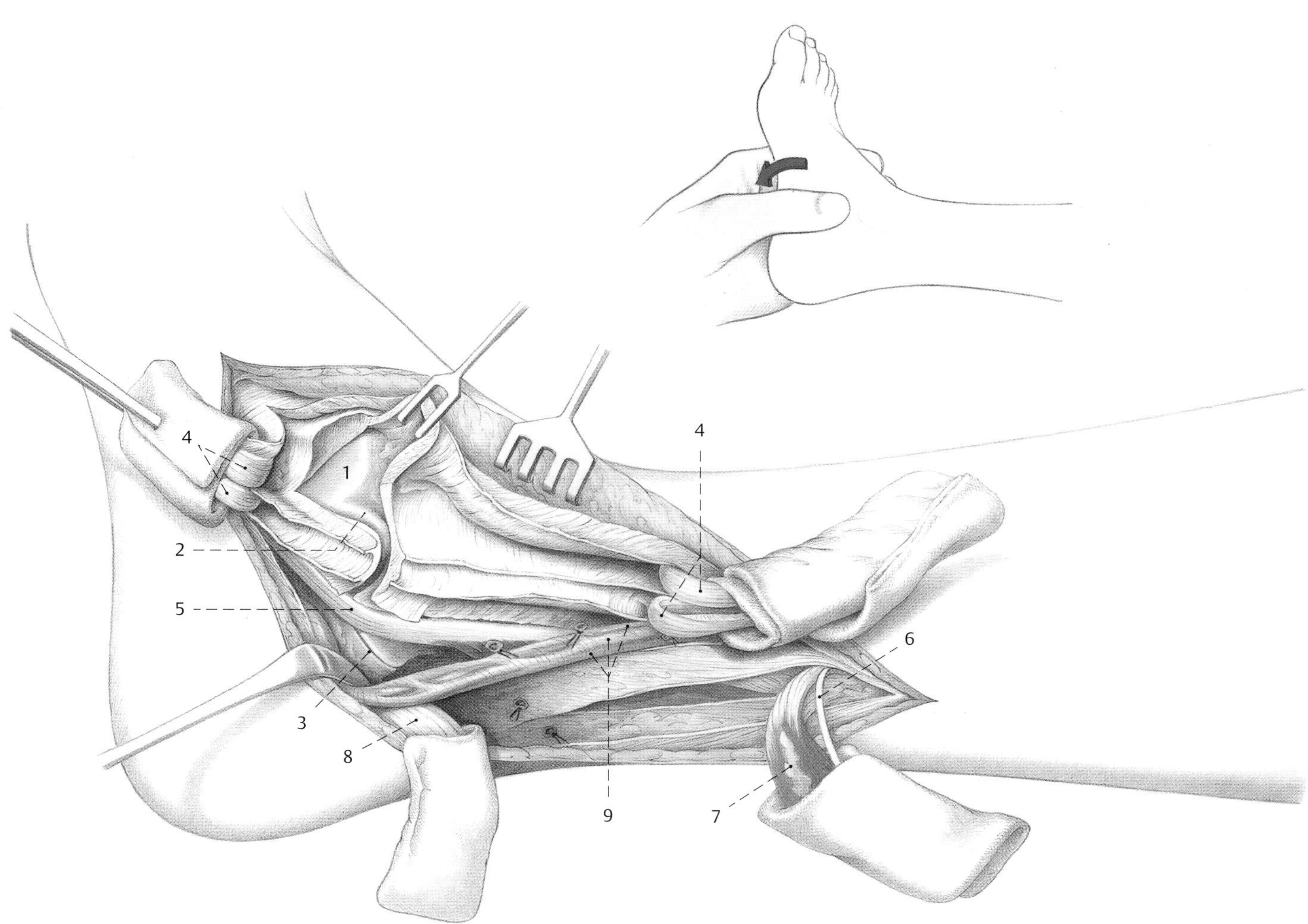

Fig. 13.34 Manual placement of the foot in pronation–eversion for exposure of the talocalcaneonavicular joint.

1 Anterior calcaneal articular surface of the talus
2 Middle calcaneal articular surface of the talus
3 Subtalar articulation
4 Tendons of tibialis posterior and flexor digitorum longus
5 Tendon of flexor hallucis longus
6 Plantaris
7 Triceps surae
8 Calcaneal tendon
9 Posterior tibial vessels and tibial nerve

13.5 Dorsolateral Approach to the Ankle Joint

R. Bauer, F. Kerschbaumer, S. Poisel

13.5.1 Principal Indications

- Simultaneous internal fixation of the fibula and a posterior avulsion fracture (Volkmann's triangle)
- Capsulotomy
- Ankle arthrodesis

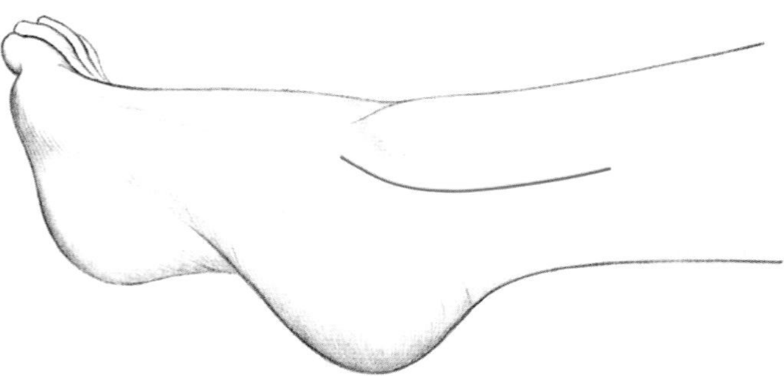

Fig. 13.35 Dorsolateral approach to the ankle joint. Skin incision (left leg).

13.5.2 Positioning and Incision

The operation may be performed with the patient placed in the prone or lateral position, or with the patient supine with the leg slightly rotated. After (optional) application of a tourniquet, the leg is draped so as to allow free movement. A skin incision approximately 10 cm long is made midway between the posterior border of the fibula and the lateral border of the Achilles tendon. The skin incision curves gently around the posterior border of the lateral malleolus (**Fig. 13.35**). After cautious splitting of the subcutaneous tissue, the small saphenous vein and the sural nerve are identified, snared, and retracted. Then the crural fascia is split over the muscle belly of flexor hallucis longus (**Fig. 13.36**). The lateral border of the fascia is grasped with forceps, and the tendon sheath of the peroneal tendons is then incised in the longitudinal direction (**Fig. 13.37**).

13.5.3 Exposure of the Ankle Joint

The peroneal tendons are retracted laterally, and the flexor hallucis longus is retracted medially (optional) with the aid of Langenbeck retractors. In the upper wound region, flexor hallucis longus, which is adherent to the fibula at this point, has to be sharply detached from its origin. Injury to the peroneal artery, which courses directly behind it, must be avoided. Smaller, transverse branches of the peroneal artery and vein are transected (**Fig. 13.38**).

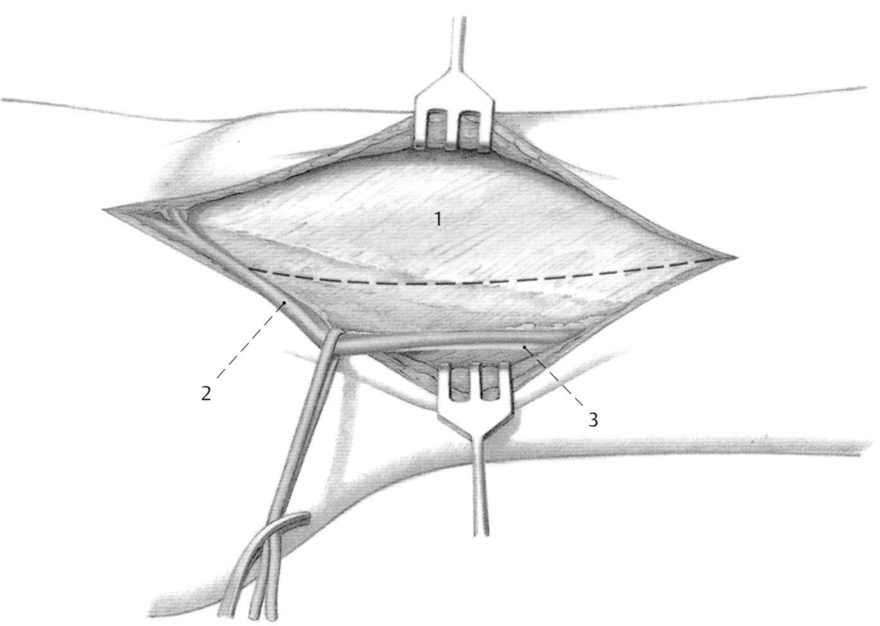

Fig. 13.36 Splitting of fascia after isolation and retraction of the sural nerve and small saphenous vein.

1 Crural fascia
2 Small saphenous vein
3 Sural nerve

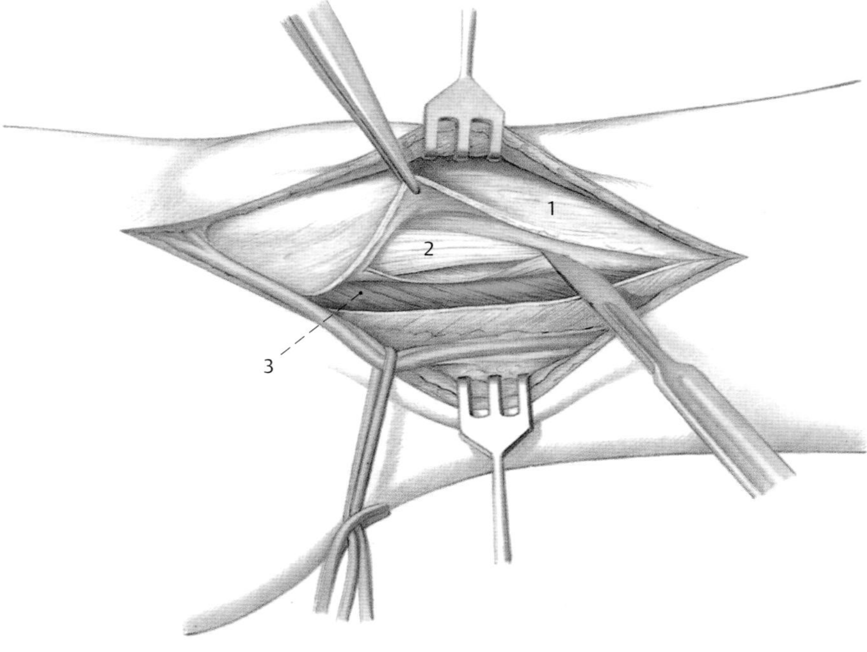

Fig. 13.37 Exposure of flexor hallucis longus and opening of the peroneal tendon sheath (optional).

1 Crural fascia
2 Peroneus longus
3 Flexor hallucis longus

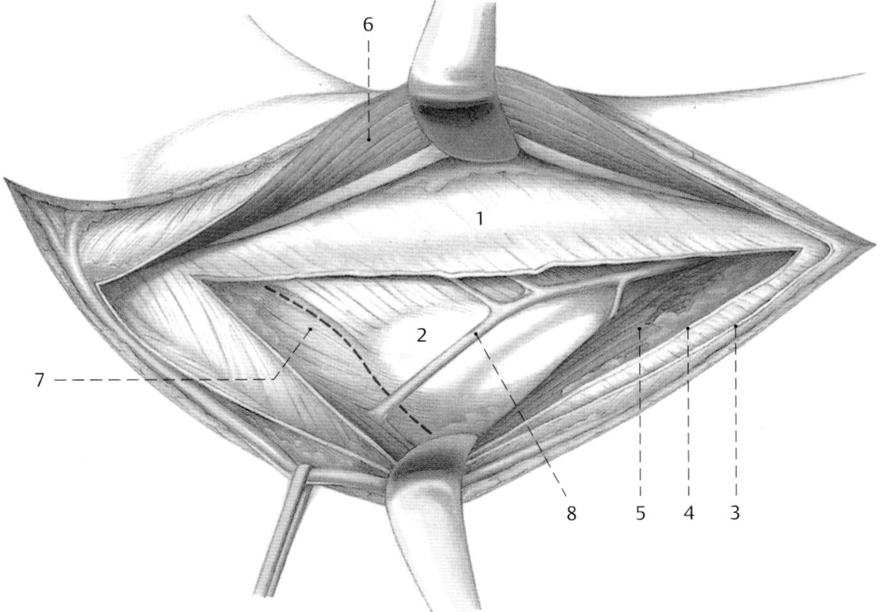

Fig. 13.38 Lateral retraction of the peroneal tendons and medial retraction of flexor hallucis longus.

1 Fibula
2 Tibia
3 Crural fascia
4 Deep crural fascia
5 Flexor hallucis longus
6 Peroneus brevis
7 Talocrural joint capsule
8 Peroneal artery

Manual redressement of the foot to the talipes calcaneus position (**Fig. 13.39**) tenses the joint capsule and allows it to be incised. After transection of the transversely running branches of the peroneal artery and vein, the latter are further mobilized medially. The posterior portion of the tibia, the fibula, and the posterior syndesmotic ligament, and the posterior portion of the talocrural joint, are now clearly exposed (**Fig. 13.40**).

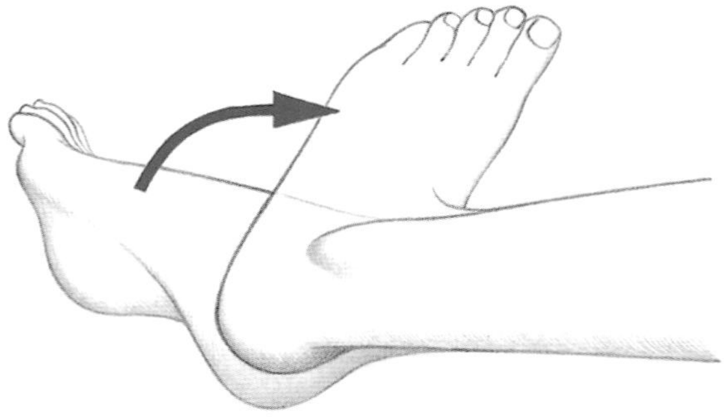

Fig. 13.39 Manual adjustment of the foot to posterior extension for stretching of the posterior joint capsule.

13.5.4 Wound Closure

After release of the tourniquet and hemostasis, the wound is closed, the capsule and the superficial crural fascia being sutured if necessary.

13.5.5 Dangers

The peroneal artery and vein may be damaged when flexor hallucis longus is stripped from the fibula.

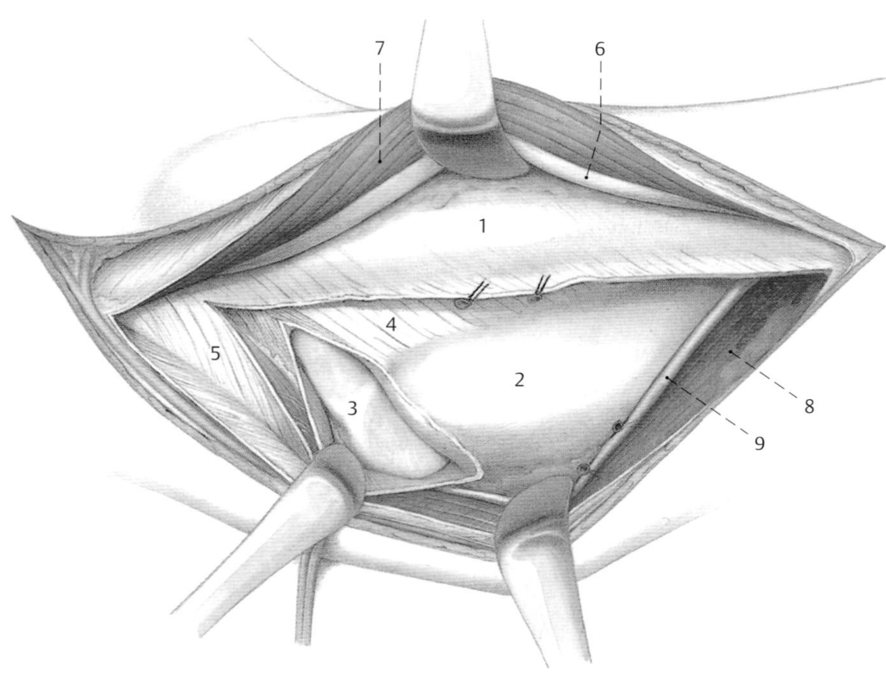

Fig. 13.40 Ligation of the transverse branches of the peroneal artery and vein, and opening of the posterior portion of ankle joint following mobilization of the peroneal artery and vein in a medial direction for clear exposure of the tibia.

1 Fibula
2 Tibia
3 Talus
4 Posterior tibiofibular ligament
5 Posterior intermuscular septum of the leg
6 Peroneus longus
7 Peroneus brevis
8 Flexor hallucis longus
9 Peroneal artery

13.6 Medial Exposure of the Ankle Joint with Osteotomy of the Medial Malleolus

R. Bauer, F. Kerschbaumer, S. Poisel

13.6.1 Principal Indications

- Osteochondritis dissecans of the talus
- Osteochondral fractures
- Talus fractures

13.6.2 Positioning and Incision

The patient is placed in the supine position. After (optional) application of a tourniquet, the leg is draped so as to allow free movement, and is rotated externally. The skin incision, approximately 10 cm in length, is begun three fingerbreadths proximally and posteriorly to the inner malleolus, and runs posterior to the malleolus in a distal and anterior direction (**Fig. 13.41**).

13.6.3 Exposure of the Ankle Joint

The fascia and the joint capsule are incised anterior and posterior to the malleolus. Posteriorly, the incision is made through the tendon sheath of tibialis posterior, which is retracted with a small hook (**Fig. 13.42**). Before osteotomy of the inner malleolus, a small stab incision is made at the tip of the malleolus. Now a small Hohmann elevator is inserted into the joint anterior and posterior to the malleolus. Then one or two holes are drilled for the insertion of malleolar screws (**Fig. 13.43**). The medial malleolus is osteotomized perpendicular to the direction of the bore, as shown in **Fig. 13.44**. The last few millimeters of the medial malleolus should be transected with a narrow osteotome since the oscillating saw causes greater chondral damage. The distal malleolar fragment is now reflected downward with a fine single-pronged hook, and at the same time the ankle is everted and abducted so that the medial and middle portion of the trochlea of the talus is clearly exposed (**Fig. 13.45**).

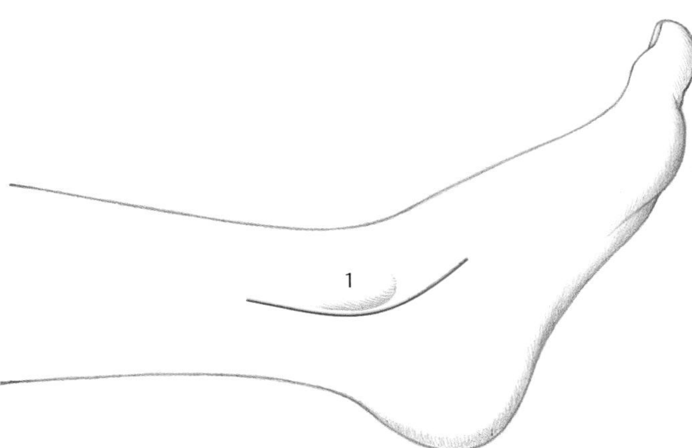

Fig. 13.41 Medial approach to the ankle joint with osteotomy of the medial malleolus. Skin incision (solid line, left leg).

1 Medial malleolus

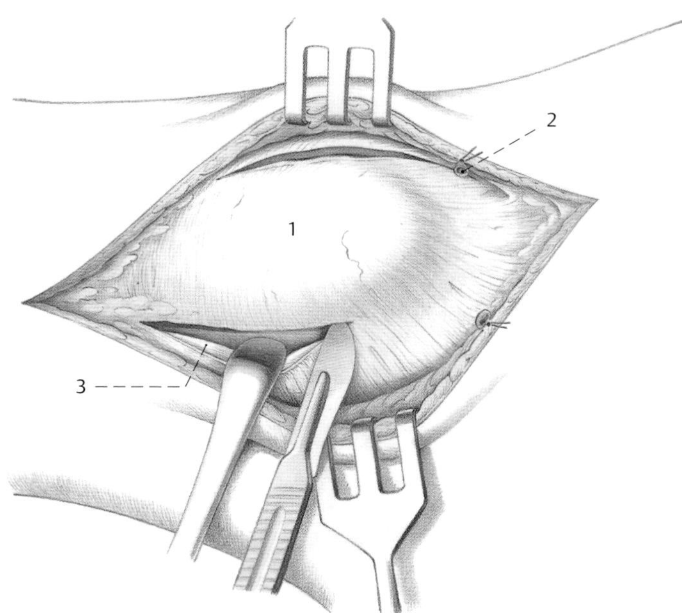

Fig. 13.42 Incision of the fascia and ankle joint capsule anterior and posterior to the medial malleolus. Posterior retraction of the tendon of tibialis posterior. Stab incision at the tip of the medial malleolus for a screw hole.

1 Medial malleolus
2 Great saphenous vein
3 Tendon of tibialis posterior

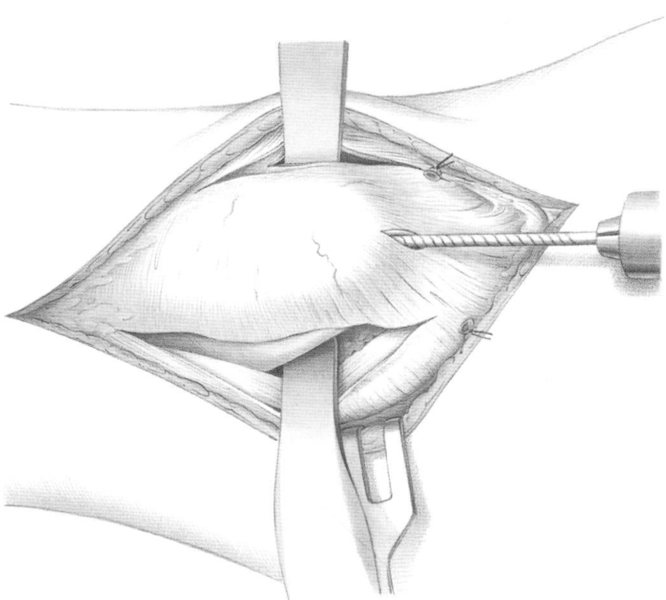

Fig. 13.43 Insertion of Hohmann elevators into the joint cavity. One or two slanting drill holes are made in the medial malleolus.

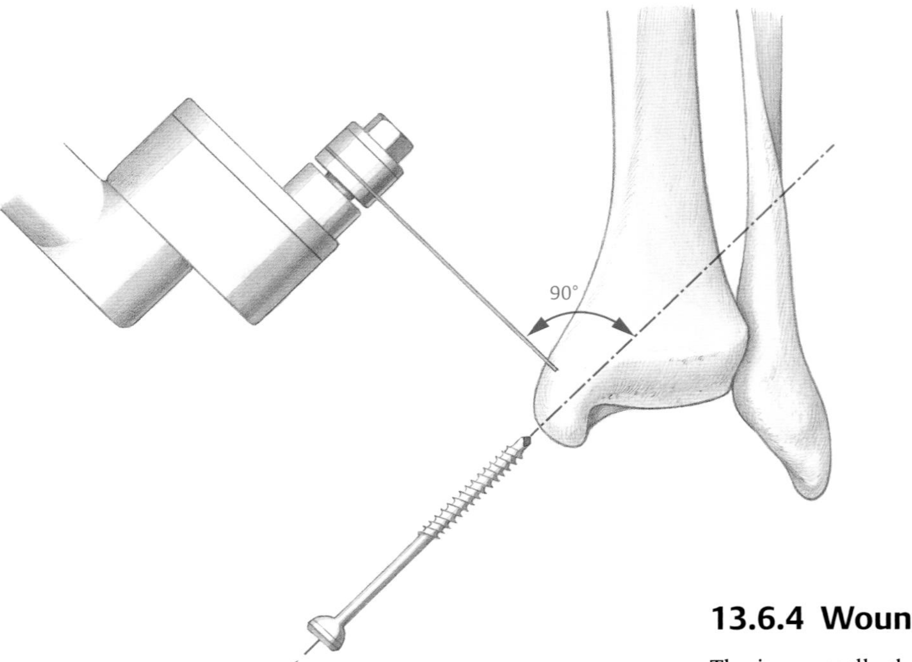

Fig. 13.44 The osteotomy of the medial malleolus should be at right angles to the plane of the screw direction.

13.6.4 Wound Closure

The inner malleolus is fixed with one or two malleolar screws. Exact apposition of the bone fragments should be assured. This is followed by suture of the tendon sheath of tibialis posterior and of the joint capsule in the anterior area (**Fig. 13.46**).

13.6.5 Note

With this approach, it is important to perform the osteotomy at the correct level. If it is done at too low a level, exposure of the trochlea of the talus will be inadequate. If the level is too high, the inferior tibial joint surface may be damaged.

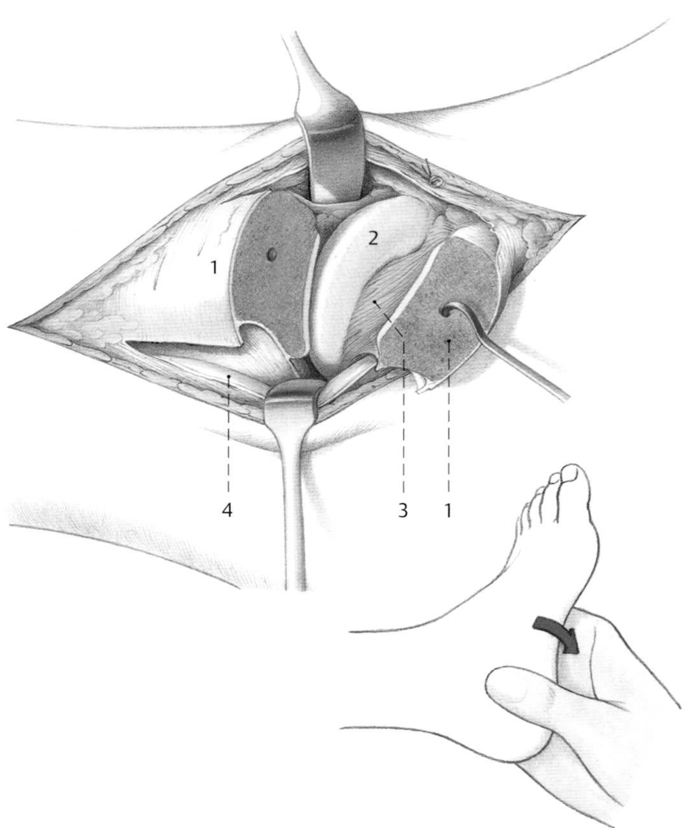

Fig. 13.45 The osteotomized distal fragment of the malleolus is reflected downward, and the foot is maximally pronated.

1 Medial malleolus
2 Medial malleolar surface of the talus
3 Deltoid ligament
4 Tendon of tibialis posterior

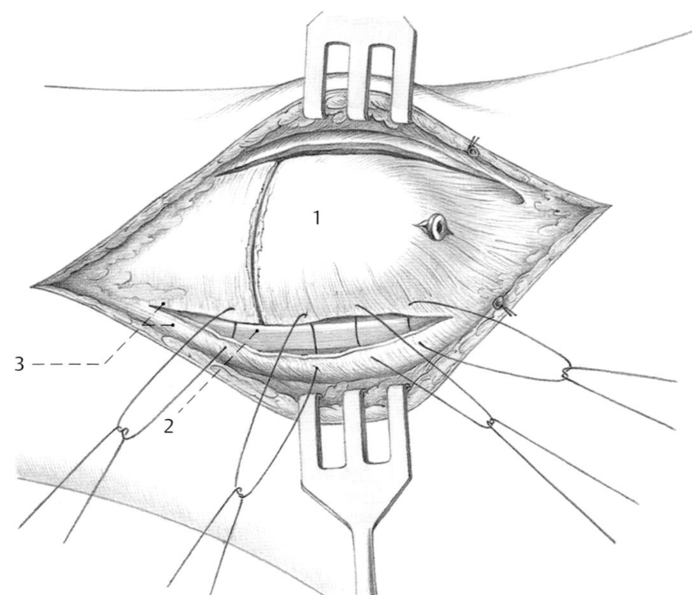

Fig. 13.46 Internal fixation of the medial malleolus with one or two malleolar screws. Suture of the capsule and tendon sheath of tibialis posterior.

1 Medial malleolus
2 Tendon of tibialis posterior
3 Tendon sheath

13.7 Arthroscopic Approaches

D. Kohn

13.7.1 Principal Indications

- Cartilage lesions
- Osteochondritis dissecans
- Intra-articular fractures
- Intra-articular loose bodies and osteophytes

13.7.2 Positioning

For ankle arthroscopy, the patient is placed in the supine position with the hip flexed to 70°. The thigh is fixed with padding beneath it. Traction is provided by a padded sterile harness (**Fig. 13.47**).

Fig. 13.47 Position for ankle arthroscopy. Traction is applied to the heel and dorsum of the foot via a padded harness. This is necessary for inspection of the posterior compartment. During inspection of the anterior compartment, the traction is reduced by turning the screw spindle.

13.7.3 Approach

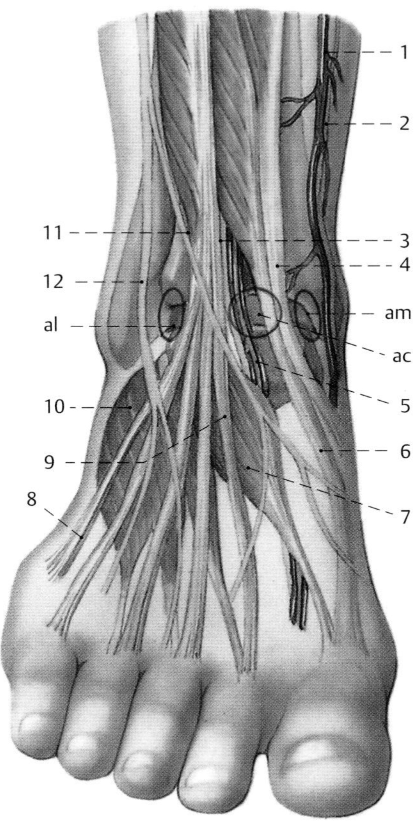

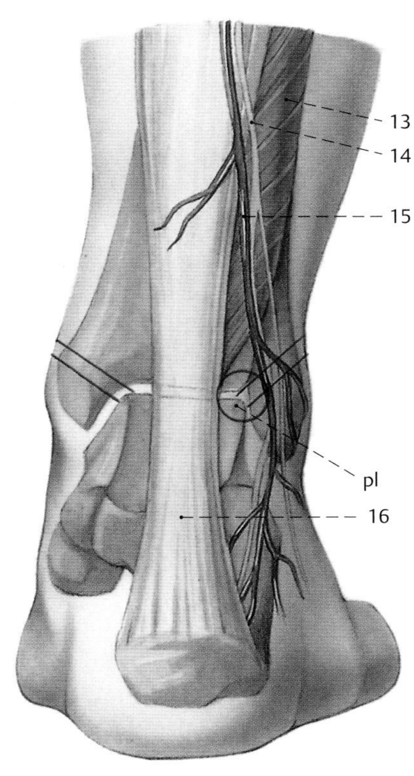

Fig. 13.48 a, b Approaches to the ankle joint. al, anterolateral; am, anteromedial; ac, anterocental; pl, posterolateral (From: Bauer R, Kerschbaumer F, Poisel S. Becken und untere Extremität. Stuttgart, Thieme; 1995. Orthopädische Operationslehre; Band 2.).

1 Great saphenous vein
2 Saphenous nerve
3 Deep peroneal nerve
4 Tendon of tibialis anterior
5 Dorsal artery of the foot
6 Tendon of extensor hallucis longus
7 Extensor hallucis brevis
8 Tendon of peroneus tertius
9 Tendons of extensor digitorum longus
10 Extensor digitorum brevis
11 Medial dorsal cutaneous nerve
12 Intermediate dorsal cutaneous nerve
13 Soleus
14 Sural nerve
15 Small saphenous vein
16 Calcaneal tendon

13.7.4 Technique

The outlines of the malleoli, the lateral border of the Achilles tendon, and the anterior ankle joint line are palpated and marked on the skin. The dorsal artery of the foot is palpated. With the foot everted and the fourth toe plantarflexed, the intermediate dorsal cutaneous nerve, a terminal branch of the superficial peroneal nerve, is marked on the lateral dorsum of the foot in slender patients. It is the most frequently injured nerve during ankle arthroscopy. The anteromedial, anterolateral, and posterolateral approaches are marked.

Arthroscopy begins with anterolateral entry to the joint (**Fig. 13.49a**), filling it with 20–30 mL Ringer lactate through a size 1 cannula. When the joint is punctured, it should be dorsiflexed to protect the cartilage surfaces of the trochlea of the talus. In most cases, some synovial membrane has to be removed to allow better visualization. A miniature burr is used and, as material is evacuated through the burr, a separate evacuation cannula is not necessary. When use of a burr is not required, a size 1 cannula placed in an otherwise unoccupied portal suffices for evacuation.

For complete inspection of the anterior and lateral parts of the joint, the optic must be switched from the anterolateral to the anteromedial approach using a switching stick (**Fig. 13.49b**). With the extension system, firm traction moves the talus sufficiently far from the tibial joint surface to allow advancement of a switching stick into the posterior joint compartment through the anteromedial portal. The stick is exchanged for a sleeve and 2.7 mm arthroscope. The posterior joint compartment can then be inspected. An additional dorsolateral portal for the optic is required in very narrow joints.

13.7.5 Wound Closure

Following ankle arthroscopy, all incisions are closed with interrupted sutures.

13.7.6 Note

The foot is placed in a prepared right-angled, padded lower leg splint for 4 days. The foot may be removed from the splint to exercise the ankle actively several times daily. No loading should occur until the ports have healed, after about a week. Depending on symptoms, full weight-bearing by the end of the second postoperative week is desirable.

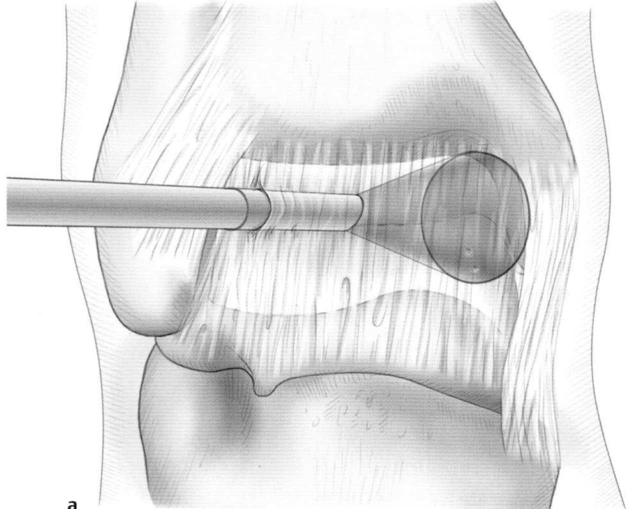

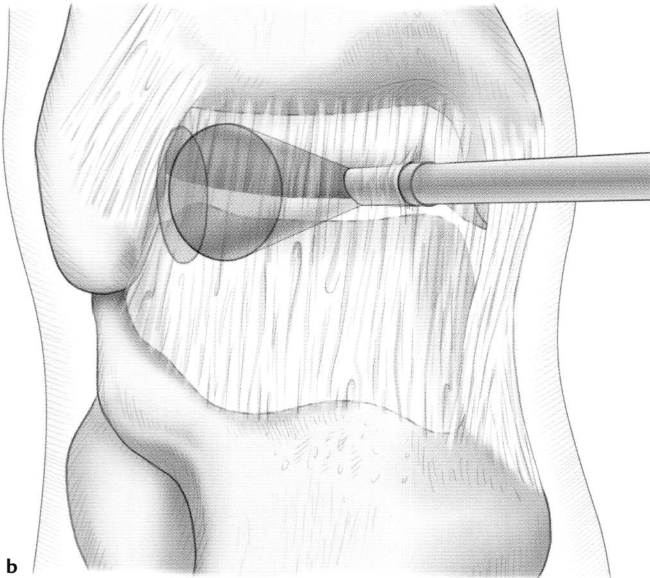

Fig. 13.49 a, b Arthroscopic inspection of the right ankle joint.

a Inspection of the anterior compartment, medial talomalleolar joint, and lateral part of the trochlea of the talus. The arthroscope is in the anterolateral portal. With plantar flexion, the central and part of the posterior trochlea become visible.
b Inspection of the posterior compartment, lateral talomalleolar joint, and medial anterior part of the trochlea of the talus. The arthroscope is in the anteromedial portal. The inserts show the arthroscopic view in the dorsolateral joint compartment (left) and lateral talomalleolar joint (right). This part of the examination is performed with traction on the foot to distract the joint. A cannula through the posterolateral portal perforates the posterior intermalleolar ligament, which reinforces the posterior joint capsule.

13.8 Medial Approach to the Medial Malleolus

R. Bauer, F. Kerschbaumer, S. Poisel

13.8.1 Principal Indications

- Fractures
- Tumors
- Osteomyelitis

13.8.2 Positioning and Incision

The patient is placed in the supine position. After (optional) application of a tourniquet, the leg is draped to allow free movement, and slightly rotated externally.

The length of the skin incision depends on the exposure required. It describes a slightly convex line anterior to the medial malleolus (**Fig. 13.50**).

13.8.3 Exposure of the Medial Malleolus

After transection of the skin and subcutaneous tissue, the great saphenous vein and the accompanying saphenous nerve are anteriorly dissected. Incision of the fascia exposes the medial malleolus (**Fig. 13.51**).

13.8.4 Wound Closure

The wound is closed by skin suture.

13.8.5 Dangers

A neuroma may form if the main branch of the saphenous nerve is cut.

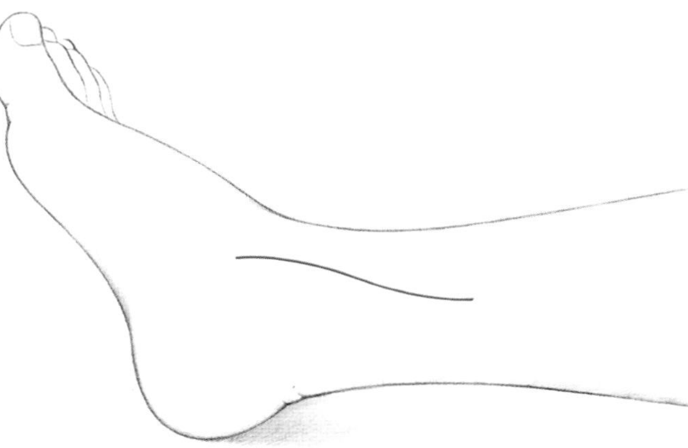

Fig. 13.50 Approach to the medial malleolus. Skin incision (right leg).

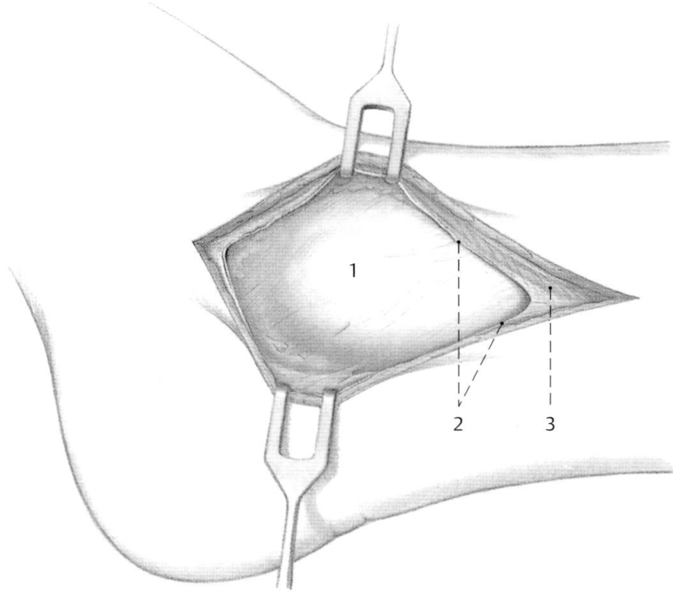

Fig. 13.51 Exposure of medial malleolus following incision of the subcutaneous tissue and fascia. Care should be taken to spare the saphenous nerve and great saphenous vein.

1 Medial malleolus
2 Crural fascia
3 Great saphenous vein

13.9 Approach to the Lateral Malleolus

R. Bauer, F. Kerschbaumer, S. Poisel

13.9.1 Principal Indications

- Fractures
- Arthrodesis of the ankle with osteotomy of the lateral malleolus
- Talofibular ligament reconstruction
- Dislocation of the peroneal tendon

13.9.2 Positioning and Incision

The patient is placed in the supine position. After (optional) application of a tourniquet, the leg is draped to allow free movement, and rotated internally. The skin incision is made just anterior to the lateral malleolus and is generally no longer than 7 cm (**Fig. 13.52**).

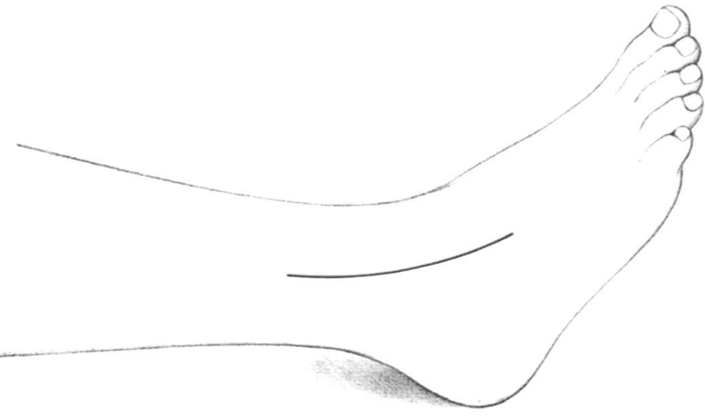

Fig. 13.52 Approach to the lateral malleolus. Skin incision (right leg).

13.9.3 Exposure of the Lateral Malleolus

After splitting the skin and subcutaneous tissue, attention must be paid to the location of the anteriorly coursing superficial intermediate dorsal cutaneous nerve, a branch of the superficial peroneal nerve (**Fig. 13.53**).

The small saphenous vein and the sural nerve lie posteriorly. If exposure of the anterior talofibular is required, the lower portion of the extensor retinaculum is split, and hereafter peroneus tertius and extensor digitorum longus are then retracted medially.

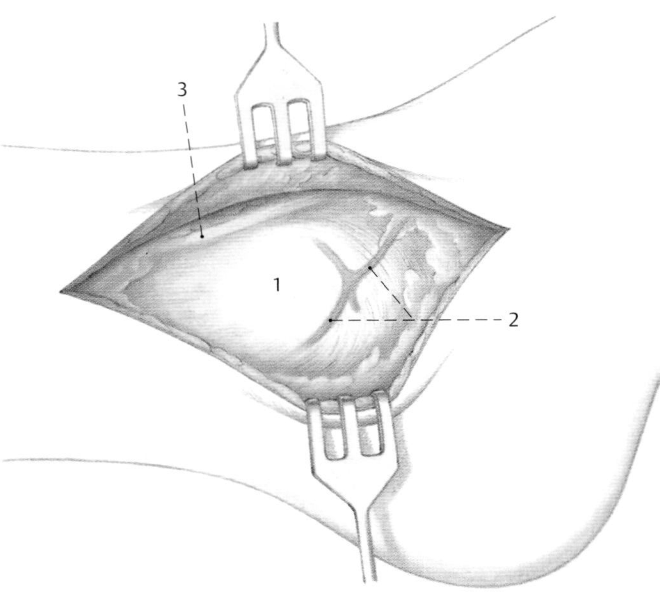

Fig. 13.53 Exposure of the lateral malleolus after splitting of the skin and fascia.

1 Lateral malleolus
2 Lateral malleolar network
3 Intermediate dorsal cutaneous nerve

13.9.4 Wound Closure

The wound is closed by means of skin sutures.

13.10 Lateral Approach to the Calcaneus

R. Bauer, F. Kerschbaumer, S. Poisel, C. J. Wirth

13.10.1 Principal Indications

- Dwyer osteotomy
- Osteomyelitis
- Tumors

13.10.2 Positioning and Incision

The patient is placed in the supine position. After (optional) application of a tourniquet, the leg is draped to remain freely movable, and is slightly rotated internally. A skin incision approximately 5 cm long is made one fingerbreadth behind the peroneal tendons, running obliquely from proximal to distal (**Fig. 13.54**).

13.10.3 Exposure of the Calcaneus

After the skin has been incised, the locations of the small saphenous vein and the sural nerve are determined. These structures are mobilized anteriorly. Now the crural fascia and the subjacent calcaneofibular ligament are transected, and the periosteum over the calcaneus is split (**Fig. 13.55**). The calcaneus may be encircled by Hohmann elevators or Langenbeck retractors. If further exposure of the calcaneus on the extensor side is needed, the peroneal tendons with their sheaths may be mobilized forward (**Fig. 13.56**).

13.10.4 Wound Closure

Wound closure is effected by suture of the calcaneofibular ligament and the fascia.

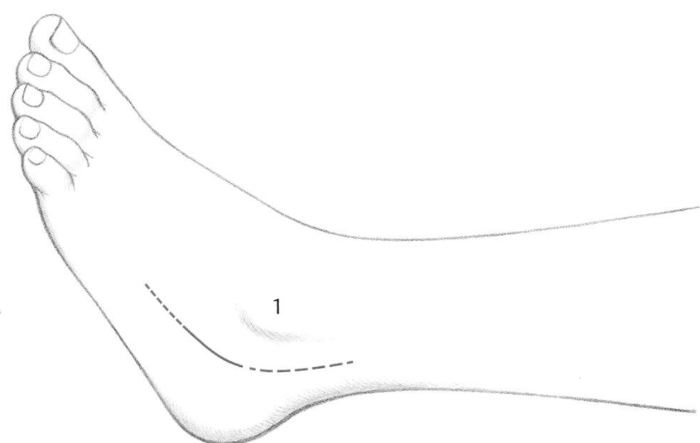

Fig. 13.54 Lateral approach to the calcaneus. Skin incision (left leg).

1 Lateral malleolus

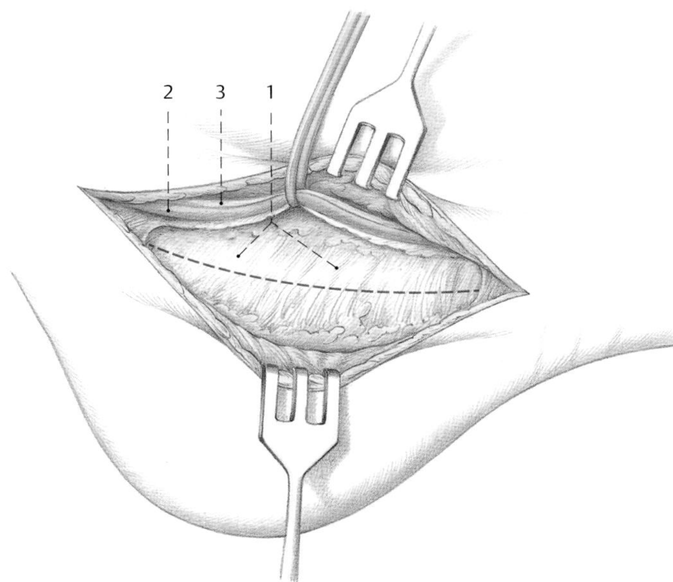

Fig. 13.55 Following dissection and retraction of the sural nerve and small saphenous vein, the fascia and periosteum behind the peroneal tendon sheath are split.

1 Crural fascia
2 Small saphenous vein
3 Lateral dorsal cutaneous nerve (sural nerve)

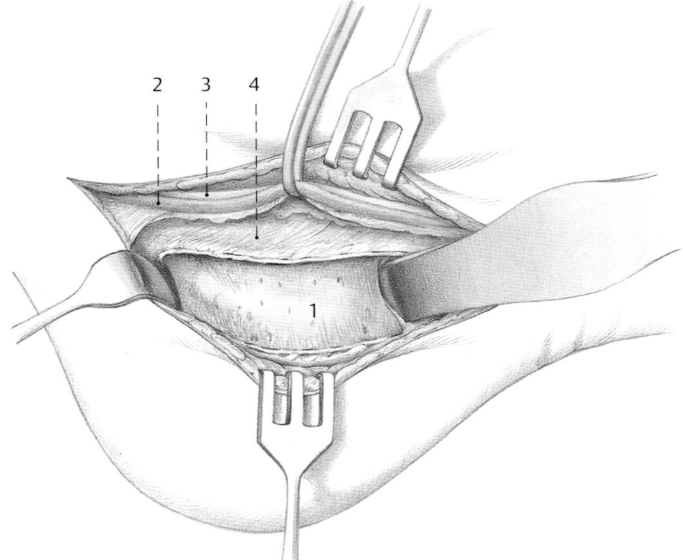

Fig. 13.56 Appearance after subperiosteal exposure of the tuberosity of the calcaneus.

1 Calcaneus
2 Small saphenous vein
3 Lateral dorsal cutaneous nerve (sural nerve)
4 Common tendinous sheath of the fibulares

13.11 Lateral Approach to the Calcaneus and Talocalcaneonavicular Joint

K. Weise, D. Höntzsch

13.11.1 Principal Indications

- Fractures
- Arthrodesis of the talocalcaneonavicular joint
- Osteotomies
- Osteomyelitis
- Tumors

13.11.2 Positioning and Incision

The patient is placed in the supine or lateral position. If the lateral position is chosen, a tunneled cushion is recommended, under which the contralateral leg is placed.

The leg to be operated on is draped so as to allow free movement. The skin incision runs behind the lateral malleolus to the calcaneus and curves 80–90° ventrally toward the fifth metatarsal (**Fig. 13.57**).

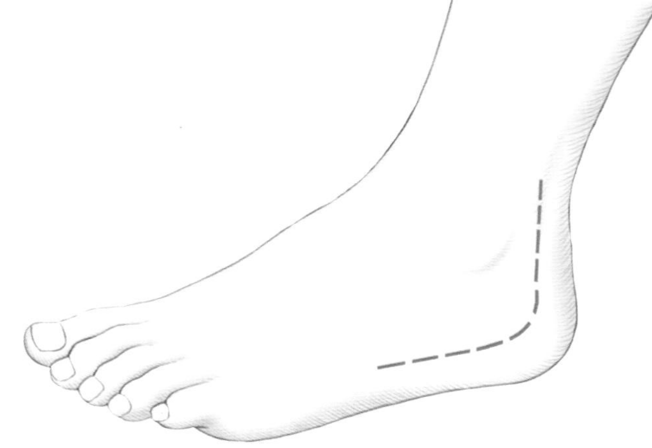

Fig. 13.57 Lateral approach to the calcaneus and talocalcaneonavicular joint. Skin incision (left leg).

13.11.3 Exposure of the Calcaneus and/or Talocalcaneonavicular Joint

After incising the skin, the position of the small saphenous vein and sural nerve should be noted. The incision is then continued directly to the periosteum of the calcaneus without dividing any other layers. The entire triangular flap is then elevated from posterior to anterior. Three or four retaining sutures are then placed through all the layers (**Fig. 13.58**).

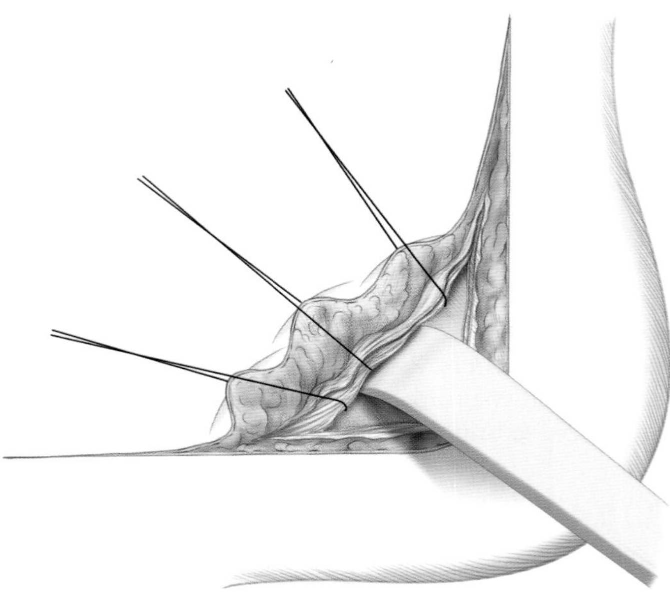

Fig. 13.58 Starting centrally, the incision is continued directly to the calcaneus. All layers remain undissected and are retracted from posterior to anterior.

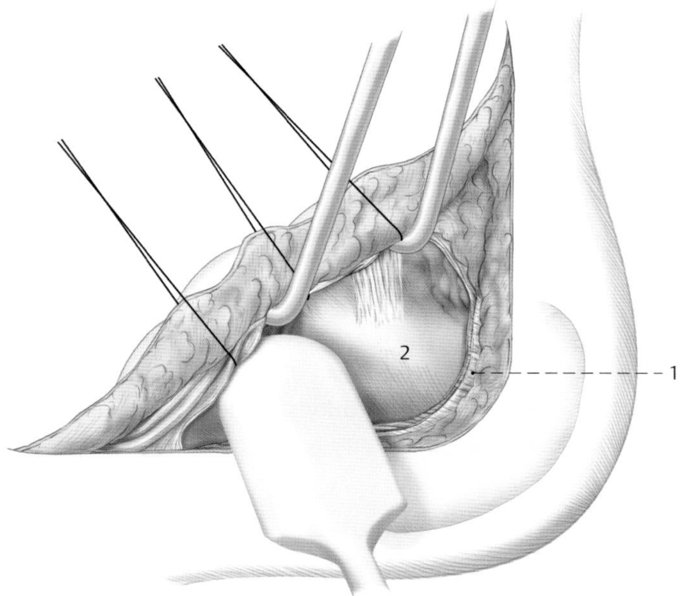

Fig. 13.59 As soon as the talocalcaneonavicular joint is reached, two or three Kirschner wires are inserted in the talus and bent by 60° so that the soft tissues can be retracted securely and without excessive pressure.

1 Periosteum
2 Calcaneus

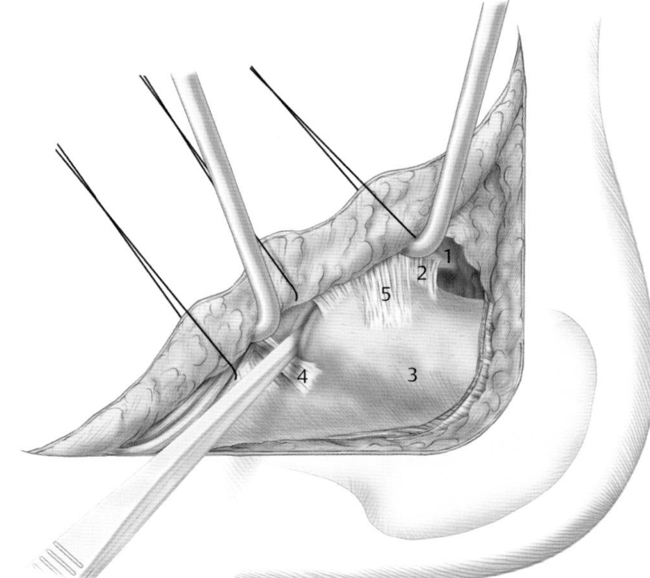

Fig. 13.60 Careful subperiosteal dissection. If necessary, the wires can be twisted and bent more.

1 Talus
2 Subtalar joint
3 Calcaneus
4 Lateral talocalcaneal ligament
5 Calcaneofibular ligament

After further mobilization and adequate exposure of the talocalcaneonavicular joint, the triangular flap is held by two or three Kirschner wires inserted into the talus (!) and then bent by 60–90° (**Fig. 13.59**).

Dissection continues until good visualization of the talocalcaneonavicular joint is obtained (**Figs. 13.60** and **13.61**).

13.11.4 Wound Closure

The subcutaneous tissue and skin are sutured over a Redon drain.

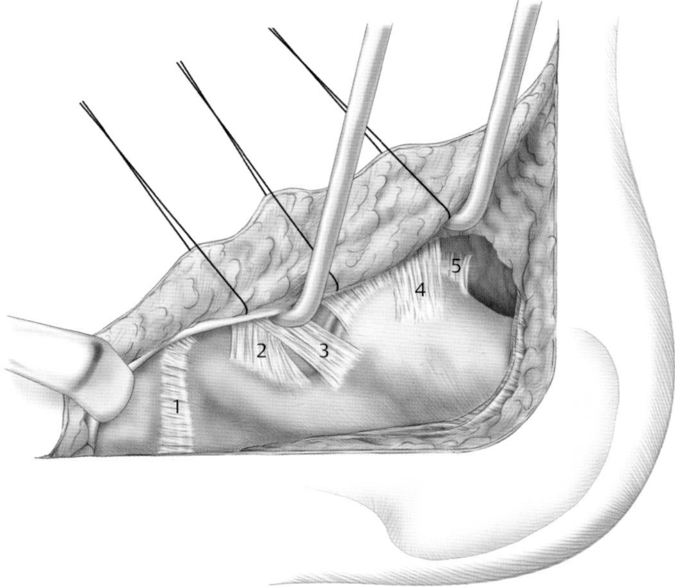

Fig. 13.61 Further dissection until the center of the talocalcaneonavicular joint can be adequately visualized from anterior to posterior.

1 Calcaneocuboid joint
2 Interosseous talocalcaneal ligament
3 Lateral talocalcaneal ligament
4 Calcaneofibular ligament
5 Subtalar joint

13.12 Medial Approach to the Calcaneus

K. Weise, D. Höntzsch

13.12.1 Principal Indications

- Fractures
- Biopsies

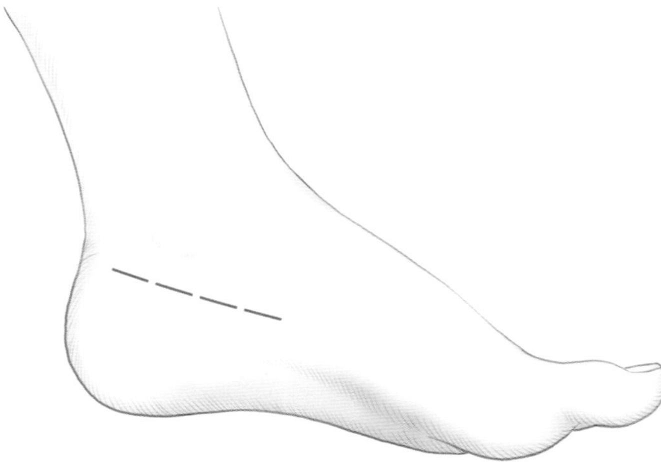

Fig. 13.62 Skin incision 2–3 cm caudal to the medial malleolus, centered over the calcaneus.

13.12.2 Positioning and Incision

The patient is placed in the supine position. The incision is made directly along the axis of the foot 2–3 cm below the medial malleolus over the center of the calcaneus (**Figs. 13.62** and **13.63**).

13.12.3 Medial Exposure of the Calcaneus

After the skin has been incised, the fascia is divided and the periosteum of the calcaneus is exposed, beginning centrally if possible. Dissection is continued in all directions as far as necessary (**Fig. 13.64**). The tendons of flexor hallucis longus and flexor digitorum longus are retracted.

13.12.4 Wound Closure

The wound is closed in layers.

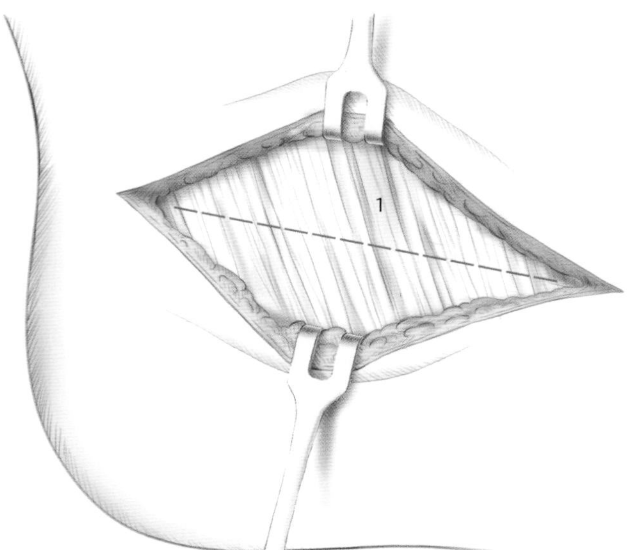

Fig. 13.63 Incision of skin and fascia over the center of the calcaneus from medial side.

1 Crural fascia

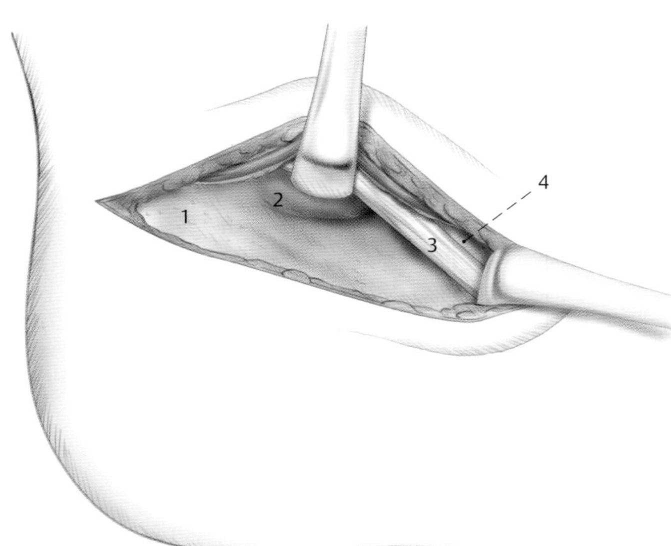

Fig. 13.64 The calcaneus is exposed down to the periosteum. During dissection in a cranial direction, the tendons of flexor hallucis longus and flexor digitorum longus are retracted cranially with a Langenbeck retractor. The anterior corner of the wound is protected with a Langenbeck retractor.

1 Calcaneus
2 Sustentaculum tali
3 Flexor hallucis longus tendon
4 Flexor digitorum longus tendon

13.13 Lateral Approach to the Talocalcaneonavicular Joint

R. Bauer, F. Kerschbaumer, S. Poisel, K. Weise, D. Höntzsch

13.13.1 Principal Indications

- Fractures, dislocations
- Corrective osteotomies
- Triple arthrodesis

13.13.2 Positioning and Incision

The patient is placed in the supine position. The skin incision begins one fingerbreadth distal and posterior to the lateral malleolus, and runs forward on the dorsum along the axis of the foot (**Fig. 13.65**). After splitting the skin and subcutaneous tissue, it is necessary to watch for the sural nerve (lateral dorsal cutaneous nerve) and the small saphenous vein in the posterior wound area, and for the intermediate dorsal cutaneous nerve in the posterior wound area (**Fig. 13.66**). The nerves, being approached from below, are snared with rubber bands. After splitting the fascia, an H-shaped incision is made in the inferior extensor retinaculum (**Fig. 13.67**).

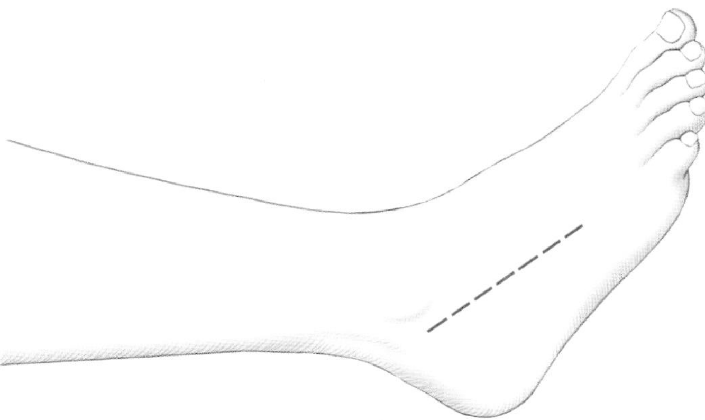

Fig. 13.65 Approach to the talocalcaneonavicular joint from the lateral side. Skin incision (right leg).

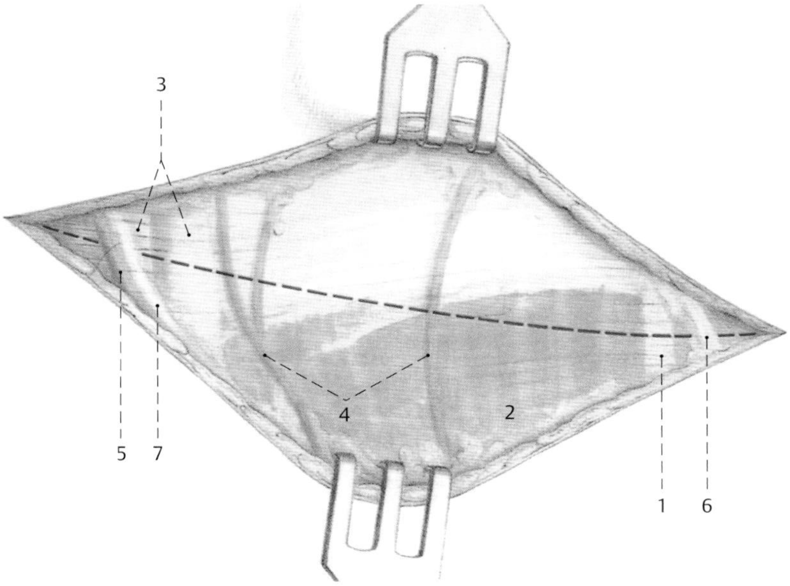

Fig. 13.66 Division of the fascia preserving the sural nerve and intermediate dorsal cutaneous nerve.

1 Tendon of extensor digitorum longus
2 Extensor digitorum brevis
3 Tendons of peroneus longus and brevis
4 Dorsal venous network of the foot
5 Small saphenous vein
6 Intermediate dorsal cutaneous nerve
7 Lateral dorsal cutaneous nerve (sural nerve)

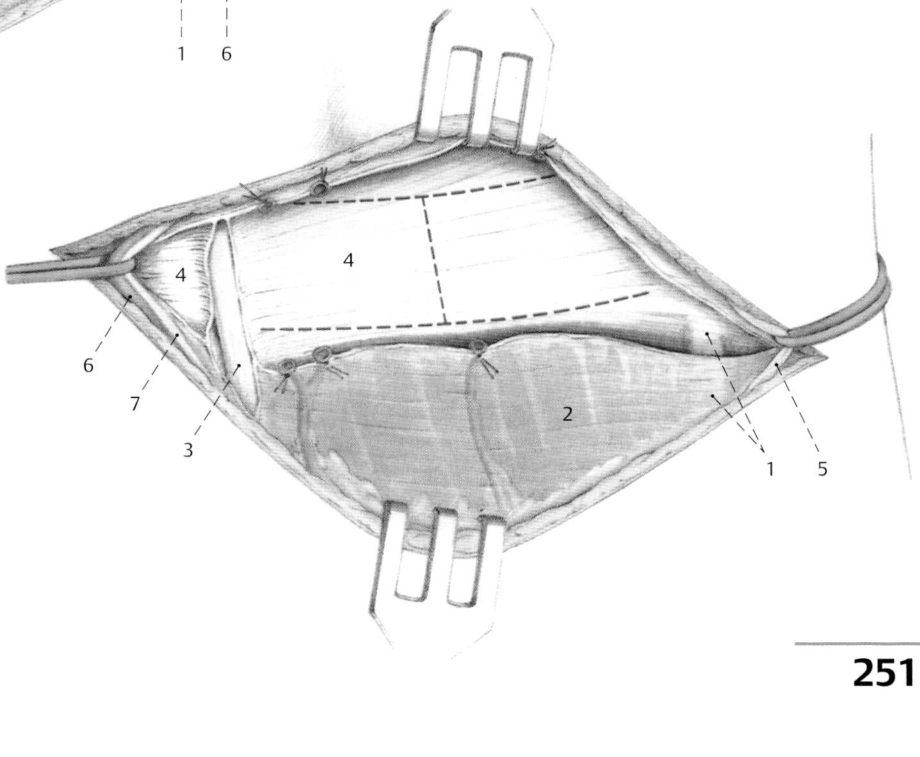

Fig. 13.67 H-incision in the inferior extensor retinaculum after transection of the transverse veins.

1 Tendon of extensor digitorum longus
2 Extensor digitorum brevis
3 Tendon of peroneus brevis
4 Inferior extensor retinaculum
5 Intermediate dorsal cutaneous nerve
6 Small saphenous vein
7 Lateral dorsal cutaneous nerve (sural nerve)

The retinaculum is dissected free of the origin of extensor digitorum brevis. The tendon sheaths of the toe extensor on one hand, and of the peroneal tendons on the other, are opened (**Fig. 13.68**). Branches of the peroneal artery over the fat of the tarsal sinus are ligated and transected. Now extensor digitorum brevis is detached from its origin and retracted distally. The tendons of the long extensor muscle should be retracted medially with a Langenbeck retractor. The fat in the tarsal sinus is removed with a scalpel.

For better exposure of the subtalar joint, a Hohmann elevator is inserted behind the talocalcaneal joint. Using a Langenbeck retractor inserted laterally beneath the calcaneocuboid articulation, the peroneal tendons are retracted in a plantar direction. Manual supination and inversion of the foot afford a clear exposure of the two parts of the talocalcaneonavicular articulations (**Fig. 13.70**).

13.13.3 Exposure of the Talocalcaneonavicular Joint

After removal of the fatty tissue from the tarsal sinus, the capsules of the subtalar joint and of the medial and lateral Chopart joint (talonavicular and calcaneocuboid articulations) are exposed (**Fig. 13.69**). T-shaped incisions are made in the joint capsules, the bifurcate ligament being transected.

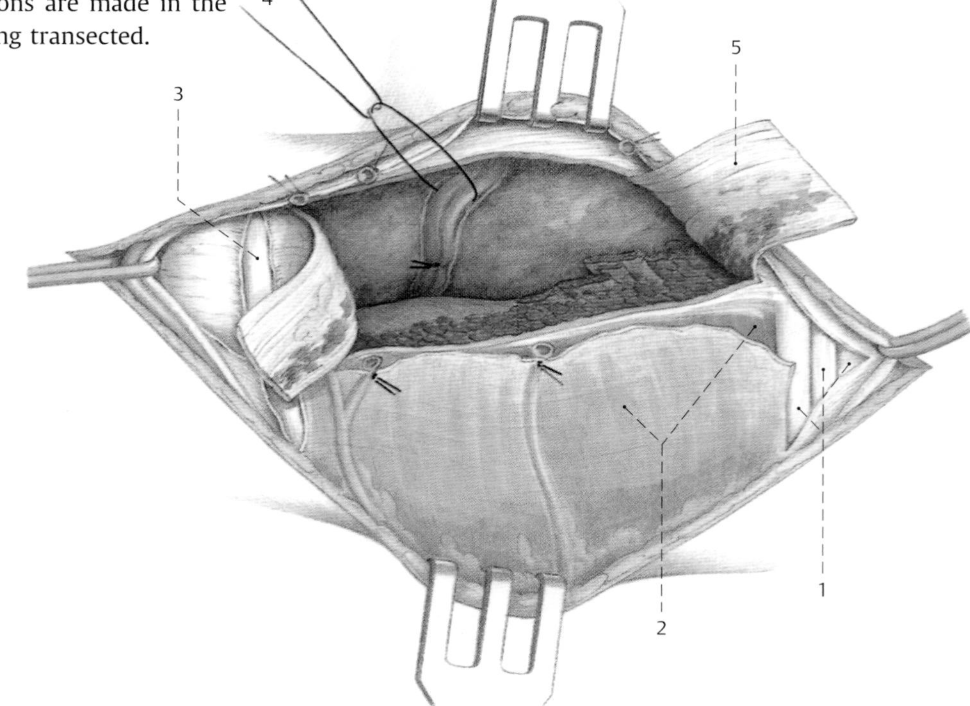

Fig. 13.68 Detachment of the retinaculum from extensor digitorum brevis. Splitting of the peroneal tendon sheath and the tendon sheath of the extensor muscles of the toes. Ligation of the perforating vessels from the peroneal artery and vein.

1 Tendons of extensor digitorum longus
2 Extensor digitorum brevis
3 Tendon of peroneus brevis
4 Perforating branch of the peroneal artery and accompanying vein
5 Inferior extensor retinaculum

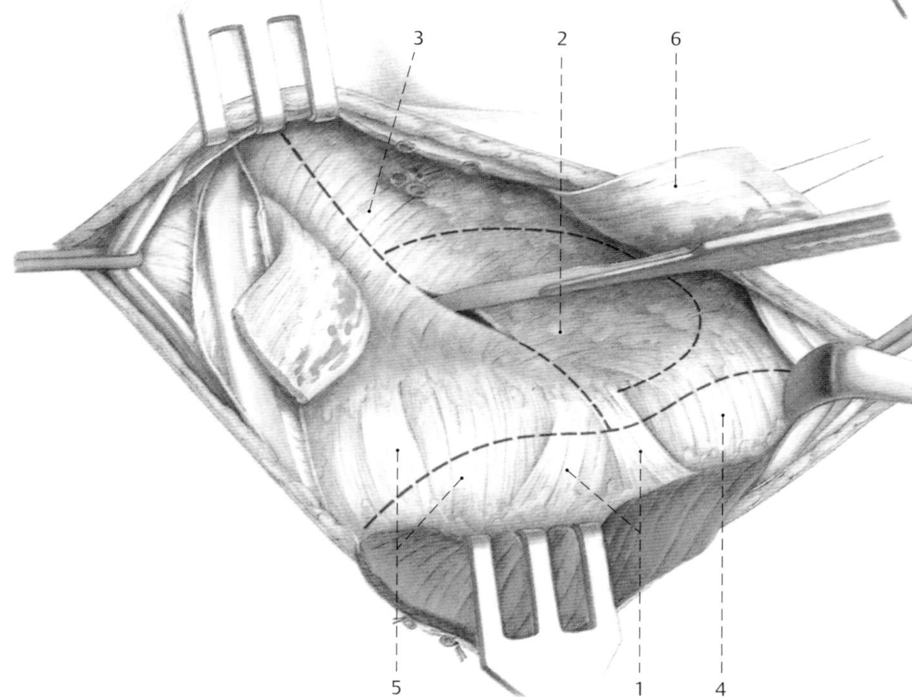

Fig. 13.69 After the removal of fat from the tarsal sinus, a T-shaped incision is made in the talocalcaneonavicular joint capsule (red dashed lines). To improve the exposure, extensor digitorum brevis is detached from its origin and distally retracted (blue dashed line).

1 Bifurcate ligament
2 Tarsal sinus
3 Lateral talocalcaneal ligament
4 Talocalcaneonavicular joint capsule
5 Calcaneocuboid joint capsule
6 Inferior extensor retinaculum

13.13.4 Wound Closure

After hemostasis, wound closure is effected by suturing the detached short extensor muscle of the toes to the joint capsule and to the lateral portion of the inferior extensor retinaculum. Subsequently, the retinaculum is sutured, and the sheaths of the common extensors and the peroneal tendons are closed.

13.13.5 Note

Exposure of the talocalcaneonavicular joint requires transection of the interosseous talocalcaneal ligament.

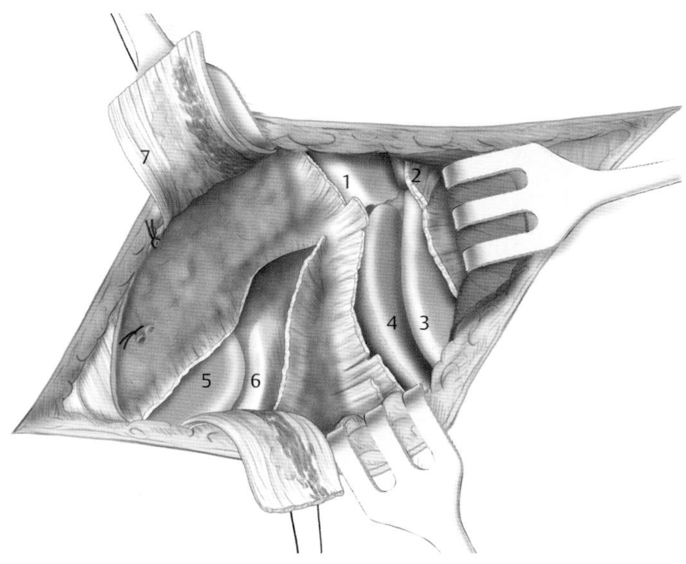

Fig. 13.70 Operative site after opening of the joint capsule. Note: A Hohmann elevator is placed behind the subtalar joint. Insertion of a Langenbeck retractor for retraction of the extensor tendons is recommended for better exposure of the talocalcaneonavicular joint.

Manual supination and inversion of the foot.
1 Head of the talus
2 Navicular bone
3 Cuboid bone
4 Cuboid articular surface of the calcaneus
5 Lateral process of the talus
6 Posterior talar articular surface
7 Inferior extensor retinaculum

13.14 Anterior Approach to the Metatarsal Joints

R. Bauer, F. Kerschbaumer, S. Poisel, K. Weise, D. Höntzsch

13.14.1 Principal Indications

- Fractures, dislocations
- Cuneiform tarsal osteotomy
- Tarsometatarsal arthrolysis
- Osteomyelitis

13.14.2 Positioning and Incision

The patient is in the supine position. A bolster is placed under the lower leg. The longitudinal skin incision is centered between the second and third metatarsals (**Fig. 13.71**).

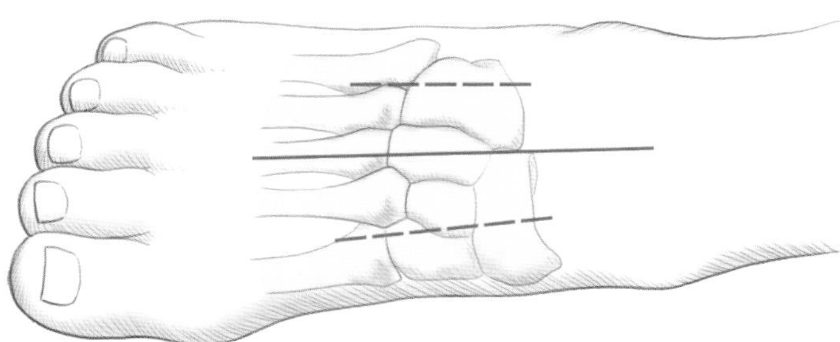

Fig. 13.71 Posterior approach to the metatarsus. Medial and lateral longitudinal incisions (dashed lines) or a transverse incision may be used (right leg).

The extrafascial cutaneous nerves coursing along the dorsum of the foot have to be preserved (**Fig. 13.72**). Any veins crossing the operative field may be ligated and transected if necessary. Following retraction of the nerves, the fascia is split parallel to the skin incision and dissected in a proximal or distal direction.

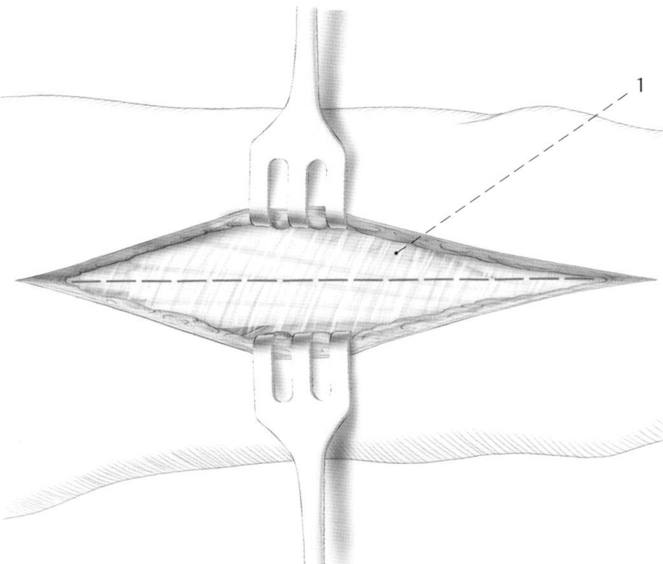

Fig. 13.72 After mobilization of the subcutaneous tissue in a proximal and distal direction, the fascia is split parallel to the skin incision, sparing the longitudinal cutaneous nerves.

1 Extensor digitorum brevis

13.14.3 Exposure of the Intertarsal Joints

The joint cavity is best located with the aid of a fine needle (**Fig. 13.73**). Now the deep peroneal nerve and the accompanying dorsal artery of the foot on the medial border of the extensor hallucis brevis are identified. They are snared together with the muscle and medially retracted if necessary. The tendons of extensor digitorum longus should also be snared and may be retracted medially or laterally if necessary. Using a raspatory, the joint capsules together with the periosteum are stripped off the dorsum of the foot.

For exposure of the calcaneocuboid joint, a Hohmann elevator is inserted beneath the extensor digitorum brevis (**Fig. 13.74**). If necessary, the lateral tarsal artery and vein crossing the operative field may be ligated and transected.

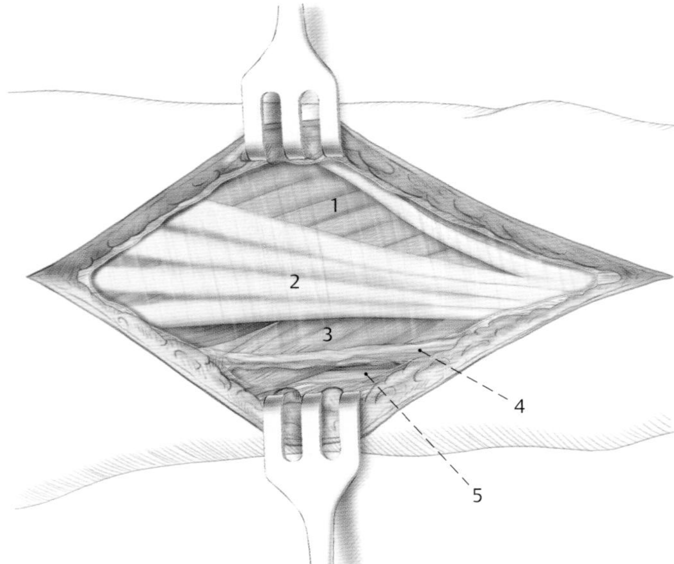

Fig. 13.73 Exposure of extensor digitorum longus and brevis as well as of the deep peroneal nerve and the dorsal artery of the foot medial to extensor hallucis brevis. The joint cavity is located with the aid of a fine needle.

1 Extensor digitorum brevis
2 Tendon sheaths of extensor digitorum longus
3 Extensor hallucis brevis
4 Medial dorsal cutaneous nerve
5 Deep peroneal nerve

13.14.4 Wound Closure

After hemostasis, the wound is closed by suture of the subcutaneous tissue and skin.

13.14.5 Dangers

Besides injury to the cutaneous nerves, this approach also entails the risk of injury or overextension of the dorsal artery of the foot and the deep branch of the peroneal nerve.

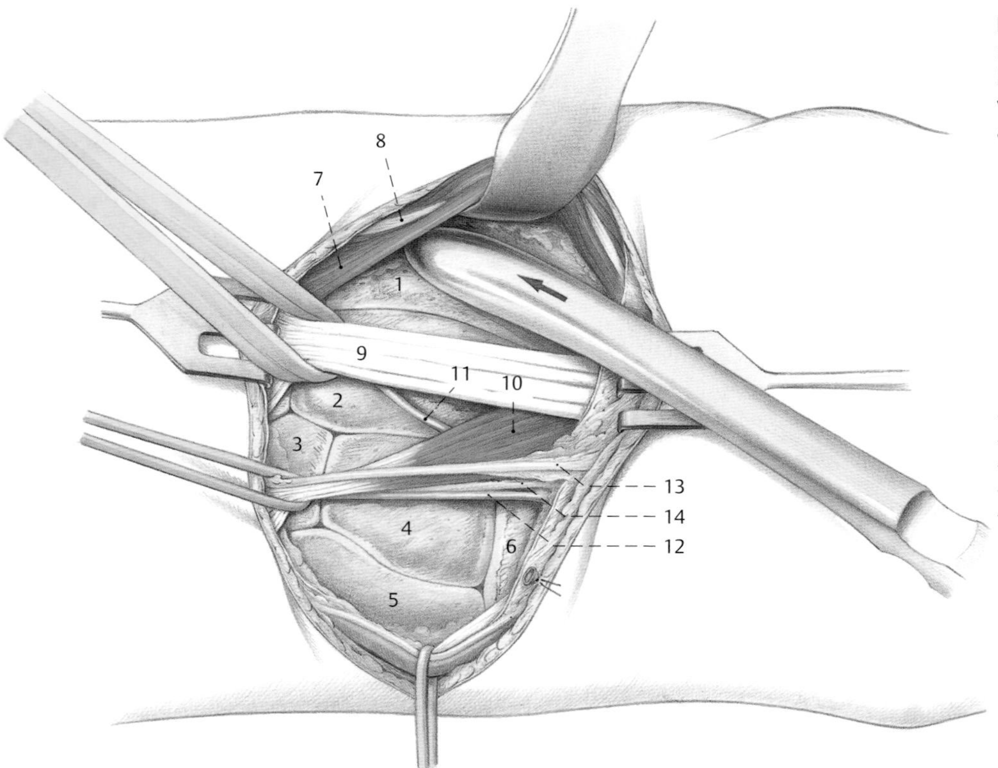

Fig. 13.74 Snaring of the extensor muscles of the toes, the neurovascular bundle, and the extensor hallucis brevis. Detachment of the joint capsule and exposure of the tarsal bones.

1 Cuboid bone
2 Lateral cuneiform bone
3 Base of the second metatarsal bone
4 Intermediate cuneiform bone
5 Medial cuneiform bone
6 Navicular bone
7 Extensor digitorum brevis
8 Peroneus tertius
9 Tendons of extensor digitorum longus
10 Extensor hallucis brevis
11 Lateral tarsal artery
12 Dorsal artery of the foot
13 Medial dorsal cutaneous nerve
14 Deep peroneal nerve

13.15 Medial Approach to the Tarsometatarsal Joints

R. Bauer, F. Kerschbaumer, S. Poisel, K. Weise, D. Höntzsch

13.15.1 Principal Indications

- Medial release for clubfoot
- Arthrodesis
- Capsulorrhaphy

13.15.2 Positioning and Incision

The patient is placed in the supine position. The leg is draped to be freely movable, and is rotated externally. The skin incision, running dorsally in a convex line, begins three fingerbreadths behind the internal malleolus, continues to the tuberosity of the navicular bone, and then passes along the first metatarsal to the metatarsophalangeal joint of the great toe (**Fig. 13.75**).

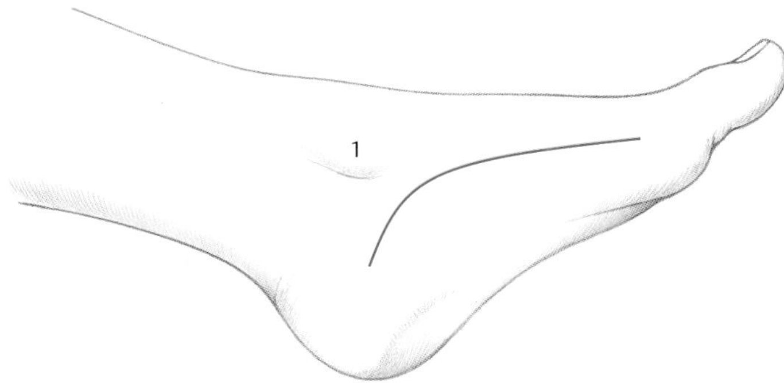

Fig. 13.75 Medial approach to the tarsal joints. Skin incision (left leg).

1 Inner malleolus

After splitting of the skin, subcutaneous tissue, and fascia, the skin flap is dissected in a plantar direction. Some transversely coursing veins are transected (**Fig. 13.76**). The abductor hallucis is partly detached from its origin on the calcaneus. The muscle is then pulled in a plantar direction (**Fig. 13.77**), care being taken to avoid injury to the branches of the medial plantar nerve supplying it. Next, the aponeurotic tendon sheath reinforcement that encloses the tendons of flexor hallucis longus and flexor digitorum longus is split. Transection of this reinforcing ligament, also known as the "master knot of Henry," is performed one fingerbreadth behind the tuberosity of the navicular bone. Now the short flexor of the great toe can be detached at its origin and retracted in a plantar direction (**Fig. 13.78**).

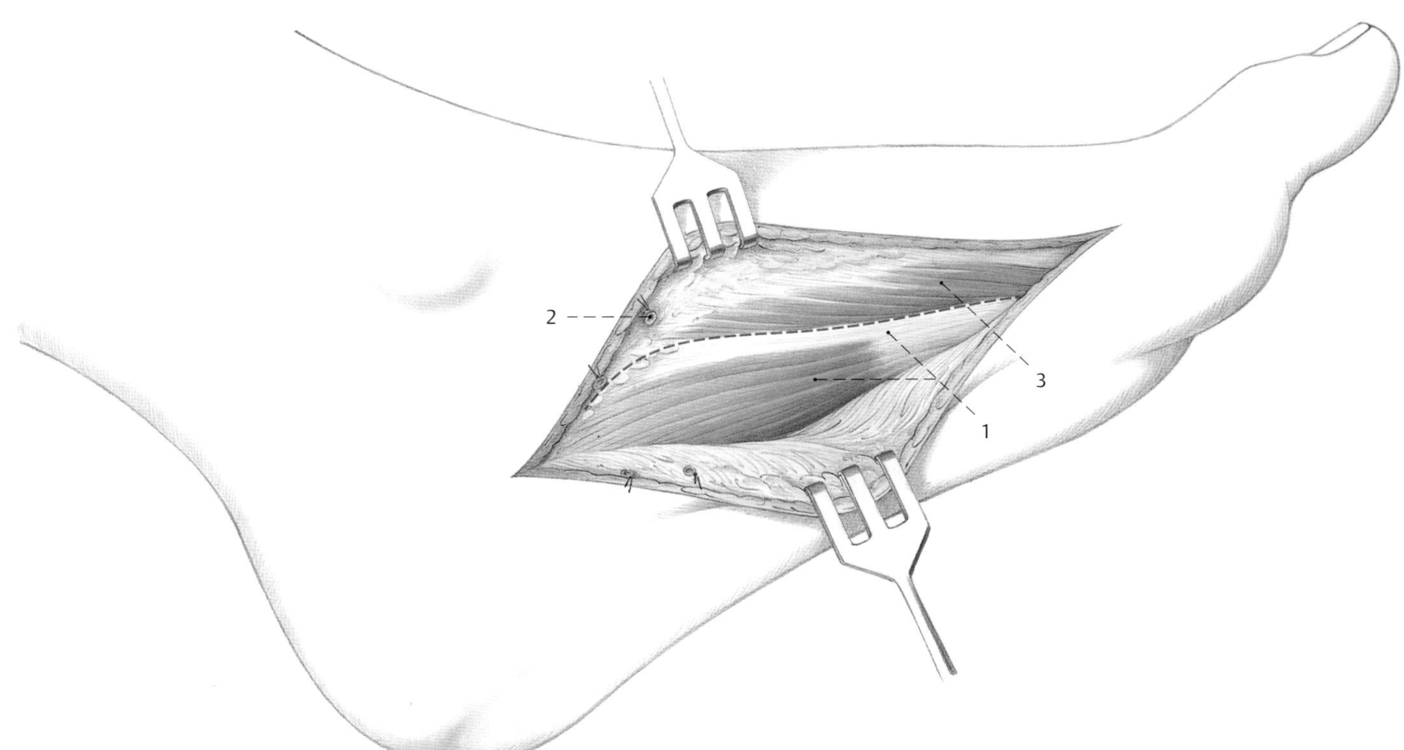

Fig. 13.76 After dissection of the skin flap in a plantar direction and splitting of the fascia, the abductor hallucis is detached from the navicular bone, the calcaneus, and flexor hallucis brevis (dashed line).

1 Abductor hallucis
2 Great saphenous vein
3 Flexor hallucis brevis

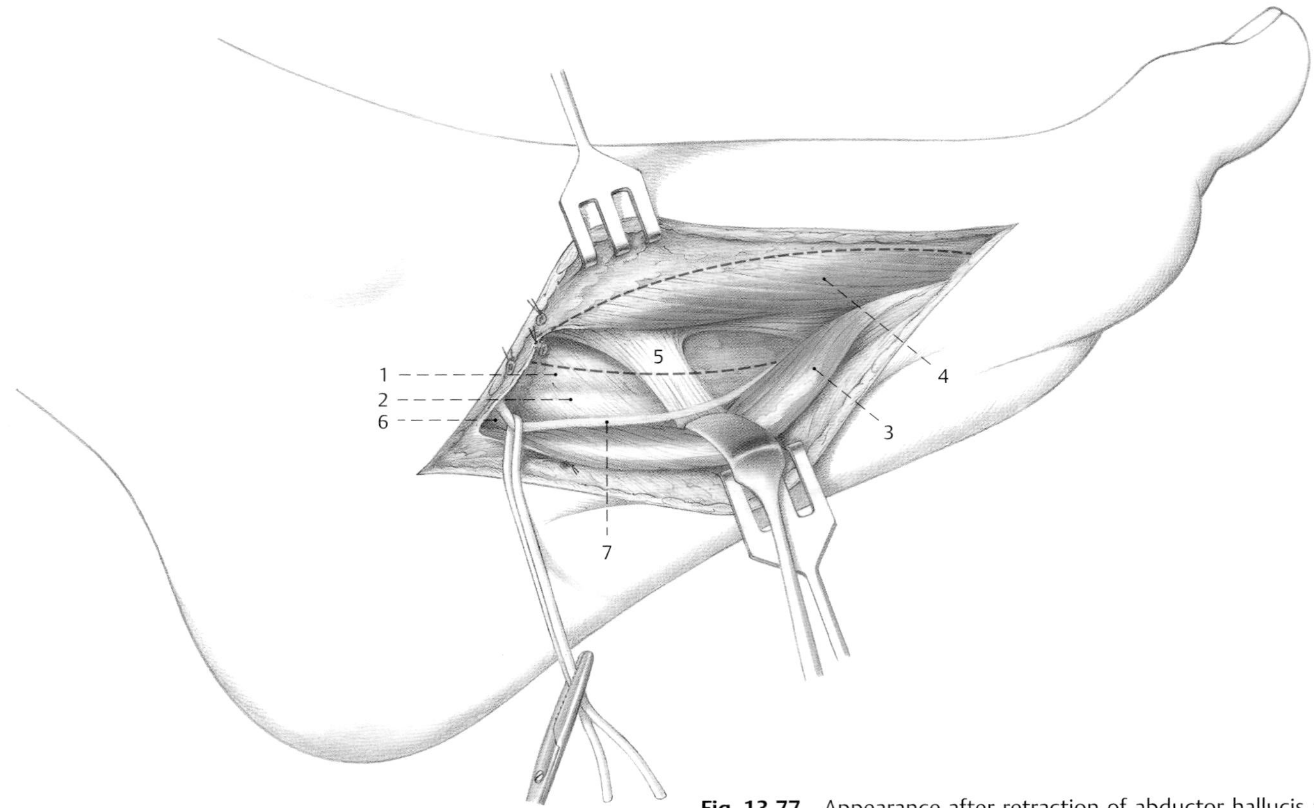

Fig. 13.77 Appearance after retraction of abductor hallucis and snaring of the medial plantar nerve. Incision of the tendon sheath over flexor hallucis longus and flexor digitorum longus ("Henry's knot").

1 Tendon sheath of flexor digitorum longus
2 Tendon sheath of flexor hallucis longus
3 Abductor hallucis
4 Flexor hallucis brevis
5 "Henry's knot"
6 Posterior tibial vein
7 Medial plantar nerve

13.15.3 Exposure of the Tarsal Joints

The tendon sheath of the tibialis posterior is split, and the tendon is tenotomized in a frontal direction. Then the joint capsules of the medial Chopart joint, the navicular cuneiform joint, and the first tarsometatarsal joint can be opened transversely. Good exposure of the joints is obtained by manual eversion of the forefoot (**Fig. 13.78**).

13.15.4 Anatomical Site

The anatomical preparation (**Fig. 13.79**) shows the course of the posterior tibial artery and vein, the tibial nerve and its distribution, and their relation to the flexor tendons.

For better exposure of the anatomical structures, abductor hallucis has been transected and retracted in a plantar direction. The tendon sheath reinforcement that secures the tendons of flexor digitorum longus and flexor hallucis longus to the longitudinal vault of the foot (Henry's knot) has already been transected. The medial neurovascular bundle passes between abductor hallucis and flexor hallucis brevis, while the lateral neurovascular bundle runs between the quadratus plantae and flexor digitorum brevis.

13.15.5 Wound Closure

Wound closure is effected following reattachment of the detached flexor hallucis brevis and abductor hallucis.

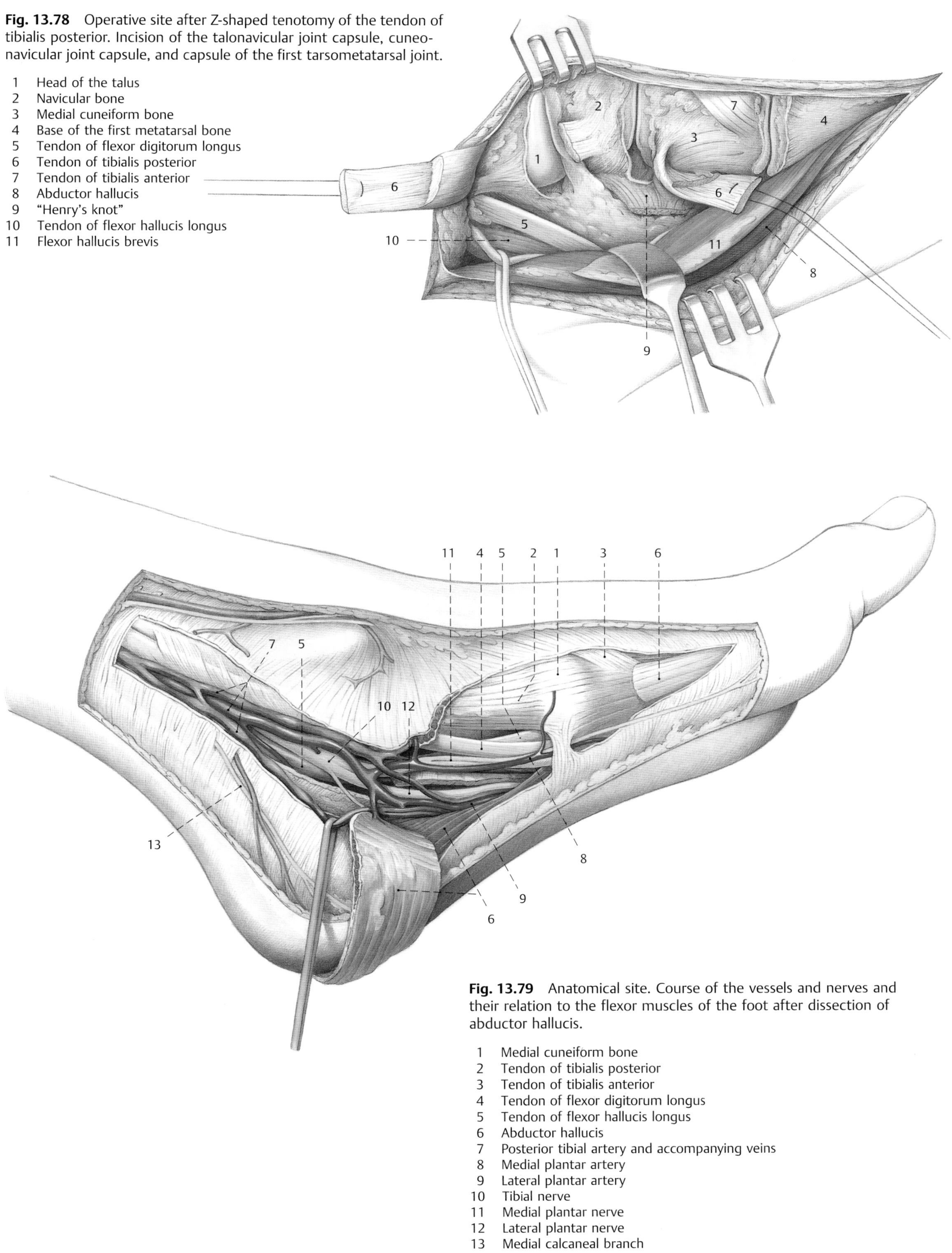

Fig. 13.78 Operative site after Z-shaped tenotomy of the tendon of tibialis posterior. Incision of the talonavicular joint capsule, cuneonavicular joint capsule, and capsule of the first tarsometatarsal joint.

1 Head of the talus
2 Navicular bone
3 Medial cuneiform bone
4 Base of the first metatarsal bone
5 Tendon of flexor digitorum longus
6 Tendon of tibialis posterior
7 Tendon of tibialis anterior
8 Abductor hallucis
9 "Henry's knot"
10 Tendon of flexor hallucis longus
11 Flexor hallucis brevis

Fig. 13.79 Anatomical site. Course of the vessels and nerves and their relation to the flexor muscles of the foot after dissection of abductor hallucis.

1 Medial cuneiform bone
2 Tendon of tibialis posterior
3 Tendon of tibialis anterior
4 Tendon of flexor digitorum longus
5 Tendon of flexor hallucis longus
6 Abductor hallucis
7 Posterior tibial artery and accompanying veins
8 Medial plantar artery
9 Lateral plantar artery
10 Tibial nerve
11 Medial plantar nerve
12 Lateral plantar nerve
13 Medial calcaneal branch

13.16 Plantar Approach to the Metatarsophalangeal Joints

R. Bauer, F. Kerschbaumer, S. Poisel, K. Weise, D. Höntzsch

13.16.1 Principal Indication

- Resection arthroplasty

13.16.2 Positioning and Incision

The patient is placed in the supine position. After draping, a bolster is placed under the lower leg. The surgeon sits at the foot of the table, while the assistant holds the patient's foot posteriorly extended. The curved skin incision runs convexly over the palpable metatarsal heads. In the presence of marked subluxation of the metatarsophalangeal joints or of callosities, a sparing oval skin incision with removal of the callosities is possible (**Fig. 13.80**). Even though this approach exposes only the second to fourth metatarsal joints, the skin incision should be extended to the first metatarsophalangeal joint so that adequate exposure of the joints may be accomplished.

The proximal skin flap has to be mobilized relatively far in the direction of the heel. Strands of the plantar aponeurosis are divided and dissected in proximal and distal directions, respectively (**Fig. 13.81**).

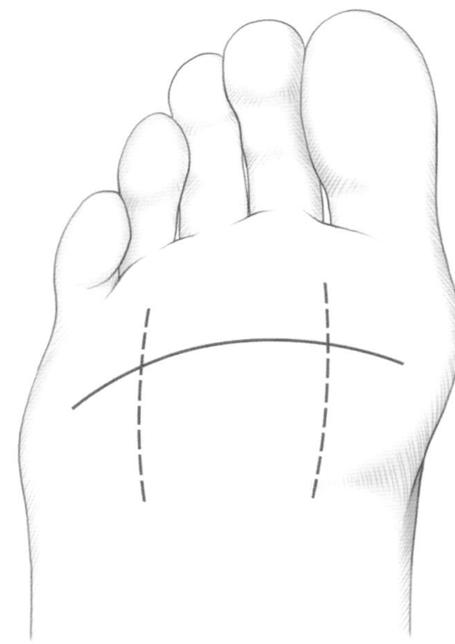

Fig. 13.80 Plantar approach to the metatarsophalangeal joints. The skin incision is optionally either convex (solid line) or longitudinal (dashed lines) (right foot).

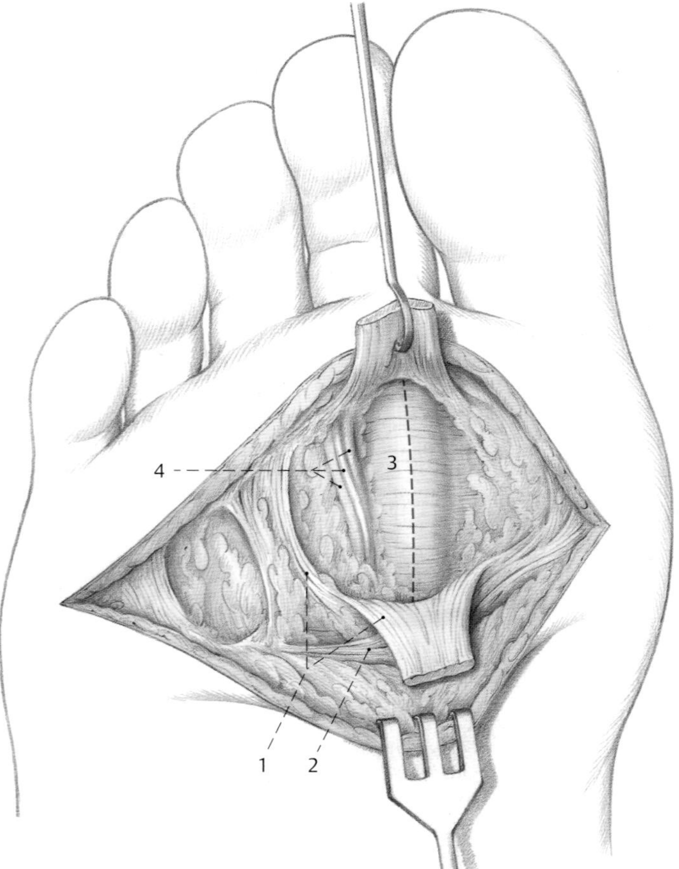

Fig. 13.81 Operative site after splitting of the skin and subcutaneous tissue. Longitudinal bands of the plantar aponeurosis have been transected and dissected in a proximal and distal direction. Incision of the flexor tendon sheath.

1 Plantar aponeurosis (longitudinal fasciculi)
2 Plantar aponeurosis (transverse fasciculi)
3 Fibrous tendon sheath of the second toe
4 Common plantar digital artery, vein, and nerve

13.16.3 Exposure of the Metatarsophalangeal Joints

After the tendon sheaths have been exposed, they are split longitudinally, and the tendons of the long and short flexor muscles of the toes are retracted medially with tendon hooks (**Fig. 13.82**). Subsequently, the deep layer of the flexor tendon sheath, the subjacent plantar metatarsal ligament, and the joint capsule are incised. For better exposure of the metatarsal head, the metaphysis of the bone is now exposed subperiosteally and held between two small Hohmann retractors (**Fig. 13.83**).

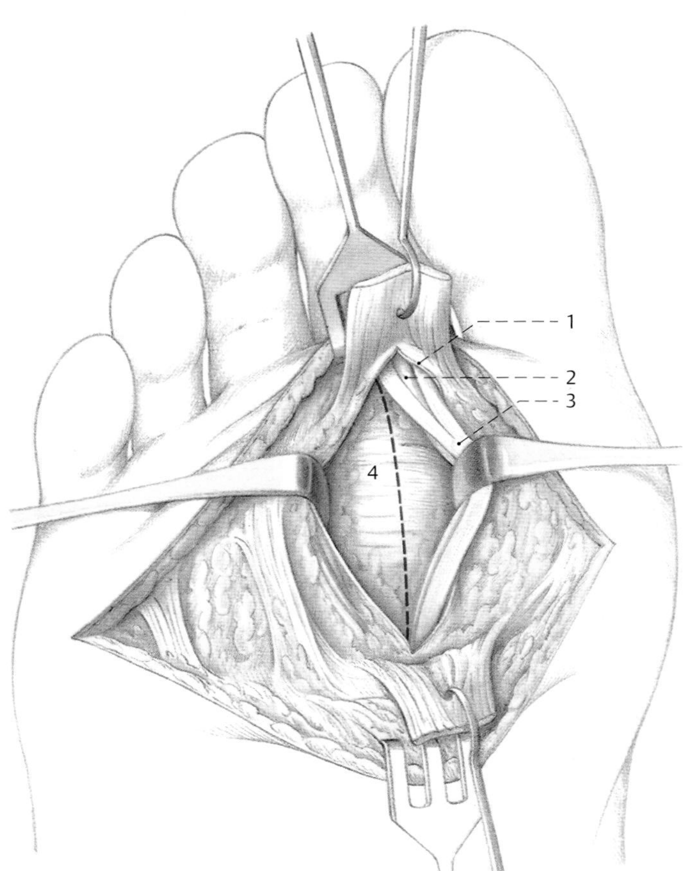

Fig. 13.82 Retraction in a medial direction of the superficial and deep flexors. Incision of the deep layer of the tendon sheath and the joint capsule.

1 Fibrous tendon sheath of the second toe
2 Tendon of flexor digitorum longus
3 Tendon of flexor digitorum brevis
4 Capsule of the first metacarpophalangeal joint

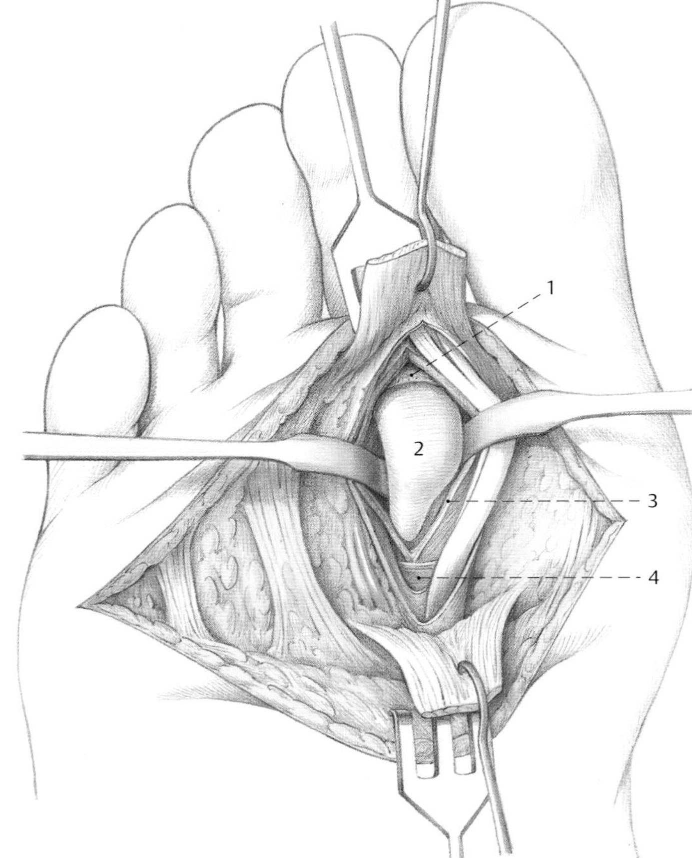

Fig. 13.83 Exposure of the second metatarsal head with small Hohmann elevators placed underneath.

1 Base of the second proximal phalanx
2 Head of the second metatarsal bone
3 Joint capsule
4 Transverse head of adductor hallucis

13.16.4 Anatomical Site

The position and course of the plantar aponeurosis and its relation to the tendon sheaths and the neurovascular bundle are illustrated in **Fig. 13.84**. The plantar aponeurosis runs from the calcaneal tuberosity over the middle portion of the sole to the toes. Proximal to the metatarsal heads, the aponeurosis divides into longitudinal and transverse bands that adhere to tendon sheaths and metatarsophalangeal joints. Transverse bands known as superficial transverse metatarsal ligaments course extrafascially and in the subcutaneous tissue. Upon surgical exposure, these should be dissected in a proximal direction together with the skin. The course of the first and fifth neurovascular bundles is extrafascial. To expose the course and distribution of the nerves and vessels, transverse fibrous bands of the plantar aponeurosis are excised in the first and fourth interdigital spaces.

Note that, by comparison with the nerves, the division of the common plantar digital arteries is considerably more distal. The tendon sheath of the second toe has been fenestrated.

13.16.5 Wound Closure

After hemostasis, skin suture generally proves sufficient. In rheumatoid arthritis, because of the frequently encountered dislocation of the flexor tendons, repositioning of the tendons and purse-string suture of the tendon sheath are recommended.

13.16.6 Dangers

If dissection of the metatarsal joints is not performed over the midline of the tendon sheath, the common plantar digital nerves or the common plantar digital arteries may be transected.

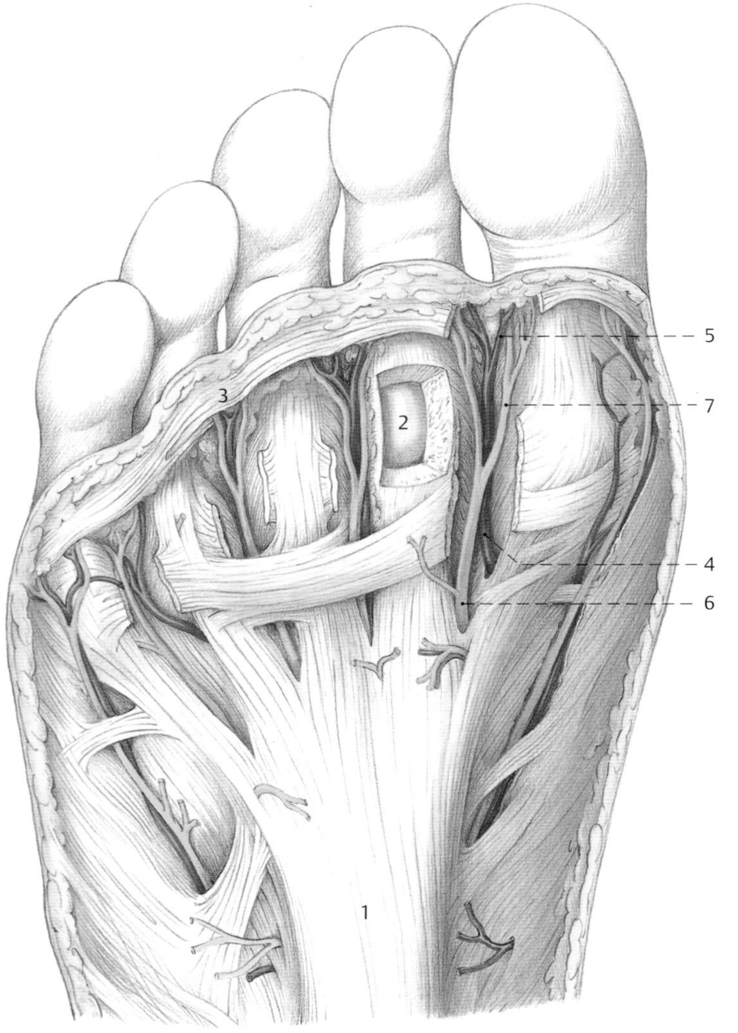

Fig. 13.84 Anatomical site. The plantar aponeurosis attaches distally to the tendon sheaths and to the metatarsophalangeal joints in the form of longitudinal and transverse fiber bundles. The tendon sheath of the second flexor tendon has been fenestrated. Note: Course and distribution of the intermetatarsal vessels and nerves.

1 Plantar aponeurosis
2 Head of the second metatarsal bone
3 Superficial transverse metatarsal ligament
4 Common plantar digital artery
5 Proper plantar digital artery
6 Common plantar digital nerve
7 Proper plantar digital nerve

13.17 Medial Approach to the Metatarsophalangeal Joint of the Great Toe

R. Bauer, F. Kerschbaumer, S. Poisel, K. Weise, D. Höntzsch

13.17.1 Principal Indications

- Hallux valgus
- Hallux rigidus

13.17.2 Positioning and Incision

The patient is placed in the supine position. After draping, the lower leg is placed on a cushion. A skin incision approximately 6 cm in length is made medially over the metatarsophalangeal joint of the great toe, or somewhat more posteriorly, and then curves along the contour of the joint (**Fig. 13.85**). If necessary (metatarsal osteotomy), the skin incision may be extended proximally.

If a McBride operation is planned, a second incision, approximately 3 cm long, is made in the first interdigital space. The skin and the subcutaneous tissue are dissected while sparing the plantar and dorsal nerves. The joint capsule is opened parallel to the skin incision (**Fig. 13.86**).

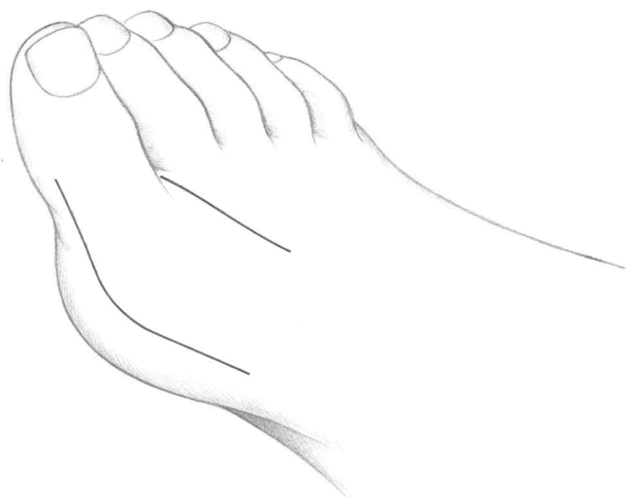

Fig. 13.85 Approach to the metatarsophalangeal joint of the great toe. Medial skin incision toward the metatarsophalangeal joint, and lateral incision for exposure of the tendon of adductor hallucis (right leg).

13.17.3 Exposure of the Joint

For clear exposure of the metatarsophalangeal joint of the great toe, the joint capsule has to be subperiosteally detached distal to the base of the proximal phalanx of the great toe and proximally behind the head of the first metatarsal bone. Subsequently, two Hohmann retractors are inserted (**Fig. 13.87**).

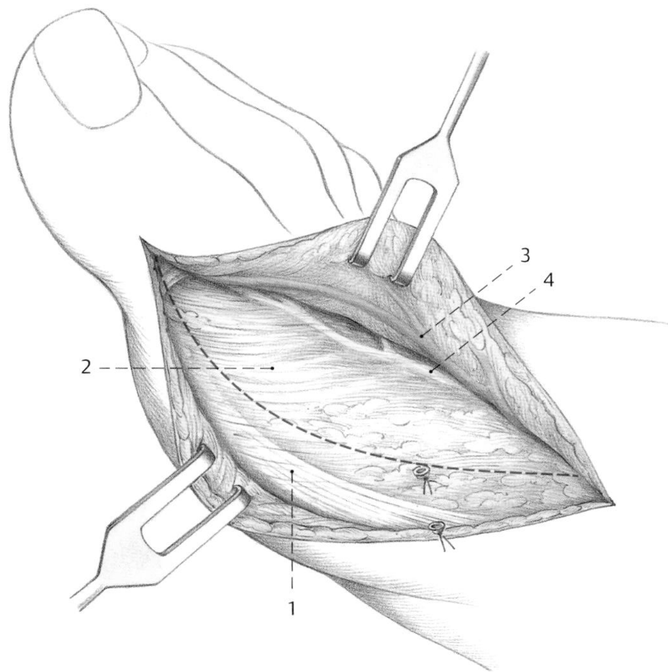

Fig. 13.86 After splitting of the skin and subcutaneous tissue, the joint capsule is incised parallel to the skin incision. Preservation of the dorsal cutaneous nerve (branch of the saphenous or medial dorsal cutaneous nerve).

1 Tendon of abductor hallucis
2 Joint capsule
3 Great saphenous vein
4 Saphenous nerve or medial dorsal cutaneous nerve

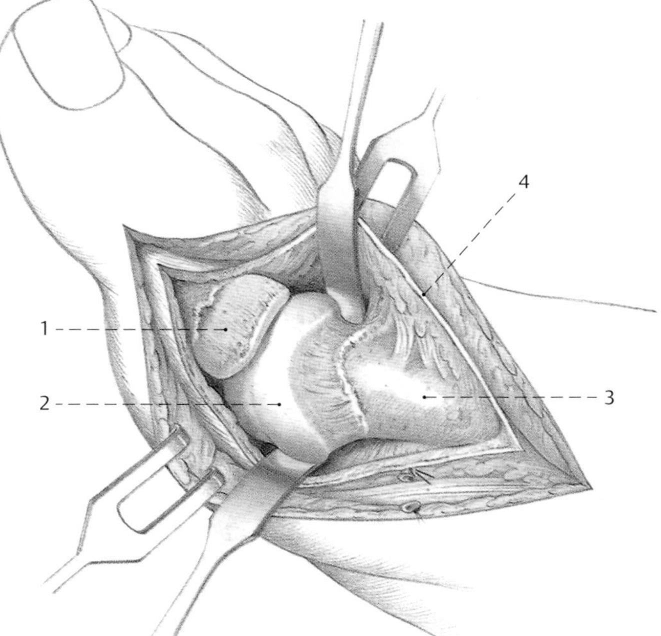

Fig. 13.87 Appearance after opening of the metatarsophalangeal joint capsule of the great toe and insertion of small Hohmann elevators.

1 Base of the first proximal phalanx
2 Head of the first metatarsal bone
3 Body of the first metatarsal bone
4 Joint capsule

13.17.4 Exposure of the Tendon of Adductor Hallucis

If tenotomy or displacement of the tendon of the adductor muscle is required, a short skin incision is made in the first intermetatarsal space. Care should be taken not to make the skin bridge between the two skin incisions too narrow. After the subcutaneous tissue and fascia have been split, the tendon of the muscle is exposed and stripped off the joint capsule and the lateral head of flexor hallucis brevis (**Fig. 13.88**). The tendon is snared with a holding suture.

If necessary, the capsule of the first metatarsophalangeal joint may, in addition, be incised transversely (**Fig. 13.89**).

13.17.5 Wound Closure

The wound closure is effected in two layers by suture of the joint capsule and skin.

13.17.6 Note

For clear exposure of the first interdigital space, the insertion of a sturdy self-retaining spreader between the first and second metatarsals, as well as manual retraction of the great toe and the other four toes with gauze strips, is recommended (**Figs. 13.88** and **13.89**).

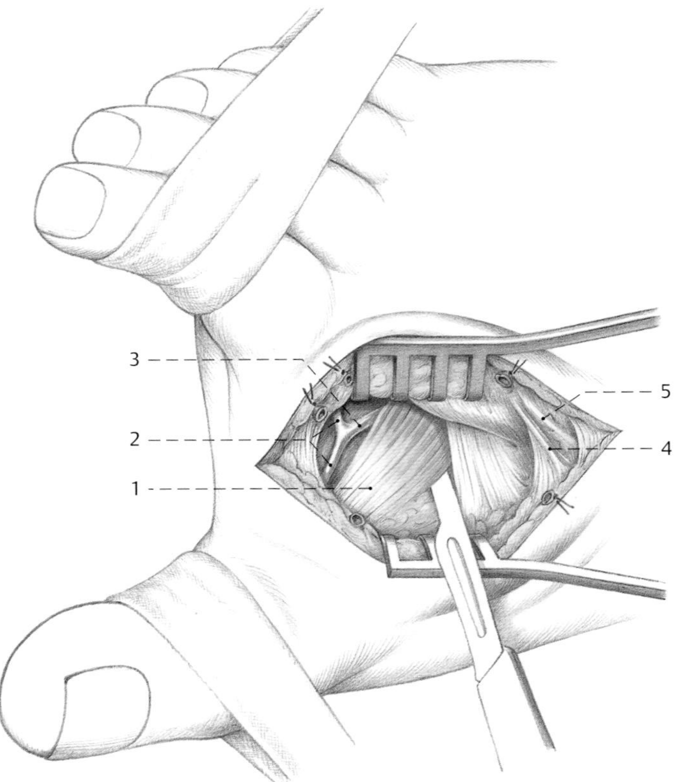

Fig. 13.88 Following incision of the first interosseous space, a self-retaining spreader is placed between the first and second metatarsal heads. The great toe and second to fourth toes are also spread. The tendon of adductor hallucis is isolated from the metatarsophalangeal joint of the great toe.

1 Adductor hallucis
2 Proper plantar digital arteries
3 Common plantar digital artery
4 Dorsal metatarsal artery I
5 Deep peroneal nerve

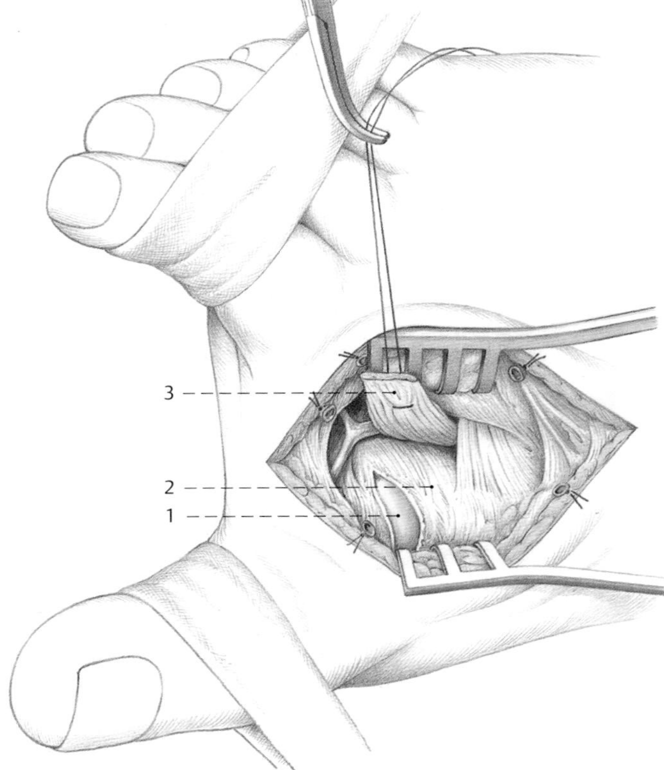

Fig. 13.89 Snaring of the tendon of adductor hallucis with a holding suture. Lateral capsulotomy of first metatarsophalangeal joint.

1 Head of the first metatarsal bone
2 Metatarsophalangeal joint capsule of the great toe
3 Tendon of adductor hallucis

13.18 Posterior Approaches to the Metatarsal Bones, Metatarsophalangeal Joint, and Interphalangeal Joint

R. Bauer, F. Kerschbaumer, S. Poisel, K. Weise, D. Höntzsch

13.18.1 Principal Indications

- Fractures
- Dislocations
- Corrective surgery

Longitudinal incisions are recommended for exposure of the metatarsal bones. The metatarsophalangeal joints are exposed from the dorsal side by a transverse incision. Isolated exposure of the fifth metatarsophalangeal joint and the interphalangeal joints is accomplished by longitudinal incisions (**Fig. 13.90**).

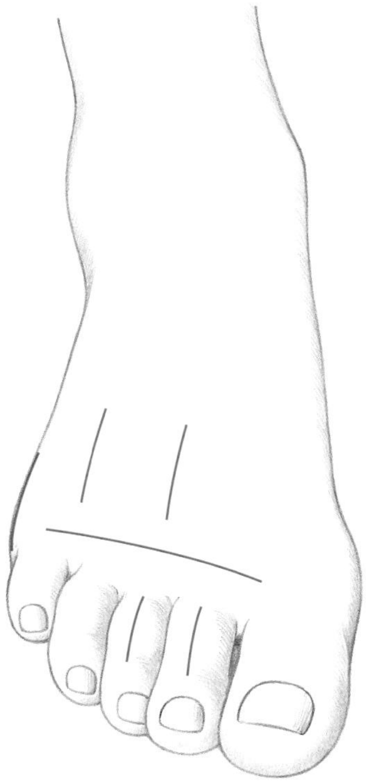

Fig. 13.90 Longitudinal incisions for exposure of the metatarsal bones, fifth metatarsophalangeal joint, and interphalangeal joints. Transverse incision for dorsal joint exposure of the second to fifth metatarsophalangeal articulations (right leg).

13.19 Plantar Approach to the Toe Flexor Tendons

C. J. Wirth

13.19.1 Principal Indication

- Flexor–extensor transfer to treat flexible claw or hammer toes

13.19.2 Positioning and Incision

Transverse incisions over the proximal phalanx and distal interphalangeal joint are recommended to access, divide, and split the long flexor tendon as two limbs (**Fig. 13.91**). These are then transferred around the proximal phalanx to the extensor side, where they are sutured.

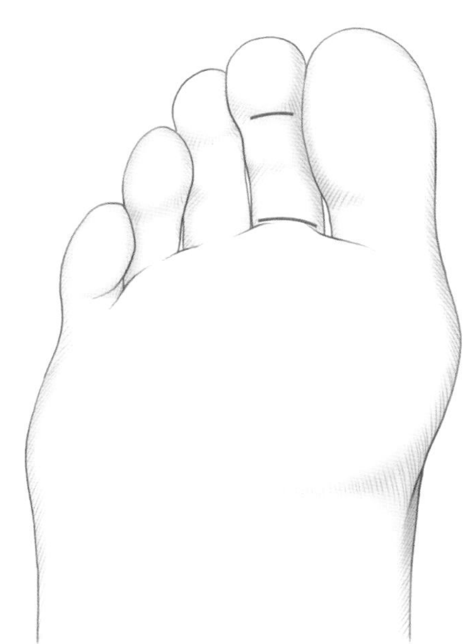

Fig. 13.91 Transverse plantar incisions over the proximal phalanx and distal interphalangeal joint for exposure of the flexor tendons (right leg).

13.20 Extensor Approach to the Second Toe

C. J. Wirth

13.20.1 Principal Indications

- Resection arthroplasty or arthrodesis of the proximal interphalangeal joint to treat contracted claw or hammer toe

13.20.2 Positioning and Incision

Via a longitudinal incision over the proximal phalanx (**Fig. 13.92**), the extensor tendon is exposed and split longitudinally (**Figs. 13.93** and **13.94**). After transverse division of the capsule of the proximal interphalangeal joint, the condyles of the proximal phalanx can be dislocated in an extensor direction by maximal plantarflexion.

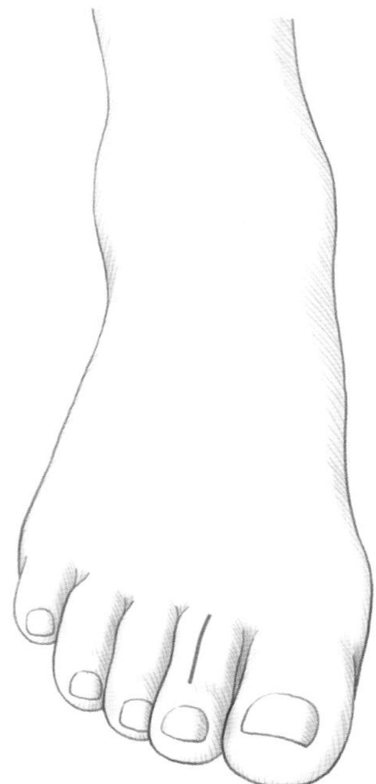

Fig. 13.92 Longitudinal incision over the extensor surface of the proximal phalanx of the second toe.

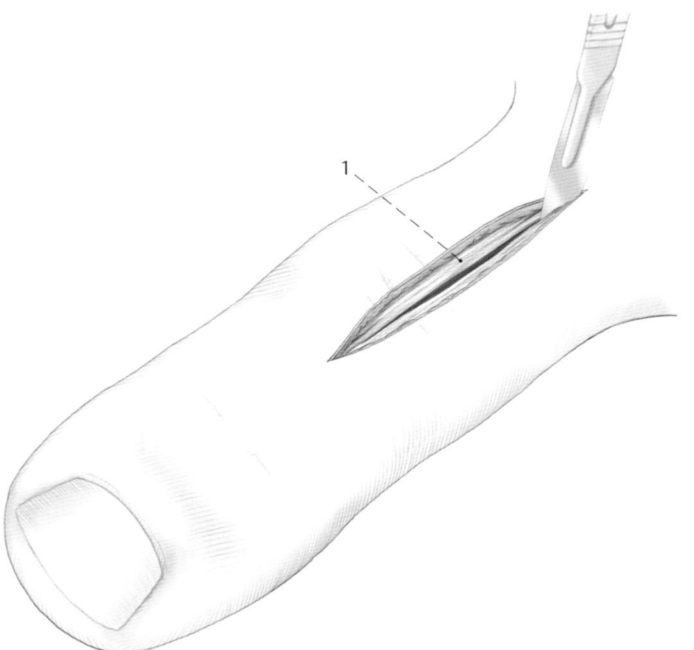

Fig. 13.93 Longitudinal splitting of the extensor tendon following longitudinal incision of skin and subcutaneous tissue.

1 Tendon of extensor digitorum longus

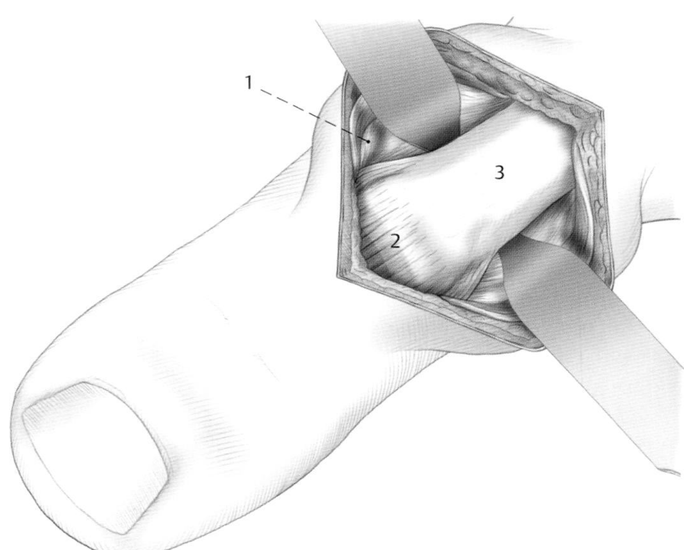

Fig. 13.94 Narrow Hohmann elevators are inserted subperiosteally under the condyles of the proximal phalanx, retracting the split bands of the extensor tendon.

1 Tendon of extensor digitorum longus
2 Proximal interphalangeal joint
3 Proximal phalanx of second toe

Further Reading: Pelvis and Lower Limb

[1] Anson BJ, McVay CB. Surgical Anatomy. Vol 1. Philadelphia: Saunders; 1971

[2] Banks SW, Laufmann H. An Atlas of Surgical Exposures of the Extremities. Philadelphia: Saunders; 1968

[3] Bauer R, Kerschbaumer F, Poisel S, Oberthaler W. The transgluteal approach to the hip joint. Arch Orthop Trauma Surg 1979;95 (1–2):47–49

[4] Berger RA, Duwelius PJ. The two-incision minimally invasive total hip arthroplasty: technique and results. Orthop Clin North Am 2004;35(2):163–172

[5] Bertin KC, Röttinger H. Anterolateral mini-incision hip replacement surgery: a modified Watson-Jones approach. Clin Orthop Relat Res 2004;429(429):248–255

[6] Bonnaire F, Muller B. Mediale Schenkelhalsfraktur im Erwachsenenalter und Osteosynthese mit der dynamischen Hüftschraube (DHS). Oper Orthop Traumatol 2001;13:121–134

[7] Cosentino R. Atlas of Anatomy and Surgical Approaches in Orthopaedic Surgery; vol 2. Springfield, IL: Thomas; 1973

[8] Engh GA, Holt BT, Parks NL. A midvastus muscle-splitting approach for total knee arthroplasty. J Arthroplasty 1997;12 (3):322–331

[9] Engh GA, Parks NL. Surgical technique of the midvastus arthrotomy. Clin Orthop Relat Res 1998; (351):270–274

[10] Fahey JJ. Surgical approaches to bones and joints. Surg Clin North Am 1949;29(1):65–76

[11] Ganz R, Gill TJ, Gautier E, Ganz K, Krügel N, Berlemann U. Surgical dislocation of the adult hip: a technique with full access to the femoral head and acetabulum without the risk of avascular necrosis. J Bone Joint Surg Br 2001;83(8):1119–1124

[12] Garden RS. The structure and function of the proximal end of the femur. J Bone Joint Surg 1991;43:576

[13] Gautier E, Ganz K, Krügel N, Gill T, Ganz R. Anatomy of the medial femoral circumflex artery and its surgical implications. J Bone Joint Surg Br 2000;82(5):679–683

[14] Grifka J, Kuster M. Orthopädie und Unfallchirurgie. Berlin: Springer; 2011

[15] Haas N, Schandelmeier P, Krettek C. Therapeutisches Konzept bei der distalen Femurfraktur mit Gelenkbeteiligung. Hefte Unfallheilkd 1990;212:179–187

[16] Halder A, Beier A, Neumann W. Mini-Subvastus-Zugang bei der Implantation von Knieendoprothesen. Oper Orthop Traumatol 2009;21(1):14–24

[17] Hardinge K. The direct lateral approach to the hip. J Bone Joint Surg Br 1982;64(1):17–19

[18] Hertel P. Frische und alte Kniebandverletzungen. Unfallchirurg 1996;99(9):686–700

[19] Hirner A, Weise K. Chirurgie. 2nd ed. Stuttgart: Thieme; 2008

[20] Hofmann AA, Plaster RL, Murdock LE. Subvastus (Southern) approach for primary total knee arthroplasty. Clin Orthop Relat Res 1991;(269):70–77

[21] Hoppenfeld S, de Boer P. Surgical Exposures in Orthopaedics. Philadelphia: Lippincott; 1984

[22] Hube R, Keim M, Mayr HO. Der Mini-Midvastus-Zugang zur Implantation von Kniegelenkendoprothesen. Oper Orthop Traumatol 2009;21(1):3–13

[23] Hughston JC. A surgical approach to the medial and posterior ligaments of the knee. Clin Orthop Relat Res 1973;(91):29–33

[24] Insall J. A midline approach to the knee. J Bone Joint Surg Am 1971;53(8):1584–1586

[25] Kerschbaumer F, Künzler S, Wahrburg J. Minimalzugang zum Hüftgelenk. Einsatzmöglichkeiten der Pfannennavigation und Robotic. In: Konermann W, Haaker R, eds. Navigation und Robotic in der Gelenk- und Wirbelsäulenchirurgie. Berlin: Springer; 2002:157–162

[26] Kinzl L. AO-Prinzipien des Frakturmanagements, Femur: Distal. Stuttgart: Thieme; 2003

[27] Kremer K, Lierse W, Platzer W, Schreiber HW, Weller S. Chirurgische Operationslehre. Band 10: Untere Extremität. Stuttgart: Thieme; 1997

[28] Krettek C, Schandelmeier P, Tscherne H. Distale Femurfrakturen. Unfallchirurg 1996;90:2

[29] Krettek C, Gerich T, Miclau T. A minimally invasive medial approach for proximal tibial fractures. Injury 2001;32(Suppl 1): SA4–SA13

[30] Letournel E. La voie ilio-inguinale. In: Méary R. Techniques Orthopédiques 1978/9. Paris: Expansion Scientifique Française; 1978

[31] Letournel E, Judet R, Elson RA. Fractures of the Acetabulum. Berlin: Springer; 1993

[32] Lüring C, Hüfner T, Kendoff D, et al. Beeinflusst der Zugangsweg die intraoperativ gemessene Beinachse in der Knieendoprothetik? Eine navigationsgestützte Studie am Kadaverknie. Unfallchirurg 2005;108(4):274–278

[33] Mast J, Jakob R, Ganz R. Planning and Reduction Technique in Fracture Surgery. Berlin: Springer; 1989.

[34] Matsen FA III. Compartmental syndrome. An unified concept. Clin Orthop Relat Res 1975;(113):8–14

[35] Matta JM, Tornetta P III. Internal fixation of unstable pelvic ring injuries. Clin Orthop Relat Res 1996;(329):129–140

[36] Matta JM, Olson SA. Surgical treatment of acetabular fractures. In: Browner B, Jupiter J, Levine AM, Trafton PG, eds. Skeletal Trauma. Philadelphia: Saunders; 1998:1181–1222

[37] Müller W. Das Knie. Berlin: Springer; 1982

[38] Mutschler W, Haas NP. Praxis der Unfallchirurgie. 2nd ed. Stuttgart: Thieme; 2004

[39] Nast-Kolb D, Ruchholtz S, Schweiberer L. Behandlung von Pipkin-Frakturen. Orthopade 1997;26(4):360–367

[40] Nicola T. Atlas operativer Zugangswege in der Orthopädie. Munich: Urban & Schwarzenberg; 1971

[41] Pichler W, Grechenig W, Tesch NP, Weinberg AM, Heidari N, Clement H. The risk of iatrogenic injury to the deep peroneal nerve in minimally invasive osteosynthesis of the tibia with the less invasive stabilisation system: a cadaver study. J Bone Joint Surg Br 2009;91(3):385–387

[42] Platzer W. Bewegungsapparat. 4th ed. Stuttgart: Thieme; 1984. Taschenatlas der Anatomie; Band 1

[43] Pohlemann T, Kiessling B, Gänsslen A, Bosch U, Tscherne H. Standardisierte Osteosynthesetechniken am Beckenring. Orthopade 1992;21(6):373–384

[44] Pohlemann T, Bosch U, Gänsslen A, Tscherne H. The Hannover experience in management of pelvic fractures. Clin Orthop Relat Res 1994;(305):69–80

[45] Repicci JA, Eberle RW. Minimally invasive surgical technique for unicondylar knee arthroplasty. J South Orthop Assoc 1999;8 (1):20–27

[46] Roth A, Layher F, Venbrocks RA. Transgluteal mini-incision. Technique and our own results [in German]. Orthopade 2006;35 (7):744–750

[47] Rüedi TP, Hochstetter AHC, Schlumpf R. Operative Zugänge zur Osteosynthese. Berlin: Springer; 1984

[48] Rüedi TP, Murphy WM. AO-Prinzipien des Frakturmanagements. Stuttgart: Thieme; 2008

[49] Schandelmaier P, Partenheimer A, Koenemann B, Grün OA, Krettek C. Distal femoral fractures and LISS stabilization. Injury 2001;32(Suppl 3):SC55–SC63

[50] Schatzker J, Tile M. The Rational of Operative Fracture Care. 2nd ed. Berlin: Springer; 1996

[51] Sculco TP, Jordan LC. The mini-incision approach to total hip arthroplasty. Instr Course Lect 2004;53:141–147

[52] Smith-Petersen MN. Approach to and exposure of the hip joint for mold arthroplasty. J Bone Joint Surg Am 1949;31A(1):40–46

[53] Tile MH, Kellam J. (2003) Fractures of the Pelvic and Acetabulum. Philadelphia: Lippincott Williams & Wilkins; 2003

[54] Tria AJ Jr, Coon TM. Minimal incision total knee arthroplasty: early experience. Clin Orthop Relat Res 2003; (416):185–190

[55] von Lanz T, Wachsmuth W. Praktische Anatomie; Band I/4. Berlin: Springer; 1972

[56] Wagner M, Schabus R. Funktionelle Anatomie des Kniegelenkes. Berlin: Springer; 1982

[57] Wahrburg J, Kerschbaumer F. Uberlegungen zum Einsatz mechatronischer Implantationshilfen bei Minimalzugängen für Hüftendoprothesen. Orthopade 2000;29(7):650–657

[58] Wenda K, Runkel M, Degreif J, Rudig L. Minimally invasive plate fixation in femoral shaft fractures. Injury 1997;28(Suppl 1):A13–A19

[59] Wohlrab D, Zeh A, Mendel T, Hein W. Quadsparing-Zugang bei Knietotalendoprothesenimplantation. Oper Orthop Traumatol 2009;21(1):25–34

[60] Zwipp H. Chirurgie des Fußes. Berlin: Springer; 1994

Shoulder and Upper Extremity

14 Scapula and Clavicle

14.1 Approach to the Clavicle and Acromioclavicular Joint

R. Bauer, F. Kerschbaumer, S. Poisel, K. Weise, K. Häringer

14.1.1 Principal Indications

- Fractures
- Pseudarthrosis
- Instability and acromioclavicular dislocation
- Inflammation, infection
- Osteoarthritis, acro-osteolysis
- Tumors

14.1.2 Positioning and Incision

The patient is placed in a semi-sitting position with an oblong cushion between the shoulder blades, and the arm is draped to allow free movement or optionally fixed to a side table. The preferred direction of the skin incision is craniocaudal (a saber cut incision). This is preferable for cosmetic reasons and to protect the medial supraclavicular nerves (**Fig. 14.1**).

The incision for exposure of the body of the clavicle is made roughly over the middle of the clavicle, while the incision for exposure of the acromioclavicular joint is barely medial to the coracoid process. The incision for access to the medial end of the clavicle follows Langer's lines transversely across the sternoclavicular joint.

Available alternatives are supraclavicular or infraclavicular transverse incisions (**Fig. 14.1**).

After the subcutaneous tissue has been transected, it is undermined and retracted (**Fig. 14.2**).

The cephalic vein lies deep in the deltopectoral groove, covered by fascia-like tissue, and is not touched in this phase of the dissection.

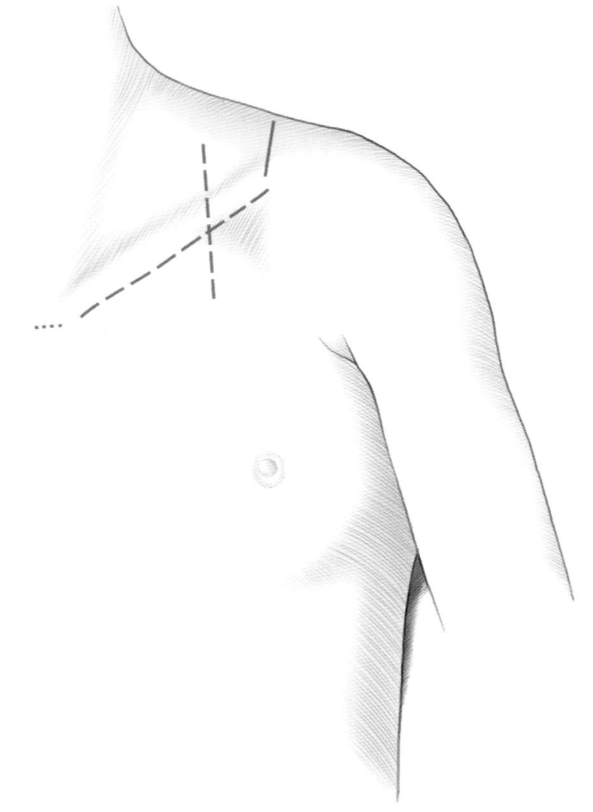

Fig. 14.1 Approach to the clavicle and acromioclavicular joint. Skin incisions (left side).

Dashed lines: Approach to the clavicle; standard approach (saber cut) along the skin crease lines or infraclavicularly.
Solid line: Approach to the acromioclavicular joint.
Dotted line: Approach to the sternoclavicular joint and for the minimally invasive insertion of an intramedullary elastic round nail.

14.1.3 Exposure of the Clavicle and Acromioclavicular Joint

The cervical fascia is now sharply detached from the posterior side of the clavicle, preserving the periosteum, and is retracted bluntly in a posterior direction together with muscle (**Fig. 14.3**).

To expose the acromioclavicular joint, a T-shaped incision is made in the trapezodeltoid fascia together with the joint capsule. By extending the incision medially by three fingerbreadths, the coracoclavicular ligaments and coracoid process may be exposed (**Fig. 14.3**).

14.1.4 Wound Closure

The opened joint capsule is sutured closed, and the detached cervical fascia is reattached to the clavicle by periosteal sutures. Suturing of the subcutaneous tissue and skin follows.

14.1.5 Dangers

Owing to the dissection of the medial parts of the deltoid muscle, the cephalic vein running in the deltopectoral groove may be injured. During dissection of the medial parts of the clavicle, the immediately subjacent subclavian vein is at risk of injury.

14.1.6 Note

Exposure of the medial part of the clavicle requires detachment of the clavicular portion of the sternocleidomastoid muscle.

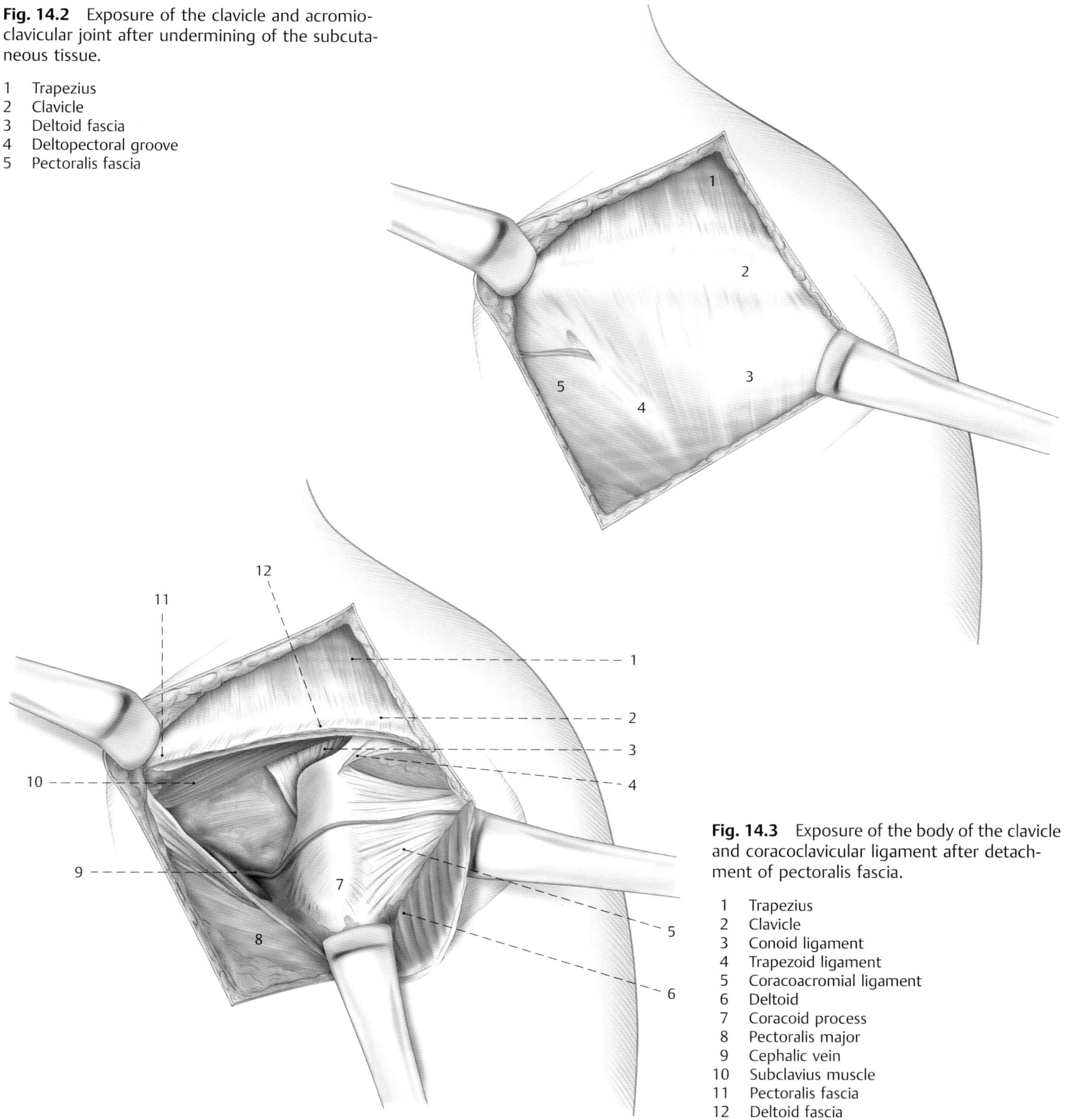

Fig. 14.2 Exposure of the clavicle and acromioclavicular joint after undermining of the subcutaneous tissue.

1 Trapezius
2 Clavicle
3 Deltoid fascia
4 Deltopectoral groove
5 Pectoralis fascia

Fig. 14.3 Exposure of the body of the clavicle and coracoclavicular ligament after detachment of pectoralis fascia.

1 Trapezius
2 Clavicle
3 Conoid ligament
4 Trapezoid ligament
5 Coracoacromial ligament
6 Deltoid
7 Coracoid process
8 Pectoralis major
9 Cephalic vein
10 Subclavius muscle
11 Pectoralis fascia
12 Deltoid fascia

14.2 Approach to the Sternoclavicular Joint

R. Bauer, F. Kerschbaumer, S. Poisel, K. Weise, K. Häringer

14.2.1 Principal Indications

- Instability and dislocations
- Fractures
- Arthritis
- Tumors
- Infections

14.2.2 Positioning and Incision

The patient is placed supine with an oblong cushion between the shoulder blades. The arm is fixed at the patient's side.

The incision follows the skin crease lines over the sternoclavicular joint, from the medial end of the clavicle to the manubrium of the sternum (**Fig. 14.4**).

After splitting of the subcutaneous tissue, the joint capsule is exposed and opened in a cruciate fashion (**Fig. 14.5**).

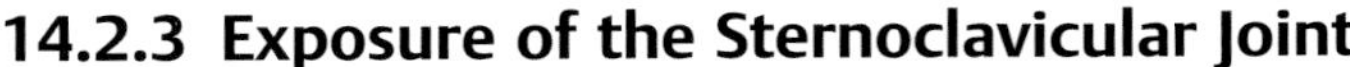

14.2.3 Exposure of the Sternoclavicular Joint

The capsular and periosteal flaps are dissected in medial and lateral directions. The clavicular part of the sternocleidomastoid muscle is dissected in a cranial direction. If broad exposure of the manubrium of the sternum is necessary, the sternal portion of the sternocleidomastoid muscle also has to be detached. This exposes the bony parts of the joint and the articular disk (**Fig. 14.6**).

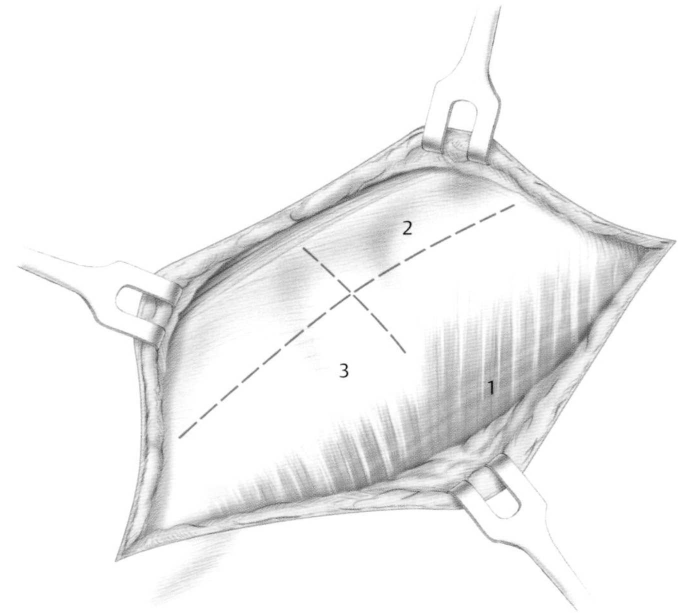

Fig. 14.5 Cruciate opening of the joint capsule.

1 Pectoralis major
2 Sternum
3 Clavicle

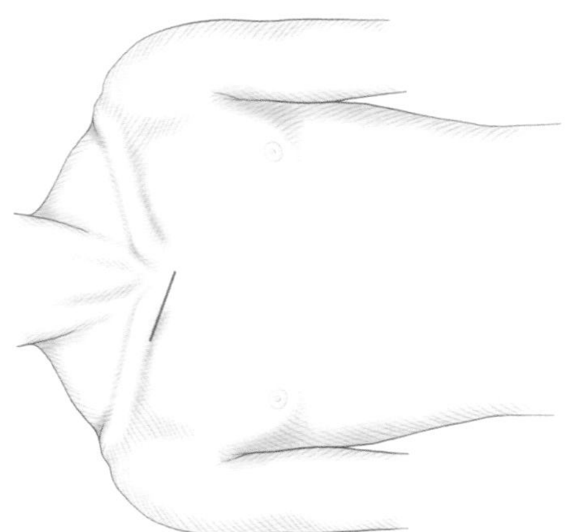

Fig. 14.4 Approach to the sternoclavicular joint. Skin incision (right side).

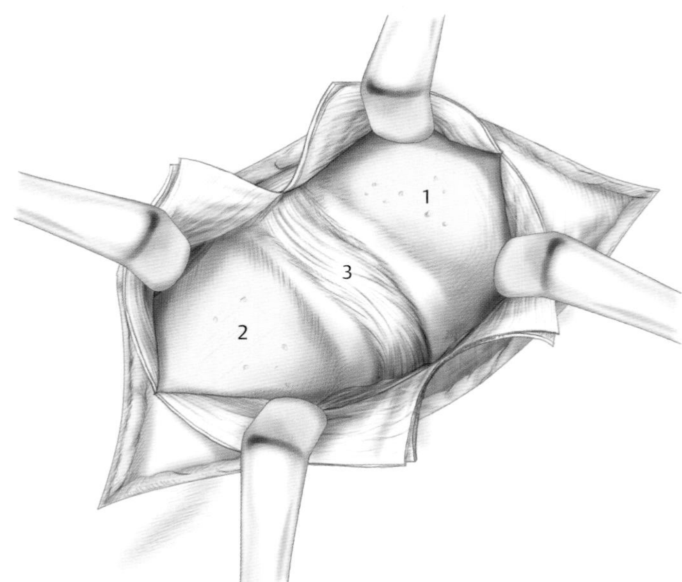

Fig. 14.6 Exposure of the sternoclavicular joint.

1 Manubrium of the sternum
2 Sternal end of the clavicle
3 Articular disk

14.3 Approach to the Scapula

R. Bauer, F. Kerschbaumer, S. Poisel, K. Weise, K. Häringer

14.3.1 Principal Indications

- Fractures
- Instability
- Tumors
- Infections
- Scapular elevation
- Exostoses

14.3.2 Positioning and Incision

The patient is placed in the prone position with a cushion under the chest. Depending on the approach, the arm is by the patient's side or abducted to 90° (**Figs. 14.7** and **14.13**).

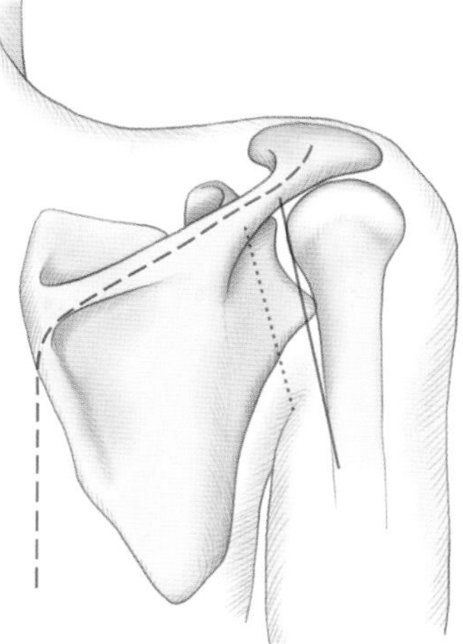

Fig. 14.7 Approach to the scapula. Skin incisions (right side, arm by patient's side).

Solid line: Rockwood approach.
Dotted line: Neer approach.
Dashed line: Judet approach.

Posterosuperior Vertical Approach (Neer)

This is the approach to the posterior glenoid rim and infraspinous fossa. With the patient's arm by his or her side, the skin incision begins over the spine of the scapula and runs approximately 12 cm in a craniocaudal direction (**Fig. 14.7**). After mobilizing the subcutaneous tissue, the deltoid is detached from the spine of the scapula leaving a rim of periosteum, and the spinal and acromial parts are dissected roughly 5 cm in a caudal direction in the intermuscular septum. The axillary nerve passes here and is protected by an anchoring suture. Following division of teres minor and infraspinatus, the nerve is retracted caudally. Separation of these muscles gives access to the posterior glenoid rim. After dissecting the muscles from the innominate tubercle, the infraspinous fossa is reached. The wound is closed by reinsertion of the muscles and continuous suture of the two parts of the deltoid.

Vertical Posterior Approach (Rockwood)

This is an alternative approach to the posterior glenoid rim. The skin incision begins 2 cm medial to the posterior border of the acromion and runs vertically over the posterior joint line to the posterior axillary fold (**Fig. 14.7**). The deltoid muscle is split bluntly in the line of its fibers as far as teres minor. Further dissection between teres minor and infraspinatus allows visualization of the posterior capsule. The axillary nerve and posterior vascular bundle must be protected. These run along the inferior border of teres minor. To extend the approach, teres minor and infraspinatus can be divided at their insertion.

Posterior Approach (Judet)

The skin incision begins slightly below the inferior angle of the scapula, runs about one fingerbreadth medial to the medial border of the scapula, and then curves over the spine of the scapula and continues as far as the acromion (**Fig. 14.7**). The incision can be extended laterally as needed for exposure of the part of the scapula involved (**Fig. 14.8**).

If the entire scapula has to be exposed posteriorly, the trapezius muscle at the spine of the scapula is first detached from lateral to medial as far the medial border. The trapezius muscle is mobilized and retracted as far as the superior angle of the scapula, care being taken to avoid injury to the accessory nerve (**Fig. 14.9**; see also **Fig. 2.32**). Exposure of the infraspinous fossa is begun by stripping the deltoid muscle from the spine of the scapula. Then, starting at the medial border of the scapula, the infraspinatus and teres major as well as the teres minor are detached subperiosteally. At the spine of the scapula, the suprascapular nerve passing through here should be preserved. At the superior angle, the levator scapulae and the rhomboid minor muscles are detached near the bone to avoid bleeding from the dorsal scapular artery. First rhomboid major and then serratus anterior are detached, also near the bone, along the medial border of the scapula. For exposure of the supraspinous fossa, supraspinatus is dissected subperiosteally from medial to lateral. Upon further dissection in a lateral direction, the suprascapular nerve and the suprascapular artery in the area of the scapular notch must be spared (**Fig. 14.10**). For exposure of the anterior aspect of the scapula, this is pulled laterally with a bone hook so that serratus anterior and subscapularis can be retracted subperiosteally (**Figs. 14.11** and **14.12**).

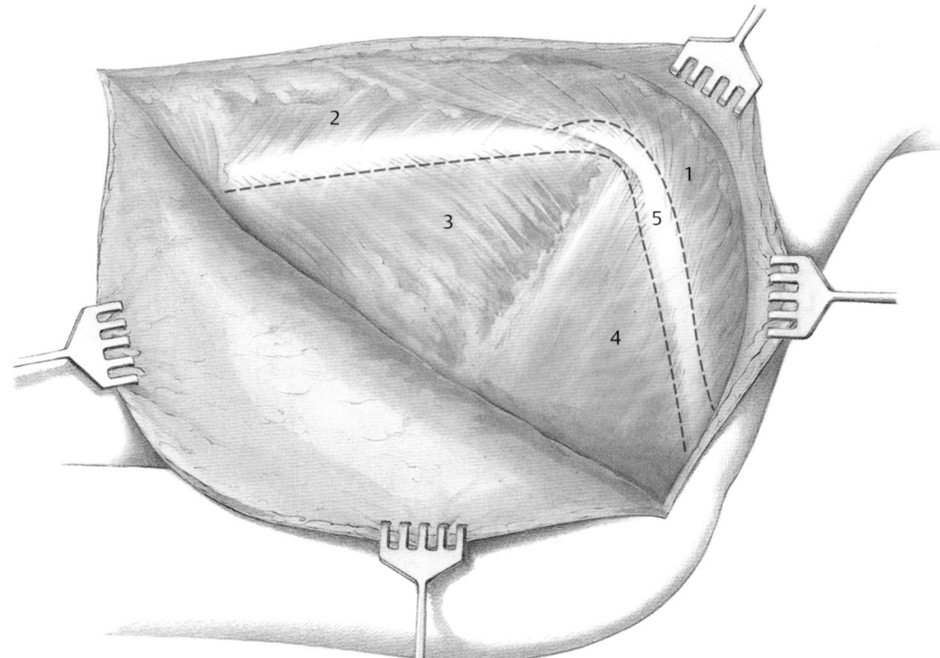

Fig. 14.8 Detachment of the scapular muscles (dashed lines).

1 Trapezius
2 Rhomboid major
3 Infraspinatus
4 Deltoid
5 Spine of the scapula

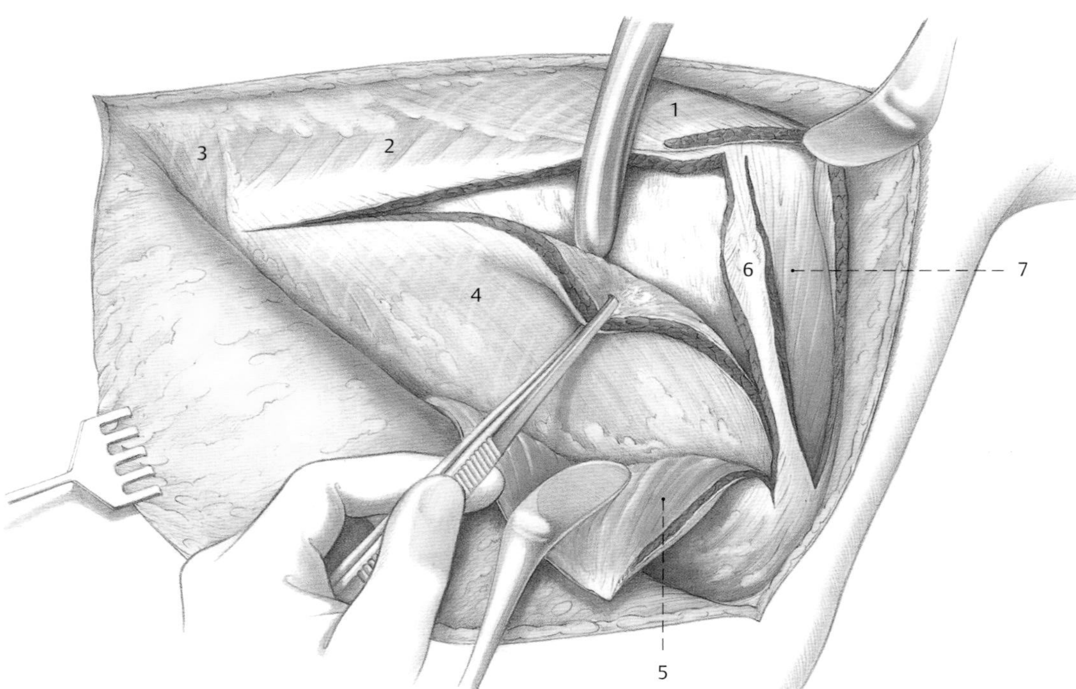

Fig. 14.9 The infraspinatus is dissected free after stripping of the trapezius and deltoid.

1 Trapezius
2 Rhomboid major
3 Latissimus dorsi
4 Infraspinatus
5 Deltoid
6 Spine of the scapula
7 Supraspinatus

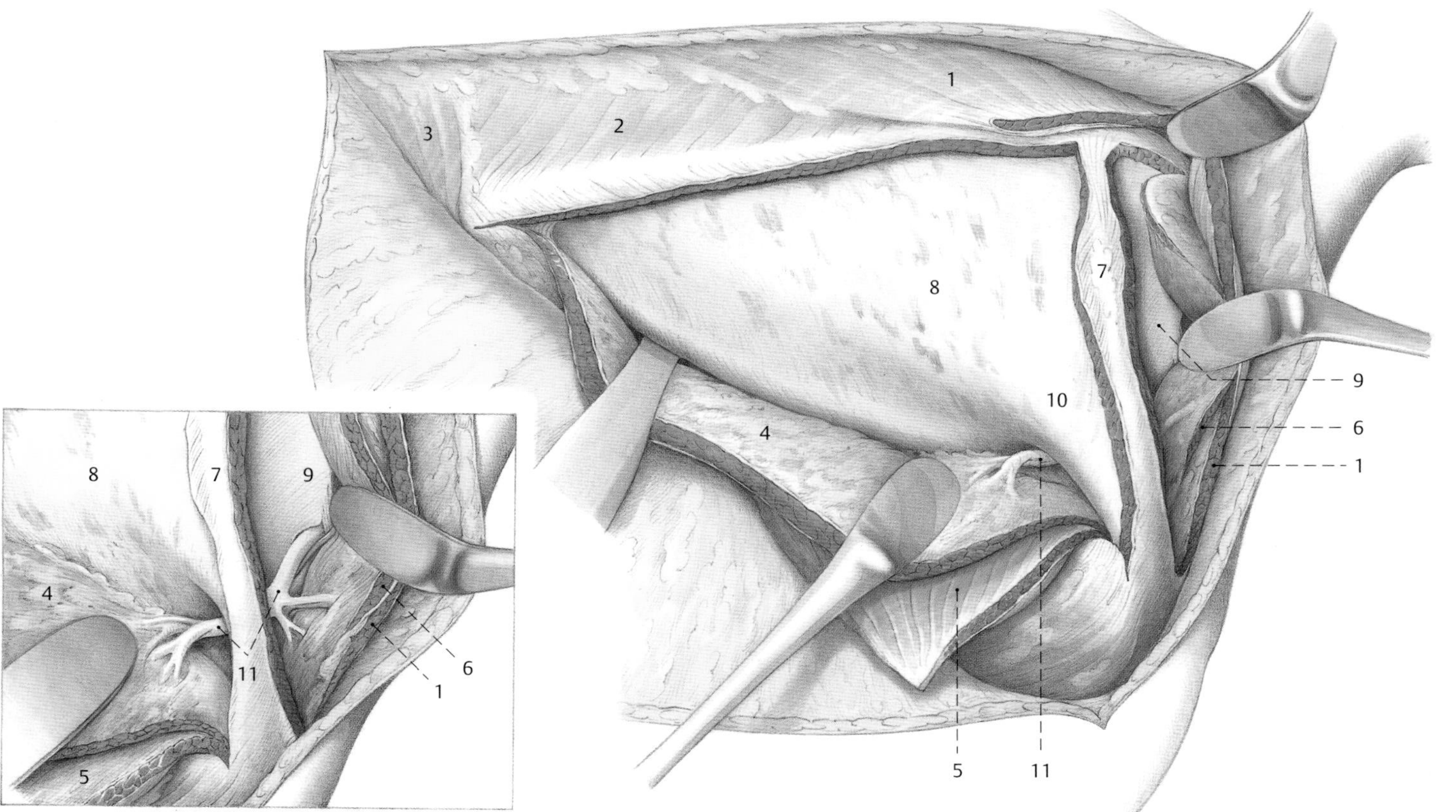

Fig. 14.10 Exposure of the posterior surface of the scapula after subperiosteal detachment of the muscles. Detail: Exposure of the course and muscular branches of the suprascapular nerve after detachment of supraspinatus and infraspinatus.

1 Trapezius
2 Rhomboid major
3 Latissimus dorsi muscle
4 Infraspinatus
5 Deltoid muscle
6 Supraspinatus
7 Spine of the scapula
8 Infraspinous fossa
9 Supraspinous fossa
10 Neck of the scapula
11 Suprascapular nerve

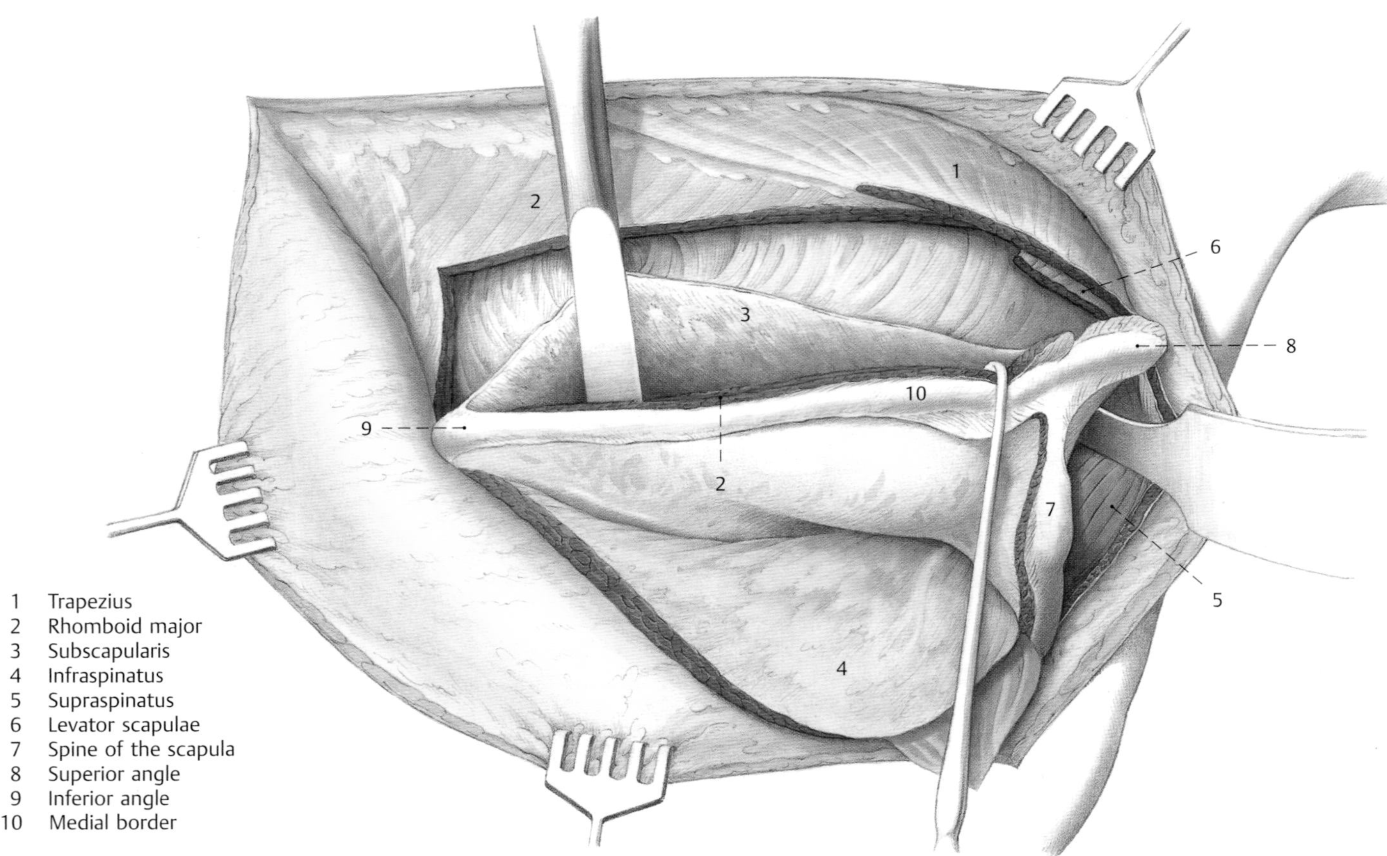

Fig. 14.11 After stripping of the trapezius and rhomboid muscles and levator scapulae, the scapula is raised with a bone hook, and subscapularis is dissected out.

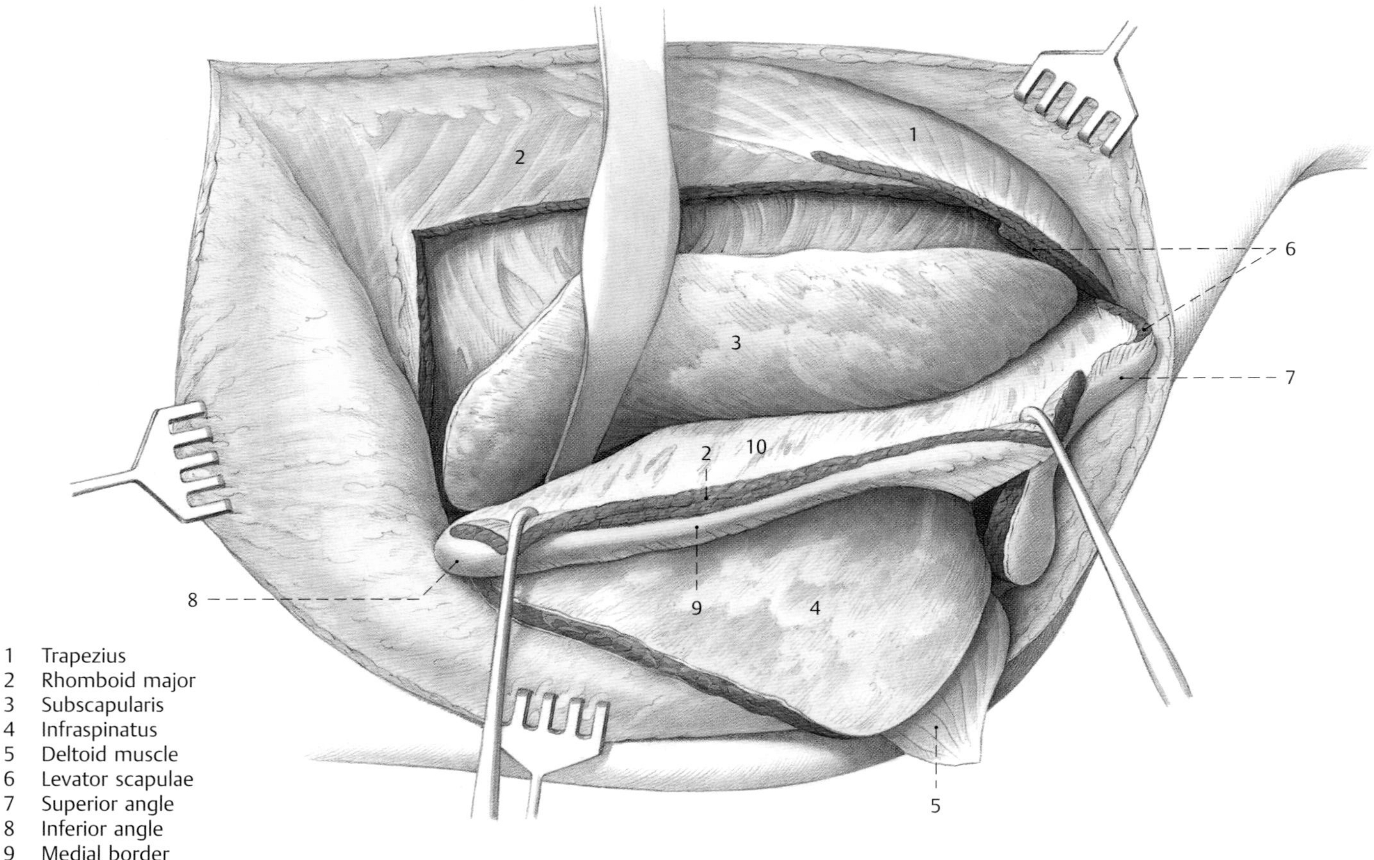

Fig. 14.12 Exposure of the costal surface of the scapula.

Posterolateral Approach (Tubiana)

This is a less traumatic approach to the lateral border of the scapula and inferior glenoid rim.

With the patient's arm abducted to 90°, the incision is made over the middle of the lateral border of the scapula parallel to the ribs (**Fig. 14.13**). After blunt dissection of teres minor and infraspinatus, the lateral border of the scapula is reached (**Fig. 14.14**). The deltoid muscle has to be mobilized for extension in a cranial direction, and the axillary nerve must be spared (**Fig. 14.15**).

To visualize the inferior part of the glenoid, teres minor is mobilized laterally, and the posterior axillary recess is opened.

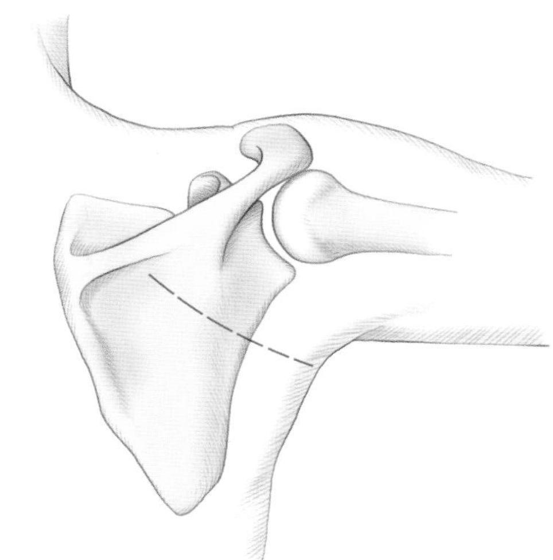

Fig. 14.13 Approach to the scapula according to Tubiana. Right side, arm abducted 90°.

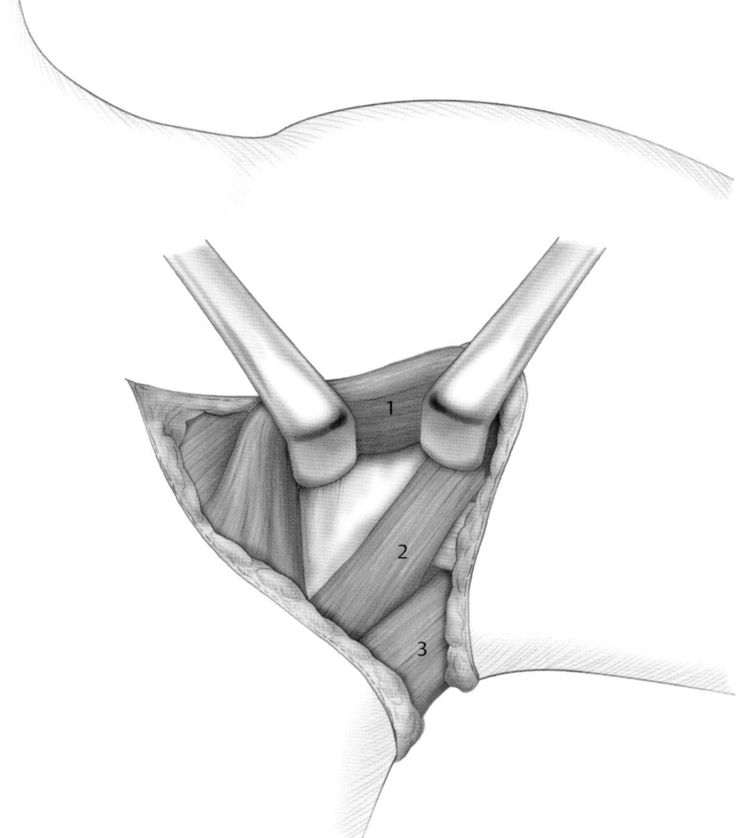

Fig. 14.14 Posterior approach to the scapula according to Tubiana. By abducting the arm, the deltoid reveals the posterior rotator cuff. Blunt dissection of the infraspinatus and teres minor.

1 Infraspinatus
2 Teres minor
3 Teres major

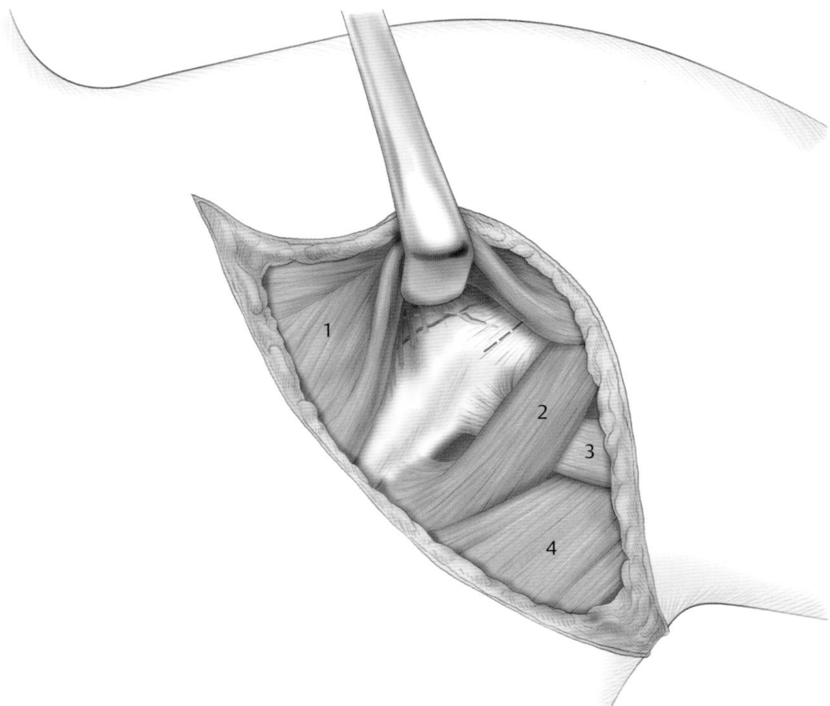

Fig. 14.15 Incision of the capsule.

1 Infraspinatus
2 Teres minor
3 Triceps brachii, long head
4 Teres major

14.3.3 Wound Closure

The detached muscle is reattached to the medial border and the spine of the scapula.

14.3.4 Dangers

The suprascapular nerve may be injured during dissection of supraspinatus and infraspinatus. Injury to the trapezius at the superior angle endangers the accessory nerve.

15 Shoulder

15.1 Anterior Approach to the Shoulder Joint

K. Weise, K. Häringer

15.1.1 Principal Indications

- Fractures
- Pseudarthrosis
- Instability and shoulder dislocations
- Injuries to the subscapularis muscle
- Inflammation, infection
- Tendon of the long head of the biceps
- Tumors

15.1.2 Positioning and Incision

The patient is placed in a semi-sitting position. Draping is done so that the arm is freely movable during the operation. At the beginning of the operation, the arm is adducted against the patient's body with the elbow flexed at a right angle (**Fig. 15.1**).

Deltopectoral Approach According to Wiedemann

The skin incision begins in the center of an imaginary line between the coracoid process and the anterior angle of the acromion, and runs caudally to the tendon of the long head of the biceps (**Fig. 15.2**).

Subcutaneous dissection on the deltoid fascia continues medially to the deltopectoral groove (**Fig. 15.3**). The clavipectoral fascia is exposed by blunt dissection through the deltopectoral

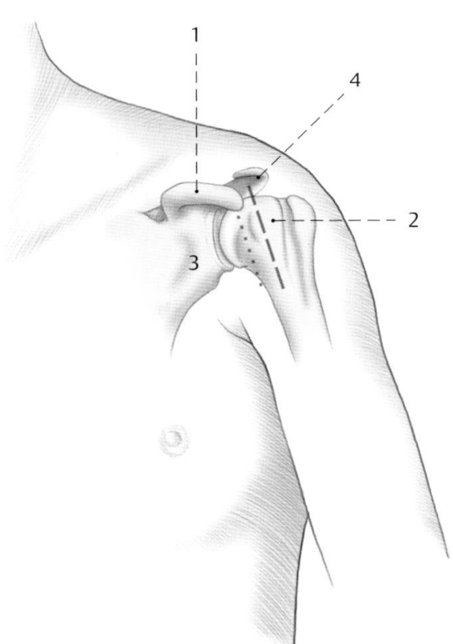

Fig. 15.1 Approaches to the anterior part of the shoulder joint (left shoulder).

Dashed line: deltopectoral approach.
Dotted line: anterior approach.
1 Coracoid process
2 Lesser tubercle
3 Neck of the scapula
4 Acromion

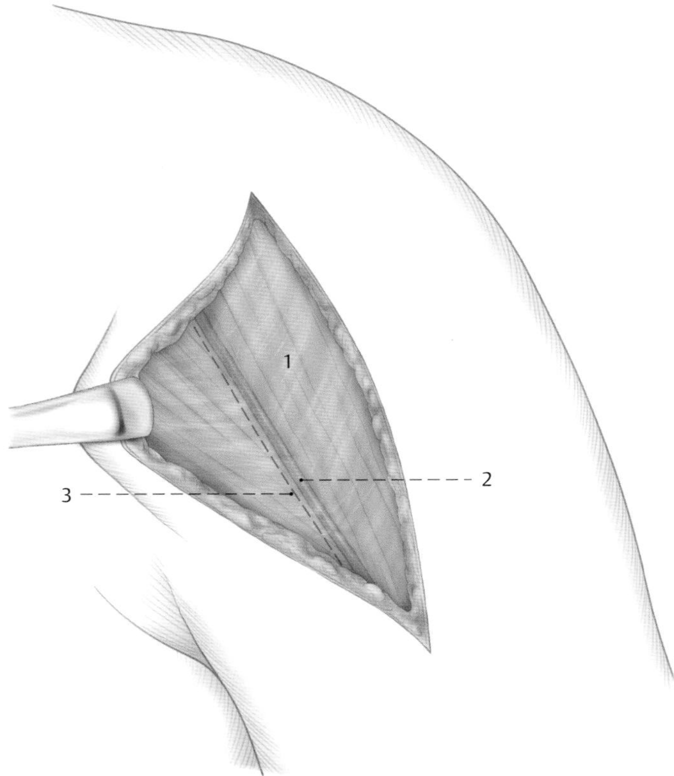

Fig. 15.2 Deltopectoral approach to the head of the humerus (left shoulder).

1 Deltoid
2 Cephalic vein
3 Deltopectoral groove

groove medial to the cephalic vein (**Fig. 15.4**). For treatment of a fracture, the deltoid is now undermined bluntly with a finger so that internal rotation of the arm provides extensive visualization of the head of the humerus.

Anterior Approach

The skin incision begins below the tip of the coracoid process and runs caudally to approximately 1 cm lateral to the axillary fold (see **Fig. 15.1**). The deltopectoral groove is sought following division of the subcutaneous tissue.

After exposure of the cephalic vein, the biceps and pectoralis major muscles are split bluntly medial to the cephalic vein (see **Fig. 15.3**). After the insertion of blunt hooks, the clavipectoral fascia, which covers the common aponeurosis of the short head of the biceps and the coracobrachialis as well as the subscapularis muscle, is visible (**Fig. 15.4**). This fascia is divided longitudinally from the coracoacromial ligament to the cranial border of the attachment of the pectoralis major tendon lateral to the short head of the biceps (**Fig. 15.5**).

The arm is externally rotated to expose the subscapularis and its transition to the tendon (**Fig. 15.6**). The lower border of the muscle is recognizable by the small vessels coursing in this area. The anterior circumflex humeral artery should be spared (**Fig. 15.7**). A curved clamp is passed from caudal to cranial beneath the tendinous portion of the subscapularis, and the muscular portion of subscapularis is snared with retaining sutures. To protect the underlying neurovascular structures, the tendon of the short head of the biceps should not be detached from the coracoid process, and coracoid osteotomy should be avoided. The tendon of subscapularis is transected across the indwelling clamp (**Fig. 15.8**).

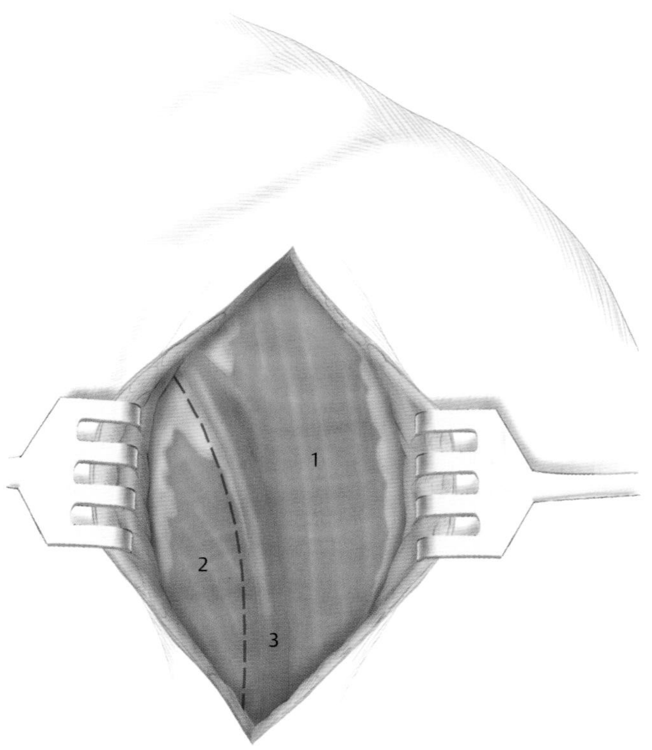

Fig. 15.3 Anterior approach to the shoulder (left shoulder).

Dashed line: deltopectoral groove medial to the cephalic vein, which acts as landmark.

1 Deltoid
2 Pectoralis major
3 Cephalic vein

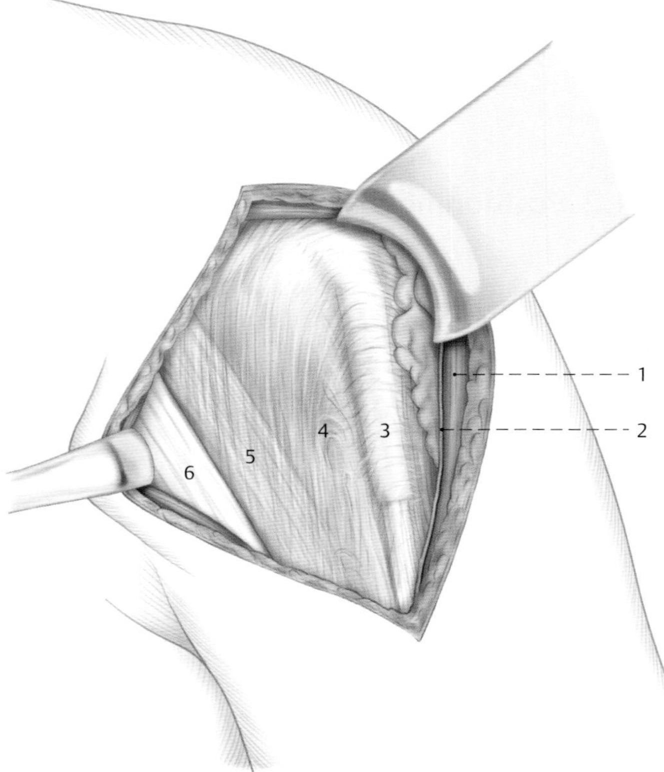

Fig. 15.4 Blunt dissection through the bicipital groove (left shoulder).

1 Deltoid
2 Cephalic vein
3 Intertubercular tendon sheath
4 Clavipectoral fascia
5 Short head of biceps brachii
6 Coracobrachialis

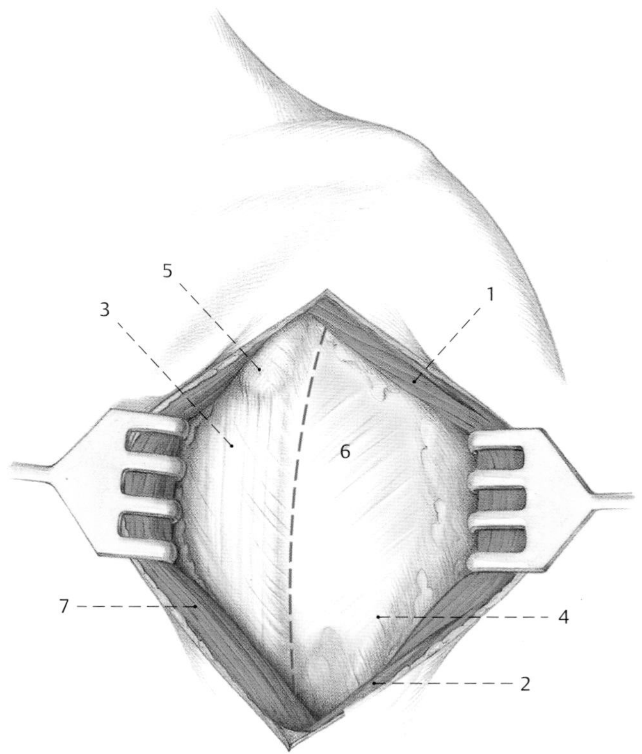

Fig. 15.5 Spreading of the deltoid lateral to the cephalic vein. Incision of the fascia next to the short head of biceps.

1 Deltoid
2 Cephalic vein
3 Short head of biceps brachii
4 Long head of biceps brachii
5 Coracoid process
6 Tendon of subscapularis
7 Pectoralis major

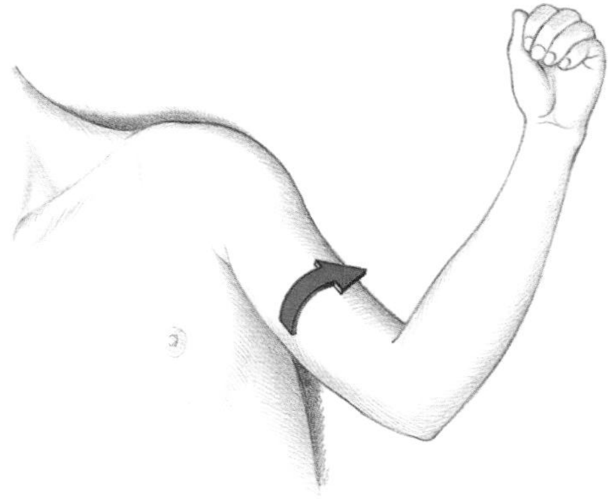

Fig. 15.6 External rotation of the upper arm.

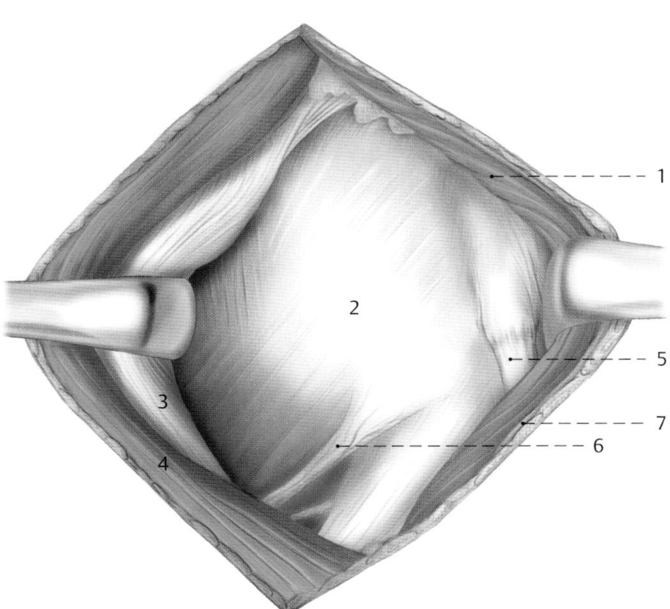

Fig. 15.7 Exposure of subscapularis after dissection through the deltopectoral groove and opening of the clavipectoral fascia.

1 Deltoid
2 Subscapularis
3 Short head of biceps brachii
4 Pectoralis major
5 Long head of biceps brachii
6 Anterior circumflex humeral artery and accompanying veins
7 Cephalic vein

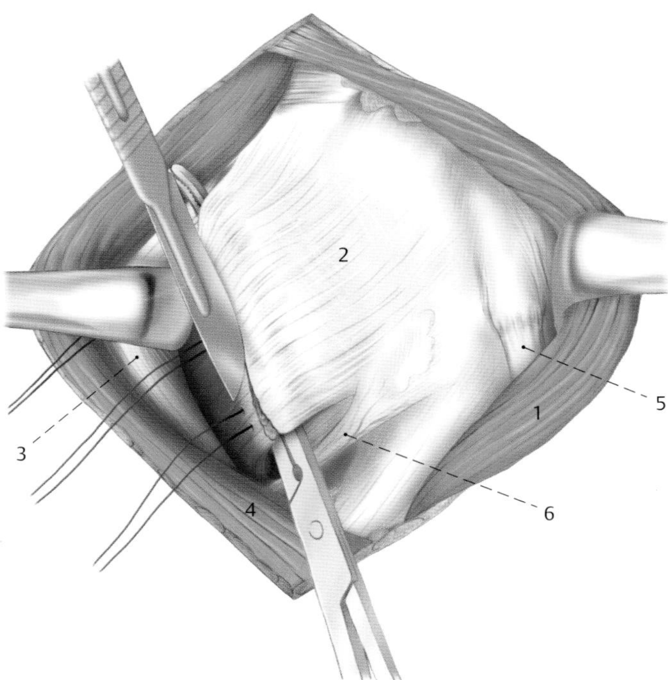

Fig. 15.8 Placement of retaining sutures and transection of subscapularis at the junction of its tendinous and muscular parts.

1 Deltoid
2 Subscapularis
3 Short head of biceps brachii
4 Pectoralis major
5 Long head of biceps brachii
6 Anterior circumflex humeral artery and accompanying veins

15.1.3 Exposure of the Shoulder Joint

As a rule, subscapularis can be readily dissected from the anterior joint capsule (**Fig. 15.9**). The joint capsule is opened alongside the glenoid lip, exposing the anterior part of the humeral head, the glenoid lip, and the neck of the scapula. To improve exposure, a small pointed Hohmann elevator may be driven into the neck of the scapula (**Fig. 15.10**). For exposure of the glenoid cavity, a specially curved humeral retractor is inserted above the posterior border of the glenoid cavity so that the humeral head can be held to the side (**Fig. 15.11**).

15.1.4 Wound Closure

The capsule is closed with the arm rotated internally by suture of the joint capsule and the subscapularis tendon. After placing Redon drains, the subcutaneous tissue and skin are sutured.

15.1.5 Dangers

The axillary nerve may be damaged in the area of the lateral axillary foramen. Unduly vigorous hook traction on the short head of the biceps or the coracobrachialis can cause injury to the branches of the musculocutaneous nerve (see **Fig. 15.12**).

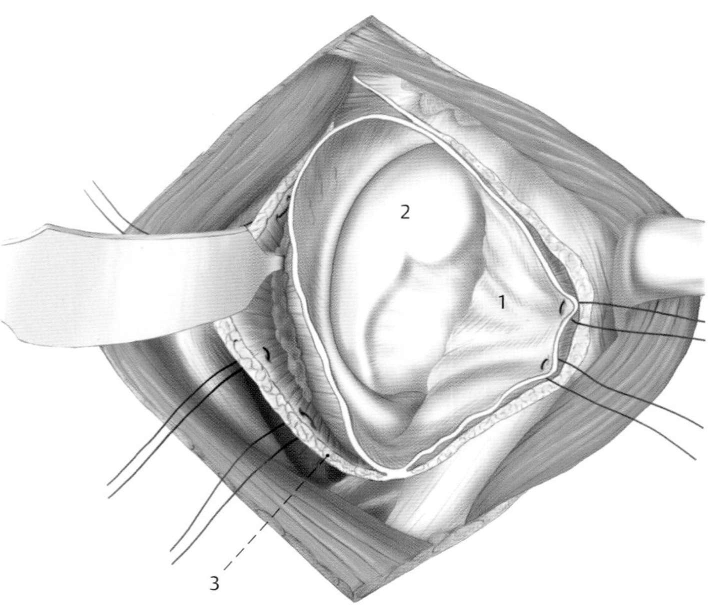

Fig. 15.10 View of the intra-articular part of the humeral head after opening the capsule.

1 Joint capsule
2 Head of humerus
3 Subscapularis

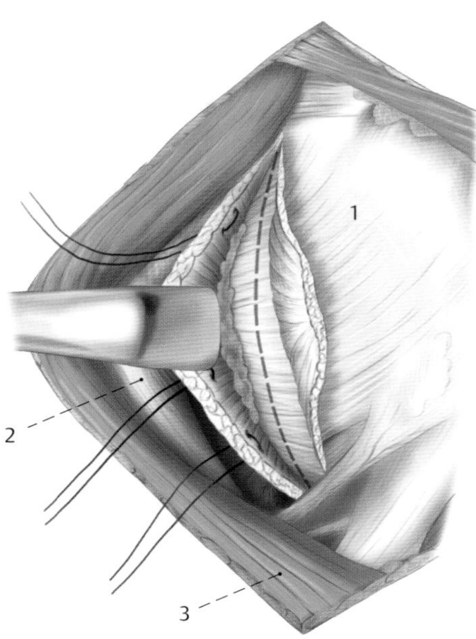

Fig. 15.9 Exposure of the joint capsule by careful dissection of the subscapularis and incision of the capsule (dashed line).

1 Subscapularis tendon
2 Short head of biceps brachii
3 Pectoralis major

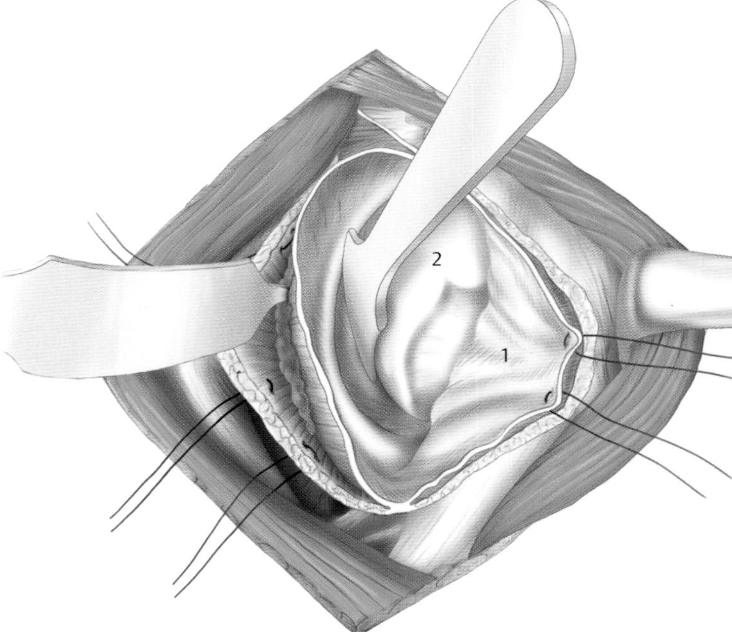

Fig. 15.11 After insertion of a humeral head retractor, the glenoid joint surface can be readily seen.

1 Joint capsule
2 Head of the humerus

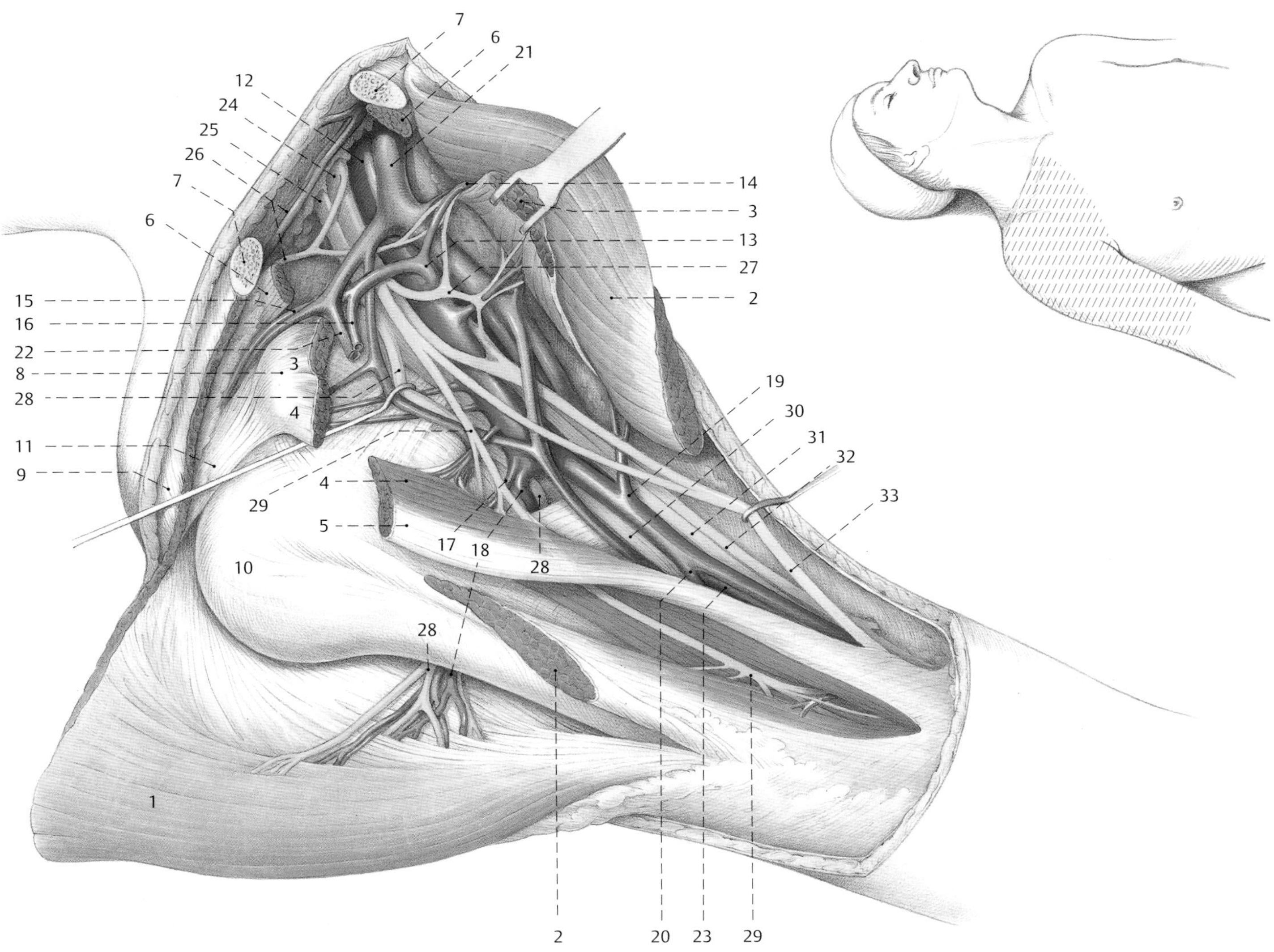

Fig. 15.12 Anatomical site. The central segment of the clavicle and subclavius, along with parts of the short head of the biceps and coracobrachialis, have been removed to expose the neurovascular bundle.

1 Deltoid
2 Pectoralis major
3 Pectoralis minor
4 Short head of biceps brachii
5 Coracobrachialis
6 Subclavius
7 Clavicle
8 Coracoid process
9 Acromion
10 Head of the humerus
11 Coracoacromial ligament
12 Axillary artery
13 Thoracoacromial artery
14 Pectoral branch of the thoracoacromial artery
15 Acromial branch of the thoracoacromial artery
16 Deltoid branch of the thoracoacromial artery
17 Anterior circumflex humeral artery
18 Posterior circumflex humeral artery
19 Brachial artery
20 Deep brachial artery
21 Subclavian vein
22 Cephalic vein
23 Brachial vein
24 Lateral cord of the brachial plexus
25 Posterior cord of the brachial plexus
26 Suprascapular artery, vein, and nerve
27 Pectoral nerves
28 Axillary nerve
29 Musculocutaneous nerve
30 Radial nerve
31 Ulnar nerve
32 Medial cutaneous nerve of the forearm
33 Median nerve

15.2 Extended Anterior Approach to the Shoulder Joint with Exposure of the Proximal Humerus

K. Weise, K. Häringer

15.2.1 Principal Indications

- Fractures of the proximal humerus
- Arthroplasty
- Tumors

15.2.2 Positioning and Incision

The patient is placed in a semi-sitting position. Draping is done so that the arm is freely movable during the operation. At the beginning of the operation, the arm is adducted against the patient's body with the elbow flexed at a right angle.

The skin incision begins in the center of an imaginary line between the coracoid process and anterior angle of the acromion, and runs caudally on the tendon of the long head of the biceps (**Fig. 15.13**) to the required length.

Subcutaneous dissection of the deltoid fascia continues medially to the deltopectoral groove. The clavipectoral fascia is exposed by blunt dissection through the deltopectoral groove medial to the cephalic vein (**Fig. 15.14**). After the insertion of blunt hooks, the clavipectoral fascia, which covers the common aponeurosis of the short head of the biceps and coracobrachialis as well as the subscapularis, is visible (**Fig. 15.4**). It is divided longitudinally from the coracoacromial ligament to the cranial border of the attachment of the pectoralis major tendon lateral to the short head of the biceps (**Fig. 15.5**). For better exposure of the humerus, the pectoralis major attachment can be notched. The short head of the biceps and the coracobrachialis are dissected bluntly and retracted medially without unduly vigorous hook traction to protect the musculocutaneous nerve. If necessary, the shoulder joint can be opened using the anterior approach described above.

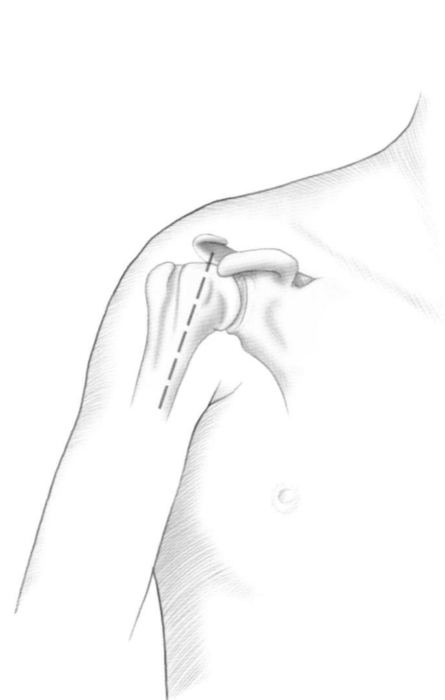

Fig. 15.13 Extended anterior approach.

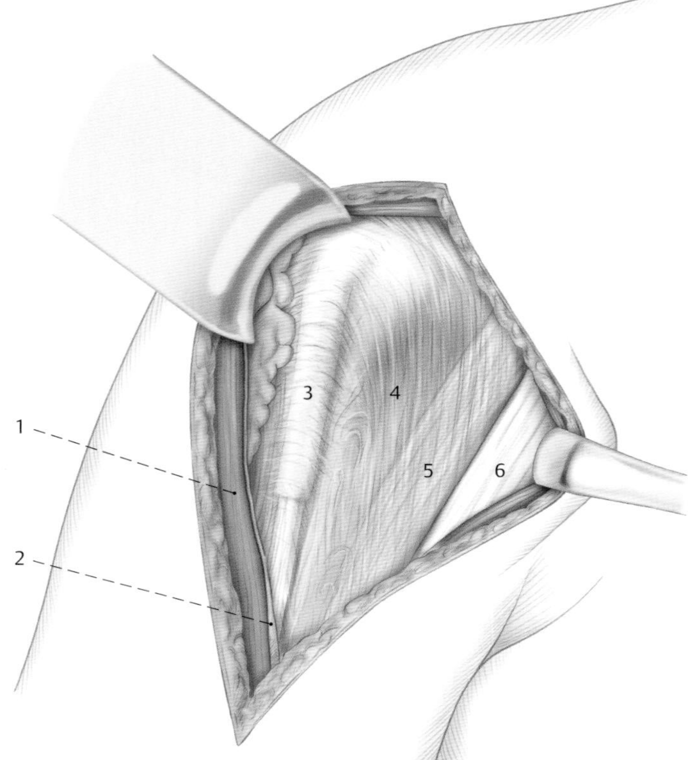

Fig. 15.14 Blunt dissection through the deltopectoral groove (right shoulder).

1 Deltoid
2 Cephalic vein
3 Intertubercular tendon sheath
4 Clavipectoral fascia
5 Short head of biceps brachii
6 Coracobrachialis

15.2.3 Wound Closure

The tendon of pectoralis major is reinserted into its origin. The gap between the deltoid and pectoralis major does not have to be closed.

15.2.4 Dangers

The axillary nerve may be damaged laterally by unduly vigorous retraction, as well as medially, where it can be seen in the interval between subscapularis and the insertion of latissimus dorsi and teres major. No retractors should therefore be inserted at this site.

15.2.5 Note

The axillary approach described in older textbooks is now used only for rare indications involving anterior instability to provide access to the inferior capsule. Dissection down to the joint is performed either below pectoralis major or between the deltoid and pectoralis major. This approach is unsuitable for the stabilizing surgical procedures in use today, which close Weitbrecht's foramen.

15.3 Anterosuperior Approach to the Shoulder Joint

K. Weise, K. Häringer

15.3.1 Principal Indications

- Rotator cuff injuries to subscapularis, supraspinatus, and infraspinatus
- Impingement
- Arthroplasty (Mackenzie approach)

15.3.2 Positioning and Incision

The patient is placed in a semi-sitting position, the arm being draped to allow free movement.

At the beginning of the operation, the adducted arm with the elbow flexed at a right angle rests against the patient's body.

Neer Approach

The skin incision begins over the acromioclavicular joint and continues along the tendon of the long head of the biceps for approximately 6 cm in caudal direction (**Fig. 15.15**). The acromioclavicular joint and deltoid muscle are exposed subcutaneously. The deltoid is then split bluntly between the clavicular and acromial parts for approximately 5 cm in caudal direction. An anchoring suture should be placed at the angle of the wound to protect the axillary nerve, which here runs transversely. After subfascial mobilization of the deltoid muscle and resection of the subdeltoid bursa, the anterior border of the acromion is reached. Acromioplasty can be performed if necessary. The subscapularis, supraspinatus, and infraspinatus muscles can be readily visualized.

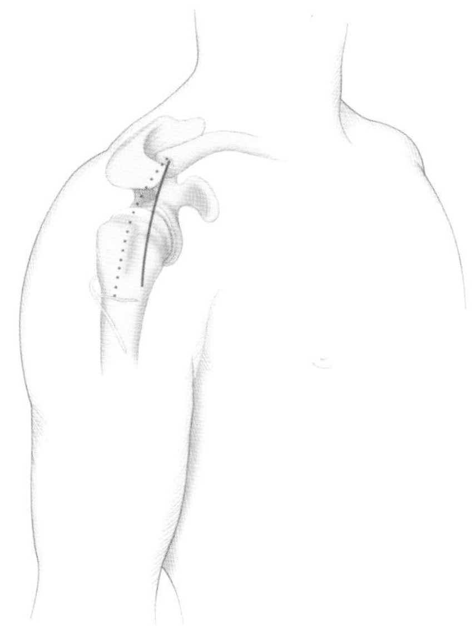

Fig. 15.15 Anterosuperior approaches.

Solid line: Neer approach.
Dotted line: Mackenzie approach.

Mackenzie Approach

The skin incision begins over the acromioclavicular joint and continues laterally over the edge of the acromion and greater tubercle for approximately 9 cm over the lateral upper arm (**Fig. 15.16**). The deltoid fascia is then split bluntly for a good 5 cm in a caudal direction, when an anchoring suture should be placed at the angle of the wound to protect the axillary nerve, which here runs transversely. For better visualization, the bony attachment of the deltoid muscle can be detached from the border of the acromion. The clavipectoral fascia is then divided, followed by blunt dissection of the short head of the biceps and the coracobrachialis, which are retracted medially with a blunt hook. Externally rotating the arm provides a good view of subscapularis (**Fig. 15.16**).

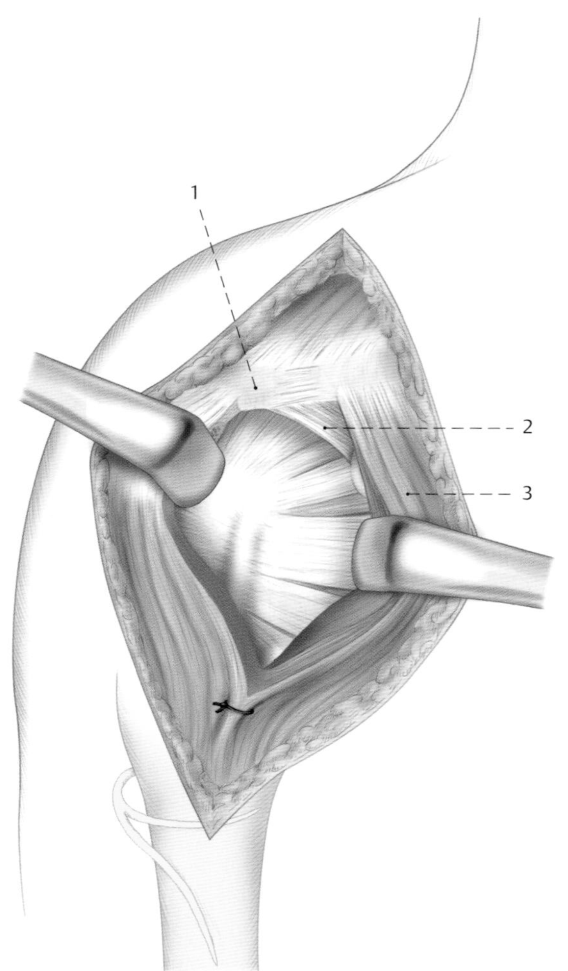

Fig. 15.16 Mackenzie approach. Splitting of the deltoid fibers for approximately 5 cm in a caudal direction, and placement of a retaining suture to protect the axillary nerve (right shoulder)

1 Acromion
2 Coracoacromial ligament
3 Deltoid

15.3.3 Wound Closure

The deltoid is closed with a continuous suture.

15.3.4 Dangers

The axillary nerve is at risk if the incision continues too far caudally.

15.4 Anterolateral Approach According to Bigliani

K. Weise, K. Häringer

15.4.1 Principal Indications

- Rotator cuff injuries to the subscapularis, supraspinatus, and infraspinatus in combination with posterior injuries
- Impingement
- Fractures of the greater tubercle

15.4.2 Positioning and Incision

The patient is placed in a semi-sitting position, the arm being draped to allow free movement. At the beginning of the operation, the adducted arm with the elbow flexed at a right angle rests against the patient's body.

The skin incision begins at the acromioclavicular joint, runs along the anterior border of the acromion to the anterior angle of the acromion, and from there continues for approximately 5 cm in a caudal direction along the deltoid fibers toward the greater tubercle (**Fig. 15.17**).

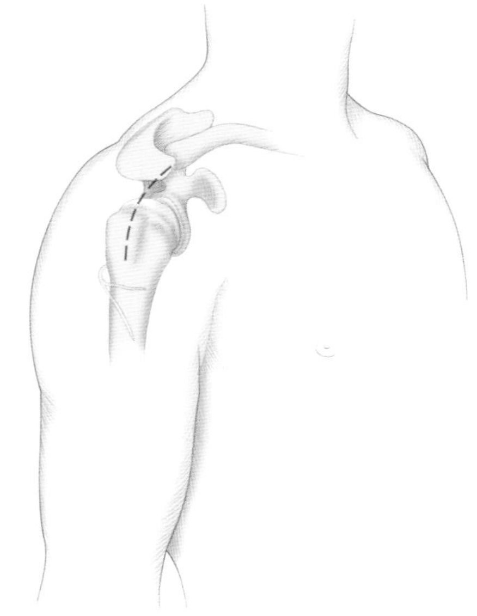

Fig. 15.17 Bigliani approach.

After subcutaneous exposure of the deltoid, the acromial part is detached subperiosteally, sparing the coracoacromial ligament (**Fig. 15.18**).

The ligament is divided separately from the acromion with a scalpel. After detaching it, the deltoid is split bluntly in the septum. An anchoring suture should be placed at the angle of the wound to protect the axillary nerve. After resection of the subdeltoid bursa and division of the ligament, the border of the acromion and cranial parts of the rotator cuff can be readily visualized (**Fig. 15.19**).

External rotation of the arm exposes the lesser tubercle and tendinous attachment of the subscapularis as well as the tendon of the long head of the biceps.

For small rotator cuff defects and if acromioplasty is not required, the mini open approach according to Levi has become popular in recent years.

The skin incision begins over the anterior border of the acromion and continues for just under 5 cm in a caudal direction toward the greater tubercle in the line of the deltoid fibers. Unlike the Bigliani approach, the deltoid muscle is not detached from the acromion but is split bluntly only in the septum. This approach does not allow acromioplasty.

15.4.3 Wound Closure

If the coracoacromial ligament and deltoid are detached, they are reattached to the acromion together with the deltoid by periosteal or transosseous suture. The deltoid is closed with a continuous suture.

15.4.4 Dangers

The axillary nerve is at risk if the incision continues too far caudally.

15.4.5 Note

The Neer anterosuperior approach gives a better cosmetic result than the Bigliani anterolateral approach as it is guided more by skin crease lines.

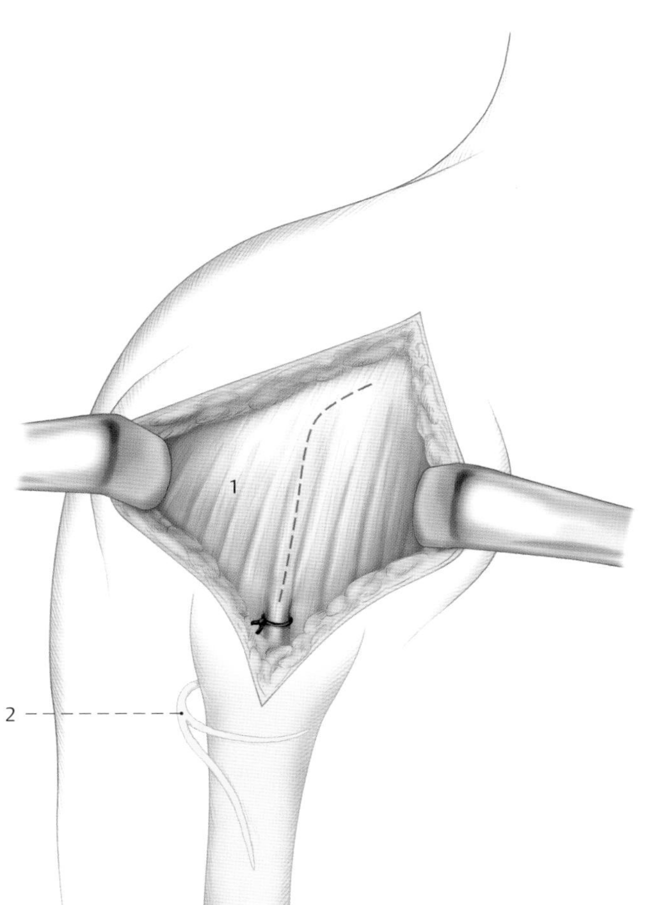

Fig. 15.18 Splitting of the deltoid.

1 Deltoid
2 Axillary nerve

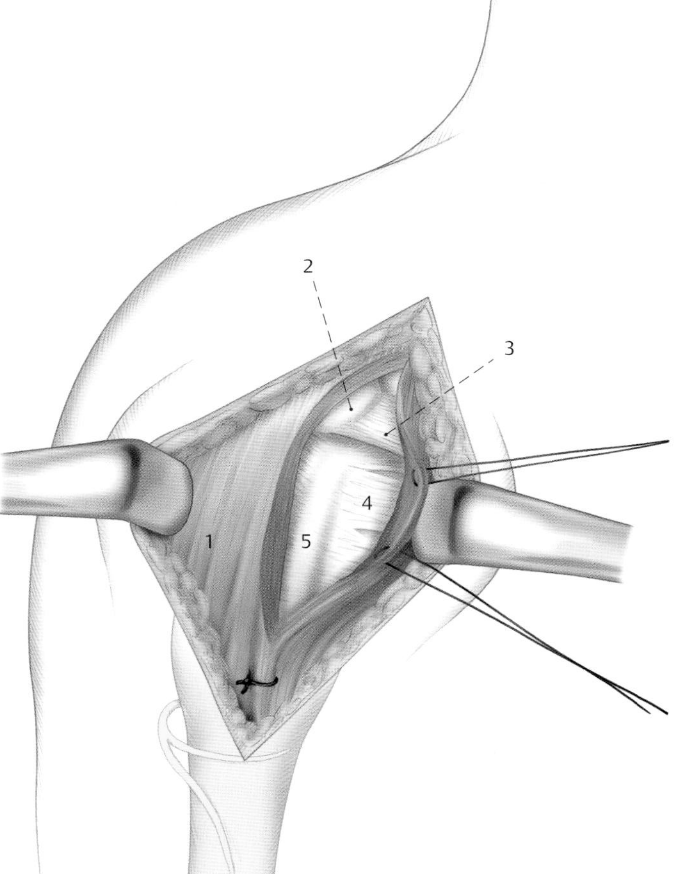

Fig. 15.19 Bigliani anterolateral approach. Exposure of the border of the acromion with cranial parts of the rotator cuff.

1 Deltoid
2 Acromion
3 Coracoacromial ligament
4 Subscapularis tendon
5 Long head of biceps brachii

15.5 Posterosuperior Approach According to Gschwend

K. Weise, K. Häringer

15.5.1 Principal Indication

- Rotator cuff injuries in the region of the supraspinatus and infraspinatus

15.5.2 Positioning and Incision

The patient is placed on his or her side, and the arm is draped to allow free movement.

The skin incision begins in the middle of the supraspinous fossa and continues laterally for approximately 5 cm somewhat anterior to the center of the acromion toward the acromial part of the deltoid (**Fig. 15.20**).

15.5.3 Exposure of the Rotator Cuff

The fascia of the trapezius and deltoid is split in the line of the fibers parallel to the skin incision. Unlike the now abandoned Debeyre approach, the muscle insertions are detached from the anterior border of the acromion with a piece of bone. After resection of the subacromial bursa, rotation of the arm provides good visualization of the cuff and, if necessary, acromioplasty can be performed.

15.5.4 Wound Closure

The detached muscles are reattached to the acromion with transosseous sutures, and the fascia is approximated with continuous sutures.

15.5.5 Dangers

The suprascapular nerve is at risk during dissection of the supraspinatus and infraspinatus, and the accessory nerve is endangered if the trapezius is injured at the superior angle.

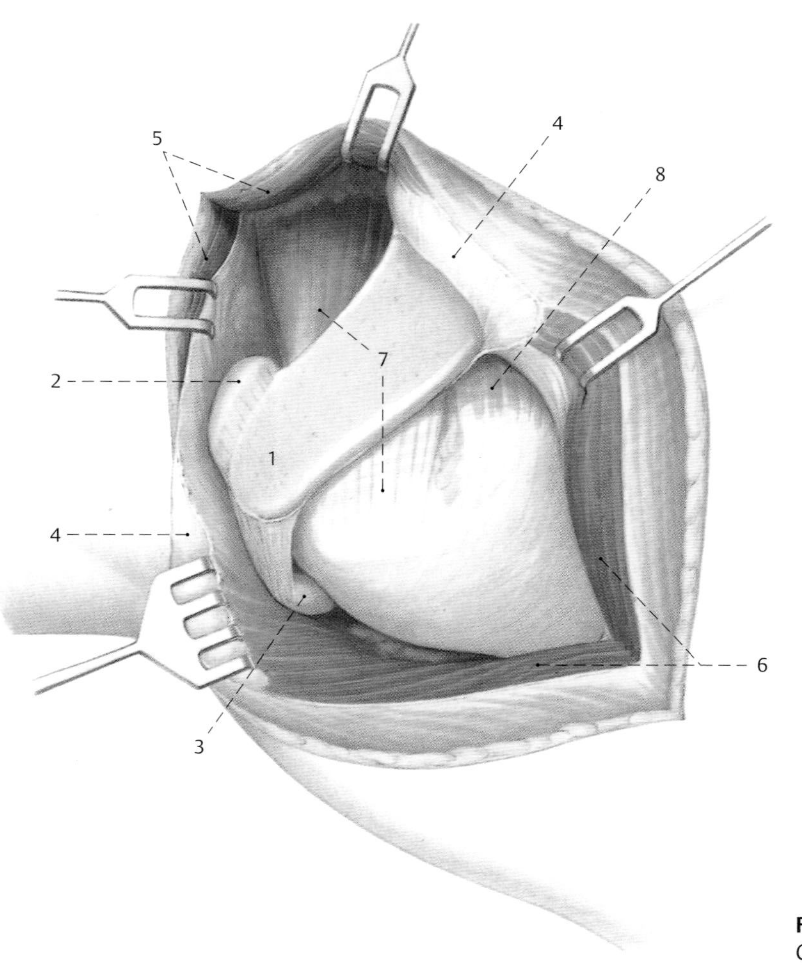

Fig. 15.20 Approach according to Kessel and Gschwend (anterolateral view).

1 Acromion
2 Clavicle
3 Coracoid process
4 Periosteum
5 Trapezius
6 Deltoid
7 Supraspinatus
8 Infraspinatus

15.6 Posterior Approach to the Shoulder Joint

K. Weise, K. Häringer

15.6.1 Principal Indications

- Posterior rotator cuff injuries
- Posterosuperior mass ruptures
- Posterior instability
- Fractures of the posterior glenoid rim

15.6.2 Positioning and Incision

If arthroscopy is performed beforehand, the patient is placed on his or her side, and the arm is draped to allow free movement. Alternatively, the patient is placed in the prone position. A pad is placed beneath the shoulder to be operated on, with the arm freely mobile so that it can be abducted to 90° if necessary with the elbow flexed over the edge of the table. For the anatomical site, see **Fig. 15.21**.

Gartsman Approach

With the patient's arm positioned alongside the body, the skin incision begins at the spine of the scapula over the cranial joint line and continues caudally for approximately 10 cm along the posterior axillary fold. After abducting the arm to 90°, the inferior border of the spinal part of the deltoid is found, and blunt dissection is continued between the deltoid and teres minor. To spare the axillary nerve, it is exposed in the lateral axillary foramen between teres major and teres minor lateral to the long head of the triceps (**Fig. 15.22**). By externally rotating the arm and inserting Hohmann hooks over the greater tubercle and under the deltoid, the insertion of supraspinatus can now be exposed. If necessary, the approach can be extended approximately 5 cm into the axilla, whereby the insertion of latissimus dorsi is elevated for latissimus transfer.

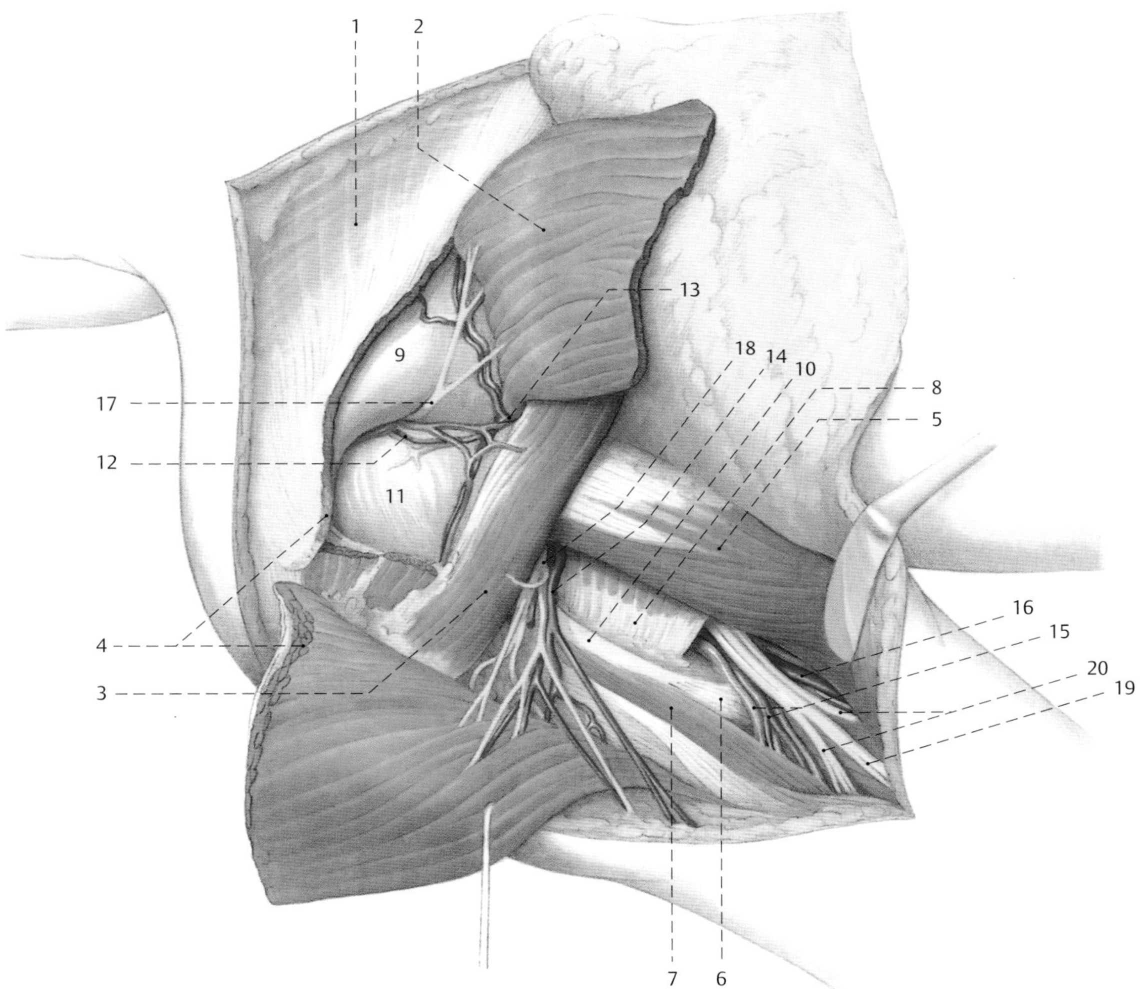

Fig. 15.21 Anatomical site. The deltoid and infraspinatus have been detached to expose the suprascapular, axillary, and radial nerves.

1 Trapezius
2 Infraspinatus
3 Teres minor
4 Deltoid
5 Long head of triceps brachii
6 Medial head of triceps brachii
7 Lateral head of triceps brachii
8 Teres major
9 Scapula
10 Humerus
11 Shoulder joint capsule
12 Suprascapular artery
13 Circumflex artery of scapula
14 Posterior circumflex humeral artery
15 Deep brachial artery and vein
16 Brachial artery
17 Suprascapular nerve
18 Axillary nerve
19 Radial nerve
20 Muscular branches of the radial nerve

Habermeyer/Herzberg Approach

The skin incision begins at the spine of the scapula over the cranial joint line, and curves over the posterior joint line for approximately 12 cm toward the inferior axillary fold. The fascia of deltoid, teres major, teres minor, and latissimus dorsi is exposed subcutaneously. To spare the axillary nerve, it is exposed in the lateral axillary foramen between teres major and teres minor lateral to the long head of the triceps (**Fig. 15.23**). The muscle belly of latissimus dorsi is now dissected bluntly from teres major as far as its tendinous insertion on the humerus. To spare the radial nerve, the tendon is divided with a scalpel with the arm abducted and internally rotated.

15.6.3 Wound Closure

The capsule is closed, the muscles are reinserted with interrupted sutures, and the deltoid is closed with a continuous suture. The gap between teres minor and infraspinatus need not be closed.

15.6.4 Dangers

The axillary nerve can be damaged by too much hook pressure in the region of the deltoid muscle on the one hand, and during dissection between the teres minor and teres major muscles on the other. In the upper corner of the wound, the suprascapular nerve that runs along the base of the acromion can be injured by too great a retraction of the infraspinatus.

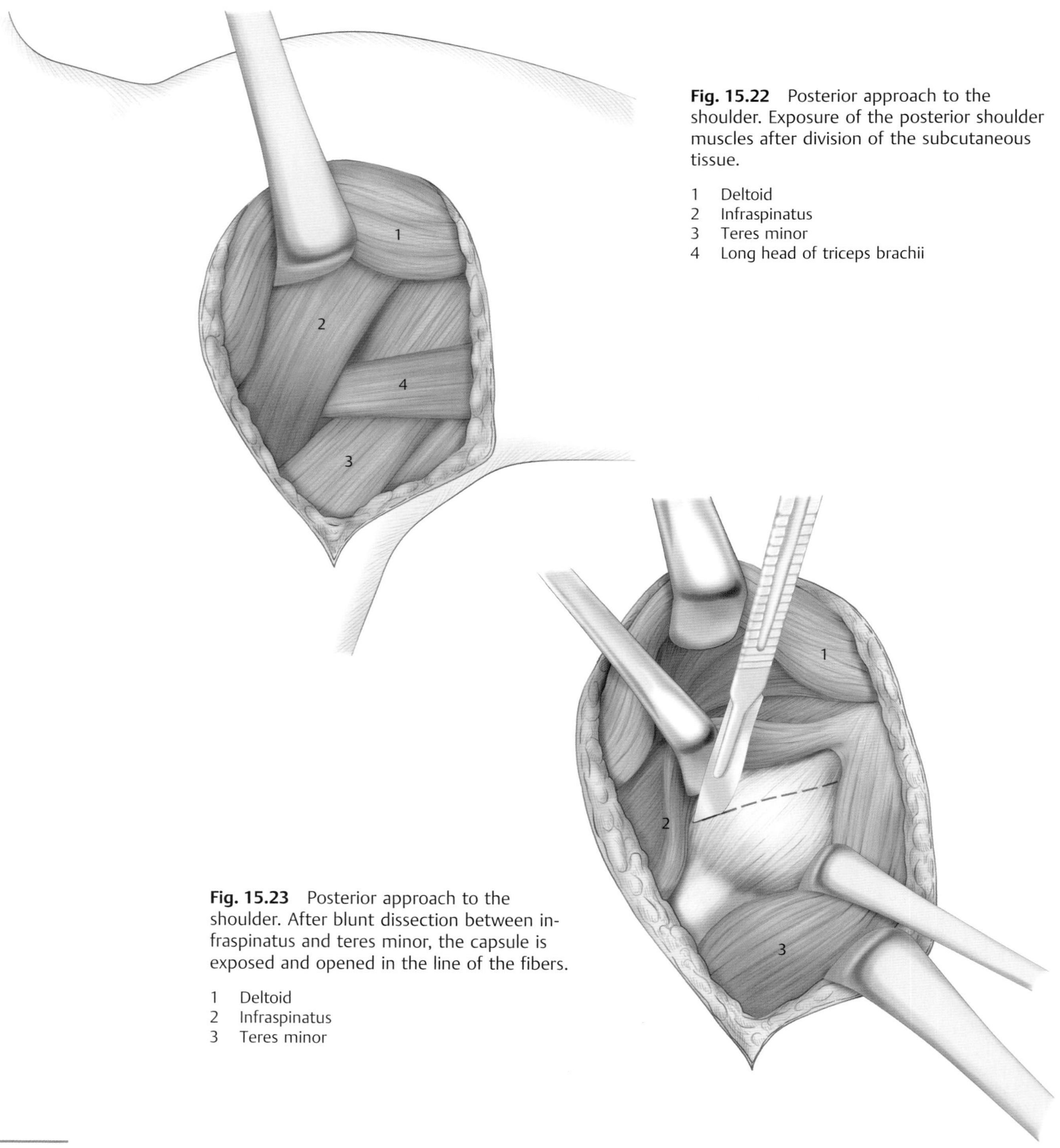

Fig. 15.22 Posterior approach to the shoulder. Exposure of the posterior shoulder muscles after division of the subcutaneous tissue.

1 Deltoid
2 Infraspinatus
3 Teres minor
4 Long head of triceps brachii

Fig. 15.23 Posterior approach to the shoulder. After blunt dissection between infraspinatus and teres minor, the capsule is exposed and opened in the line of the fibers.

1 Deltoid
2 Infraspinatus
3 Teres minor

15.7 Arthroscopic Approach to the Shoulder

D. Kohn

15.7.1 Principal Indications

- Shoulder instability
- Impingement syndromes
- Arthritis of the acromioclavicular joint
- Rotator cuff injuries

15.7.2 Positioning

There are two competing methods, each with its advantages and disadvantages. We use the lateral position with a vacuum mattress and arm harness (**Fig. 15.24**). The upper body is tilted 30° posteriorly, which brings the glenoid cavity into the horizontal position. The operator works "as if on a plate." The arm is placed in 45° of abduction and 15° of anteversion, and is held in a harness. Abduction of 20° is better for access to the subacromial space and the acromioclavicular joint. A padded roll must be placed in the contralateral axilla to prevent overstretching of the brachial plexus on that side. Longitudinal traction with a weight of 5 kg (up to 7.5 kg for muscular patients) is applied to the arm. Symptoms due to overstretching of the brachial plexus are likely if the weight exceeds 10 kg.

The alternative position, preferred by some surgeons, is the beach chair position (**Fig. 15.25**). The patient's arm is draped to allow free movement and is placed on a draped sterile arm support.

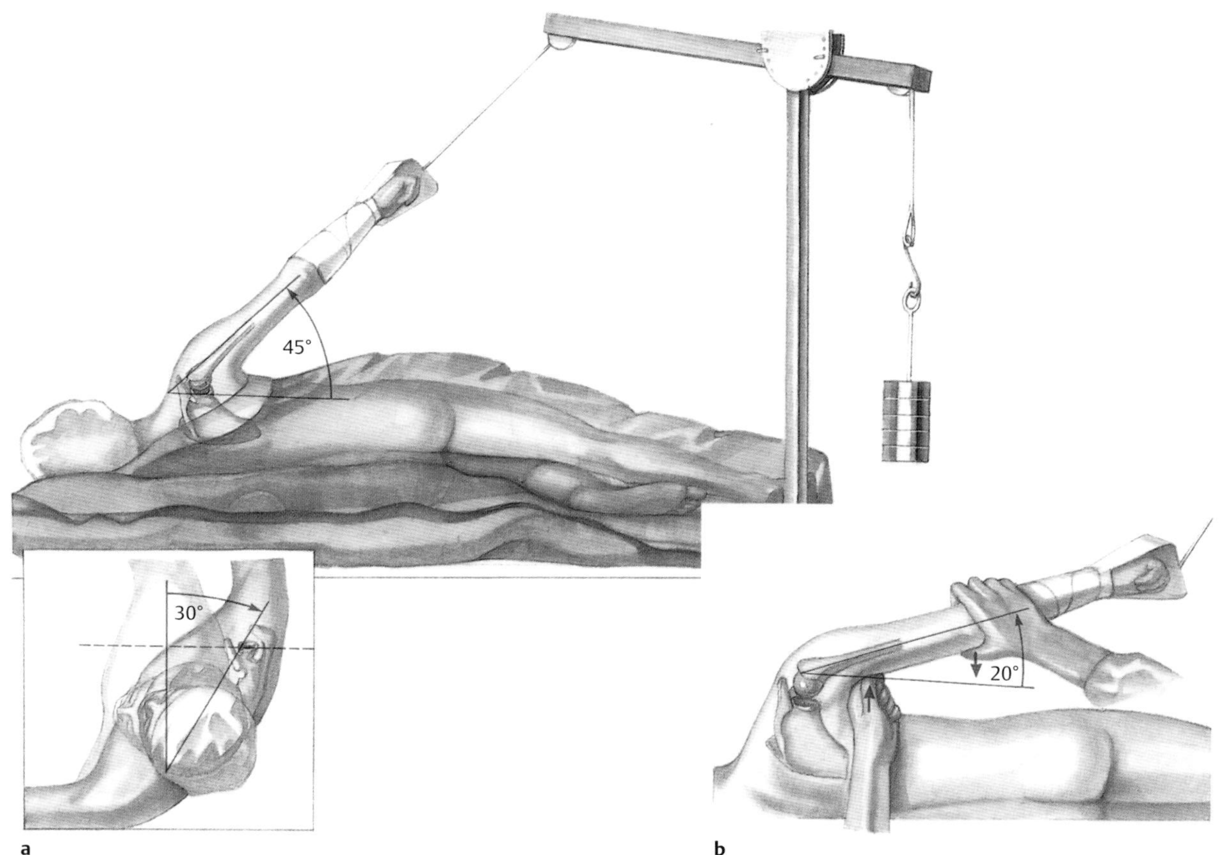

Fig. 15.24 a, b Lateral position for arthroscopy of the glenohumeral joint, subacromial bursa and acromioclavicular joint. (From: Bauer R, Kerschbaumer F, Poisel S. Schulter und obere Extremität. Stuttgart, Thieme; 1997. Orthopädische Operationslehre; Band 3.)

a Patient in the lateral position with the upper body tilted 30° posteriorly. This brings the glenoid cavity into the horizontal position (detail).
b In operations on the anterior wall of the joint, the humeral head is elevated from the glenoid cavity by the assistant.

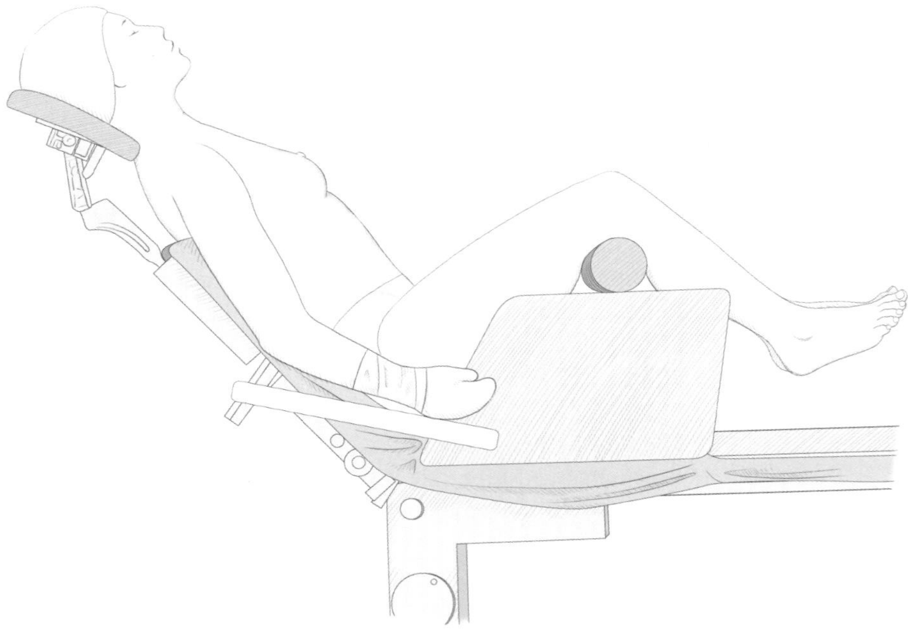

Fig. 15.25 Beach chair position. The forearm rests on an arm board, and the elbow "floats" freely above the arm board. The elbow must not be in contact with the board.

15.7.3 Approaches

The strong periarticular soft tissues make clinical palpation of the shoulder and arthroscopy access difficult. The approaches are long, and a special puncturing technique is required. Furthermore, the important suprascapular, axillary, and musculocutaneous nerves are located in the vicinity of the portals. If the cephalic vein is injured, it must be exposed and ligated. The posterior approach is the most important portal to the joint and subacromial bursa (**Fig. 15.26a**). Shoulder arthroscopy begins with introduction of the arthroscope at this site.

Approaches to the shoulder are defined by the following bony landmarks:

- Posterior approach: 2 cm distal and medial to the posterosuperior angle of the acromion
- Superior approach: in the "bay" formed by the spine of the scapula, acromion, and lateral end of the clavicle
- Lateral approach: in an extension of the anterior border of the clavicle 4 cm lateral to the lateral border of the acromion

Other approaches (**Fig. 15.26b**) are defined by intra-articular landmarks and are created either from within outward using a Wissinger rod, or in the opposite direction by first probing with a long needle.

This is the anterior approach in the triangle between the anterior labrum, the upper border of the subscapularis, and the biceps tendon, with the anterior superior portal (**Fig. 15.27**) in the angle between the upper border of subscapularis, the anterior labrum, and the anterior border of the supraspinatus tendon.

The anterior inferior portal is close to the musculocutaneous nerve and brachial plexus. Its use is therefore less advisable.

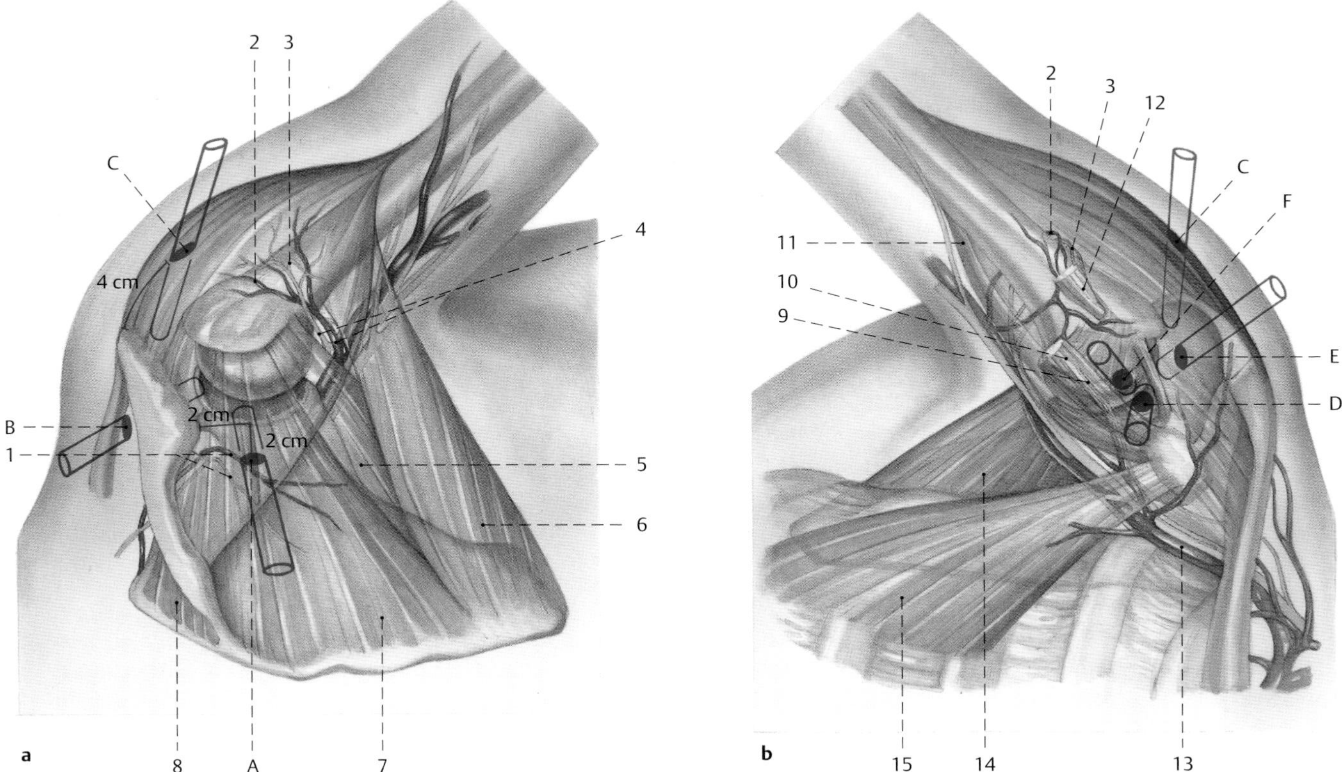

Fig. 15.26 a, b Approaches with the lateral decubitus position. (From: Bauer R, Kerschbaumer F, Poisel S. Schulter und obere Extremität. Stuttgart, Thieme; 1997. Orthopädische Operationslehre; Band 3.)

A Posterior approach
B Superior approach
C Lateral approach
D Anterior approach
E Anterosuperior approach
F Anteroinferior approach

1 Suprascapular artery and nerve
2 Posterior circumflex humeral artery, muscular branch
3 Axillary nerve, deltoid branch
4 Posterior circumflex humeral artery and axillary nerve
5 Teres minor
6 Teres major
7 Infraspinatus
8 Supraspinatus
9 Musculocutaneous nerve
10 Short head of biceps brachii
11 Coracobrachialis
12 Long head of biceps brachii
13 Axillary artery
14 Subscapularis
15 Pectoralis minor

a Posterior view.
b Anterior view.

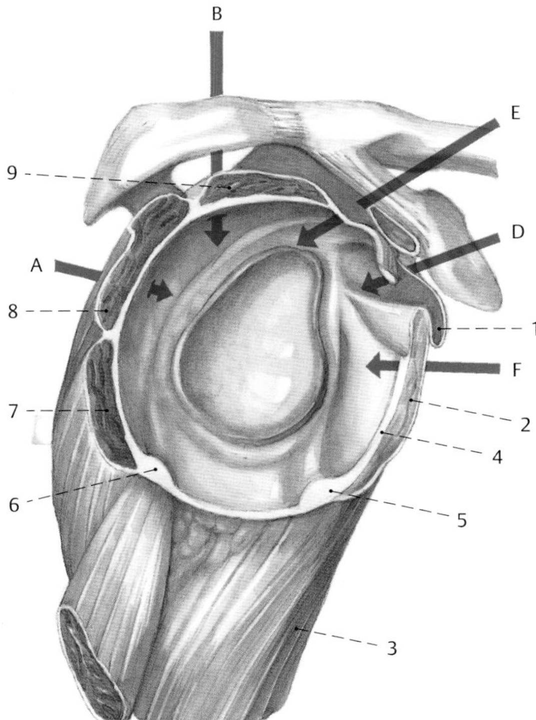

Fig. 15.27 Summary of approaches, with the joint opened laterally, after removal of the head of the humerus. (From: Bauer R, Kerschbaumer F, Poisel S. Schulter und obere Extremität. Stuttgart, Thieme; 1997. Orthopädische Operationslehre; Band 3.)

1 Subcoracoid bursa
2 Tendon of subscapularis
3 Subscapularis
4 Middle glenohumeral ligament
5 Inferior glenohumeral ligament, anterior part
6 Inferior glenohumeral ligament, posterior part
7 Teres minor
8 Infraspinatus
9 Supraspinatus
A–F Approaches, see **Fig. 15.28**

15.7.4 Incision

The bony contours are drawn (**Fig. 15.28**). The arm is internally rotated by the assistant, and the soft depression corresponding to the posterior approach is palpated. An 8 mm skin incision is made in the line of the skin creases. The left index finger is placed on the tip of the coracoid process (**Fig. 15.29**), and the muscle is penetrated with a sharp trocar inserted into the trocar sleeve until the firm resistance of the joint capsule is met. The sharp trocar is exchanged for a blunt one, which is used to palpate the angle formed by the glenoid rim and the head of the humerus (**Fig. 15.30**). The trocar is then pushed into this angle, aiming toward the tip of the coracoid process. The arthroscope is introduced into its sleeve. Following visual identification of the joint space, it is filled with Ringer lactate at a pressure of 50 mmHg.

For diagnostic arthroscopy, an outflow cannula must next be introduced through the superior approach. The cranial "bay" is palpated, and a stab incision is made at its center. A long size 1 needle is inserted, directed toward the tip of the arthroscope. The arthroscope's line of vision is in a cranial direction to ensure that the needle penetrates the capsule before injuring the biceps tendon (**Fig. 15.31**). When the needle is correctly positioned, it is replaced by the larger outflow cannula. The procedure continues with a steady flow of fluid through the joint.

Before introducing the palpating hook, diagnostic arthroscopy is performed. However, the approach for the palpating hook is described here: the arthroscope is advanced into the triangle formed by the superior border of the subscapularis tendon, biceps tendon, and labrum. The long needle punctures the skin where it is transilluminated, the arthroscope is with-

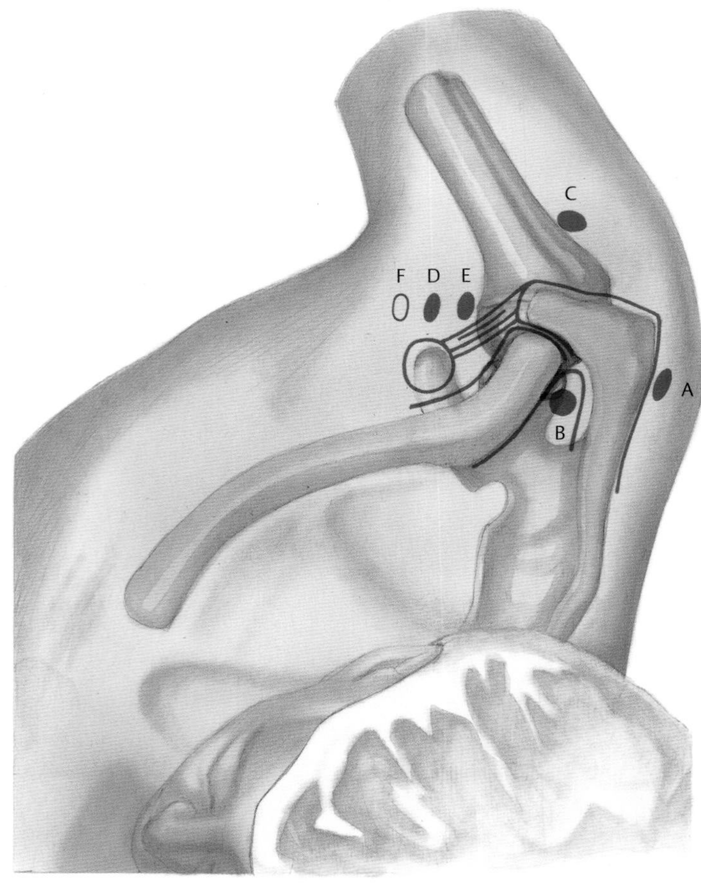

Fig. 15.28 The palpable bony contours and the planned approaches are drawn. (From: Bauer R, Kerschbaumer F, Poisel S. Schulter und obere Extremität. Stuttgart, Thieme; 1997. Orthopädische Operationslehre; Band 3.)

A Posterior approach
B Superior approach
C Lateral approach
D Anterior approach
E Anterosuperior approach
F Anteroinferior approach

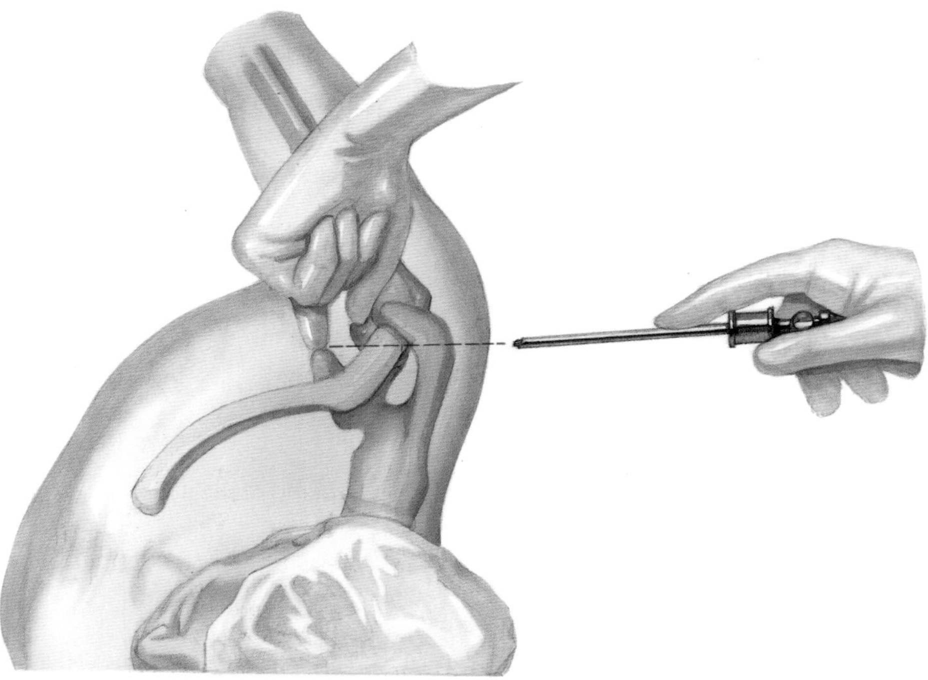

Fig. 15.29 Posterior approach. This points toward the tip of the coracoid process. (From: Bauer R, Kerschbaumer F, Poisel S. Schulter und obere Extremität. Stuttgart, Thieme; 1997. Orthopädische Operationslehre; Band 3.)

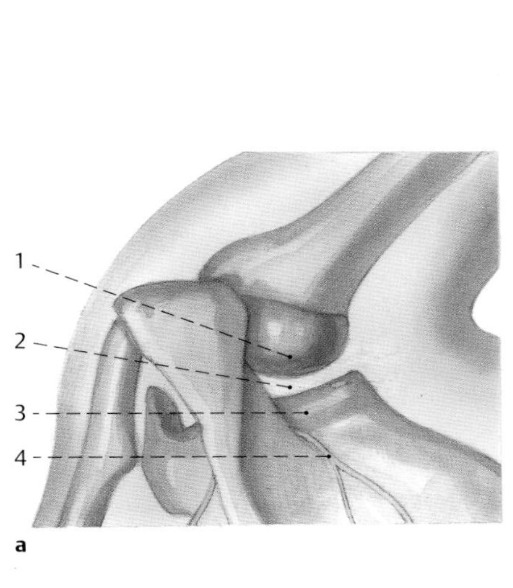

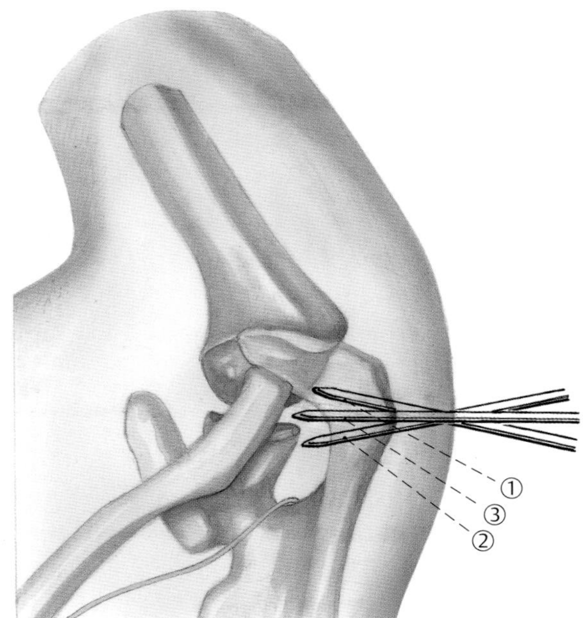

Fig. 15.30 a, b Posterior approach. (From: Bauer R, Kerschbaumer F, Poisel S. Schulter und obere Extremität. Stuttgart, Thieme; 1997. Orthopädische Operationslehre; Band 3.)

a 1 Head of the humerus
2 Joint line
3 Glenoid cavity
4 Suprascapular nerve

b Head of humerus ① and glenoid rim ② are palpated with the blunt trocar. The entry portal to the joint is between them ③.

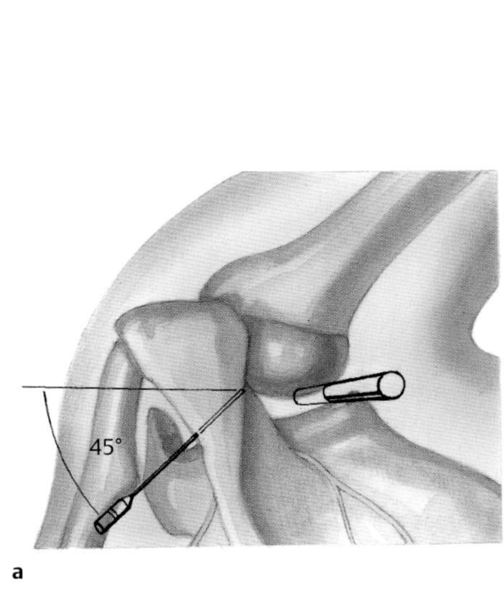

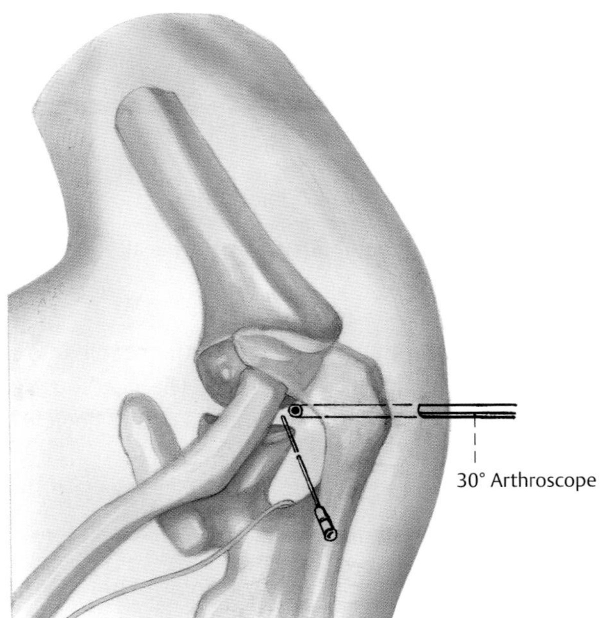

Fig. 15.31 a, b Introduction of outflow cannula under arthroscopic vision. (From: Bauer R, Kerschbaumer F, Poisel S. Schulter und obere Extremität. Stuttgart, Thieme; 1997. Orthopädische Operationslehre; Band 3.)

a Posterior view.
b Cranial view.

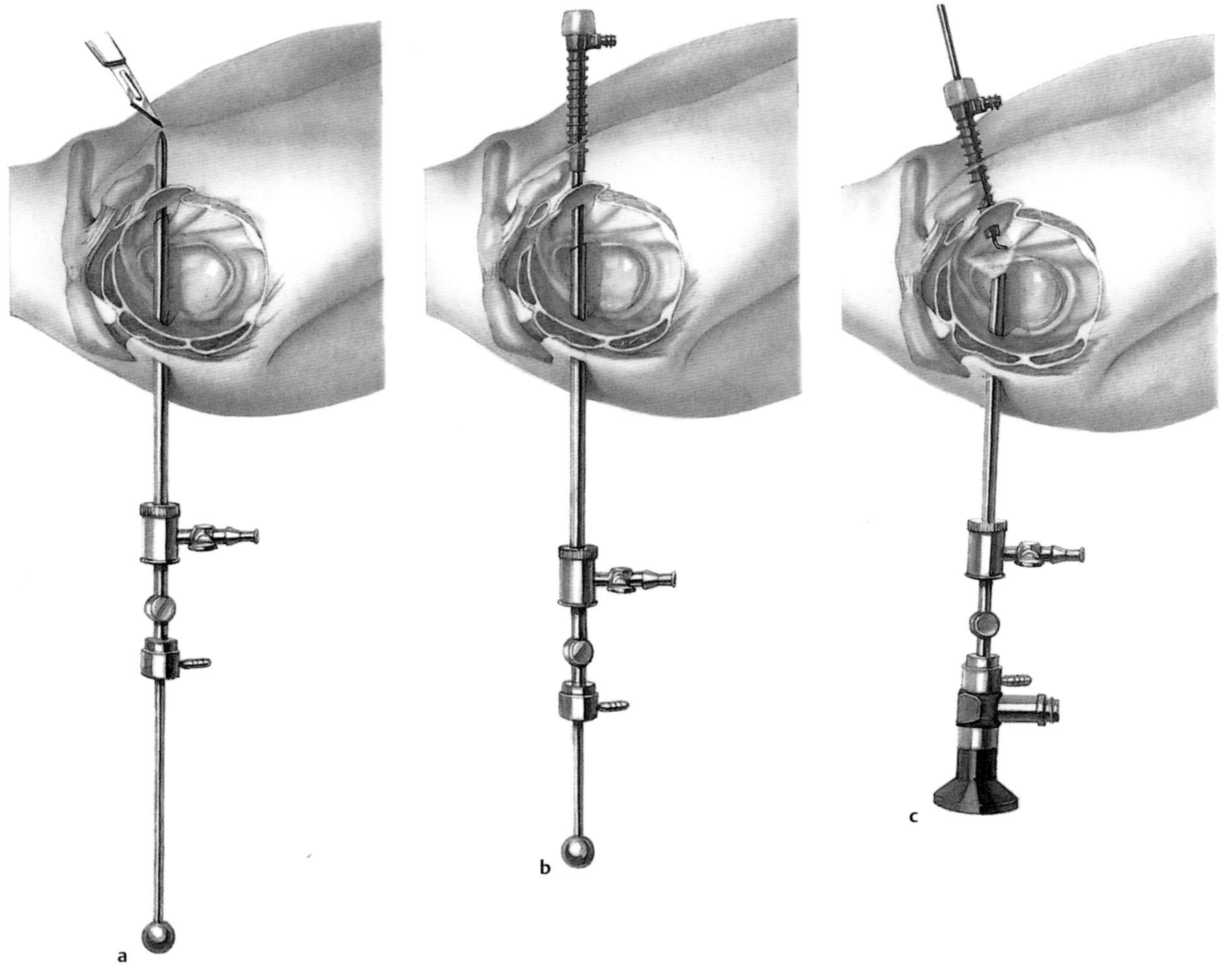

Fig. 15.32 a–c Creating the anterior approach using a Wissinger rod. (From: Bauer R, Kerschbaumer F, Poisel S. Schulter und obere Extremität. Stuttgart, Thieme; 1997. Orthopädische Operationslehre; Band 3.)

a Counterincision.
b Insertion of the working cannula.
c Insertion of the arthroscope and palpating hook.

drawn 1 cm, and the penetration of the needle into the "anterior shoulder triangle" is observed. The needle is removed, a stab incision is made, and the long palpating hook is advanced.

Figure 15.32 shows an alternative way to create the anterior approach.

After inspecting the shoulder joint, the arthroscope is switched to the subacromial space: the optic is exchanged for a blunt trocar. The trocar is withdrawn from the joint, but not through the deltoid. The fingers of the left hand palpate the surface of the acromion (**Fig. 15.33**). The posterior angle of the acromion is palpated with the blunt trocar. The trocar is then pushed between the acromion and the rotator cuff. The instrument is advanced, moving it to and fro, until the coracoacromial ligament can be felt as definite resistance.

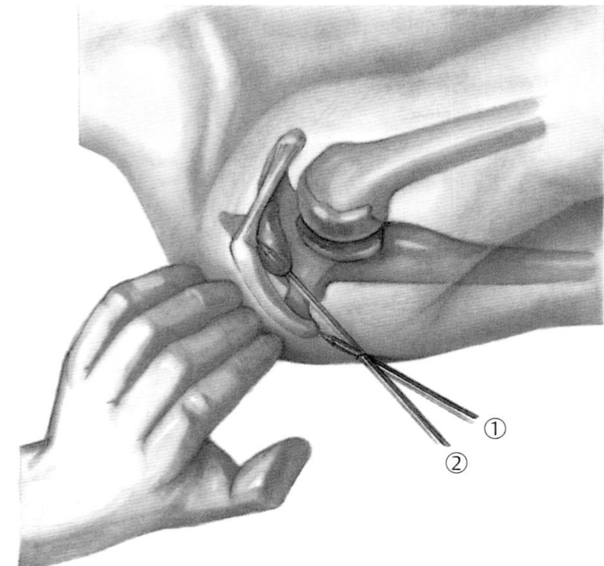

Fig. 15.33 Moving the trocar sleeve to the subacromial space. (From: Bauer R, Kerschbaumer F, Poisel S. Schulter und obere Extremität. Stuttgart, Thieme; 1997. Orthopädische Operationslehre; Band 3.)

Palpating the acromion ①
and inserting the instrument ②.

16 Humerus

16.1 Proximal Approach to the Humerus

K. Weise, K. Häringer

16.1.1 Principal Indications

- Fractures
- Pseudarthrosis

16.1.2 Positioning and Incision

The patient is placed in the beach chair position on the shoulder table. The arm is draped to allow free movement during the operation, with good access to the shoulder.

The skin incision begins at the anterior border of the acromion and runs laterally for approximately 3 cm over the anterior angle of the acromion to the deltoid (**Fig. 16.1**). The deltoid is split subcutaneously from the anterior border of the acromion (**Fig. 16.2**). The fibers of the deltoid are retracted cautiously in an anterior direction. Opening the subacromial bursa exposes the rotator cuff; this is snared with retaining sutures and then divided between the sutures in the line of its fibers, together with the capsule. This provides a clear view of the head of the humerus (**Fig. 16.3**).

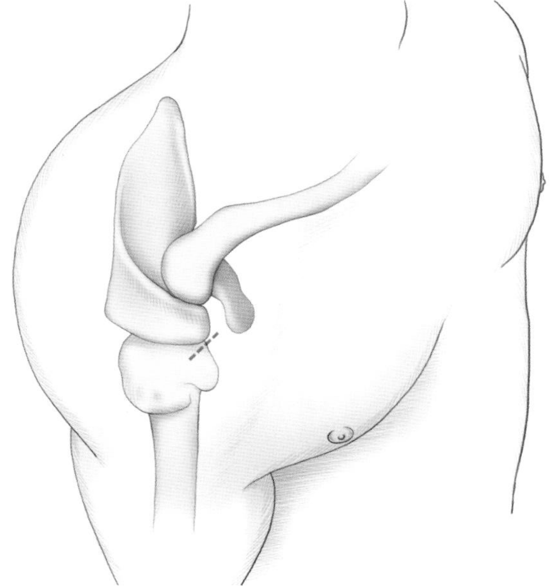

Fig. 16.1 Superior approach for anterograde nailing. Skin incision (right shoulder, oblique view from above)

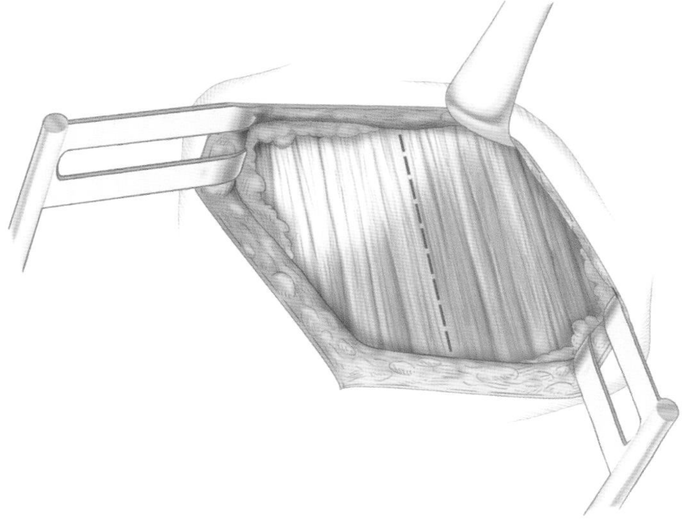

Fig. 16.2 Splitting of the deltoid in the line of its fibers.

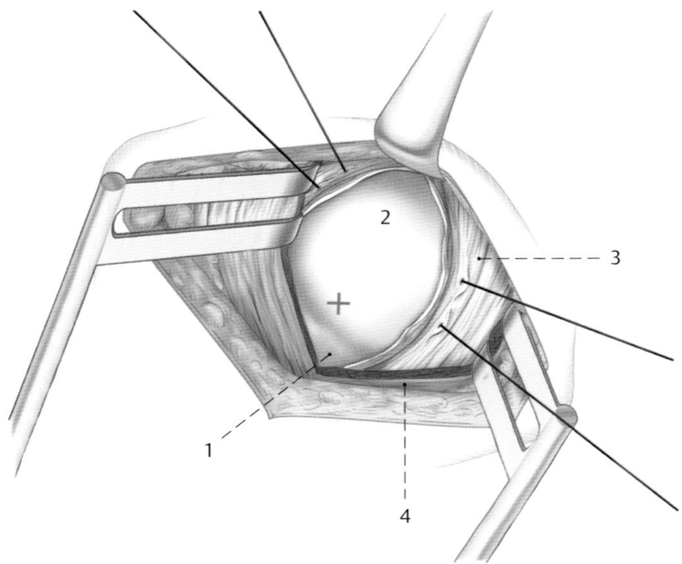

Fig. 16.3 Nail entry site at the highest point of the head of humerus.

1 Greater tubercle
2 Head of humerus
3 Supraspinatus tendon
4 Deltoid
Cross: entry site.

16.1.3 Wound Closure

After an intra-articular Redon drain has been positioned, the rotator cuff is sutured, and the divided parts of the deltoid are reattached with interrupted sutures.

16.1.4 Note

The entry site for proximal medullary nailing is most easily obtained if the arm is freely mobile and hanging down.

16.2 Posterior Approach to the Humerus

K. Weise, K. Häringer

16.2.1 Principal Indications

- Fractures
- Pseudarthrosis
- Tumors
- Inflammation

16.2.2 Positioning and Incision

The patient is placed in the prone position with the upper arm abducted and the elbow flexed. A pad is placed beneath the shoulder. Draping should allow the arm to be moved freely.

The skin incision begins on the posterior aspect 3 cm distal to the acromion and continues to the tip of the olecranon (**Fig. 16.4**). After transection of the subcutaneous tissue, the triceps fascia is divided in the center proximally from the olecranon, and the triceps muscle is then dissected bluntly with a finger and divided sharply from the distal humerus (**Fig. 16.5**). The radial nerve and deep brachial artery can be palpated in the depth of the wound, passing from proximal

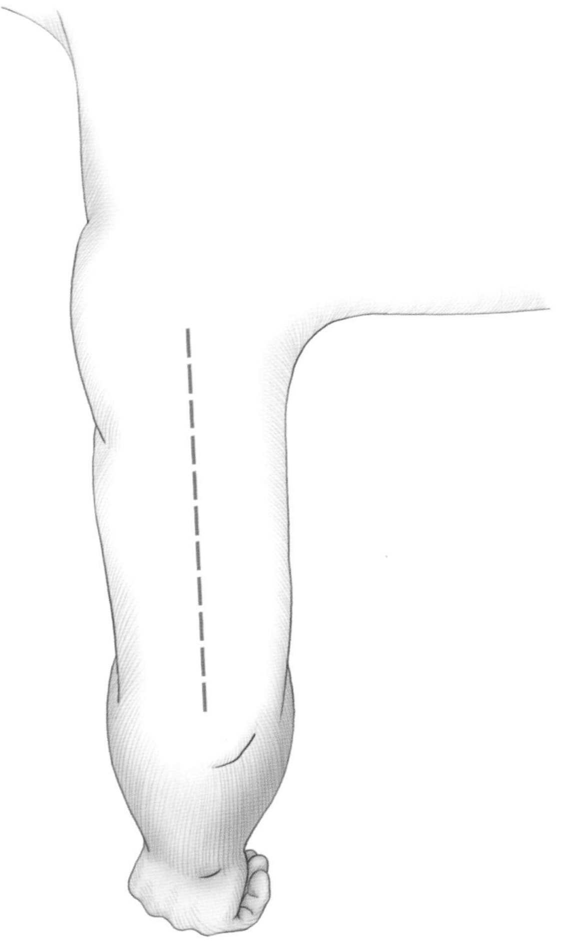

Fig. 16.4 Posterior approach to the humerus, skin incision.

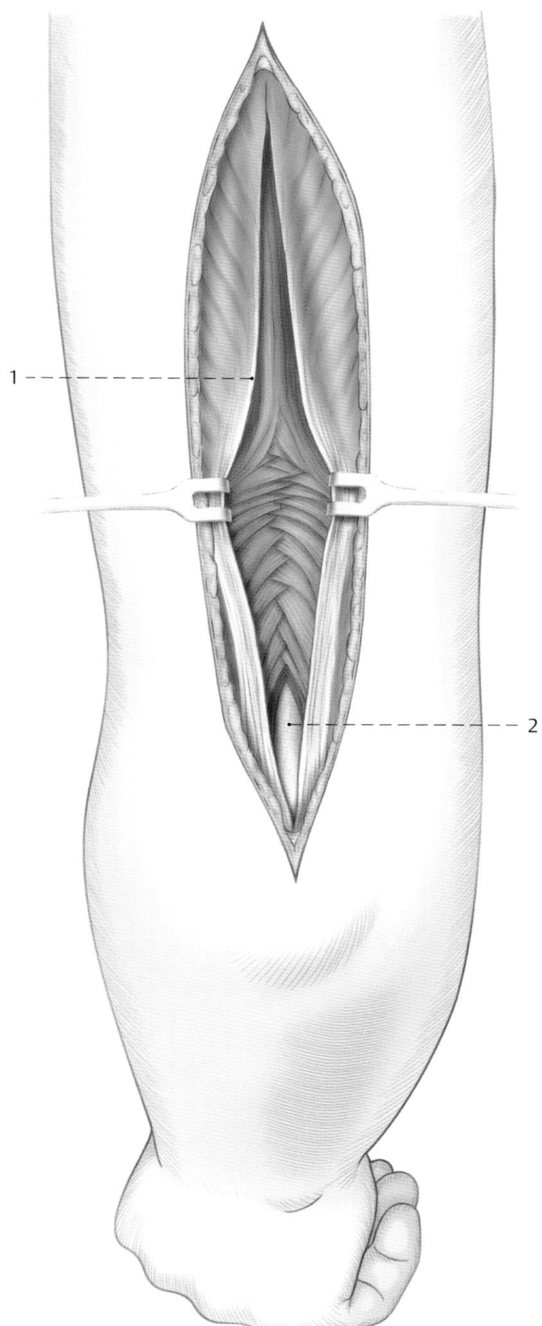

Fig. 16.5 Splitting of the triceps.

1 Triceps brachii
2 Humerus

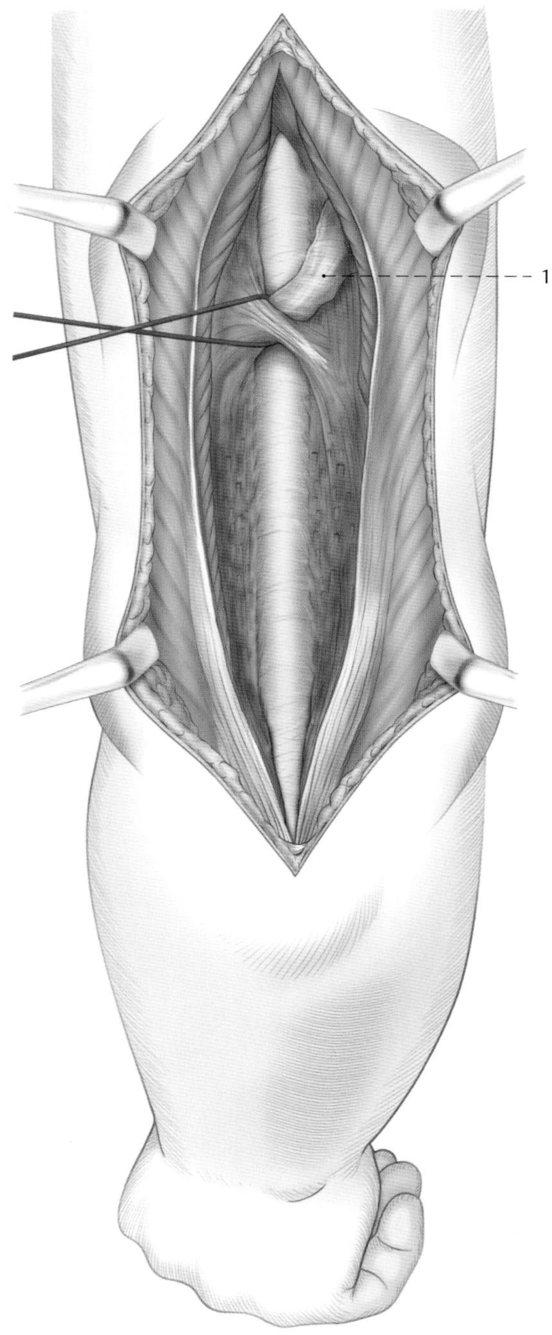

Fig. 16.6 Exposure of the radial nerve with its accompanying vessels.

1 Radial nerve

and medial to distal and lateral. The neurovascular bundle is snared from below and retracted laterally with cautious traction (**Fig. 16.6**). The triceps is then further dissected proximal to this, bluntly at first and then with a raspatory. The neurovascular bundle can be undermined with the raspatory, cautiously retracting it in the medial and distal direction.

16.2.3 Exposure of the Radial Nerve

If exposure of the radial nerve is desired, the lateral intermuscular septum together with the remainder of the adherent medial head of the triceps is split with scissors from proximal to distal, which brings the radial nerve clearly into view.

16.2.4 Anatomical Site

The back of the humerus is covered by a superficial and a deep layer of the triceps. The superficial layer consists of the long and the lateral heads of the triceps, which unite distally at the common tendon insertion. Distal to the sulcus of the radial nerve, nearly the entire posterior aspect of the humerus is covered by the medial head of the triceps. The radial nerve and the accompanying deep brachial artery run in a distal direction in the sulcus of the radial nerve and pierce the lateral intermuscular septum, reaching the flexor side of the upper arm (**Fig. 16.7**). A cross-section of the posterior approach is shown schematically in **Fig. 16.8**.

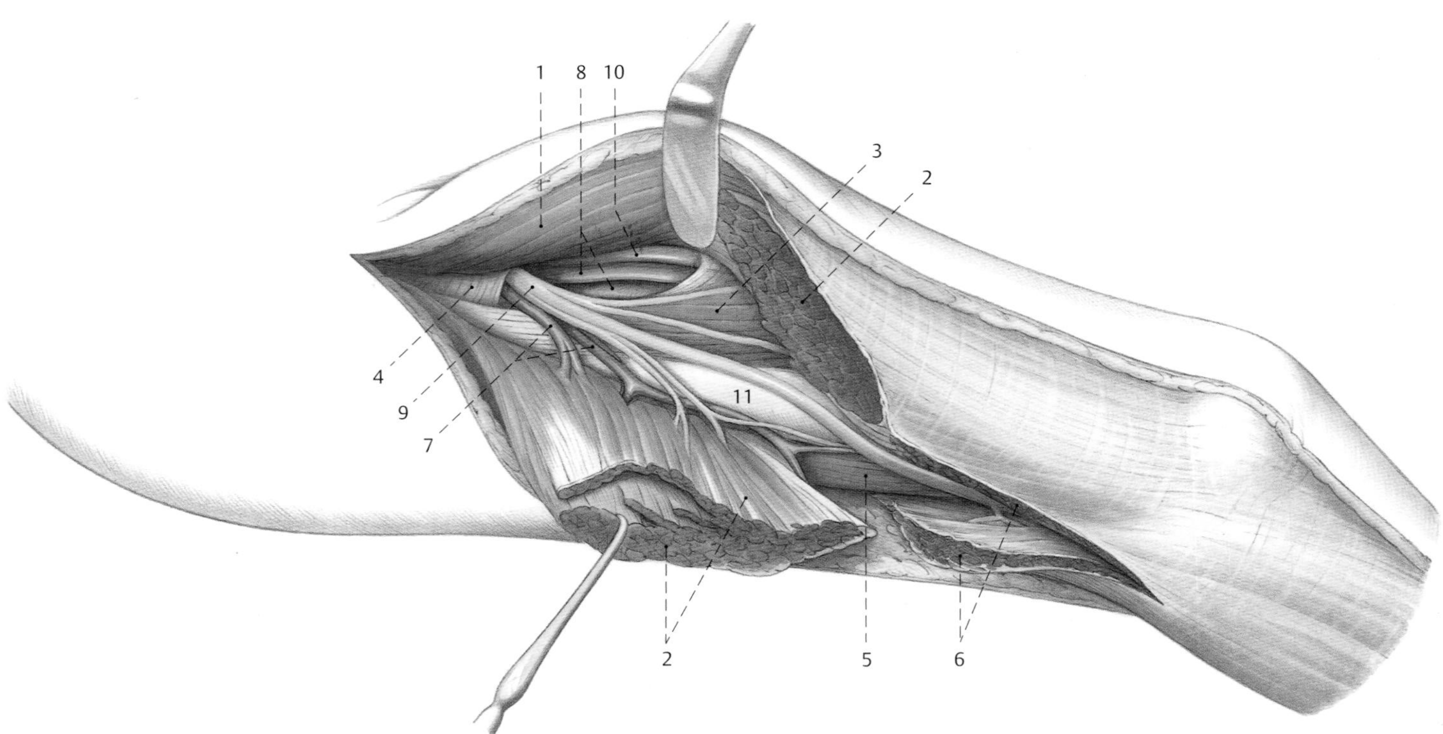

Fig. 16.7 Anatomical site of the medial and posterior aspects of the humerus with the radial nerve. For better exposure of the radial nerve, the lateral head of triceps has been transected. Note also the position and course of the ulnar nerve and of the brachial artery medial to the triceps.

1 Long head of triceps brachii
2 Lateral head of triceps brachii
3 Medial head of triceps brachii
4 Tendon of latissimus dorsi
5 Brachialis
6 Brachioradialis
7 Deep brachial artery and vein
8 Brachial artery and vein
9 Radial nerve
10 Ulnar nerve
11 Body of humerus

16.2.5 Wound Closure

The triceps fascia is closed with a continuous suture after insertion of a Redon drain.

16.2.6 Dangers

The radial nerve on the lateral side and the ulnar nerve on the medial distal side may be damaged during dissection of the humerus (**Fig. 16.8**; see also **Fig. 16.21**). Before splitting the deep-lying medial head of the triceps, care should be taken not to injure the muscular branches issuing from the radial nerve. In the proximal wound region, the cutaneous branches emerging at the distal end of the deltoid muscle must be spared.

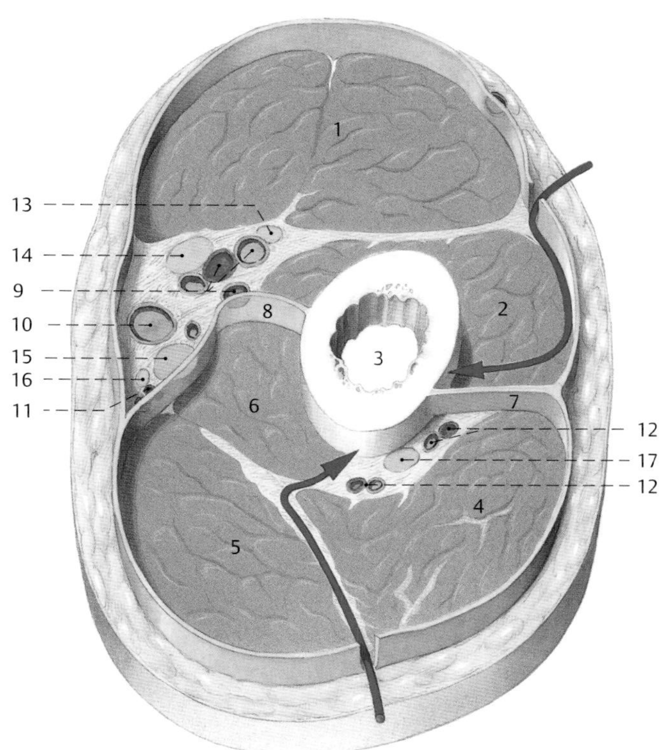

Fig. 16.8 Anatomical site. Schematic cross-section through the proximal upper arm. The posterior and lateral approaches are identified by arrows (right arm, view from proximal side).

1 Biceps brachii
2 Brachialis
3 Humerus
4 Lateral head of triceps brachii
5 Long head of triceps brachii
6 Medial head of triceps brachii
7 Lateral intermuscular septum
8 Medial intermuscular septum
9 Brachial artery and accompanying veins
10 Basilic vein
11 Superior ulnar collateral artery and vein
12 Deep brachial artery and vein
13 Musculocutaneous nerve
14 Median nerve
15 Ulnar nerve
16 Medial cutaneous nerve of forearm
17 Radial nerve

16.3 Distal Posterior Approach to the Humerus

K. Weise, K. Häringer

16.3.1 Principal Indications

- Fractures
- Pseudarthrosis

16.3.2 Positioning and Incision

The patient is placed in the prone position with the arm abducted and the elbow flexed. A pad is placed beneath the shoulder. Draping should allow the arm to be moved freely (**Fig. 16.9**). The skin incision begins approximately 7 cm proximal to the tip of the olecranon on the back of the upper arm and continues in a straight line to the tip of the olecranon. After transection of the subcutaneous tissue, the triceps fascia is opened, the muscle is split bluntly, and the olecranon fossa is exposed using a raspatory (**Fig. 16.10**).

The medullary cavity is opened in the fossa by three drill holes, which are combined into a single hole with a burr (**Fig. 16.11**).

16.3.3 Wound Closure

The triceps fascia is closed with a continuous suture.

16.3.4 Dangers

The ulnar nerve is at risk on the medial side when wound hooks or Hohmann elevators are inserted.

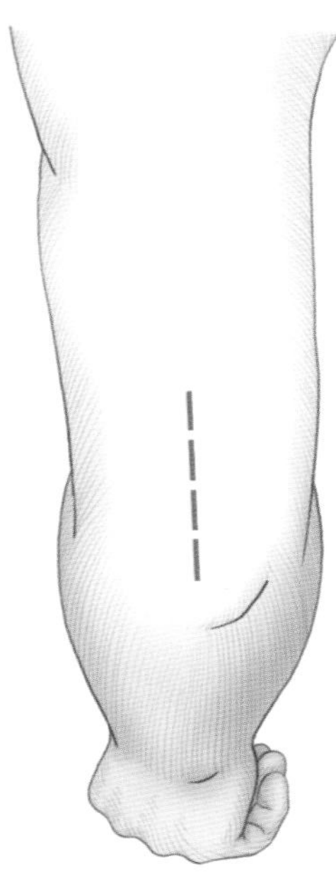

Fig. 16.9 Posterior approach to the medullary cavity for retrograde nailing.

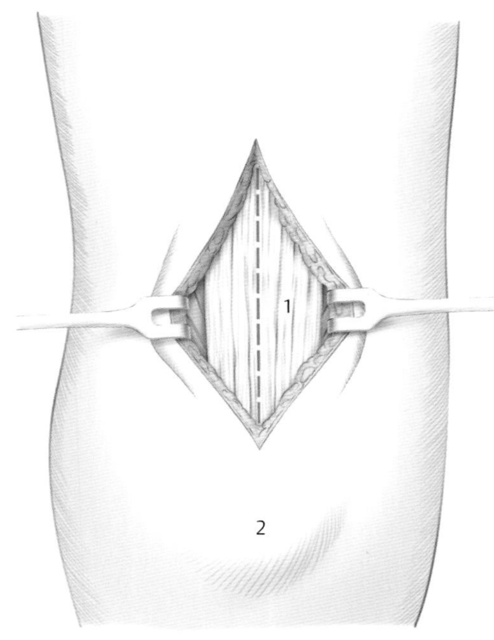

Fig. 16.10 Splitting of triceps tendon.

1 Triceps brachii tendon
2 Olecranon

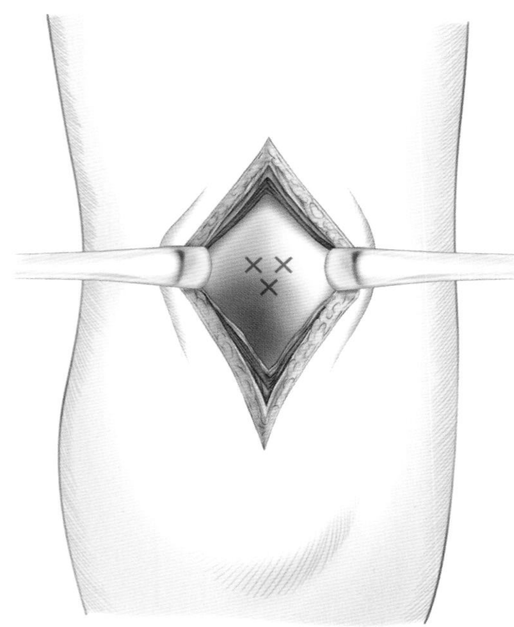

Fig. 16.11 Drill marks for opening the medullary cavity.

16.4 Anterior Approach to the Humerus

R. Bauer, F. Kerschbaumer, S. Poisel, C. J. Wirth

16.4.1 Principal Indications

- Tumors
- Inflammation

The anterior approach is considered to be a standard approach for exposure of the proximal and middle parts of the shaft. Internal fixation using a plate cannot be performed as readily from the anterior as from the posterior side because of the shape of the humerus. A plate can generally be applied laterally, in which case the insertions or origins of the deltoid and brachialis must be detached.

16.4.2 Positioning and Incision

The patient is placed supine with a pad under the shoulder and the forearm adducted (**Fig. 16.12**). In some cases, the upper arm may also be abducted and placed on an arm board. The skin incision begins distal to the tip of the coracoid process, continues distally alongside the deltopectoral groove on the lateral side of the biceps, and ends medially at the level of the elbow. After splitting of the subcutaneous tissue, the fascia is divided from proximal to distal over the deltopectoral groove lateral to the biceps. The deltoid muscle and the cephalic vein are laterally dissected (**Fig. 16.13**).

Now the humeral insertion of the pectoralis major is identified. For clear exposure of the humerus, temporary detachment of the pectoralis major tendon is helpful (**Fig. 16.14**). After the insertion of stay sutures, the tendon may be transected over a grooved director or a curved clamp. Transection of the tendon is not absolutely necessary, however; the humerus may also be exposed on the lateral side of the tendon insertion.

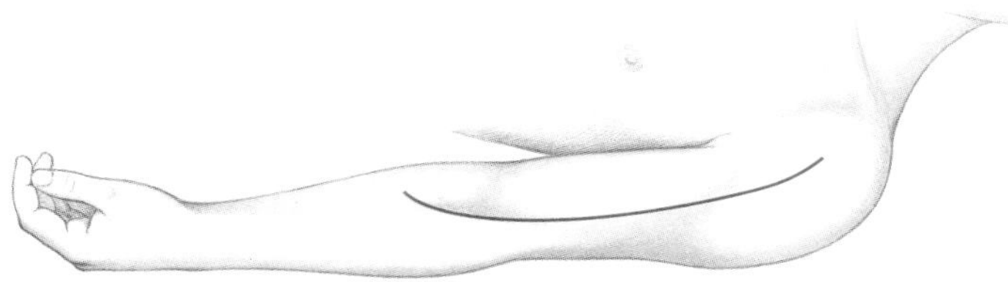

Fig. 16.12 Anterior approach to humerus (left side). Skin incision (solid line).

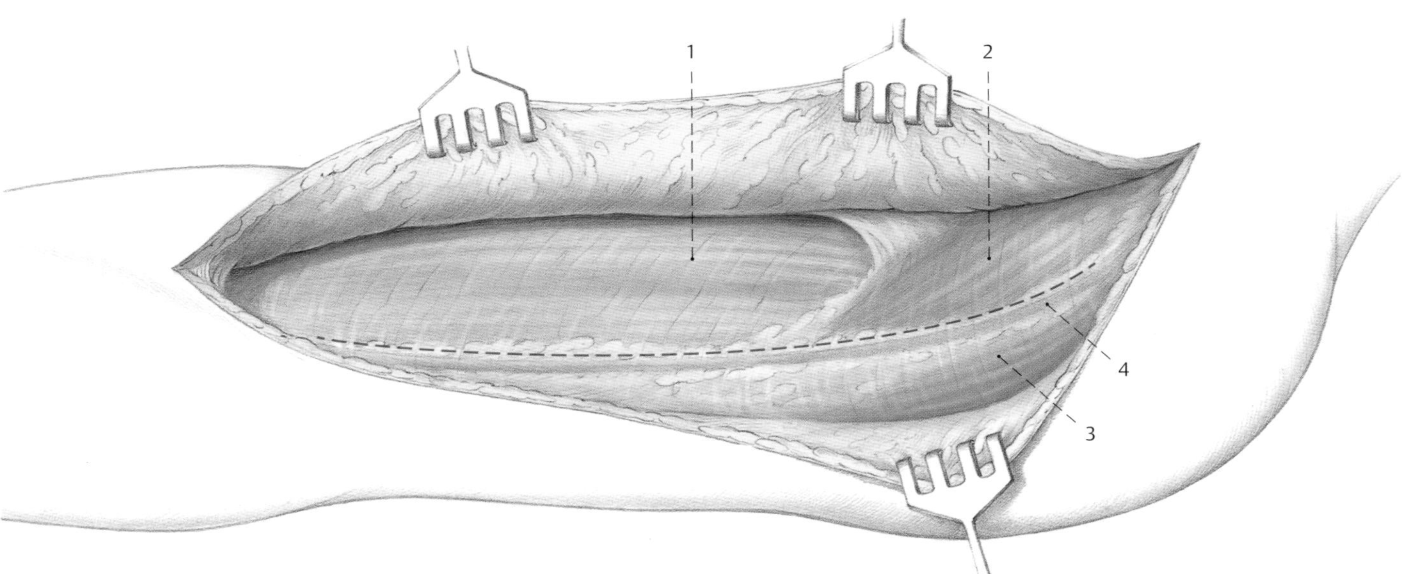

Fig. 16.13 Splitting of the fascia medial to the cephalic vein.

1 Biceps brachii
2 Pectoralis major
3 Deltoid
4 Cephalic vein

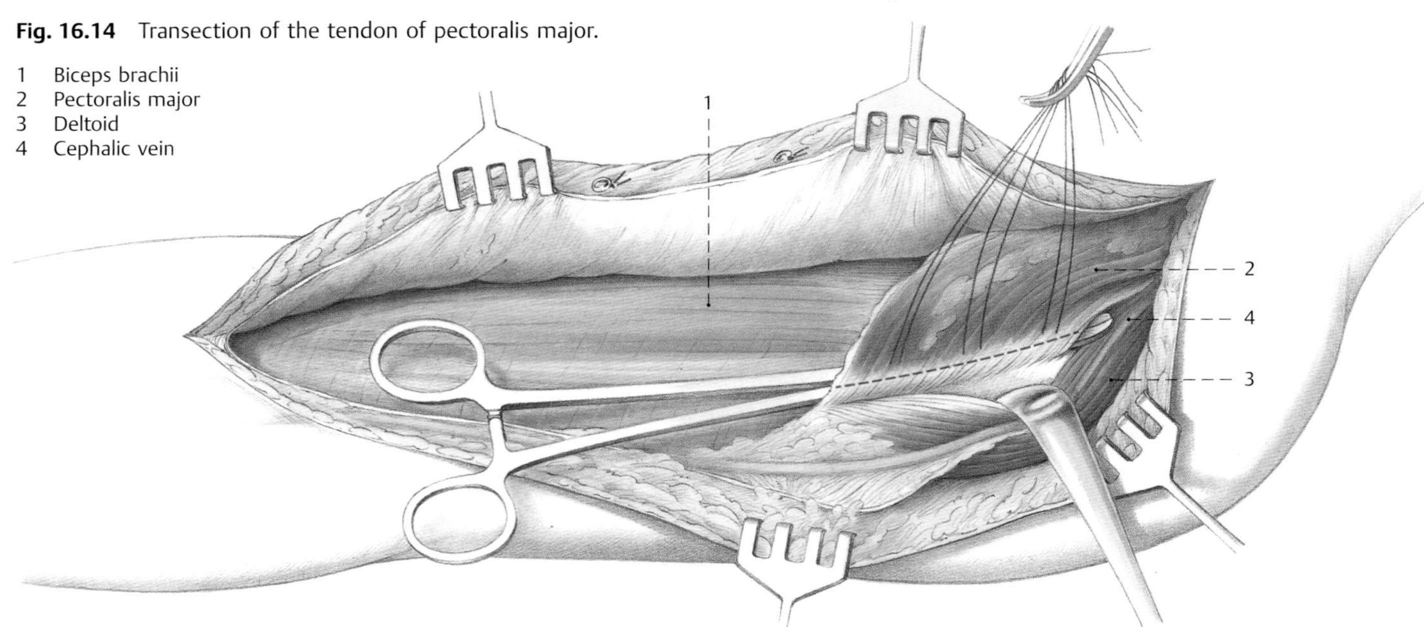

Fig. 16.14 Transection of the tendon of pectoralis major.

1 Biceps brachii
2 Pectoralis major
3 Deltoid
4 Cephalic vein

16.4.3 Anterior Exposure of the Humerus

Medial retraction of the biceps brings into view the subjacent brachialis. This muscle is transected down to the bone about one fingerbreadth lateral to the midline in a longitudinal direction, the point of the scalpel being aimed toward the middle of the humeral shaft (the neural supply of the medial portion of brachialis is via the musculocutaneous nerve, whereas the lateral portion of this muscle is supplied by the radial nerve). Transection by diathermy is inadvisable owing to the immediate proximity of the radial nerve (**Fig. 16.15**). For more distal exposure of the humerus, flexion at the elbow joint is recommended to relax the brachialis muscle. When dissecting the humerus, Langenbeck retractors rather than

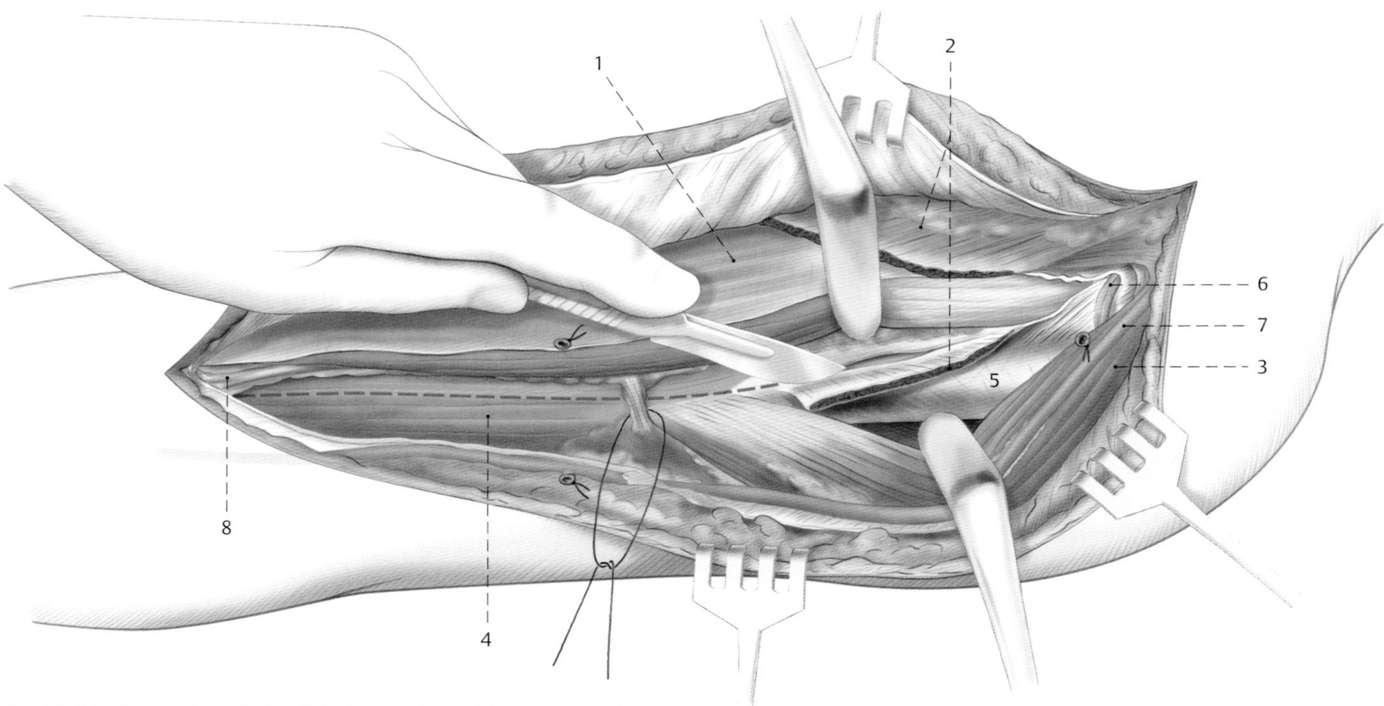

Fig. 16.15 Retraction of the deltoid in a lateral direction, and division of brachialis as far as the periosteum of the humerus (dashed line). The tendon attaching pectoralis major to the bone is left intact for later reinsertion.

1 Biceps brachii
2 Pectoralis major
3 Deltoid
4 Brachialis
5 Body of the humerus
6 Anterior circumflex humeral vessels
7 Cephalic vein
8 Lateral cutaneous nerve of forearm

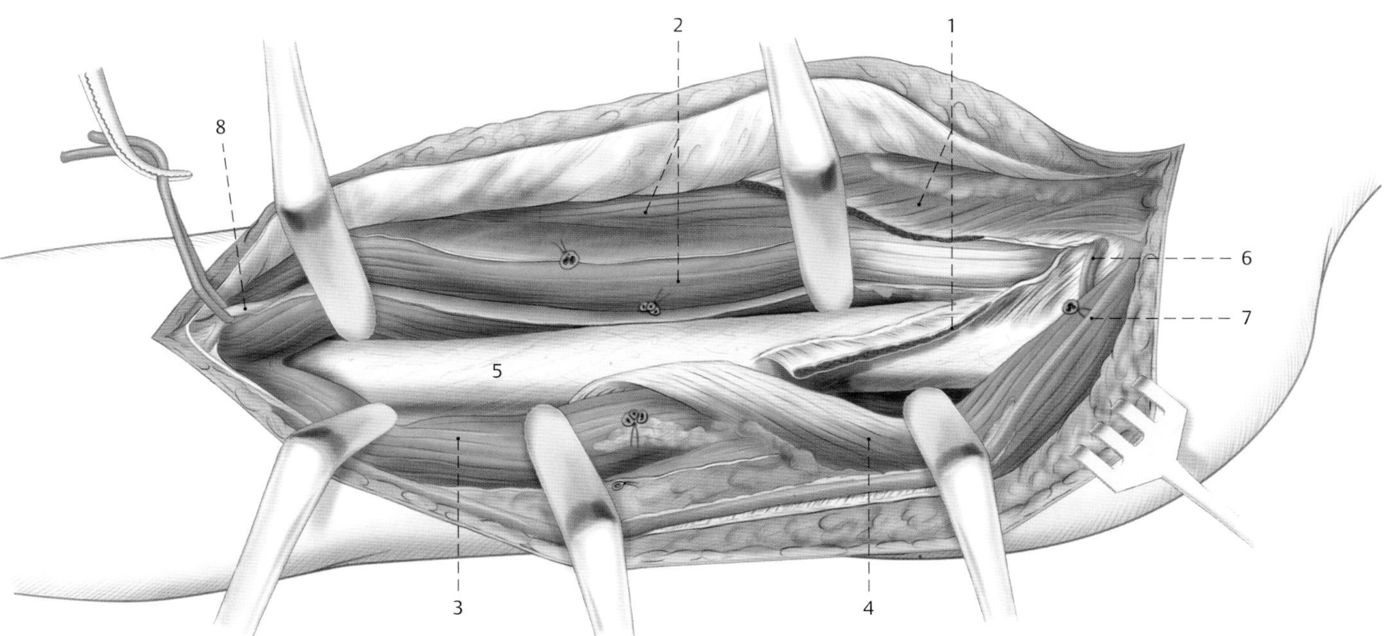

Fig. 16.16 Operative site after exposure of the medial and proximal areas of the humeral shaft.

1 Pectoralis major
2 Biceps brachii
3 Brachialis
4 Deltoid
5 Body of the humerus
6 Anterior circumflex humeral vessels
7 Cephalic vein
8 Lateral cutaneous nerve of forearm

Hohmann elevators should be placed on the lateral side of the bone distal to the insertion of the deltoid so that the radial nerve may be protected (**Fig. 16.16**). If necessary, this approach may also be used to open the shoulder joint capsule anteriorly (see Section 5.1, **Figs. 15.6–15.11**).

16.4.4 Exposure of the Neurovascular Bundle

If exposure of the neurovascular bundle in the bicipital groove is required, the fascia is bluntly dissected with scissors over the neurovascular bundle on the medial side of the short head of the biceps and the coracobrachialis (**Fig. 16.17**). Traction exerted on the coracobrachialis and biceps with a Langenbeck retractor should be moderate so that damage to the musculocutaneous nerve is avoided. If necessary, the median nerve, lying closest to the surface, may be undermined and snared. This nerve overlies the brachial artery and vein and, in the greatest depth, the ulnar nerve (**Fig. 16.18**). The radial nerve can also be exposed in the upper region of the wound.

16.4.5 Dissection of the Radial Nerve

If exposure of the radial nerve is required, this may be accomplished according to Henry one fingerbreadth distal to the insertion of the deltoid by splitting the brachialis longitudinally (**Fig. 16.19**). The radial nerve then becomes visible in the depth between the bands of fibers of the triceps (**Fig. 16.20**).

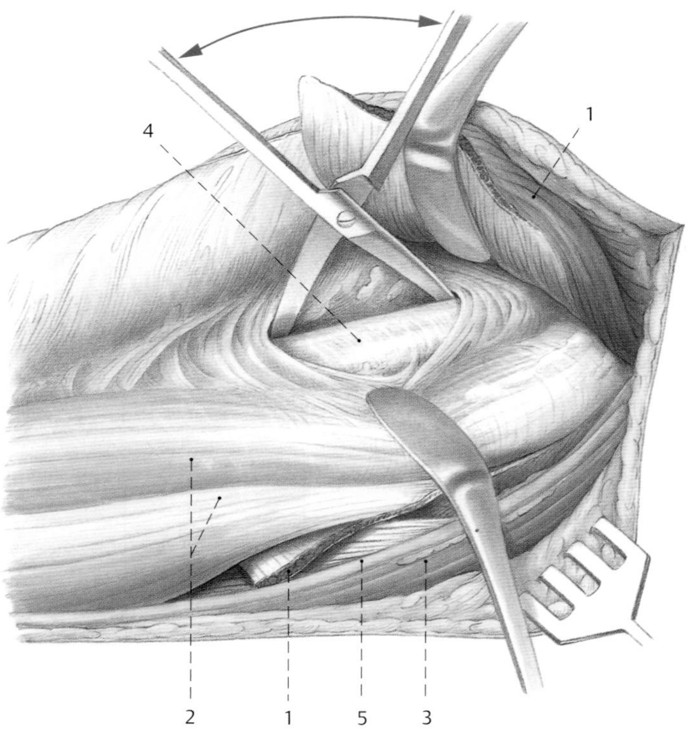

Fig. 16.17 Exposure of the neurovascular bundle medial to biceps and coracobrachialis.

1 Pectoralis major
2 Biceps brachii
3 Deltoid
4 Neurovascular bundle
5 Cephalic vein

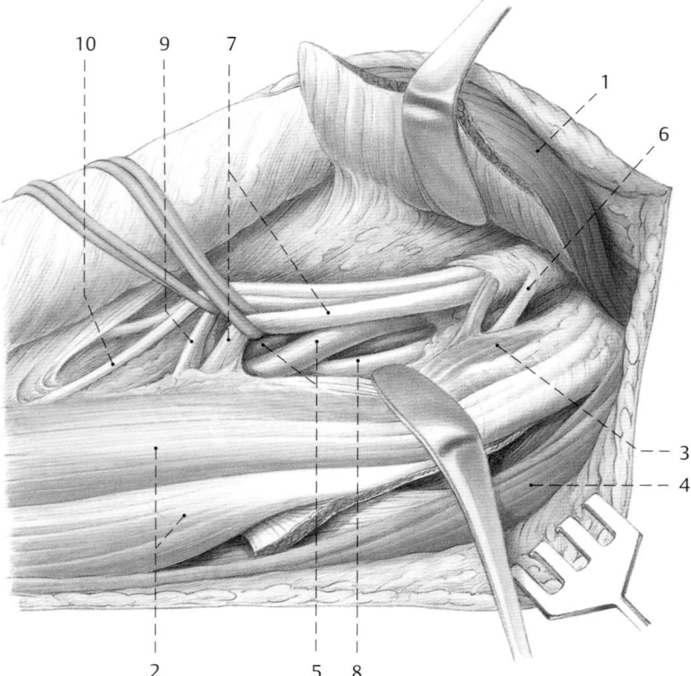

Fig. 16.18 Operative site after encirclement and snaring of the median and ulnar nerves. Exposure of the brachial artery and vein, and radial and musculocutaneous nerves.

1 Pectoralis major
2 Biceps brachii
3 Coracobrachialis
4 Deltoid
5 Brachial vessels
6 Musculocutaneous nerve
7 Median nerve
8 Radial nerve
9 Ulnar nerve
10 Medial cutaneous nerve of forearm

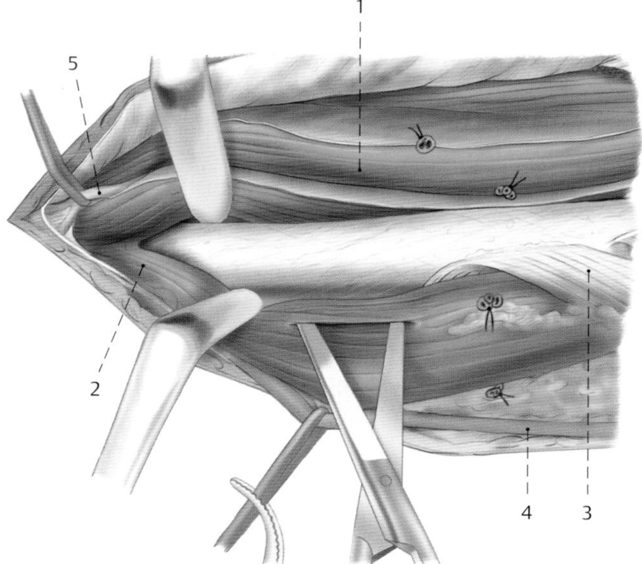

Fig. 16.19 Splitting of brachialis and triceps for exposure of the radial nerve.

1 Biceps brachii
2 Brachialis
3 Deltoid
4 Cephalic vein
5 Lateral cutaneous nerve of forearm

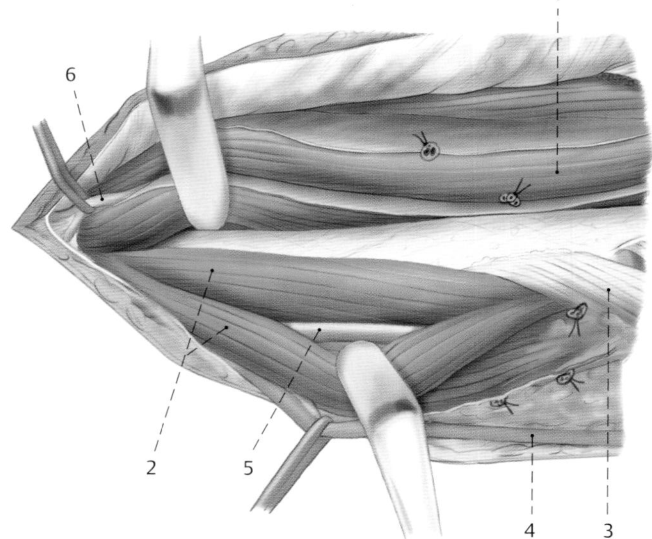

Fig. 16.20 Exposure of the radial nerve.

1 Biceps brachii
2 Brachialis
3 Deltoid
4 Cephalic vein
5 Radial nerve
6 Lateral cutaneous nerve of forearm

16.4.6 Anatomical Site

Figure 16.21 presents the course of the musculocutaneous nerve and its relation to the biceps, coracobrachialis, and brachialis.

Note the course of the brachial artery together with the median nerve, of the deep brachial artery with the radial nerve, and of the superior ulnar collateral artery with the ulnar nerve behind the medial intermuscular septum.

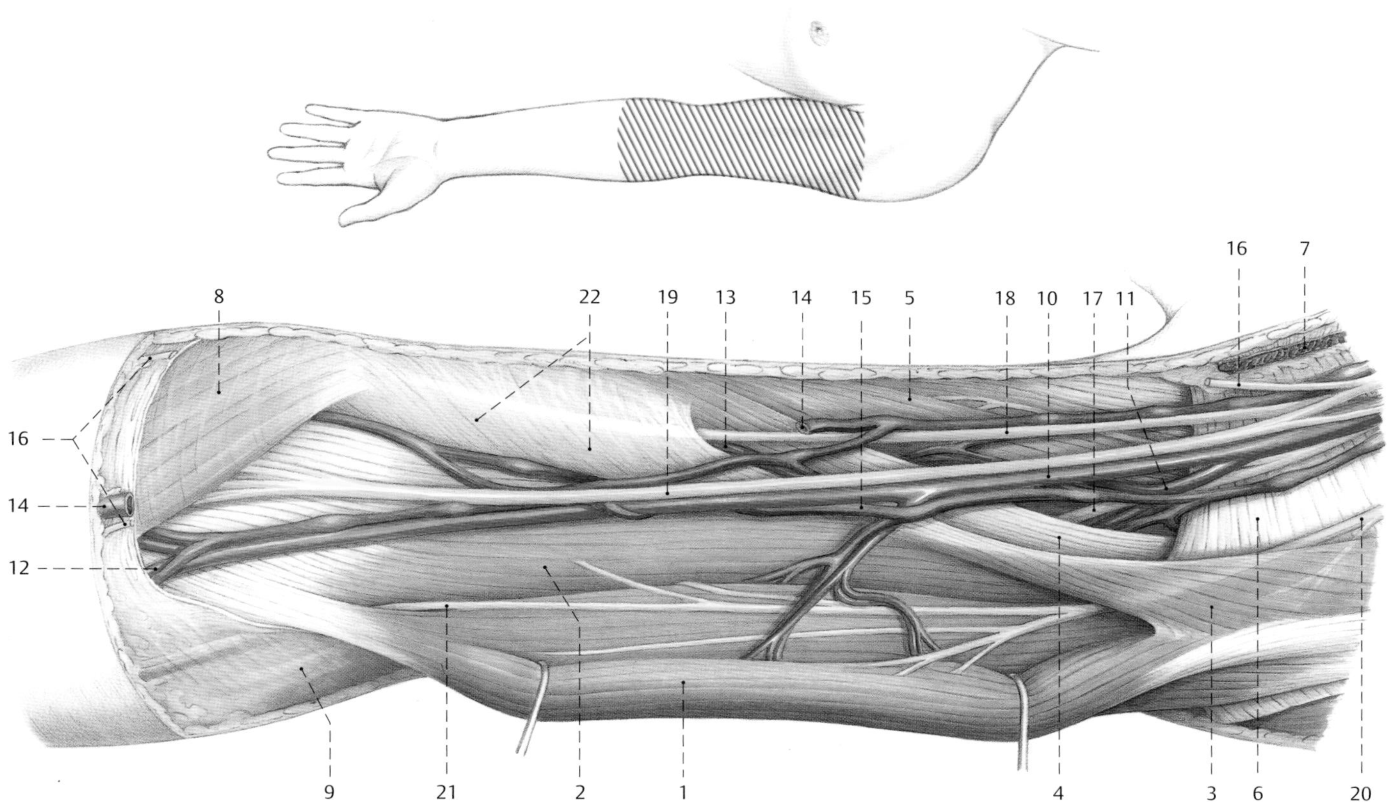

Fig. 16.21 Anatomical site of the anterior and medial aspects of the upper arm. Note the direction and course of the musculocutaneous nerve, and the origin of a muscular branch for innervation of the medial half of brachialis. The ulnar nerve is anterior to the triceps and posterior to the medial intermuscular septum.

1 Biceps brachii
2 Brachialis
3 Coracobrachialis
4 Medial head of triceps brachii
5 Long head of triceps brachii
6 Latissimus dorsi
7 Pectoralis major
8 Common head of the flexor muscles
9 Brachioradialis
10 Brachial artery
11 Deep brachial artery
12 Radial artery
13 Superior ulnar collateral artery
14 Basilic vein
15 Brachial vein
16 Medial cutaneous nerve of forearm
17 Radial nerve
18 Ulnar nerve
19 Median nerve
20 Musculocutaneous nerve
21 Lateral cutaneous nerve of forearm
22 Medial intermuscular septum

16.5 Lateral Approach to the Humerus

R. Bauer, F. Kerschbaumer, S. Poisel, K. Weise, K. Häringer

16.5.1 Principal Indications

- Fractures
- Pseudarthrosis
- Tumors
- Inflammation

16.5.2 Positioning and Incision

The patient is placed in the supine position. The arm lies next to the side of the body and may be supported if necessary. The skin incision begins two fingerbreadths proximal to the insertion of the deltoid and runs to the elbow as far laterally as the palpable belly of the brachioradialis (**Fig. 16.22**).

Following transection of the fascia (**Fig. 16.23**), the plane between the brachialis on the one hand, and the triceps (proximal) and brachioradialis (distal) on the other hand, is developed (**Fig. 16.24**).

The radial nerve is sought and exposed between the brachialis and brachioradialis in the distal corner of the wound (**Fig. 16.25**).

Dissection of muscles on the shaft of the humerus (**Fig. 16.26**).

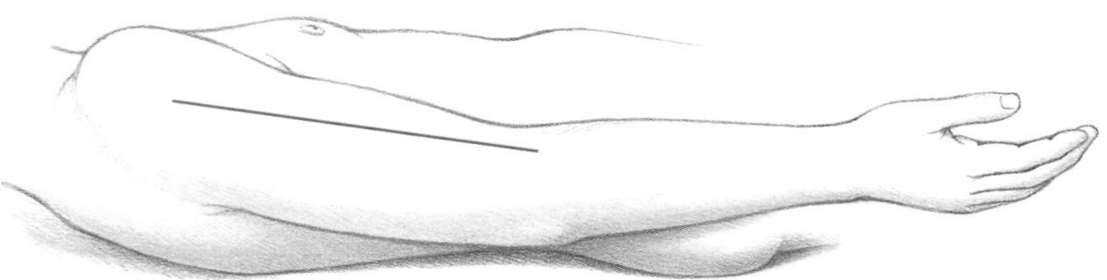

Fig. 16.22 Lateral approach to the humerus (right side). Skin incision (solid line).

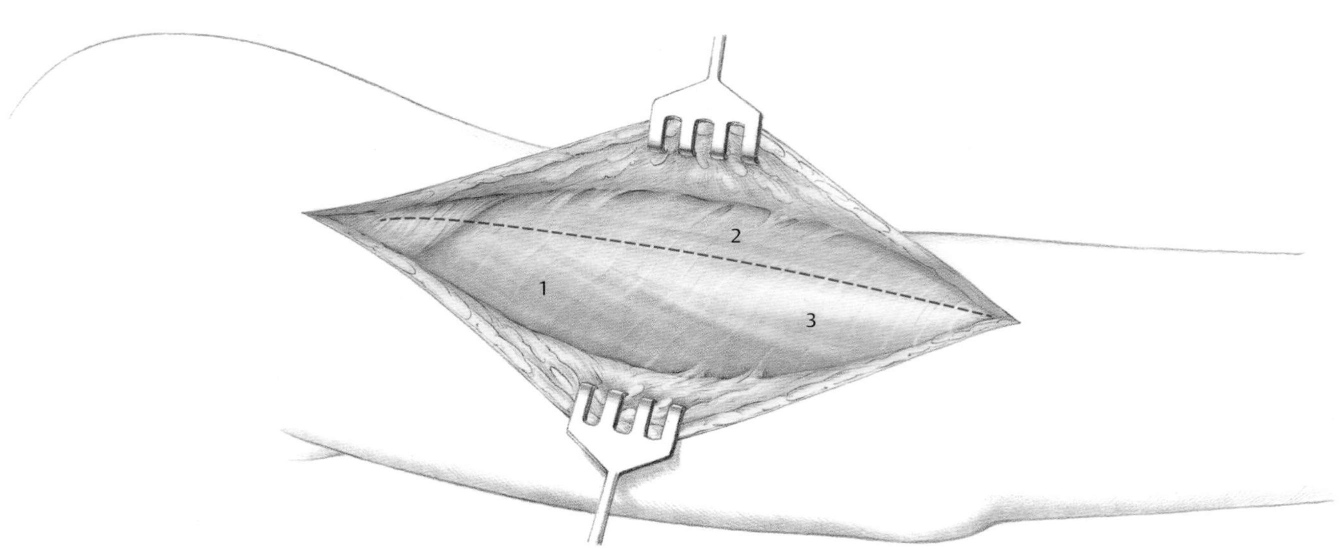

Fig. 16.23 Splitting of fascia between the brachialis, triceps, and brachioradialis.

1 Triceps brachii
2 Brachialis
3 Brachioradialis

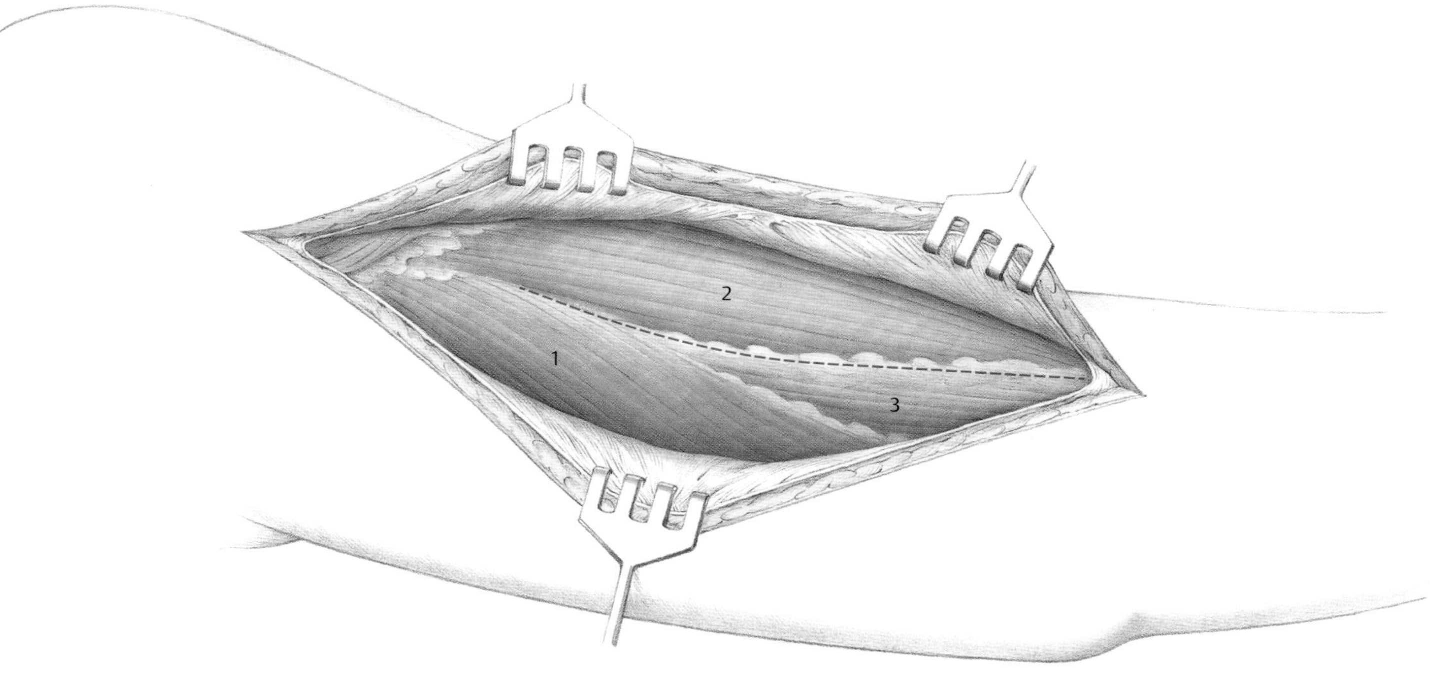

Fig. 16.24 Dissection of the layer between brachialis, triceps, and brachioradialis (lateral bicipital groove).

1 Triceps brachii
2 Brachialis
3 Brachioradialis

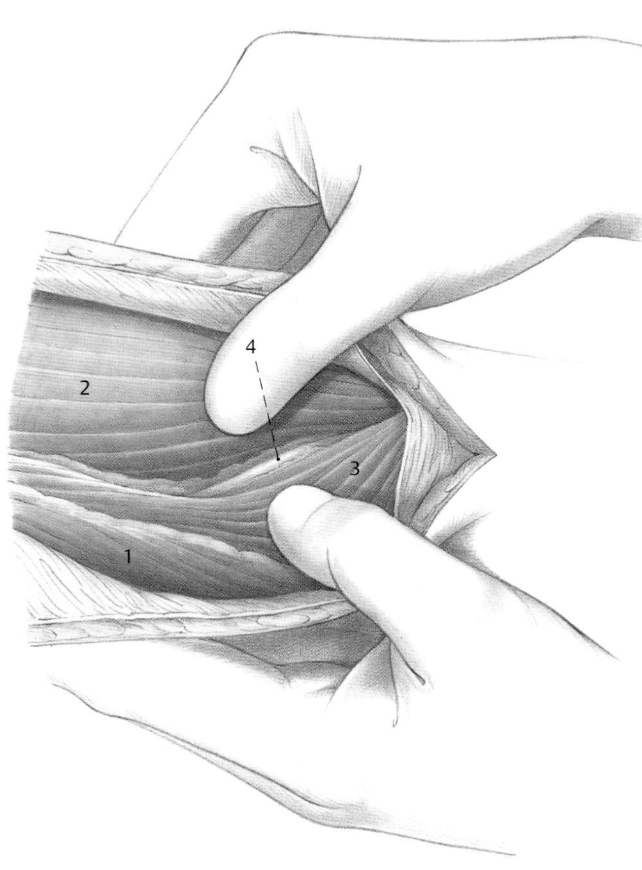

Fig. 16.25 Exposure of the radial nerve between brachialis and brachioradialis.

1 Triceps brachii
2 Brachialis
3 Brachioradialis
4 Radial nerve

16.5.3 Exposure of the Humeral Shaft

After snaring the radial nerve, the humeral shaft anterior to the lateral intermuscular septum is exposed by means of a raspatory (**Fig. 16.27**). Exposure of the bone in a proximal direction is limited by a muscular branch of the radial nerve.

16.5.4 Extension of the Incision

If necessary, the lateral approach can be combined with the deltopectoral approach to the shoulder, providing an anterolateral approach. The incision may be extended distally for exposure of the anterior portion of the distal third of the humerus and the elbow joint, proceeding along the brachioradialis beyond the elbow.

16.5.5 Wound Closure

The detached brachialis is reattached to the lateral intermuscular septum with a continuous suture.

16.5.6 Dangers

If retractors or Hohmann elevators are inserted in the distal wound area, the radial nerve is at risk.

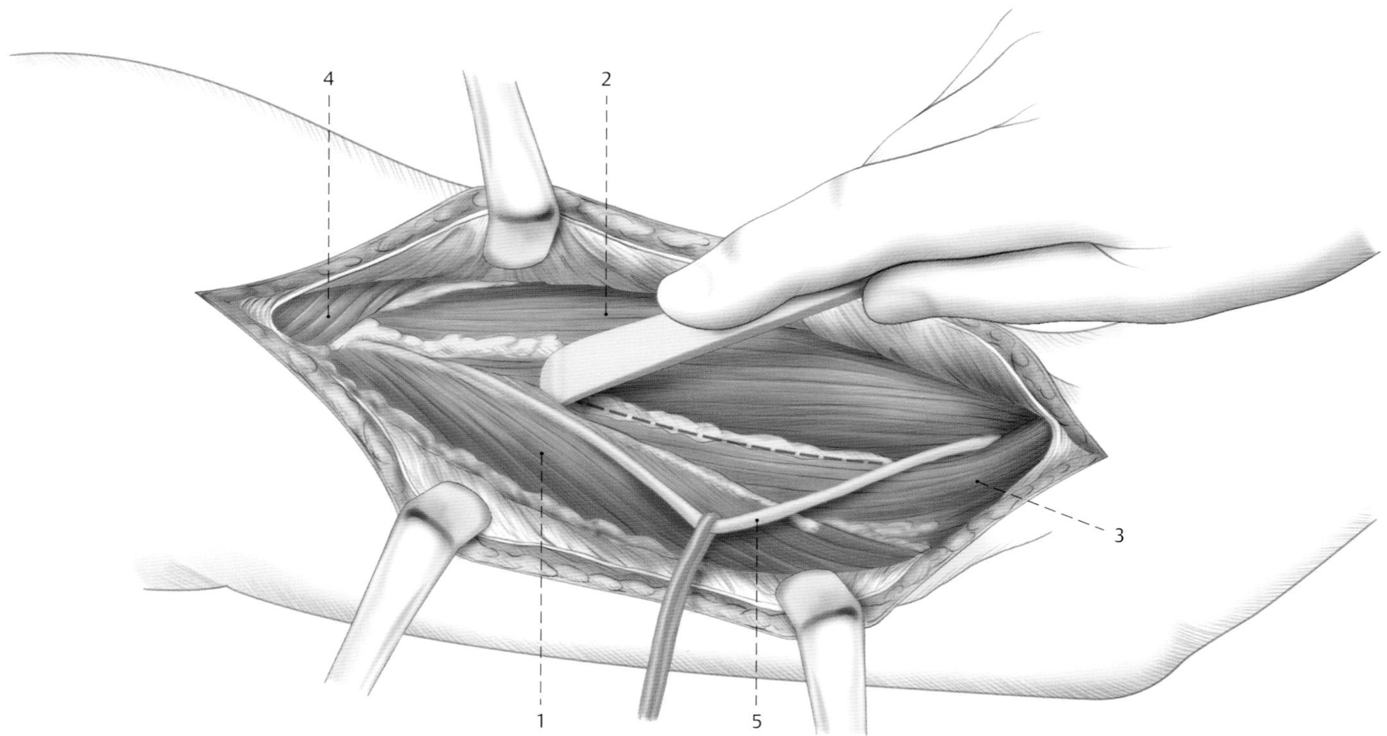

Fig. 16.26 Periosteal incision lateral to the brachialis.

1 Triceps brachii
2 Brachialis
3 Brachioradialis
4 Deltoid
5 Radial nerve

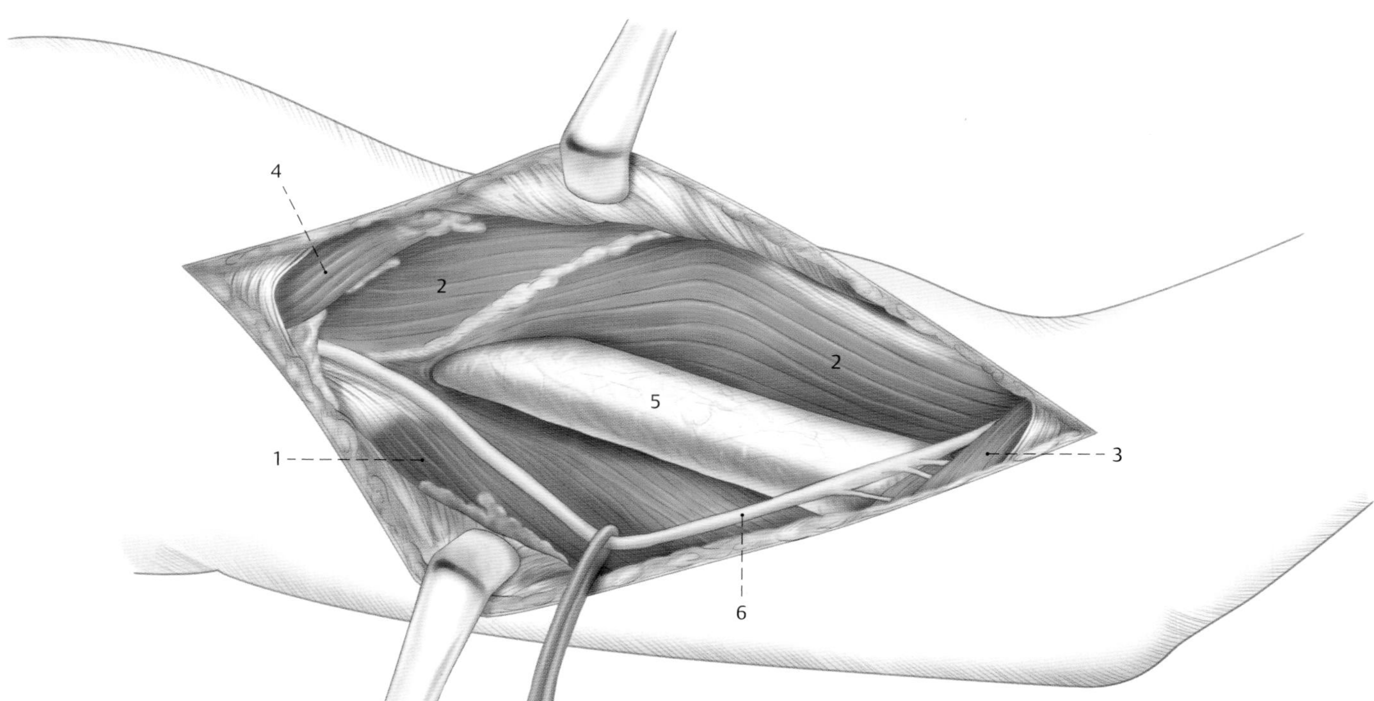

Fig. 16.27 Exposure of the humeral shaft with the elbow flexed and the forearm supinated.

1 Triceps brachii
2 Brachialis
3 Brachioradialis
4 Deltoid
5 Body of the humerus
6 Radial nerve

16.6 Medial Approach to the Humerus

R. Bauer, F. Kerschbaumer, S. Poisel, C. J. Wirth

The medial approach permits exposure of the middle third of the shaft.

16.6.1 Principal Indications

- Injuries to the neurovascular bundle
- Revision surgery when skin conditions are poor laterally

16.6.2 Positioning and Incision

The patient is placed in the supine position, with the arm abducted 90° and resting on a support. The skin incision runs in a straight line from the anterior axillary fold at the inferior border of pectoralis major to the medial epicondyle of the humerus (**Fig. 16.28**). After splitting of the subcutaneous tissue, the fascia of the upper arm is incised on the flexor side of the medial intermuscular septum (**Fig. 16.29**). The posteriorly situated ulnar nerve is identified and dissected free, the septum being split in a slightly distal direction (**Fig. 16.30**).

16.6.3 Exposure of the Humerus

Following ligation of several fairly small, transversely running vessels (**Fig. 16.31**), the periosteum and muscle are dissected in anterior and posterior directions so that the middle third of the shaft is clearly exposed (**Fig. 16.32**).

16.6.4 Extension of the Approach

The incision may be extended distally to expose the medial epicondyle of the humerus and the elbow joint from the medial side.

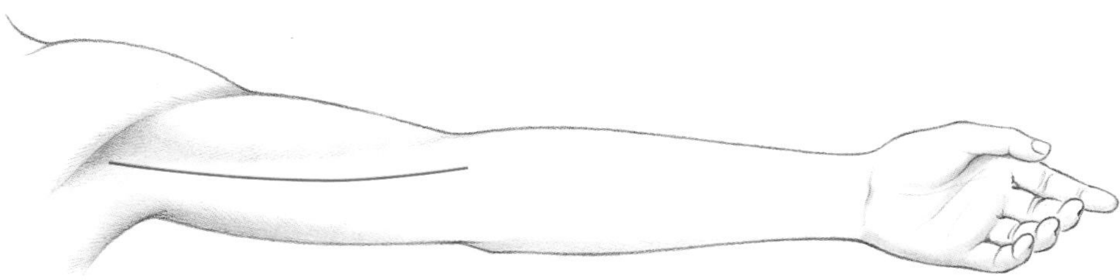

Fig. 16.28 Medial approach to humerus (left side). Skin incision (solid line).

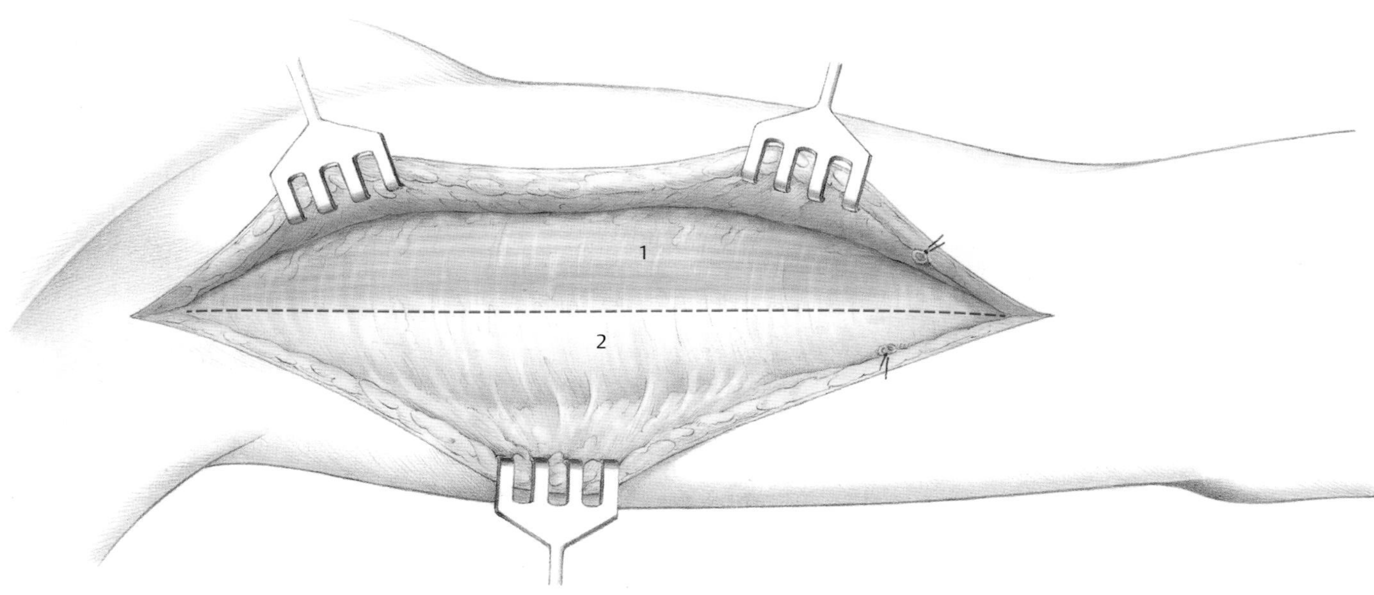

Fig. 16.29 Splitting of the fascia at the posterior margin of the biceps (medial bicipital grooves, dashed line).

1 Biceps brachii
2 Neurovascular bundle

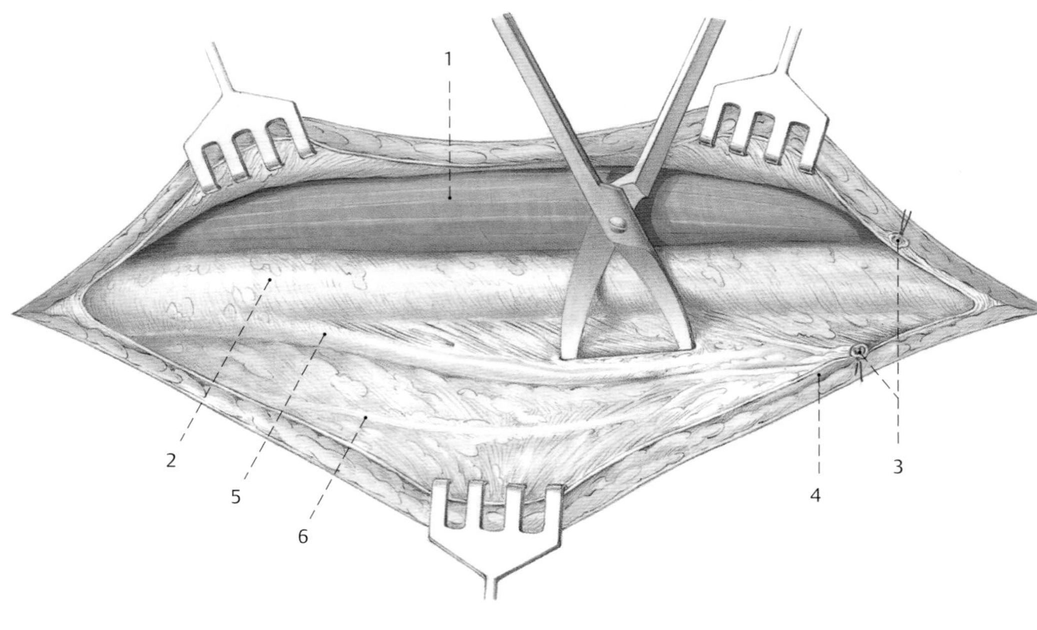

Fig. 16.30 Identification of the ulnar nerve.

1 Biceps brachii
2 Neurovascular bundle
3 Median cubital vein
4 Basilic vein
5 Ulnar nerve
6 Medial cutaneous nerve of forearm

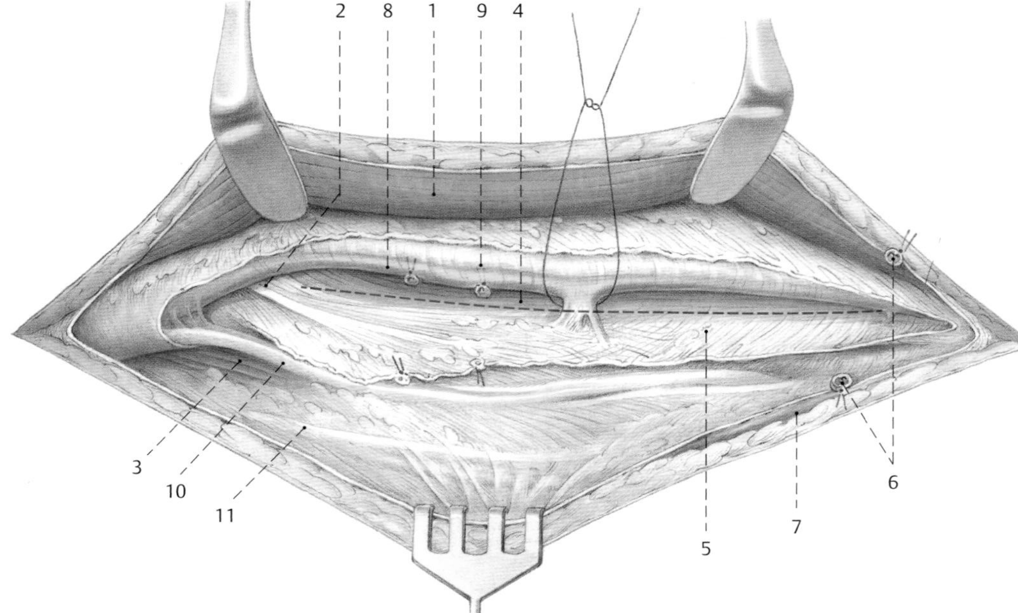

Fig. 16.31 Ligation and transection of transversely running vessels anterior to the medial intermuscular septum. Periosteal incision between triceps and brachialis (dashed line).

1 Biceps brachii
2 Medial head of triceps
3 Long head of triceps
4 Brachialis
5 Medial intermuscular septum
6 Median cubital vein
7 Basilic vein
8 Brachial vein
9 Median nerve
10 Ulnar nerve
11 Medial cutaneous nerve of forearm

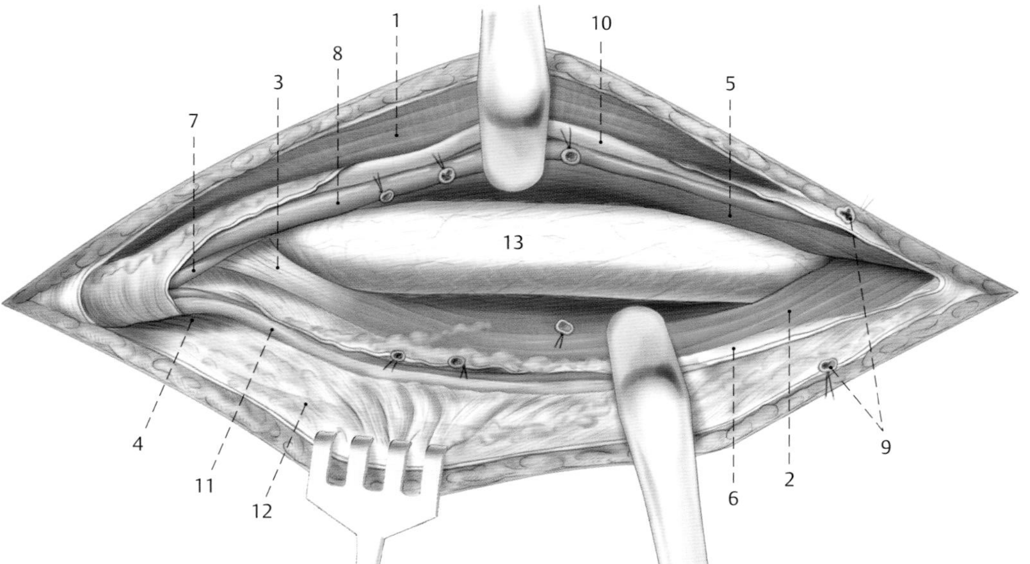

Fig. 16.32 Exposure of the middle of the humeral shaft.

1 Biceps brachii
2 Triceps brachii
3 Medial head of triceps brachii
4 Long head of triceps brachii
5 Brachialis
6 Medial intermuscular septum
7 Brachial artery
8 Brachial vein
9 Median cubital vein
10 Median nerve
11 Ulnar nerve
12 Medial cutaneous nerve of forearm
13 Humerus

16.6.5 Anatomical Site

(**Fig. 16.33**)

The medial, lateral, and posterior approaches to the middle and distal portions of the humerus are shown schematically in cross-section. In the medial and lateral approaches, the bone is exposed on the anterior side of the intermuscular septum, the ulnar and radial nerve, respectively, being retracted posteriorly.

16.6.6 Wound Closure

The brachialis is approximated to the medial intermuscular septum. Closure is otherwise effected in conventional fashion.

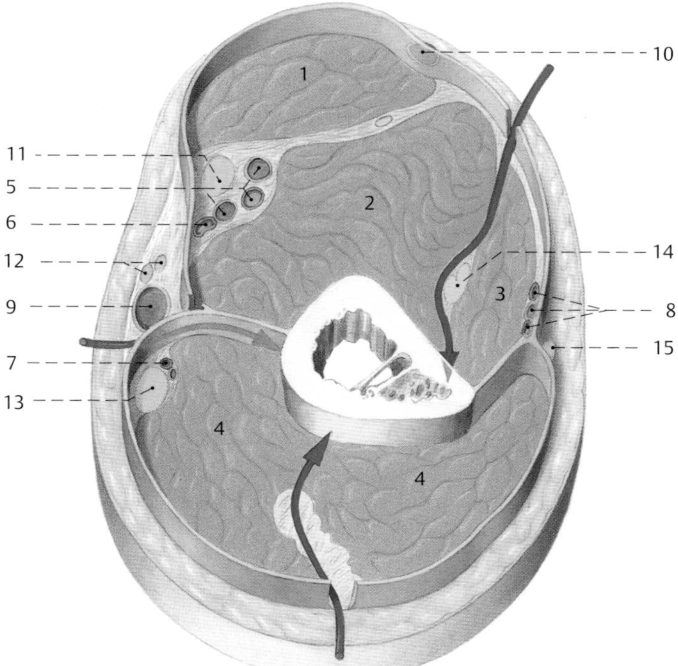

Fig. 16.33 Anatomical site. The schematic cross-section between the middle and distal third of the upper arm shows the medial, lateral, and posterior approaches (arrows) (right arm, proximal view).

1 Biceps brachii
2 Brachialis
3 Brachioradialis
4 Triceps brachii
5 Brachial artery and accompanying veins
6 Inferior ulnar collateral artery
7 Superior ulnar collateral artery and vein
8 Radial collateral artery and accompanying veins
9 Basilic vein
10 Cephalic vein
11 Median nerve
12 Medial cutaneous nerve of forearm
13 Ulnar nerve
14 Radial nerve
15 Posterior cutaneous nerve of forearm

17 Elbow

Four approaches to the elbow joint are described: the posterior approach with three variants, the lateral, the medial, and the anterior approaches.

For smaller operations, either the lateral or the medial and, in special cases, the anterior approach may be chosen.

For major operations on the elbow joint, the posterior approach is most suitable because it gives access to the entire posterior side of the elbow joint.

17.1 Posterior Approach to the Elbow Joint

K. Weise, K. Häringer

17.1.1 Principal Indications

- Fractures
- Pseudarthrosis
- Posttraumatic malpositions
- Arthroplasty

17.1.2 Positioning and Incision

The patient is placed in the prone position with a cushion under the chest. After (optional) application of a tourniquet, the arm is draped to allow free movement, and is placed in abduction on a small side table or an upper arm rest. The supporting table should not be too long so that the elbow can be flexed over 90° during the operation.

The skin incision begins 10 cm proximally to the tip of the olecranon and curves radially alongside the olecranon to a point 10 cm distal to its tip over the posterior margin of the ulna (**Fig. 17.1**). After dividing the subcutaneous tissue, the ulnar nerve is identified where it emerges from the triceps and is exposed as it passes through the ulnar groove, and then is snared and retracted (**Fig. 17.2**).

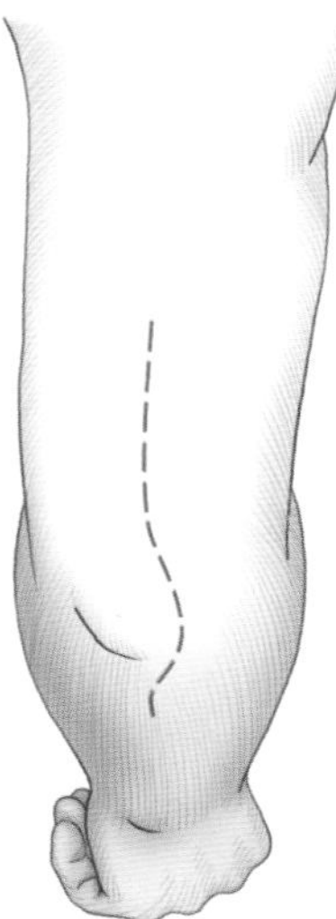

Fig. 17.1 Approach to the elbow joint (right side). Skin incision.

Paratricipital Approach

This approach is used for extra-articular fractures.

A window to the humerus is dissected medial and lateral to the triceps, and the muscle is pushed off the humerus with a raspatory.

The triceps is then mobilized medially from the olecranon and lateral to the anconeus muscle (**Figs. 17.3** and **17.4**).

After division of the medial collateral ligament, the ulna can be dislocated by maximal pronation using the **Alonso-Llames technique** (triceps-on), providing access to the humeral joint surface.

In the **Bryan-Morrey technique**, the triceps is initially mobilized, and the forearm fascia merging with the joint capsule is incised for approximately 6 cm (**Fig. 17.5**). With the elbow flexed 30°, the two structures are retracted together from the olecranon using a raspatory, starting medially (**Fig. 17.6**).

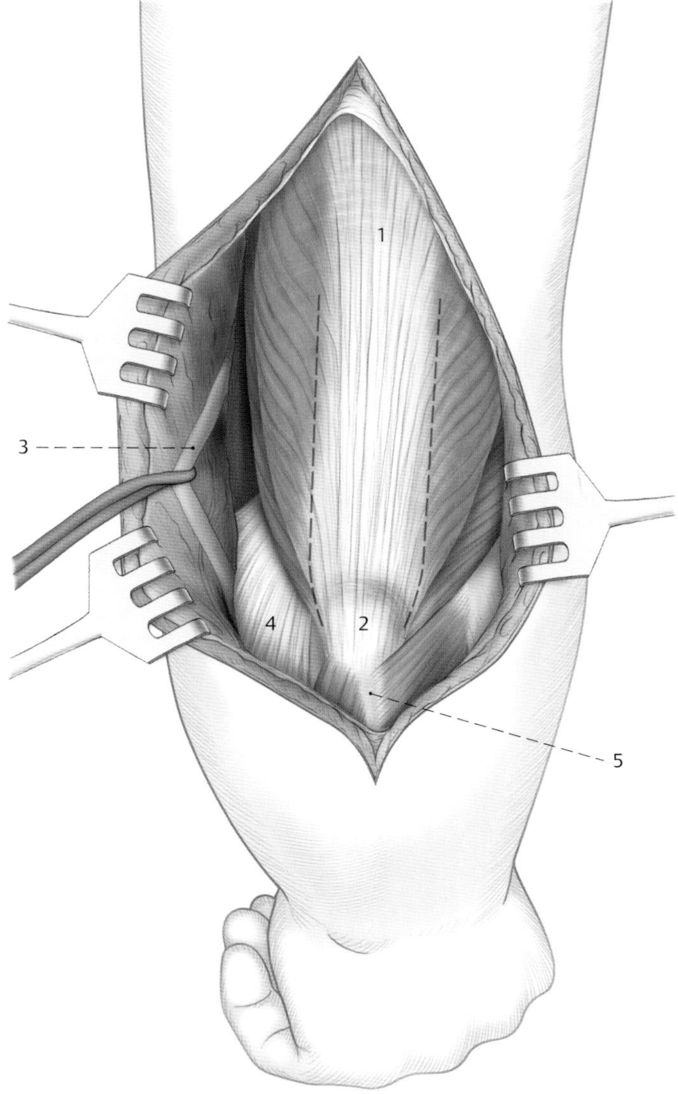

Fig. 17.2 Paratricipital approach medial and lateral to the triceps. The ulnar nerve is identified and snared.

1 Triceps brachii
2 Olecranon
3 Ulnar nerve
4 Forearm flexor muscles
5 Antebrachial fascia

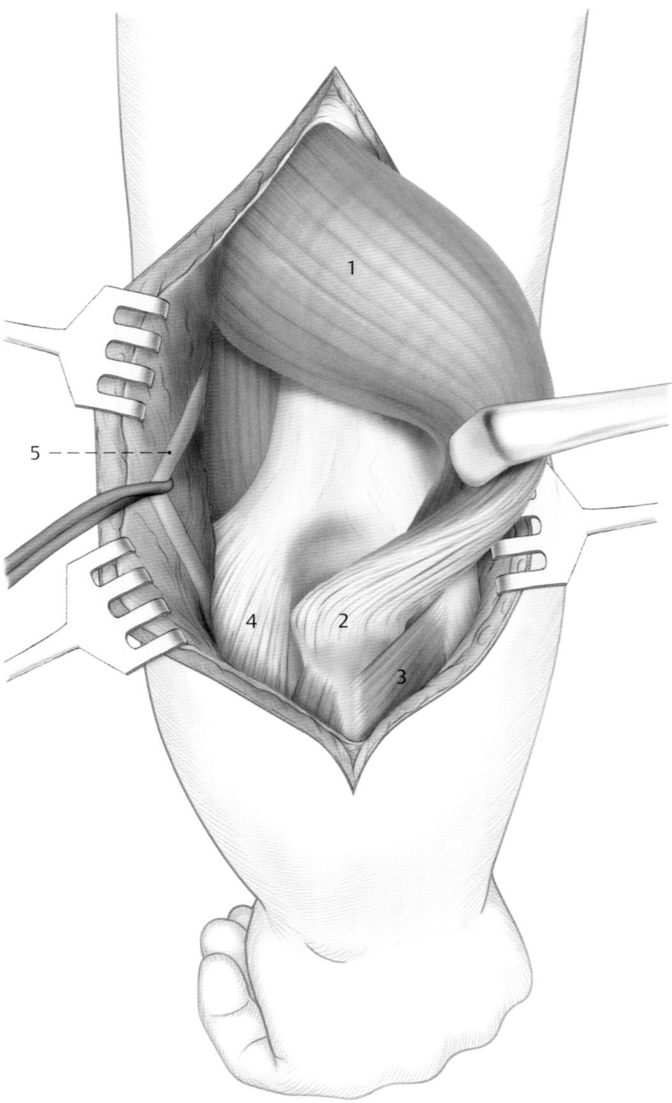

Fig. 17.3 Paratricipital approach to the medial epicondyle.

1 Triceps brachii
2 Olecranon
3 Anconeus
4 Forearm flexor muscles
5 Ulnar nerve

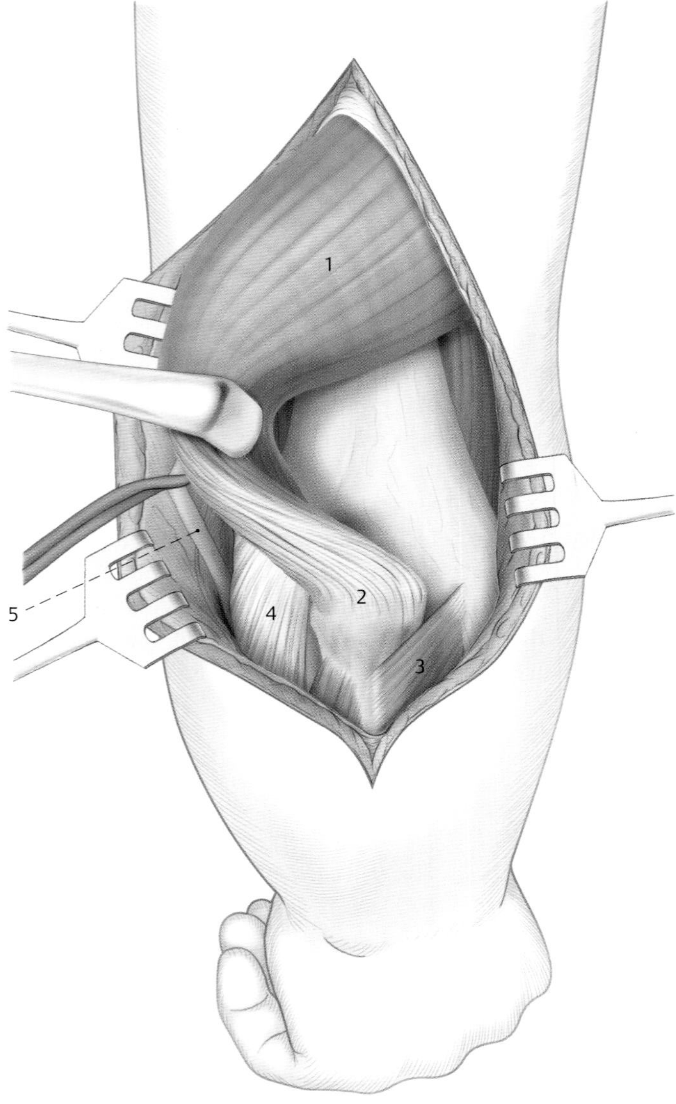

Fig. 17.4 Paratricipital approach to the lateral epicondyle.

1 Triceps brachii
2 Olecranon
3 Anconeus
4 Forearm flexor muscles
5 Ulnar nerve

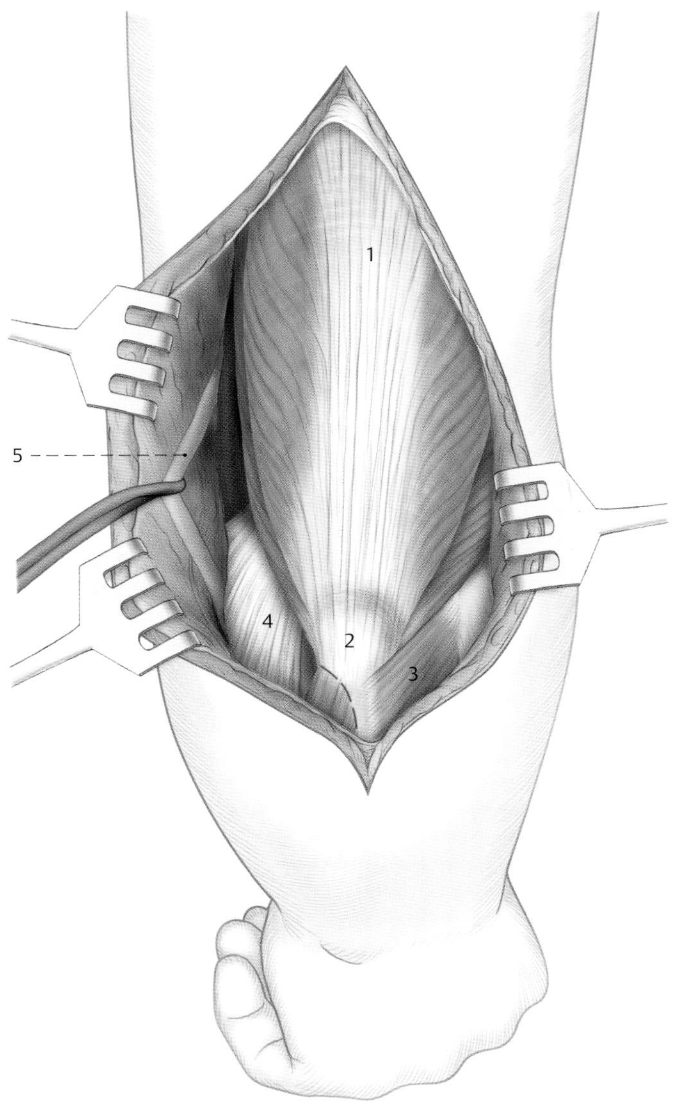

Fig. 17.5 Incision of antebrachial fascia using the Bryan-Morrey technique.

1 Triceps brachii
2 Olecranon
3 Anconeus
4 Forearm flexor muscles
5 Ulnar nerve

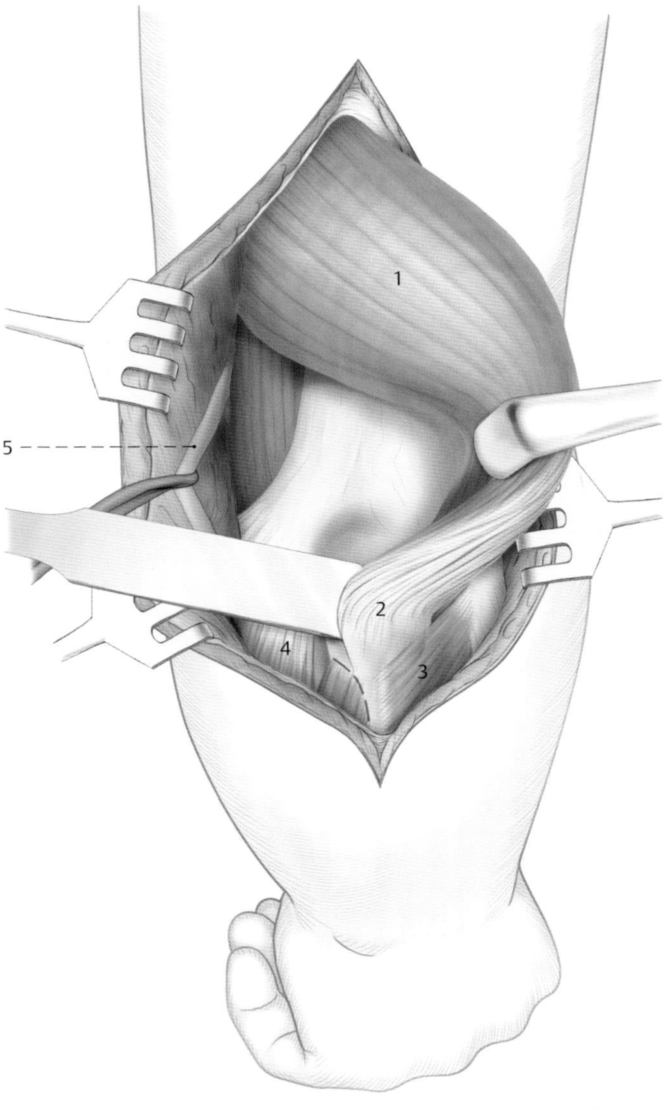

Fig. 17.6 Retraction of triceps and the antebrachial fascial from the olecranon starting medially using the Bryan-Morrey technique.

1 Triceps brachii
2 Olecranon
3 Anconeus
4 Forearm flexor muscles
5 Ulnar nerve

Straight Splitting of the Triceps

The common triceps tendon is split down the middle from approximately 10 cm proximal to the olecranon as far as the tip of the olecranon (**Fig. 17.7**), and the muscle is retracted bluntly to either side (**Fig. 17.8**). It is then retracted from the joint capsule using a raspatory. This provides a good view of the distal humerus (**Fig. 17.9**).

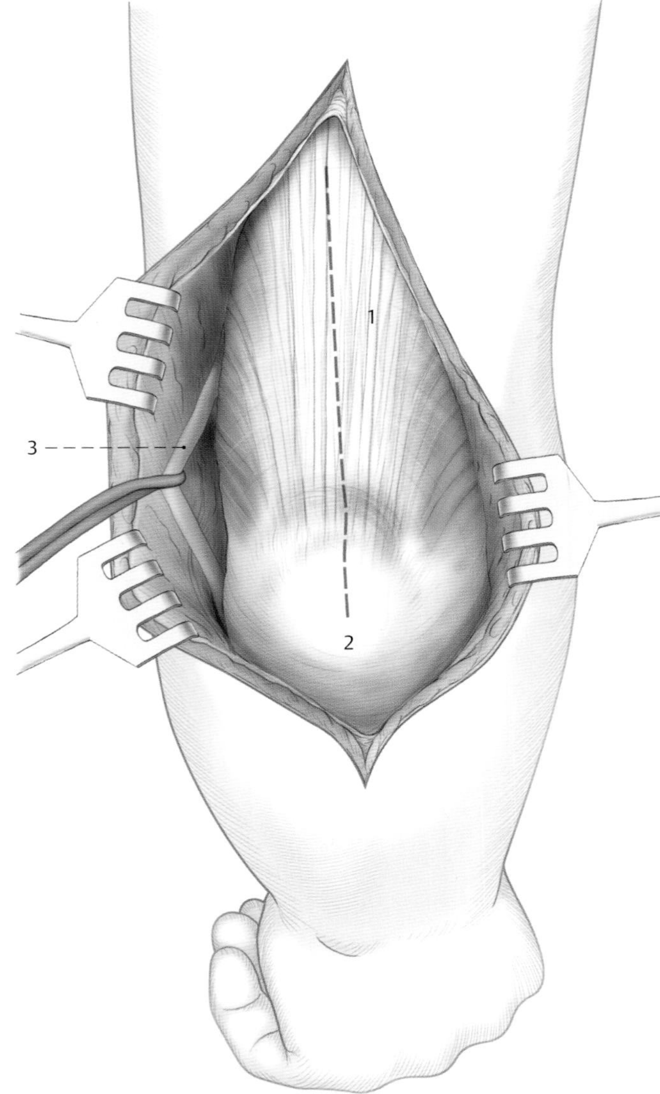

Fig. 17.7 Straight splitting of the triceps, fascial incision.

1 Triceps brachii
2 Olecranon
3 Ulnar nerve

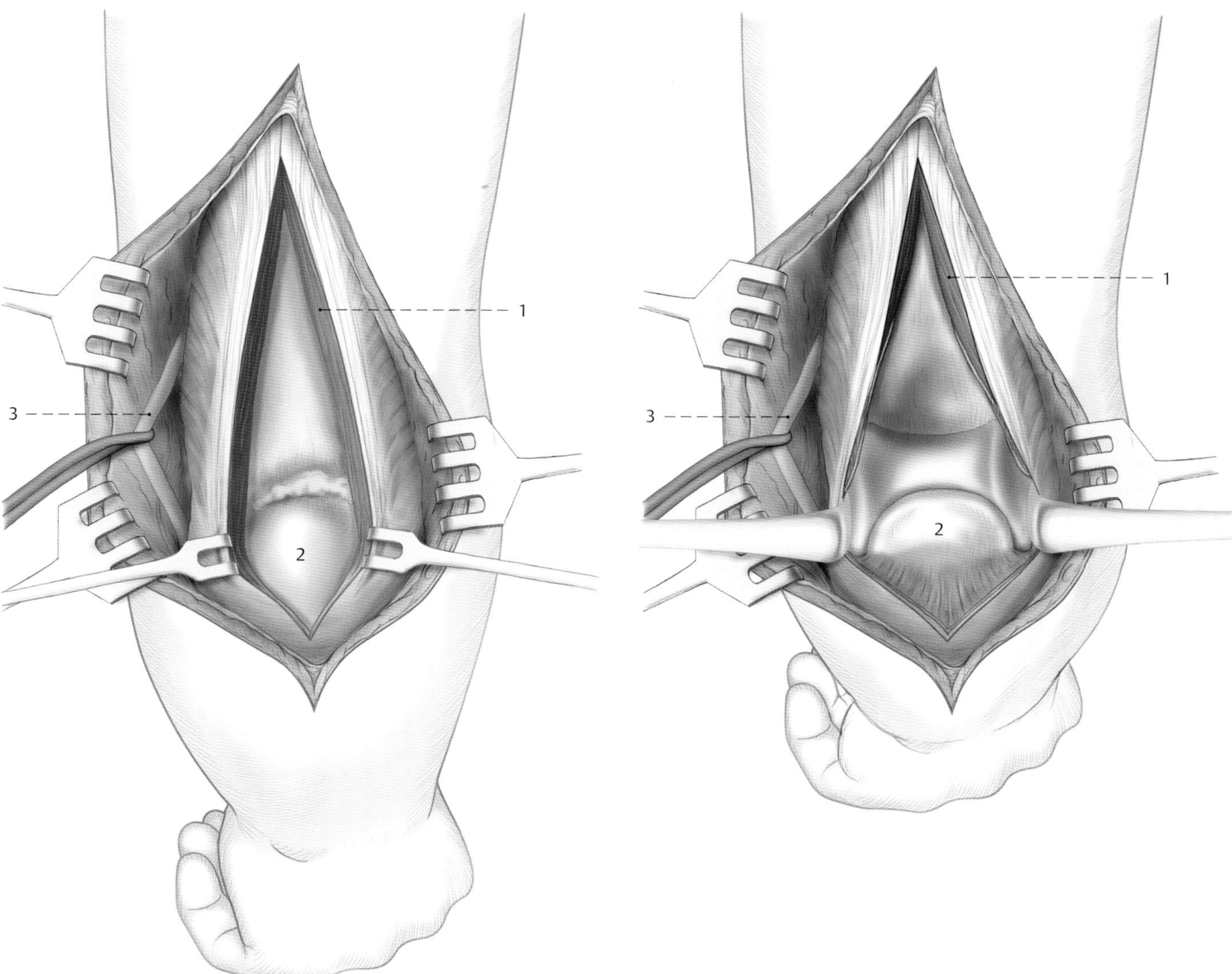

Fig. 17.8 Straight splitting of the triceps, exposure of the distal humerus.

1 Triceps brachii
2 Olecranon
3 Ulnar nerve

Fig. 17.9 Straight splitting of the triceps, exposure of the trochlea where possible with joint flexion.

1 Triceps brachii
2 Olecranon
3 Ulnar nerve

Osteotomy of Olecranon

This approach is suitable for C-fractures of the distal humerus.

After a radial incision over the olecranon and extension of the approach by up to 10 cm distally along the border of the ulna, the proximal ulna is exposed. A V-shaped incision is made in the periosteum distal to the olecranon (**Fig. 17.10**), a V is cut in the ulna with a saw, and the olecranon is then lifted out with a chisel. The triceps tendon with the olecranon and adherent posterior parts of the joint capsule is now dissected in a proximal direction so that the trochlea of the humerus can be readily visualized (**Fig. 17.11**). The entire circumference of the trochlea can be exposed by further flexion of the elbow and opening of the capsule in an ulnar and radial direction. The olecranon can be reattached, for example, by tension banding (**Fig. 17.12**).

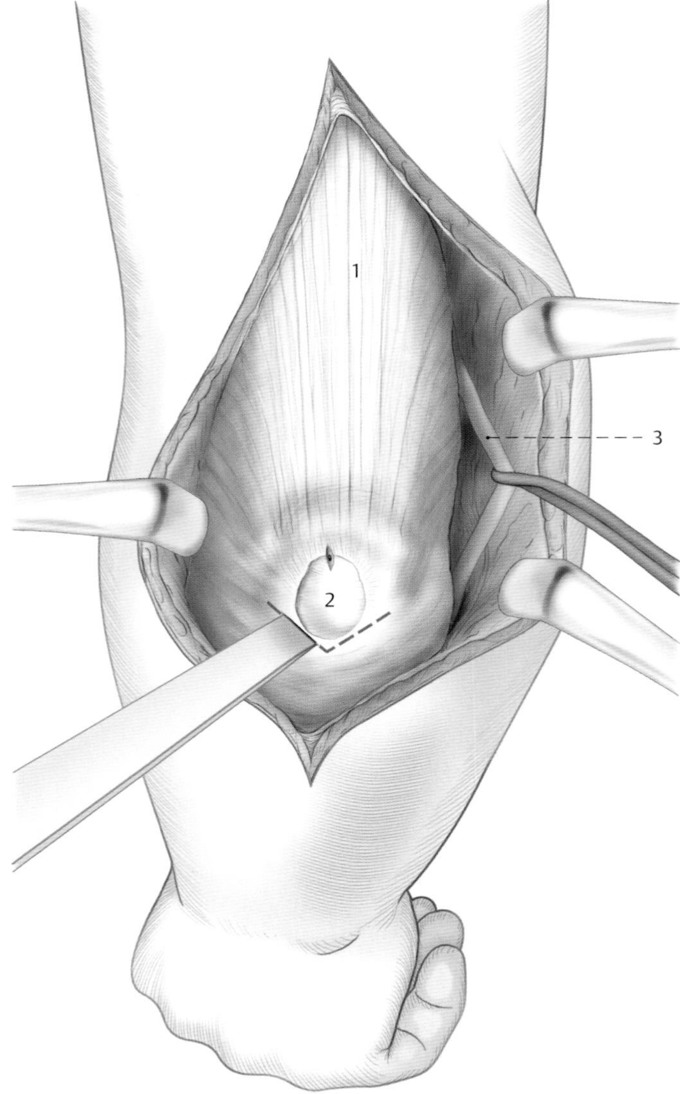

Fig. 17.10 V-shaped osteotomy of the olecranon (left arm).

1 Triceps brachii
2 Olecranon
3 Ulnar nerve

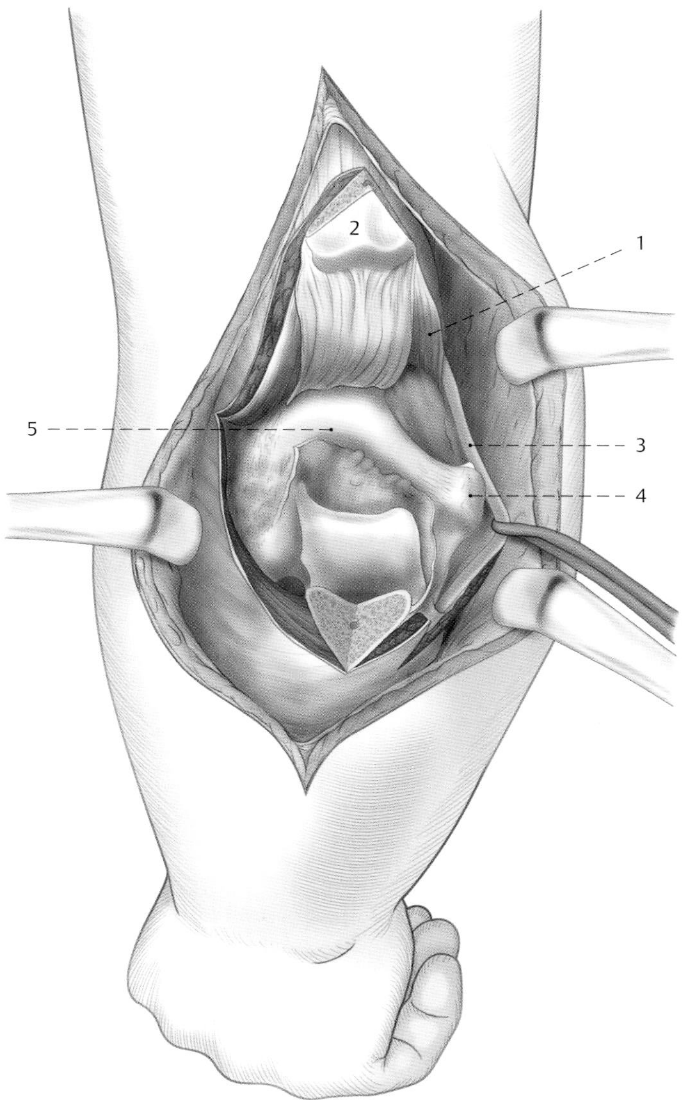

Fig. 17.11 The olecranon with the detached triceps is retracted cranially.

1 Triceps brachii
2 Olecranon
3 Ulnar nerve
4 Medial epicondyle
5 Humerus

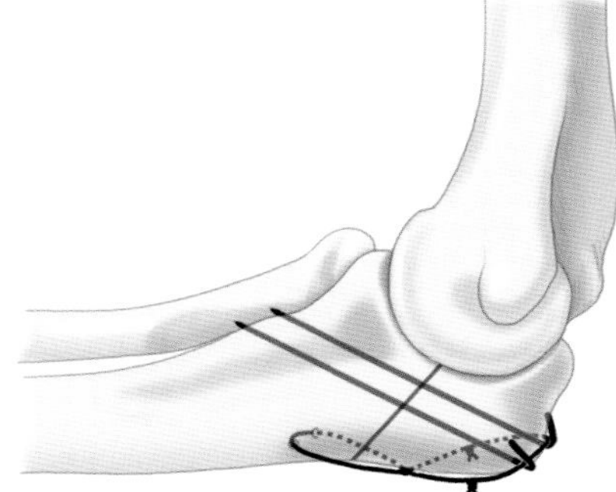

Fig. 17.12 Internal fixation of the olecranon with tension banding.

17.1.3 Extension of the Approach

Improved intra-articular visualization can be obtained by subperiosteal detachment of the anconeus from the ulna and division of the medial collateral ligament.

17.1.4 Wound Closure

After insertion of a Redon drain and tension banding of the olecranon (**Fig. 17.12**), the triceps is reattached with a continuous suture. The anconeus and ligaments are reattached with transosseous sutures.

17.1.5 Dangers

The deep branch of the radial nerve is at risk during dissection of the proximal ulna.

There is a danger of injury to the ulnar nerve when the medial condyle is exposed. It is therefore advisable to expose the nerve over a length of approximately 8 cm and snare it. It is identified proximally between the medial head of triceps and the medial intermuscular septum (arcade of Struthers), and the septum is split. From here it is followed as far as the Osborne arcade, which spans the head of the humerus and the ulnar head of flexor carpi ulnaris. This arcade is also split. The accompanying vessels, especially the motor branch to flexor carpi ulnaris, should be spared.

17.2 Lateral Approach to the Elbow Joint

R. Bauer, F. Kerschbaumer, S. Poisel, K. Weise, K. Häringer

17.2.1 Principal Indications

- Fractures of the radial epicondyle
- Fractures and dislocations of the head of the radius
- Instability
- Osteochondritis dissecans
- Synovectomy
- Inflammation

17.2.2 Positioning and Incision

The patient is placed supine with a pad under the shoulder. The arm is draped to allow free motion and may rest on the patient's body or on a small side table. The skin incision begins three fingerbreadths proximal to the radial epicondyle and continues in a straight line three fingerbreadths over the head of the radius in a distal and posterior direction (**Fig. 17.13**).

The fascia between the ulnar extensor of the wrist and the anconeus is split subcutaneously, and the incision is continued in a more proximal direction behind the radial epicondyle (**Fig. 17.14**). The muscle bellies of the extensor carpi ulnaris and anconeus are spread out so that the underlying capsule comes into view.

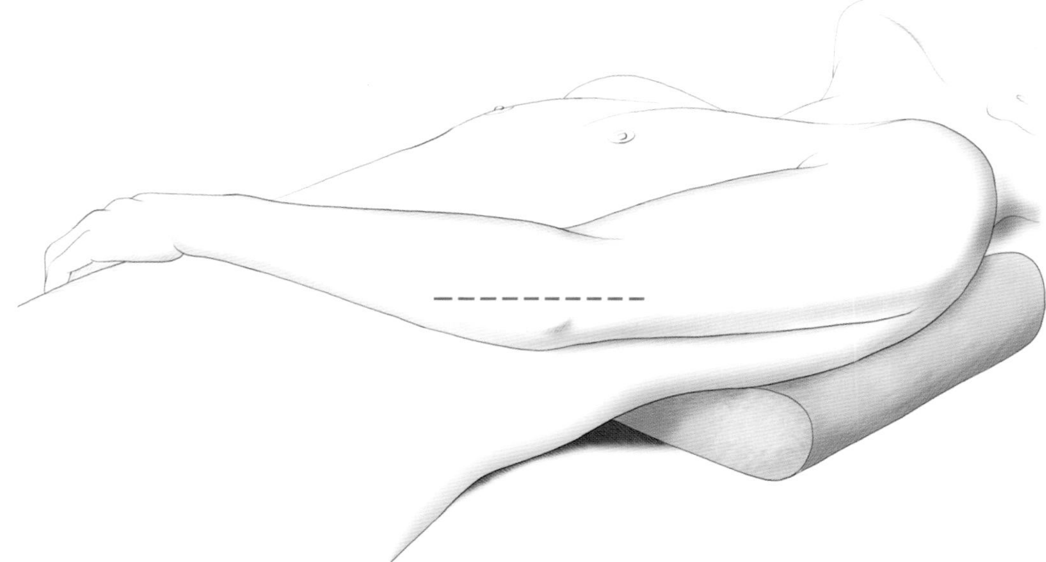

Fig. 17.13 Lateral approach to the elbow joint (left arm).

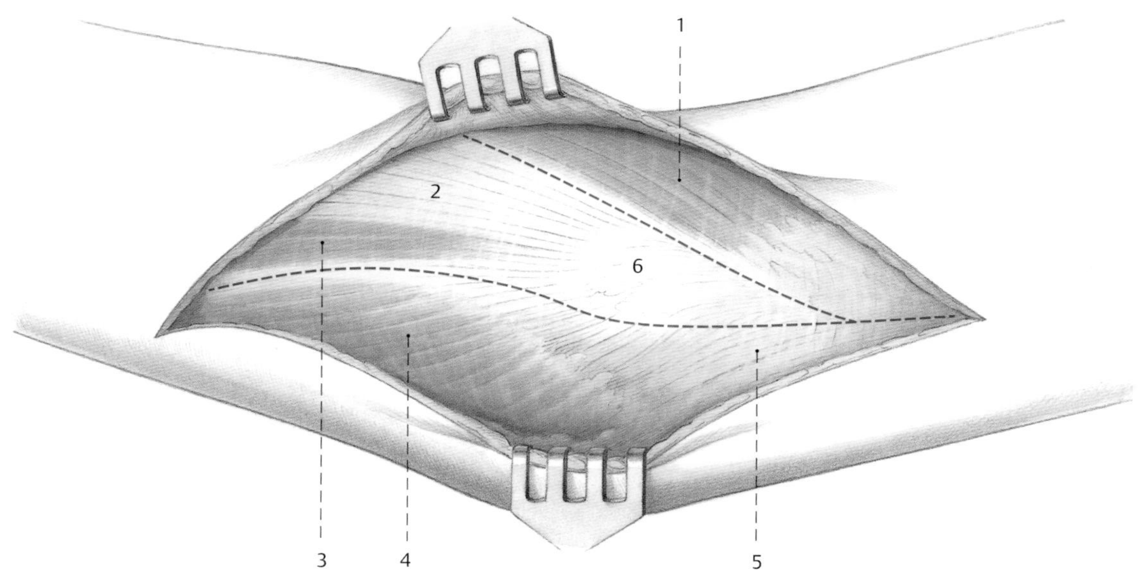

Fig. 17.14 Incision between extensor carpi ulnaris and anconeus for exposure of the posterior parts of the joint. Incision between extensor digitorum and the radial extensors for exposure of the anterior aspect of the joint.

1 Extensor carpi radialis longus
2 Extensor digitorum
3 Extensor carpi ulnaris
4 Anconeus
5 Tendon of triceps brachii
6 Lateral epicondyle of humerus

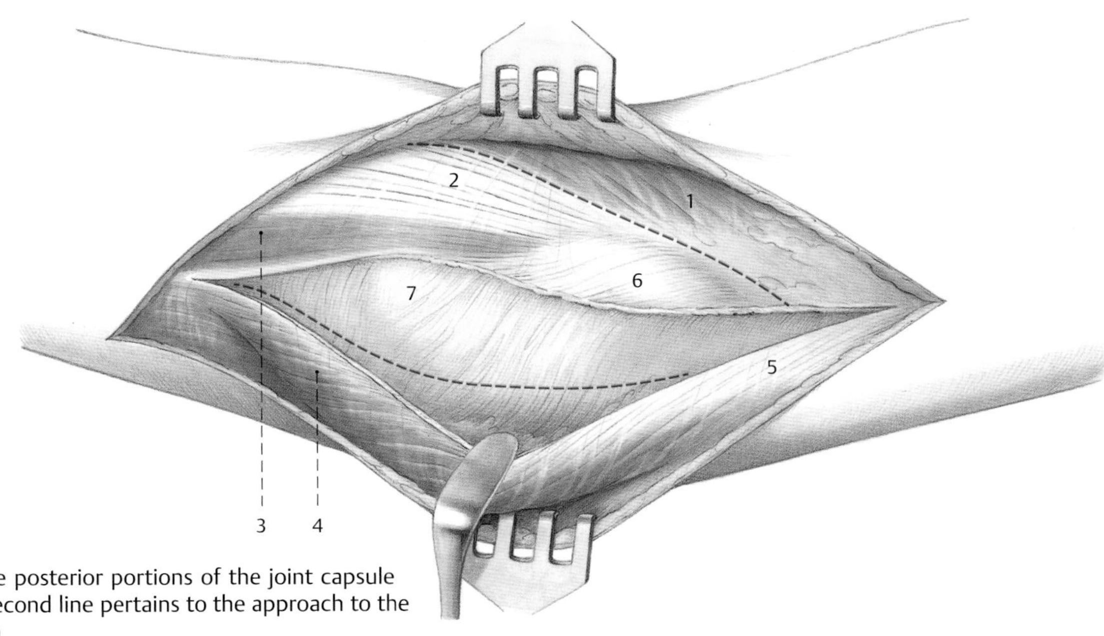

Fig. 17.15 Opening of the posterior portions of the joint capsule (lower dashed line). (The second line pertains to the approach to the anterior parts of the joint.)

1 Extensor carpi radialis longus
2 Extensor digitorum
3 Extensor carpi ulnaris
4 Anconeus
5 Tendon of triceps brachii
6 Lateral epicondyle of humerus
7 Head of radius

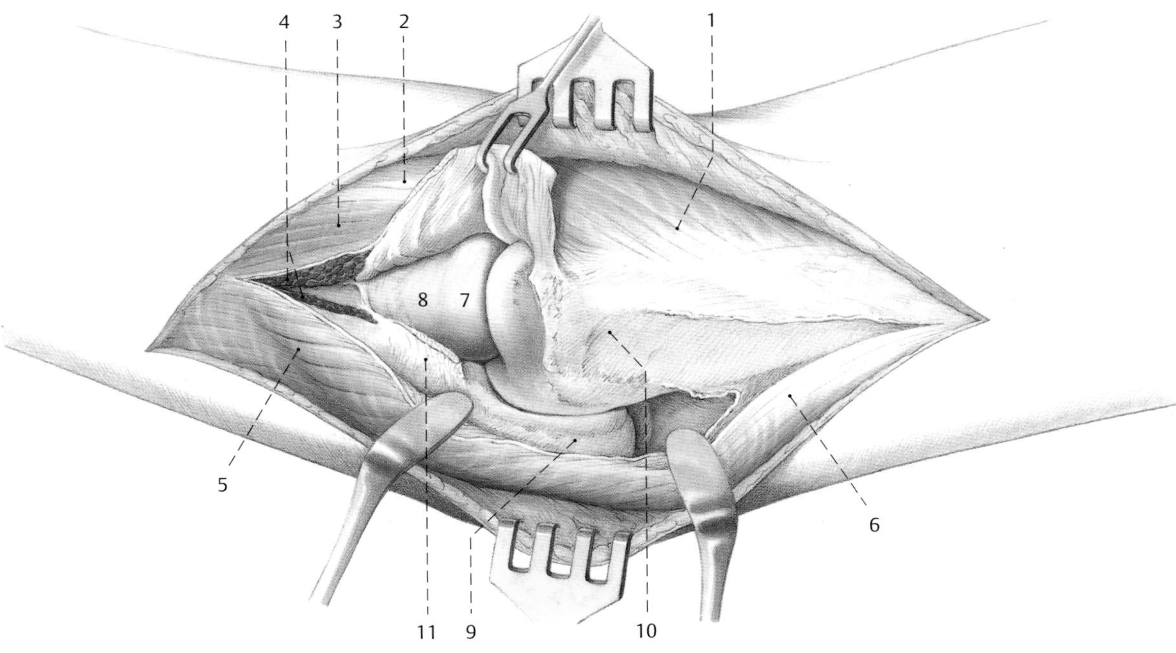

Fig. 17.16 Exposure of the head of the radius, capitulum of the humerus, olecranon, and olecranon fossa. The radial collateral ligament has not been detached.

1 Extensor carpi radialis longus
2 Extensor digitorum
3 Extensor carpi ulnaris
4 Supinator
5 Anconeus
6 Triceps brachii
7 Head of the radius (articular circumference)
8 Neck of the radius
9 Olecranon
10 Lateral epicondyle of the humerus
11 Annular ligament of the radius

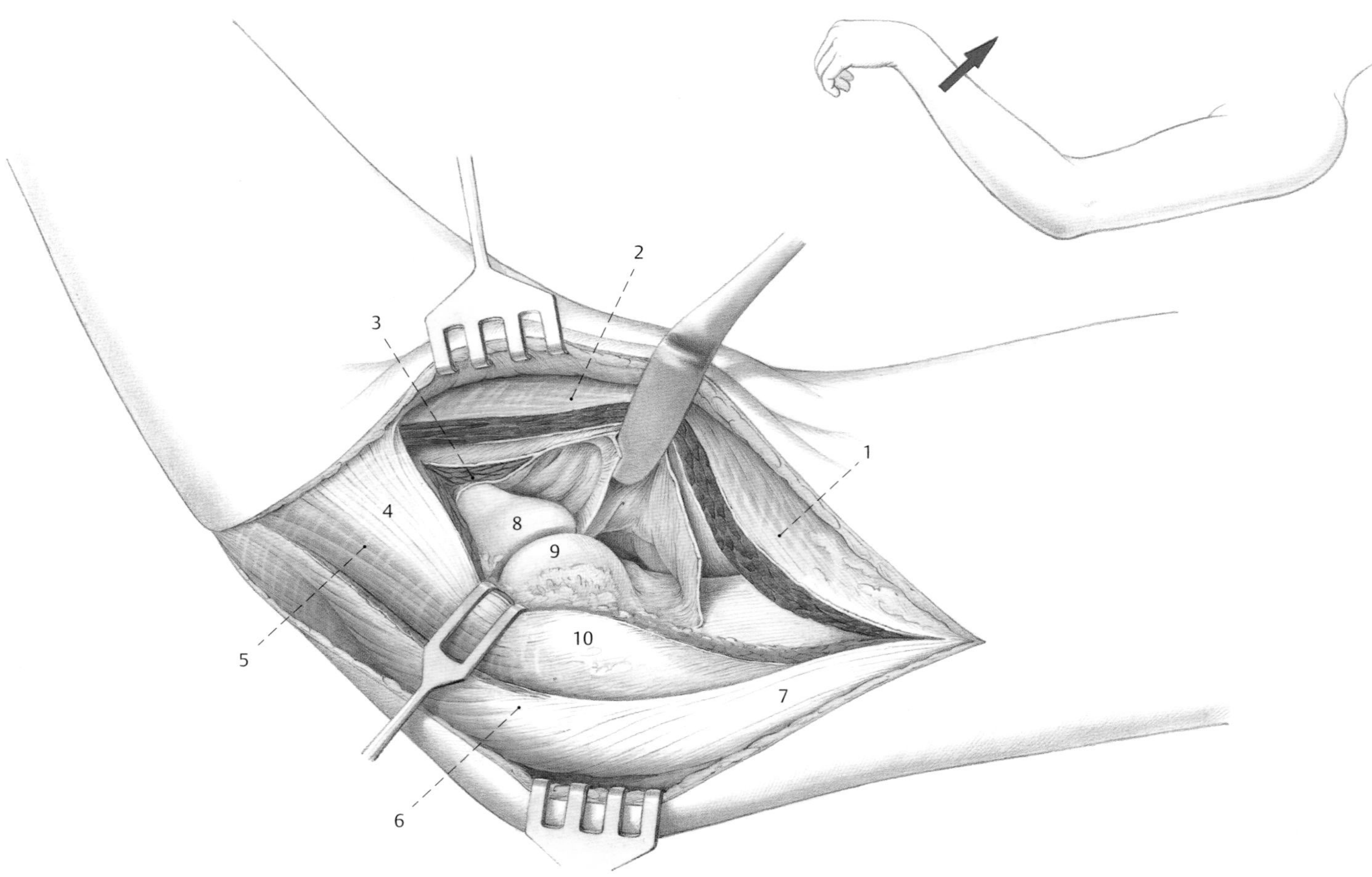

Fig. 17.17 With the elbow flexed, the radial extensor muscles are transected, and the anterior portions of the joint are opened.

1 Brachioradialis
2 Extensor carpi radialis longus
3 Supinator
4 Extensor digitorum
5 Extensor carpi ulnaris
6 Anconeus
7 Triceps brachii
8 Head of the radius (articular circumference)
9 Capitulum of the humerus
10 Lateral epicondyle of the humerus

17.2.3 Exposure of the Elbow Joint

Two retaining sutures are placed in the joint capsule, and the capsule is then split longitudinally (**Fig. 17.15**). With the elbow joint extended, the following components of the joint can be viewed: the head of the radius with the annular ligament of the radius, the capitulum of the humerus with the radial part of the trochlea, and the lateral portion and tip of the olecranon (**Fig. 17.16**). With the elbow slightly flexed, the olecranon fossa is also revealed by this approach. If, in addition, exposure of the anterior parts of the joint is required, a second incision may be made between extensor digitorum and extensor carpi radialis brevis and longus (**Fig. 17.17**). This incision runs distally on the flexor side anterior to the lateral epicondyle of the humerus. The origins of extensor carpi radialis brevis and extensor carpi radialis longus may be detached from the humerus close to the bone, care being taken not to damage the posterior cutaneous nerve of the forearm. After retraction of the radial extensor muscles on the flexor side, the joint capsule may be opened. With the elbow flexed, a Langenbeck retractor is inserted beneath the anterior joint capsule, allowing exposure of the anterior portion of the head of the radius, the capitulum of the humerus, the lateral part of the humeral trochlea, and the lateral portion of the coronoid process.

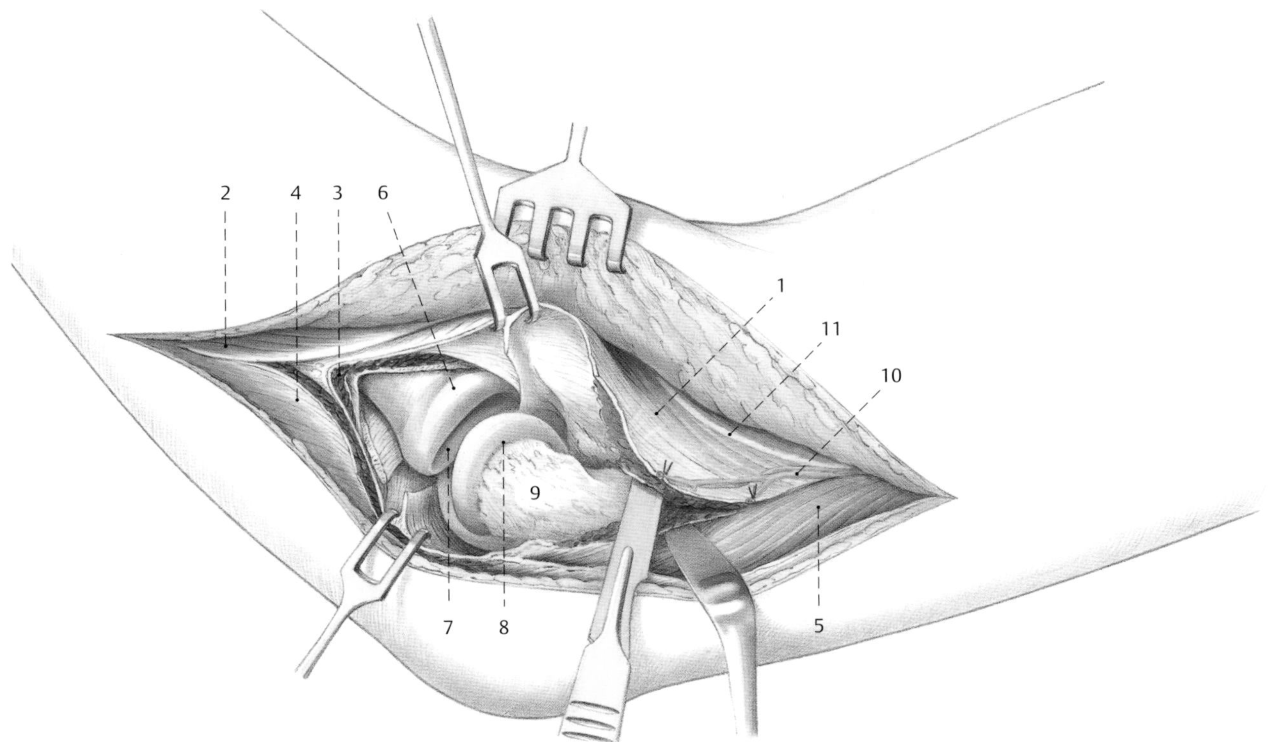

Fig. 17.18 Extended lateral approach. After incision between the extensor carpi ulnaris and anconeus, the capsule is opened and the radial collateral ligament at the lateral epicondyle of the humerus is detached. The muscle should not be stripped more than a handbreadth proximal to the lateral epicondyle of the humerus (radial nerve!).

1 Brachioradialis
2 Extensor carpi ulnaris
3 Supinator
4 Anconeus
5 Triceps brachii
6 Head of the radius (articular circumference)
7 Articular fovea
8 Capitulum of the humerus
9 Lateral epicondyle of the humerus
10 Radial collateral artery and vein
11 Posterior cutaneous nerve of forearm

17.2.4 Extension of the Lateral Approach with Detachment of the Radial Collateral Ligament

If a wider exposure is desired in the lateral approach to begin with, for example for arthroplastic operations, the joint capsule together with the origin of the radial collateral ligament may be detached from the lateral humeral epicondyle via the posterior incision between extensor carpi ulnaris and anconeus (**Fig. 17.18**). The extensor muscles on the humerus can be stripped as far as a handbreadth proximal to the lateral epicondyle of the humerus without injuring the radial nerve. At the same time, the posterior cutaneous nerve of the forearm should be spared in this approach. Distally, the annular ligament of the radius and the supinator can be detached from the ulna with the forearm pronated. The slightly flexed elbow is reflected laterally so that the joint becomes clearly visible as far as the medial epicondyle of the humerus (**Fig. 17.19**).

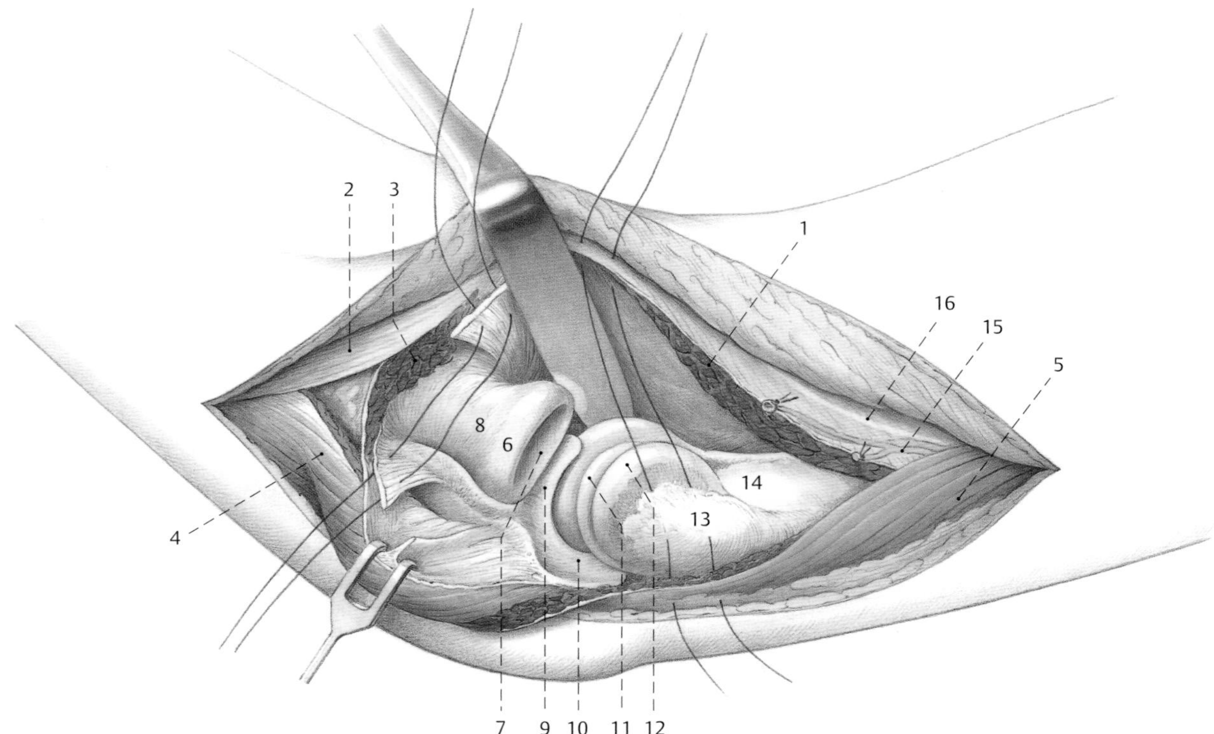

Fig. 17.19 All parts of the joint are exposed in this position. Wound closure is effected by transosseous reinsertion of the radial collateral ligament and suture of the annular ligament.

1 Brachioradialis
2 Extensor carpi ulnaris
3 Supinator
4 Anconeus
5 Triceps brachii
6 Head of radius (articular circumference)
7 Articular facet
8 Neck of radius
9 Coronoid process
10 Olecranon
11 Trochlea of the humerus
12 Capitulum of the humerus
13 Lateral epicondyle of the humerus
14 Coronoid fossa
15 Radial collateral artery and vein
16 Posterior cutaneous nerve of forearm

17.2.5 Wound Closure

The origin of the radial collateral ligament should be attached to the lateral epicondyle of the humerus with transosseous sutures. The annular ligament of the radius is likewise reconstructed. The extensor muscles of the forearm are approximated to the triceps or anconeus.

17.2.6 Dangers

When the extended lateral approach with detachment of the collateral ligament is used, the radial nerve or its branches can be damaged at two points: proximally during detachment of the radial forearm muscles, and distally in the area of the supinator if this has not been stripped from the ulna close to the bone with the forearm pronated.

17.3 Medial Approach to the Elbow Joint

R. Bauer, F. Kerschbaumer, S. Poisel, K. Weise, K. Häringer

17.3.1 Principal Indications

- Fractures of the medial humeral epicondyle
- Instability
- Osteochondritis dissecans
- Synovectomy
- Inflammation
- Ulnar groove syndrome
- Lengthening of the flexor muscles in cerebral palsy

17.3.2 Positioning and Incision

The patient is placed in the supine position. The arm is draped to allow free movement, abducted, and placed on an arm table. The surgeon sits at the axillary side of the arm. The skin incision may curve alternatively in front of or behind the medial humeral epicondyle and has a length of 10 cm (**Fig. 17.20**). Subcutaneously, the medial cutaneous nerves of the arm and forearm are at risk of injury on the flexor side. Behind the medial intermuscular septum, first the fascia covering the ulnar nerve is split, and then the ulnar nerve is exposed and snared. The dissection extends as far as the sulcus of the ulnar nerve. Then, with the elbow flexed, the sail-shaped aponeurosis between the humeral and ulnar origins of flexor carpi ulnaris is split in a longitudinal direction so that the ulnar nerve can be dissected and snared in this area as well. The motor branches supplying flexor carpi ulnaris must be spared (**Figs. 17.21** and **17.22**).

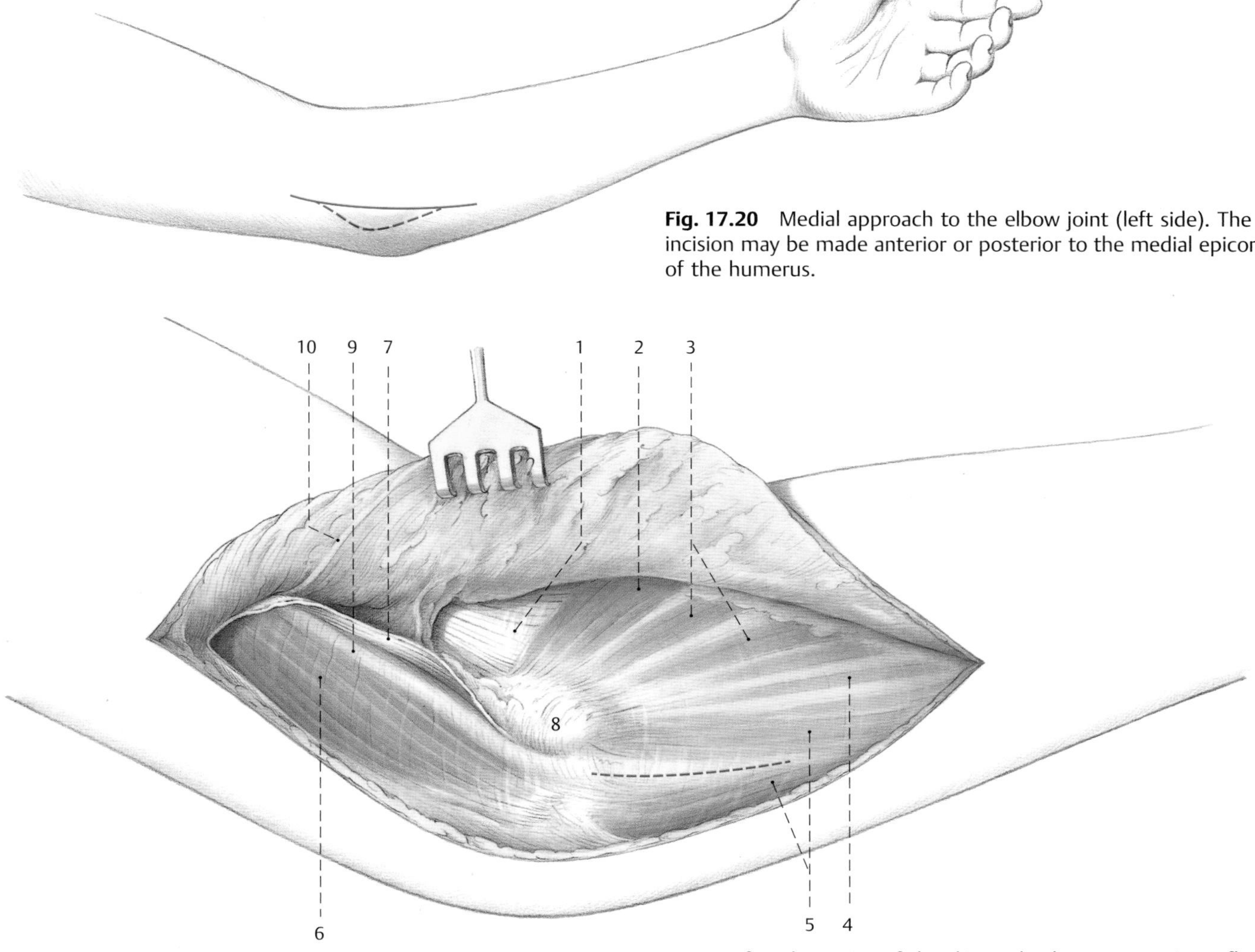

Fig. 17.20 Medial approach to the elbow joint (left side). The skin incision may be made anterior or posterior to the medial epicondyle of the humerus.

Fig. 17.21 After dissection of the skin and subcutaneous tissue flap sparing the cutaneous nerves, the fascia over the ulnar nerve is split.

1 Brachialis
2 Pronator teres
3 Flexor carpi radialis
4 Palmaris longus
5 Flexor carpi ulnaris
6 Triceps brachii
7 Medial intermuscular septum
8 Medial epicondyle of humerus
9 Ulnar nerve
10 Medial cutaneous nerve of forearm

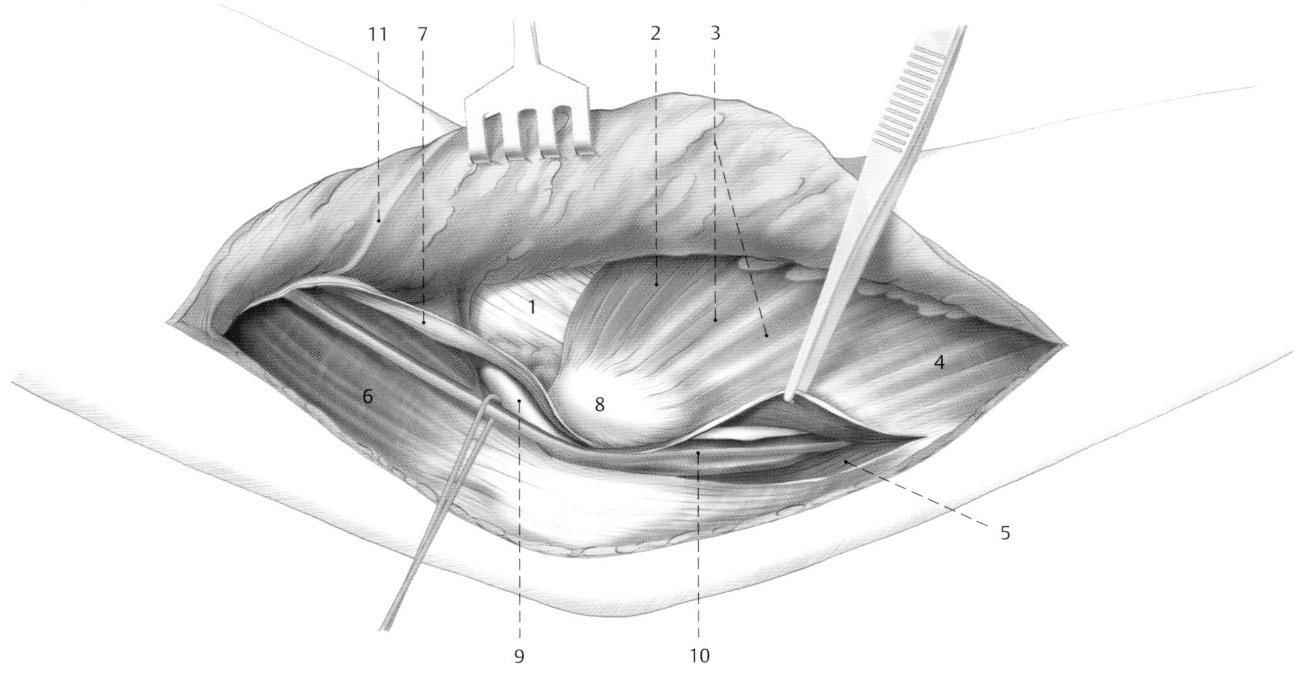

Fig. 17.22 Exposure and snaring of the ulnar nerve.

1 Brachialis
2 Pronator teres
3 Extensor carpi radialis
4 Palmaris longus
5 Flexor carpi ulnaris
6 Triceps brachii
7 Medial intermuscular septum
8 Medial epicondyle of the humerus
9 Sulcus of the ulnar nerve
10 Ulnar nerve
11 Medial cutaneous nerve of forearm

17.3.3 Exposure of the Elbow Joint

Medial arthrotomy may be performed either by detachment of the antebrachial flexors from the medial epicondyle of the humerus or by osteotomy of the epicondyle. Following transection of the medial intermuscular septum, the tip of the medial epicondyle together with the forearm flexor muscles may be retracted distally. Care should be taken not to overextend the motor branches of the median and ulnar nerves. For better exposure of the joint, the elbow is flexed and the ulnar nerve retracted anteriorly. This permits visualization of the coronoid process, the olecranon, and the trochlea of the humerus.

17.3.4 Extension of the Approach

A proximal extension of the approach for exposure of the distal end of the humerus can be obtained by subperiosteal dissection of the brachialis and triceps (**Figs. 17.23** and **17.24**).

Distal extension of the approach is not possible on account of the neural supply of the forearm flexors by the median and ulnar nerves.

17.3.5 Wound Closure

The osteotomized medial epicondyle is reattached with a tension band or tension screw.

17.3.6 Dangers

Excessive distal mobilization of the detached antebrachial flexor muscles with the tip of the epicondyle can lead to partial denervation of the forearm flexor muscles by overextension and rupture of the motor branches. Use of retractors on the anterior side of the brachialis endangers the median nerve.

17.3.7 Note

In case a displacement of the ulnar nerve on the flexor side should prove necessary, the group of forearm flexors has to be mobilized distally. After closure of the medial joint capsule, the ulnar nerve may be transposed between the anterior side of the joint capsule and the forearm flexor muscles. Then the tip of the medial epicondyle is reattached to the humerus.

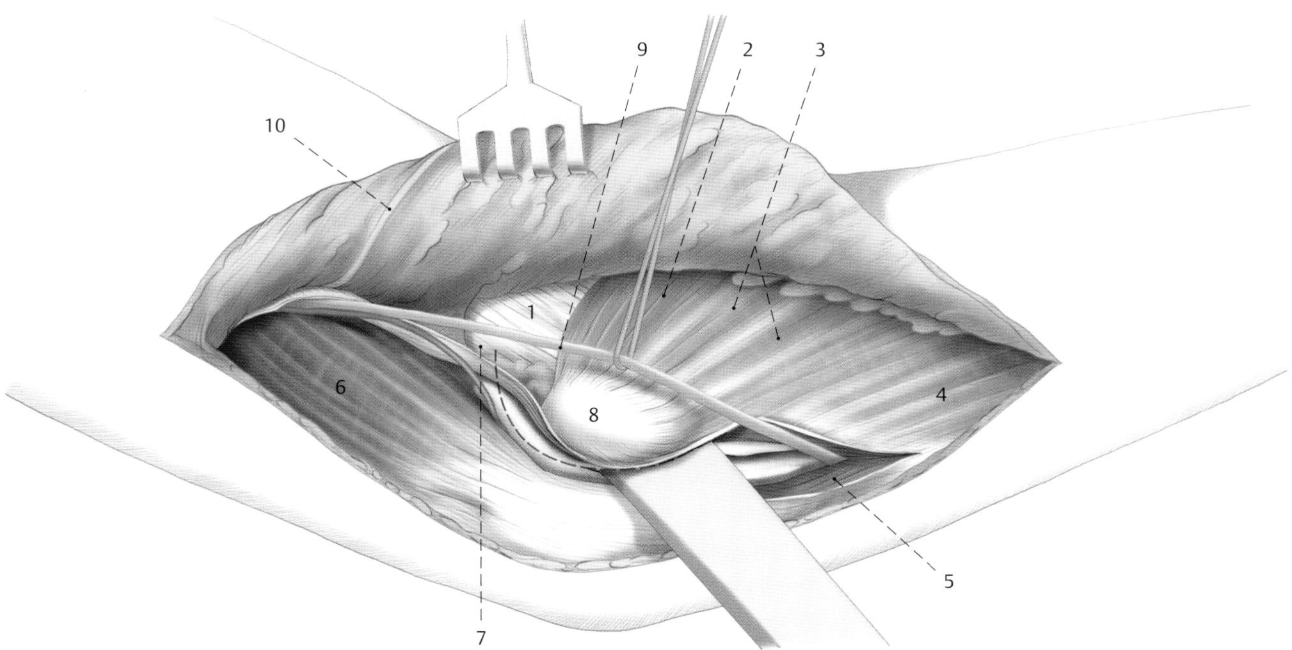

Fig. 17.23 After forward retraction of the ulnar nerve, a drill hole is made, and the medial epicondyle of the humerus is then osteotomized.

1 Brachialis
2 Pronator teres
3 Flexor carpi radialis
4 Palmaris longus
5 Flexor carpi ulnaris
6 Triceps brachii
7 Medial intermuscular septum
8 Medial epicondyle of the humerus
9 Ulnar nerve
10 Medial cutaneous nerve of forearm

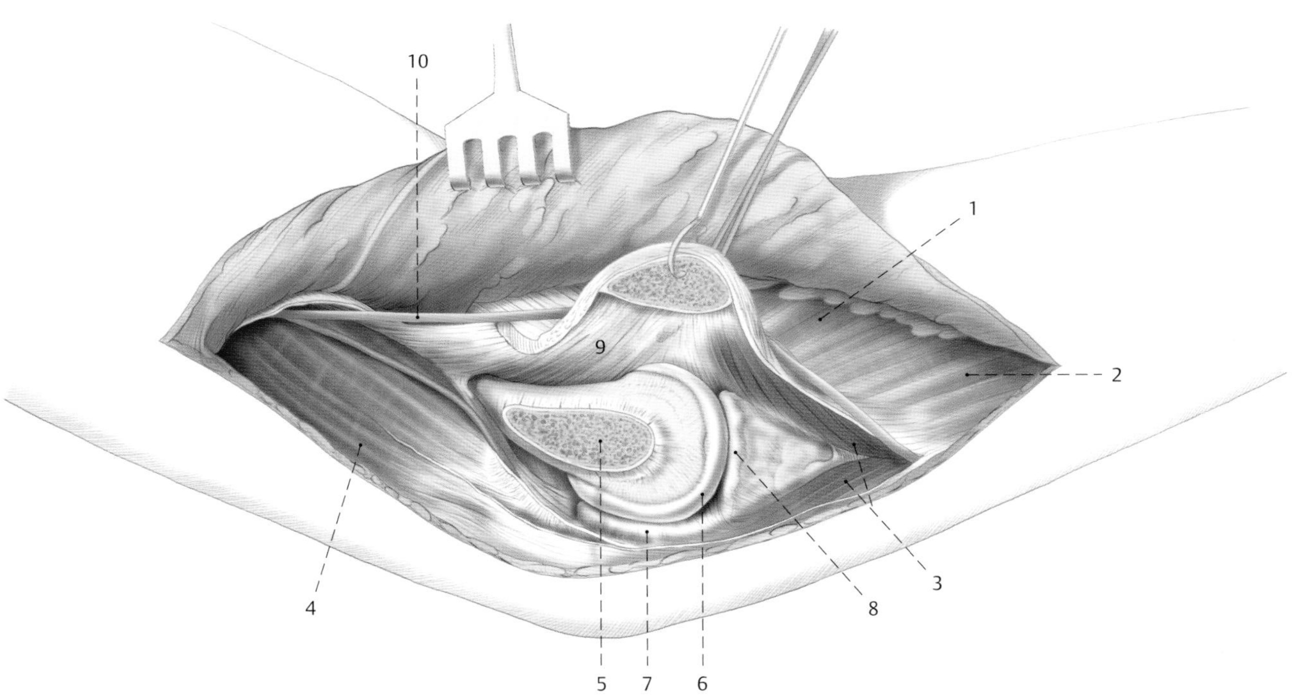

Fig. 17.24 Exposure of the incised elbow joint from the medial side after osteotomy of the medial epicondyle of humerus.

1 Flexor carpi radialis
2 Palmaris longus
3 Flexor carpi ulnaris
4 Triceps brachii
5 Medial epicondyle of the humerus
6 Trochlea of the humerus
7 Olecranon
8 Coronoid process
9 Elbow joint capsule
10 Ulnar nerve

17.4 Anterior Approach to the Elbow Joint

R. Bauer, F. Kerschbaumer, S. Poisel, K. Weise, K. Häringer

17.4.1 Principal Indications

- Fractures of the coronoid process
- Osteochondritis dissecans
- Ruptures of the distal biceps tendon
- Radial nerve compression syndromes
- Dislocations

17.4.2 Positioning and Incision

The patient is placed in the supine position. The arm is draped to allow free movement, abducted, and placed on an arm table. The elbow is extended and the forearm supinated. An S-shaped incision is begun in the groove between the brachialis and brachioradialis, and is continued in a distal direction over the elbow bend (**Fig. 17.25**). Exposure of the fascia requires the ligation of several transversely running veins. The lateral cutaneous nerve of the forearm is at risk subcutaneously. After exposure of the nerve, the fascia is completely split in a longitudinal direction, and the plane between brachioradialis and brachialis is identified (**Fig. 17.26**). Retraction of both muscles brings into view the radial nerve with its division into the superficial and deep branches. The radial recurrent artery with its branches is found in the medial wound region. This vessel should be exposed, ligated, and transected. Now the space between the forearm flexors medially and the forearm extensors laterally can be exposed with the aid of retractors (**Fig. 17.27**).

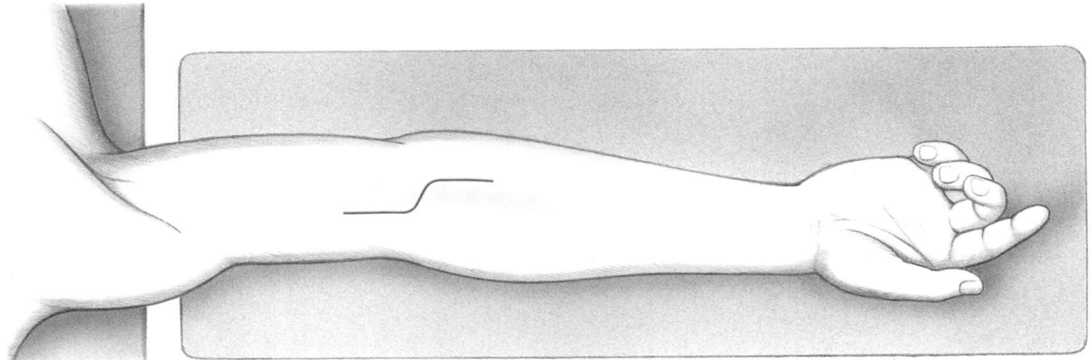

Fig. 17.25 Anterior approach to the elbow joint (right side). Skin incision (solid line).

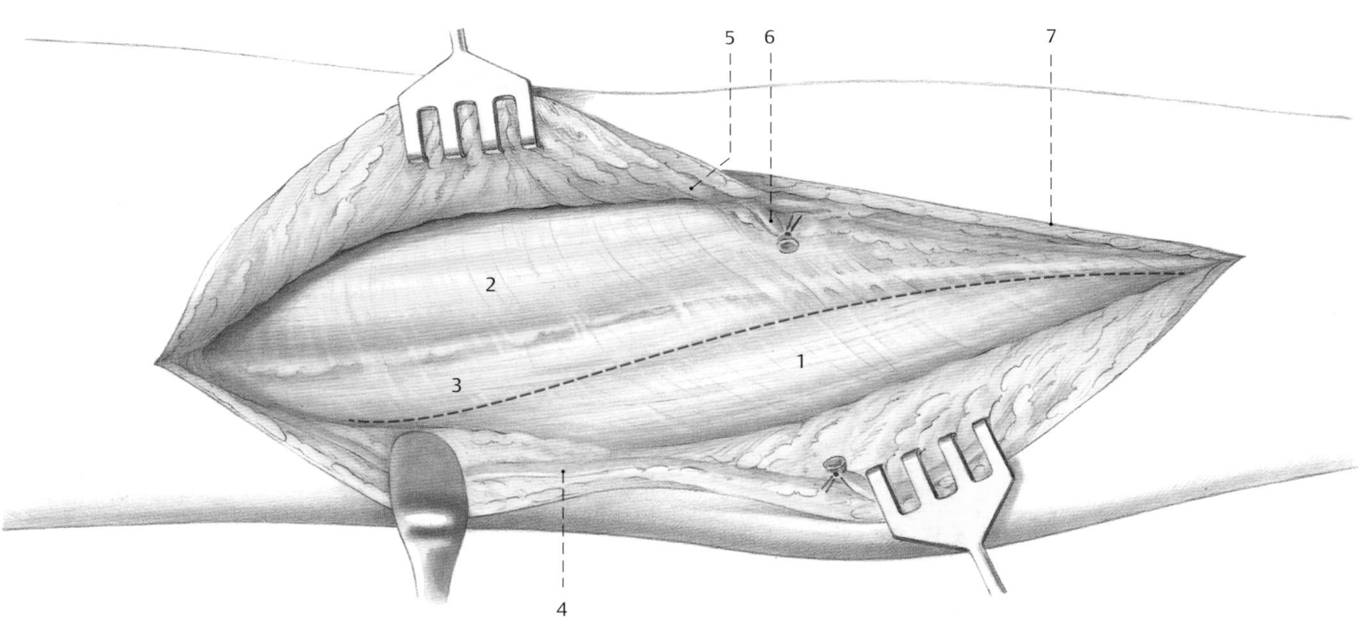

Fig. 17.26 Ligation and transection of the subcutaneous veins, exposure of the lateral cutaneous nerve of the forearm, and splitting of the fascia (dashed line).

1 Brachioradialis
2 Biceps brachii
3 Brachialis
4 Cephalic vein
5 Basilic vein
6 Median cubital vein
7 Lateral cutaneous nerve of forearm

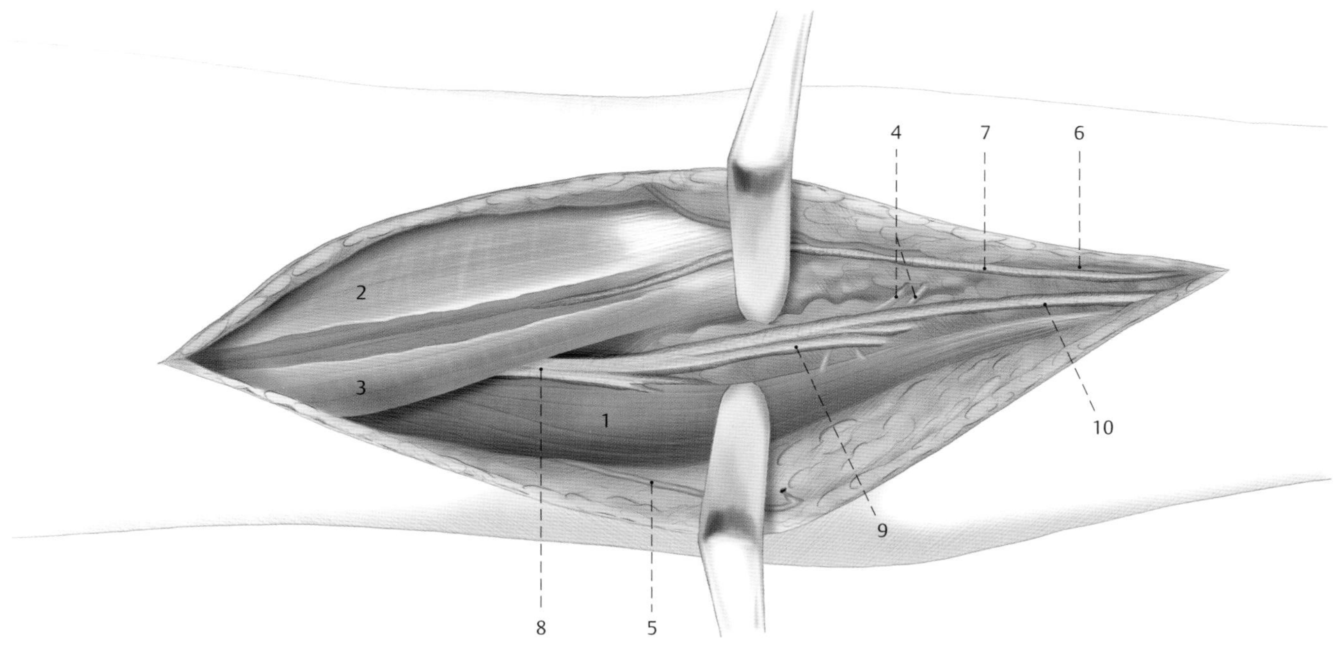

Fig. 17.27 Exposure of the radial nerve between brachialis and brachioradialis.

1 Brachioradialis
2 Biceps brachii
3 Brachialis
4 Radial recurrent artery and vein
5 Cephalic vein
6 Basilic vein
7 Lateral cutaneous nerve of forearm
8 Radial nerve
9 Deep branch of the radial nerve
10 Superficial branch of the radial nerve

17.4.3 Exposure of the Joint

At maximal supination of the forearm, first the bicipitoradial bursa at the insertion of the biceps tendon on the radial tuberosity is incised. The supinator is now detached as far ulnarly as possible, and the annular ligament of the radius and the joint capsule are then opened in longitudinal direction (**Fig. 17.28**). For better exposure, a Langenbeck retractor may be introduced beneath the brachialis while the elbow is slightly flexed. A small Hohmann elevator is passed under the head of the radius. In this way, the humeral capitulum, the radial portion of the trochlea of the humerus, and the head and neck of the radius are clearly visualized (**Fig. 17.29**).

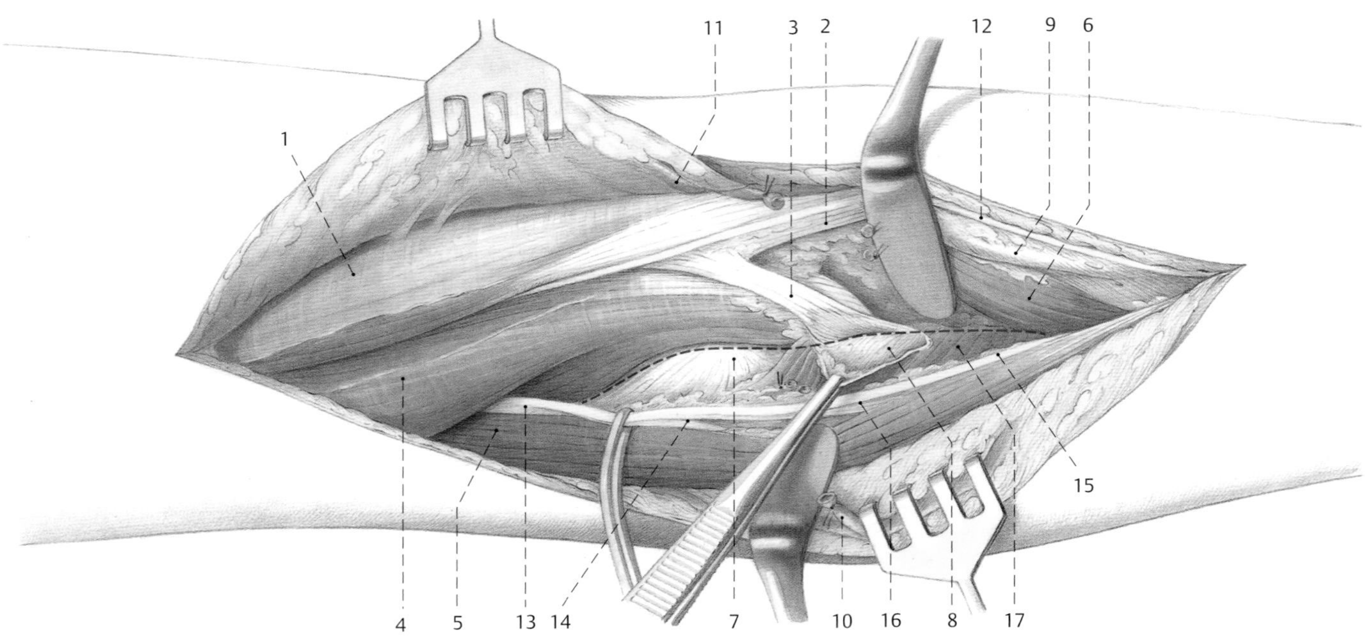

Fig. 17.28 Following ligation of the radial recurrent artery and supination of the forearm, the supinator muscle is detached from the radial tuberosity and the joint capsule is opened (dashed line).

1 Biceps brachii
2 Aponeurosis of biceps brachii
3 Tendon of biceps brachii
4 Brachialis
5 Brachioradialis
6 Pronator teres
7 Elbow joint capsule
8 Bicipitoradial bursa
9 Radial vessels
10 Cephalic vein
11 Basilic vein
12 Lateral cutaneous nerve of forearm
13 Radial nerve
14 Deep branch of the radial nerve
15 Superficial branch of the radial nerve
16 Muscular branch of the radial nerve
17 Supinator

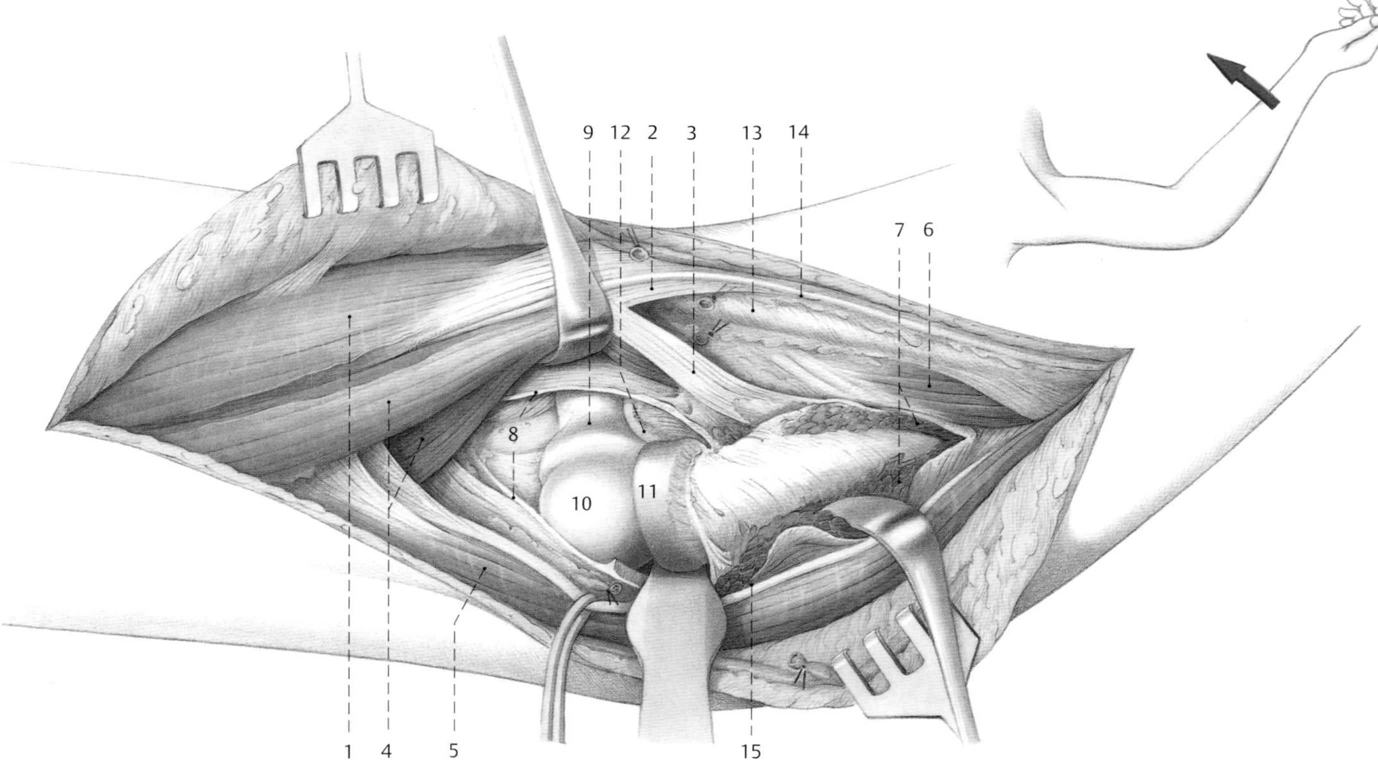

Fig. 17.29 Exposure of the capitulum of the humerus and the proximal end of the radius with the joint incised and flexed.

1 Biceps brachii
2 Aponeurosis of biceps brachii
3 Tendon of biceps brachii
4 Brachialis
5 Brachioradialis
6 Pronator teres
7 Supinator
8 Elbow joint capsule
9 Trochlea of the humerus
10 Capitulum of the humerus
11 Head of the radius (articular circumference)
12 Coronoid process of the ulna
13 Radial vessels
14 Lateral cutaneous nerve of forearm
15 Superficial branch of the radial nerve

17.4.4 Extension of the Approach with Transection of Brachialis

Transection of brachialis occasionally proves necessary in flexion contractures of the elbow joint. In such cases, the brachial artery and the median nerve have to be identified and medially retracted. The brachialis is exposed at its musculotendinous junction, and a curved clamp is passed beneath it from the lateral side. A V-shaped incision is made in the tendinous part, and the tendon is transected (**Fig. 17.30**). The subjacent joint capsule can now be incised transversely. In this way, a complete extension of the elbow can usually be obtained. Now the trochlea of the humerus as well as the coronoid process are well exposed (**Fig. 17.31**).

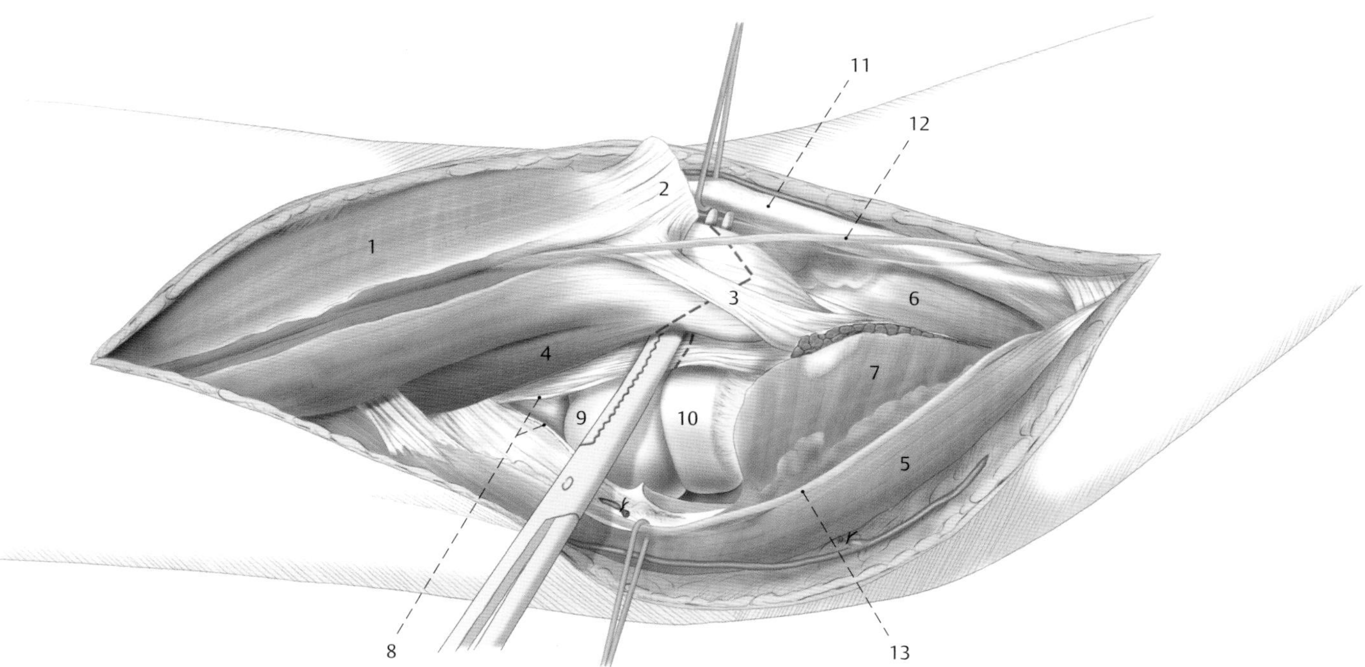

Fig. 17.30 Following exposure and retraction of the brachial artery and the median nerve, the tendon of brachialis is transected, and the joint capsule is opened (dashed line).

1 Biceps brachii
2 Aponeurosis of biceps brachii
3 Tendon of biceps brachii
4 Brachialis
5 Brachioradialis
6 Pronator teres
7 Supinator
8 Elbow joint capsule
9 Capitulum of the humerus
10 Head of radius (articular circumference)
11 Radial vessels and median nerve
12 Lateral cutaneous nerve of forearm
13 Superficial branch of the radial nerve

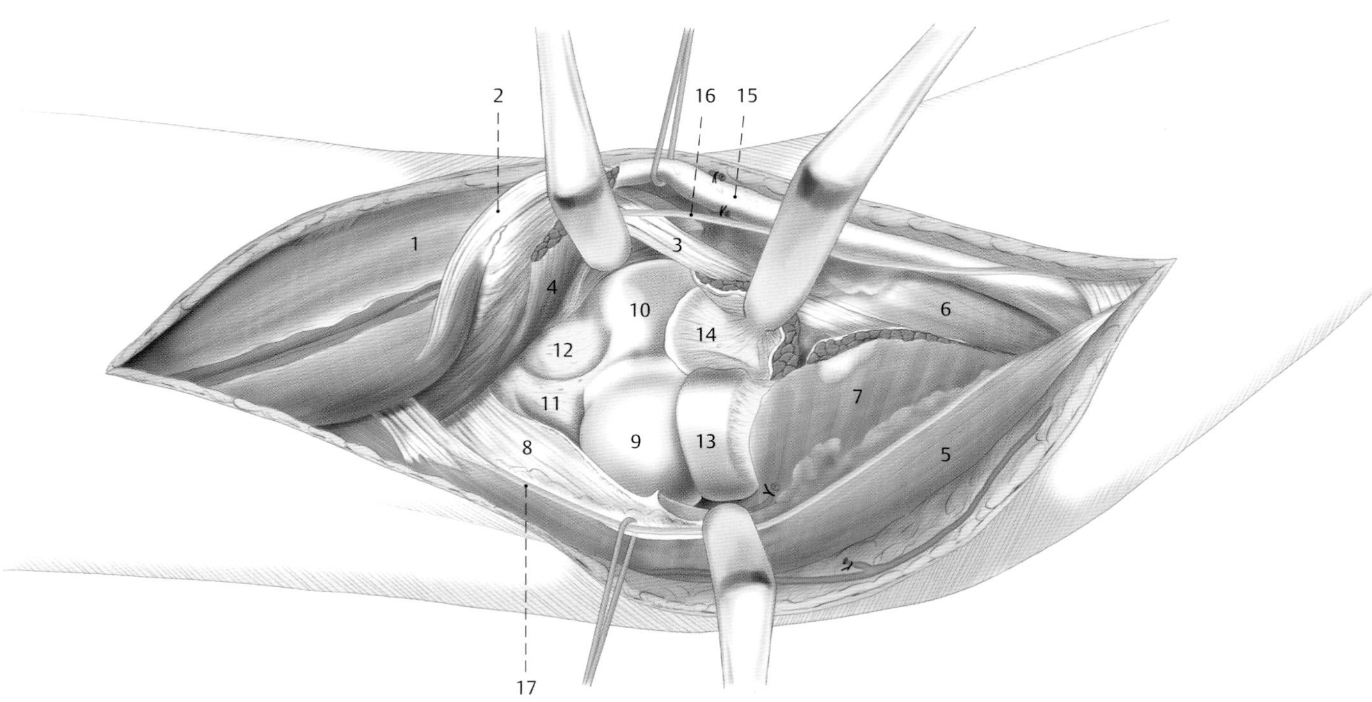

Fig. 17.31 Exposure of the trochlea of the humerus and the coronoid process after transection of the tendon of brachialis.

1 Biceps brachii
2 Aponeurosis of biceps brachii
3 Tendon of biceps brachii
4 Brachialis
5 Brachioradialis
6 Pronator teres
7 Supinator
8 Elbow joint capsule
9 Capitulum of the humerus
10 Trochlea of the humerus
11 Radial fossa
12 Coronoid fossa
13 Head of the radius (articular circumference)
14 Coronoid process of the ulna
15 Radial vessels and median nerve
16 Lateral cutaneous nerve of forearm
17 Superficial branch of the radial nerve

17.4.5 Anatomical Site

The course of the radial artery and median nerve is shown on the flexor side of the elbow and forearm. For better exposure of the muscular branches of the median nerve, the humeral head of pronator teres and the flexor digitorum superficialis have been detached from the radius. The relation of the median nerve to the various layers of the forearm flexor muscles also points to possible locations of proximal median nerve compression syndromes (**Fig. 17.32**).

17.4.6 Wound Closure

With the enlarged approach, the tendon of the brachialis is sutured in the extended position by V–Y reconstruction. The joint capsule is closed, and the supinator muscle is reinserted.

17.4.7 Dangers

The deep branch of the radial nerve can be damaged if detachment of the supinator from the neck of the radius is not done directly on the radial tuberosity with the forearm supinated. The lateral cutaneous nerve of the forearm can be injured on splitting the fascia and should therefore always be identified and exposed. In the enlarged approach, the brachial artery and the median nerve have to be exposed and retracted before transection of the brachialis to avoid damage.

17.4.8 Note

In case a displacement of the ulnar nerve on the flexor side should prove necessary, the group of forearm flexors has to be mobilized distally. After closure of the medial joint capsule, the ulnar nerve may be transposed between the anterior side of the joint capsule and the forearm flexor muscles. Then the tip of the medial epicondyle is reattached to the humerus.

A 2–3 cm transverse incision in the elbow usually suffices for reattaching the distal biceps tendon without the aid of a suture anchor.

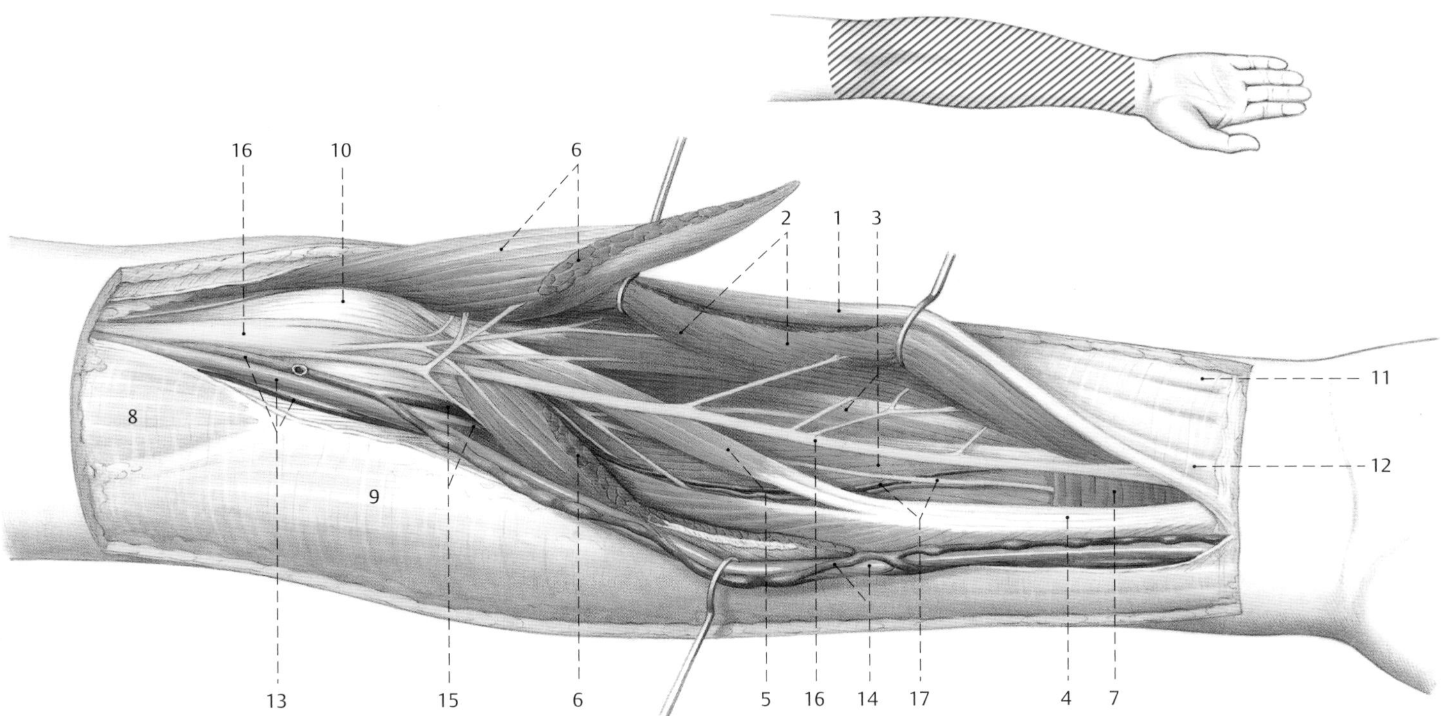

Fig. 17.32 Anatomical site. Note the position and course of the median nerve and its muscular branches. The humeral head of pronator teres and the flexor digitorum superficialis have been detached from the radius.

1 Flexor carpi radialis
2 Flexor digitorum superficialis
3 Flexor digitorum profundus
4 Flexor pollicis longus
5 Humeral head of flexor pollicis longus (var.)
6 Pronator teres
7 Pronator quadratus
8 Biceps brachii
9 Brachioradialis
10 Brachialis
11 Flexor carpi ulnaris
12 Palmaris longus
13 Brachial artery and accompanying veins
14 Radial artery and accompanying veins
15 Ulnar artery and accompanying veins
16 Median nerve
17 Anterior interosseous vessels and nerve

17.5 Approaches for Elbow Arthroscopy

D. Kohn

17.5.1 Principal Indications

- Unexplained pain and blockade despite imaging
- Prior to open surgery
- Removal of loose bodies
- Synovectomy
- Arthrolysis

17.5.2 Positioning

We prefer the supine position with the patient's arm suspended and freely mobile (**Fig. 17.33**) as this allows clear visualization of the structures on the flexor side of the joint. An assistant is essential to stabilize the elbow in space. Other authors prefer the prone or the lateral decubitus position, which provides better access to the posterior side of the joint and more stable fixation of the arm (**Fig. 17.34**). The position of the surgical and anesthetic team does not depend on the patient's position.

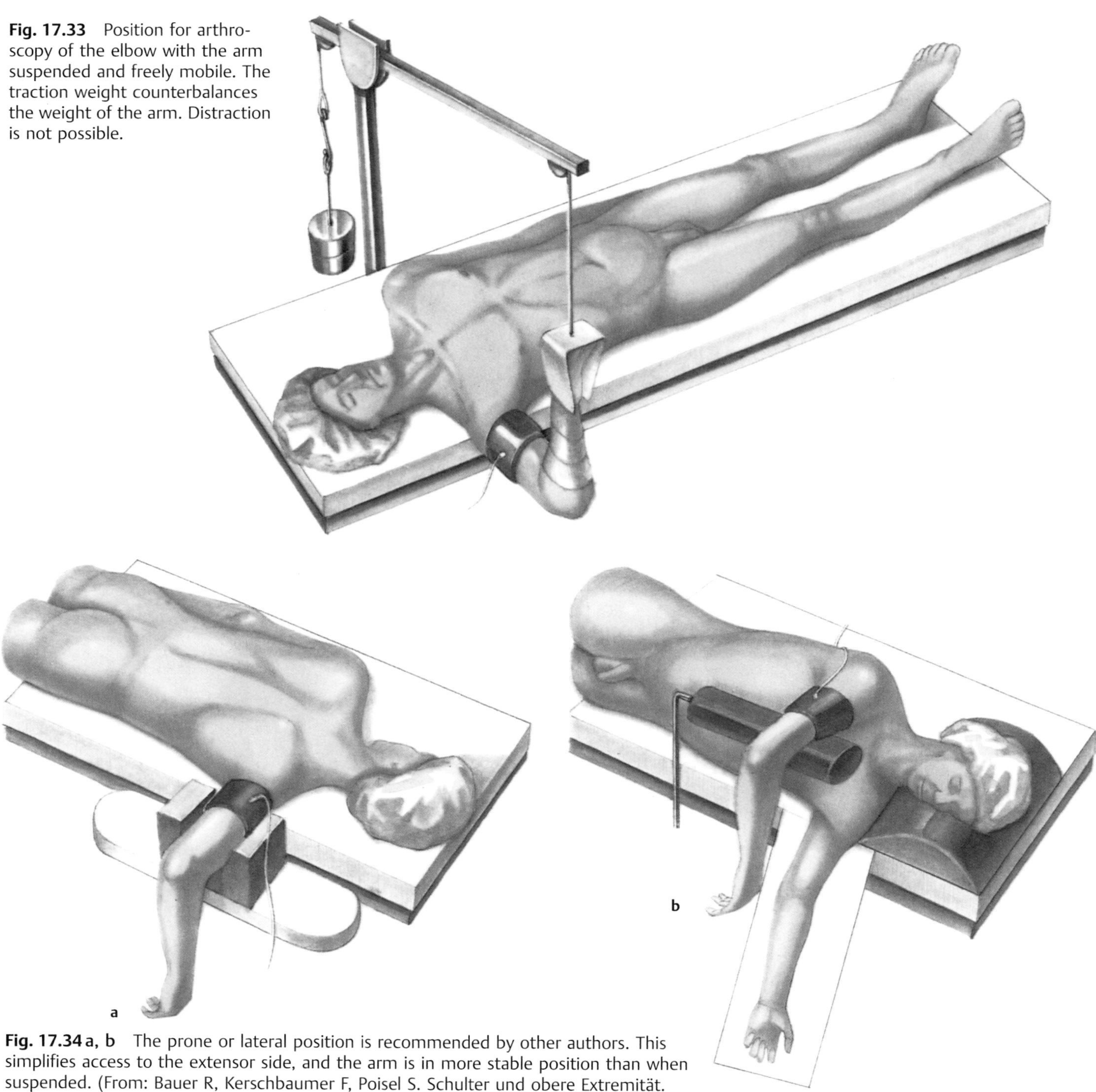

Fig. 17.33 Position for arthroscopy of the elbow with the arm suspended and freely mobile. The traction weight counterbalances the weight of the arm. Distraction is not possible.

Fig. 17.34 a, b The prone or lateral position is recommended by other authors. This simplifies access to the extensor side, and the arm is in more stable position than when suspended. (From: Bauer R, Kerschbaumer F, Poisel S. Schulter und obere Extremität. Stuttgart, Thieme; 1997. Orthopädische Operationslehre; Band 3.)

a Prone position.
b Lateral position.

17.5.3 Approaches

All approaches to the elbow are defined by bony landmarks. The approaches are created only after the joint has been filled, as the safe distance from neurovascular structures is greater when the joint is tensely filled. The joint is punctured at the center of the triangle formed by the tip of the olecranon, the head of the radius, and the radial epicondyle (**Fig. 17.35**). As with the ankle, the sensory nerve branches must be spared by a special technique when opening portals for the elbow as there is no adequate safe distance. The incision is made in an elevated skin fold. The path of the trocar and trocar sleeve is prepared with a clamp. The synovial capsule is penetrated with a blunt trocar.

Further approaches (**Fig. 17.36**) are made either from without inward using the same technique as at the ankle because of the proximity of sensory nerves (**Fig. 17.37**), or from within outward (**Fig. 17.38**)

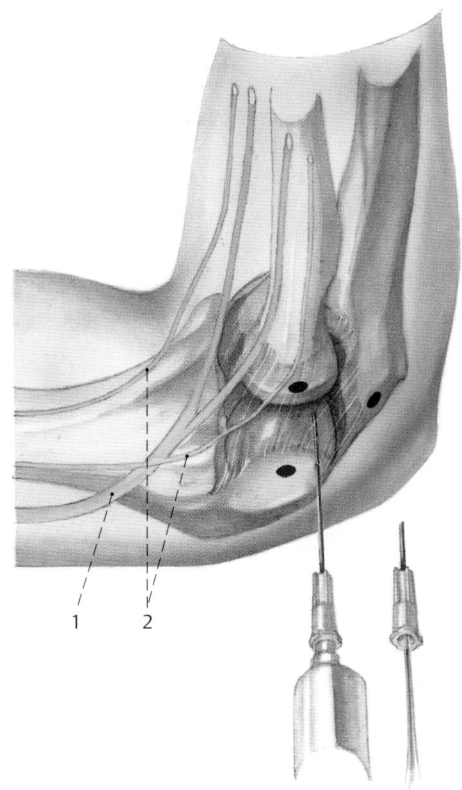

Fig. 17.35 Puncture of the elbow and filling it via the posteroradial approach. A free backflow of fluid from the needle confirms that it is in the correct intra-articular position. (From: Bauer R, Kerschbaumer F, Poisel S. Schulter und obere Extremität. Stuttgart, Thieme; 1997. Orthopädische Operationslehre; Band 3.)

1 Radial nerve
2 Lateral cutaneous nerve of forearm

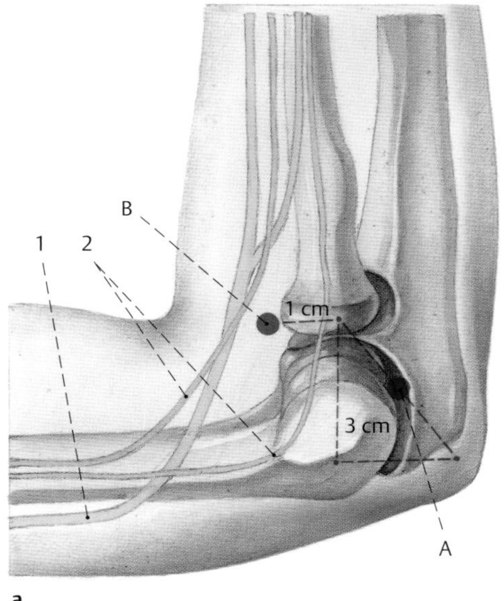

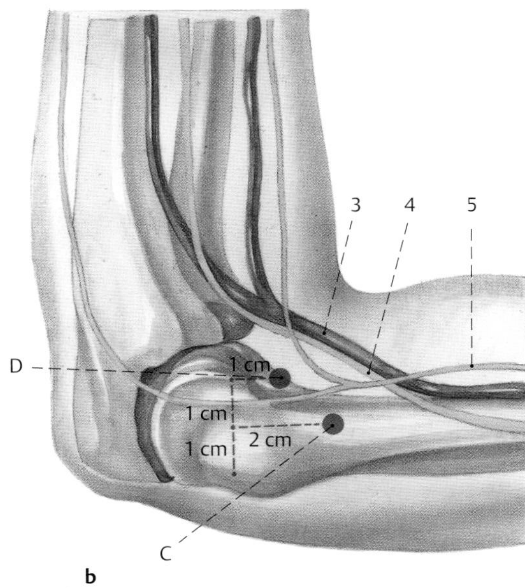

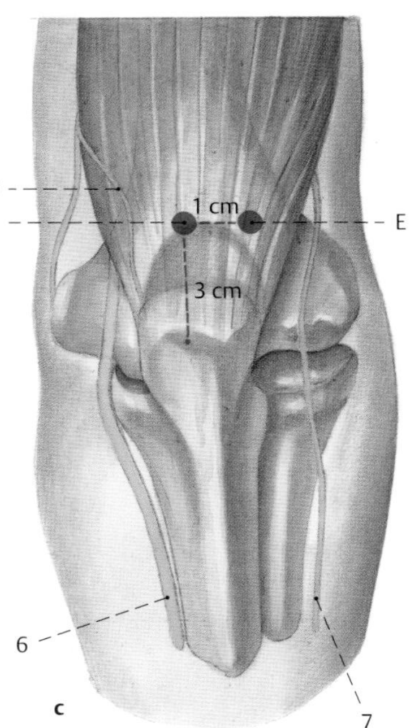

Fig. 17.36 a–c Approaches. (From: Bauer R, Kerschbaumer F, Poisel S. Schulter und obere Extremität. Stuttgart, Thieme; 1997. Orthopädische Operationslehre; Band 3.)

1 Radial nerve
2 Lateral cutaneous nerve of forearm
3 Brachial artery
4 Median nerve
5 Medial cutaneous nerve of forearm
6 Ulnar nerve
7 Posterior cutaneous nerve of forearm

a Radial.
A Posteroradial
B Anteroradial
b Ulnar.
C Superoulnar
D Anteroulnar
c Posterior.
E Posterolateral
F Posterocentral

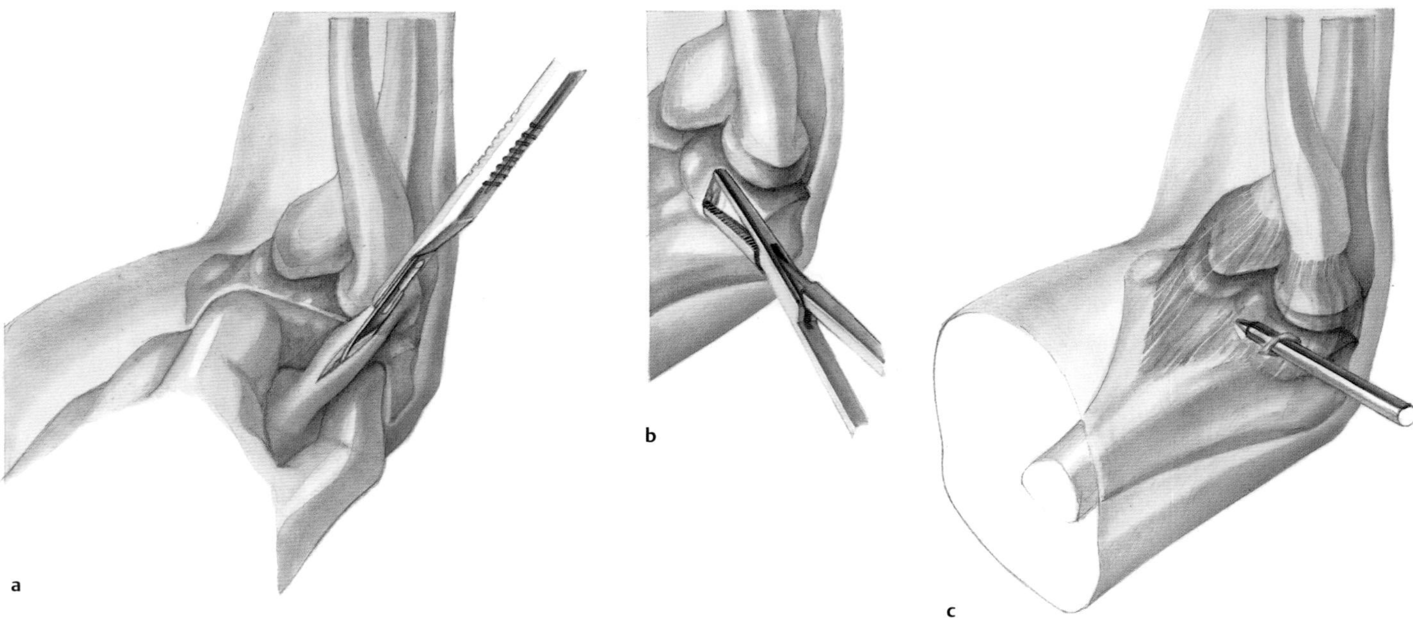

Fig. 17.37 a–c Technique for sparing sensory nerve branches when opening the approaches. (From: Bauer R, Kerschbaumer F, Poisel S. Schulter und obere Extremität. Stuttgart, Thieme; 1997. Orthopädische Operationslehre; Band 3.)

a The incision is made in an elevated skin fold.
b The path of the trocar sleeve is prepared with a small blunt clamp.
c The joint capsule is penetrated with a blunt trocar/trocar sleeve.

17.5.4 Wound Closure

Following removal of the arthroscopy instruments, the wound is closed by skin sutures. The tourniquet should be released before the end of the operation so that hemostasis can take place and a Redon drain can be inserted if necessary.

17.5.5 Dangers

Injury to cutaneous nerves, neurovascular structures (brachial artery and median nerve), or the ulnar nerve and radial nerve may occur. Ulnar approaches are contraindicated if the ulnar nerve has previously been transposed anteriorly.

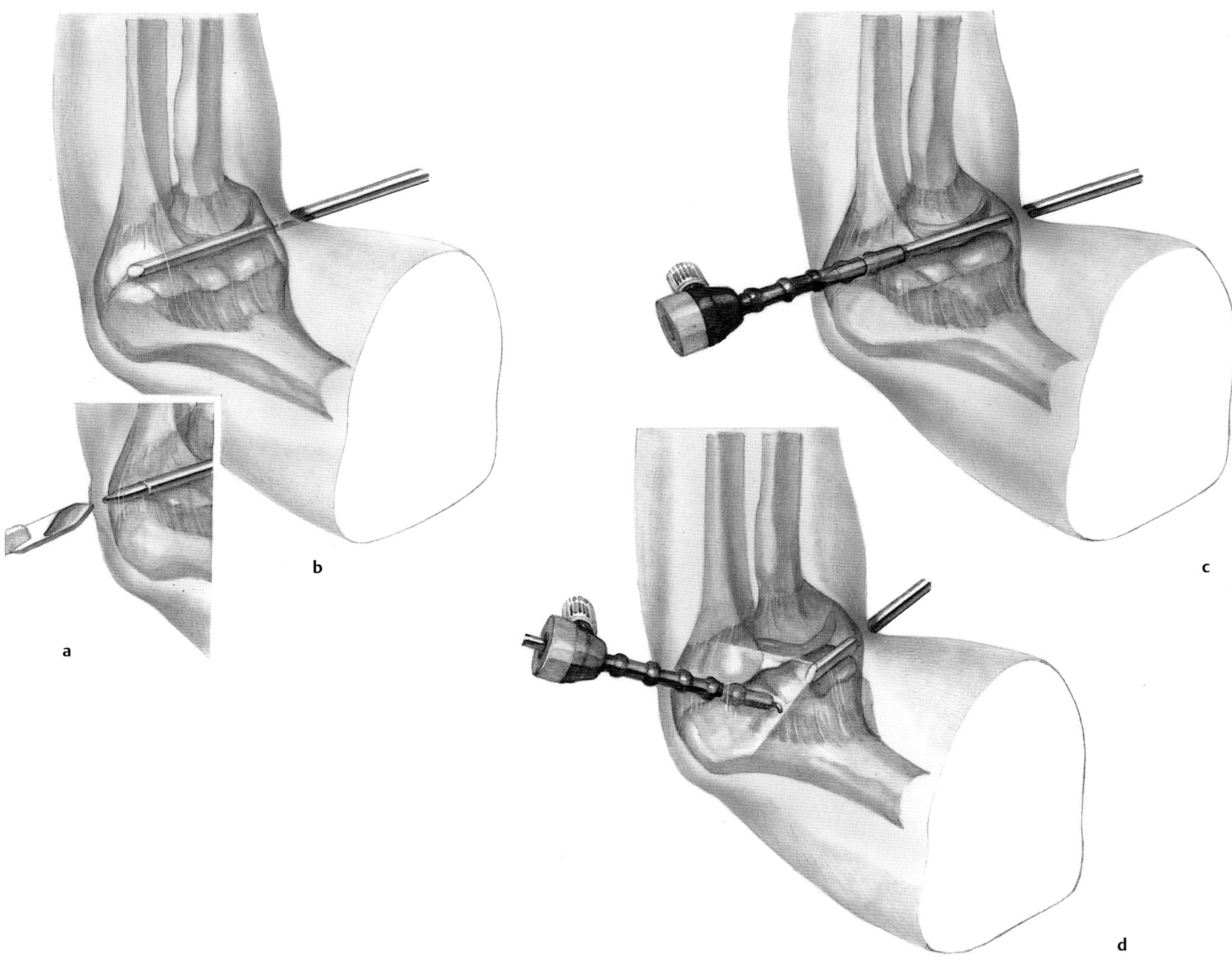

Fig. 17.38 a–d Creation of the anteroulnar approach from an existing anteroradial approach. (From: Bauer R, Kerschbaumer F, Poisel S. Schulter und obere Extremität. Stuttgart, Thieme; 1997. Orthopädische Operationslehre; Band 3.)

a The arthroscope is advanced transversely through the joint cavity and placed on the ulnar wall of the joint.
b The sharp trocar is introduced, and the medial capsule and skin are perforated after a counterincision.
c A working cannula is attached, and the trocar is replaced with the arthroscope.
d The arthroscope is withdrawn and the palpating hook is placed in the working cannula.

18 Forearm

18.1 Anterior Approach to the Radius According to Henry

R. Bauer, F. Kerschbaumer, S. Poisel

Exposure of the proximal two-thirds of the radius and of the humeroradial joint.

18.1.1 Principal Indications

- Fractures of the radius
- Dislocation of the head of the radius
- Rupture of the biceps tendon
- Inflammation
- Tumors

18.1.2 Positioning and Incision

The patient is placed in the supine position, and the abducted forearm rests on a side table. After application of a tourniquet, the arm is draped to allow free movement. The skin incision is started a handbreadth proximal to the elbow bend between the palpable biceps tendon and the lateral forearm extensors. The incision curves over the elbow joint and continues distally as far as the styloid process of the radius (**Fig. 18.1**). After transection of the skin, the transversely running superficial veins are transected and ligated. The lateral cutaneous nerve of the forearm has to be spared and retracted medially when the fascia is transected.

The biceps tendon is exposed on its lateral side, and the fascia is split in a distal direction along the course of the brachioradialis. This muscle is now laterally retracted, while the flexor muscles of the forearm are retracted in a medial direction (**Fig. 18.2**). Proximally, the radial nerve is revealed between the brachialis and brachioradialis. For exposure of the proximal portion of the radius, the radial recurrent artery has to be exposed, ligated, and transected. The forearm is supinated, the bicipitoradial bursa at the radial tuberosity is incised, and the proximal end of the radius is exposed just at the insertion of the biceps tendon. The supinator is separated subperiosteally and retracted in a lateral direction together with the deep branch of the radial nerve. Further incision, proximally and distally, is made along the dashed line in **Fig. 18.2**. If possible, the insertion of pronator teres should not be detached.

18.1.3 Exposure of the Radius

The forearm should now be pronated (**Fig. 18.3**), as a result of which the posterior portion of the radius becomes readily visible. If necessary, the distal portion of the radius may also be exposed. The use of Hohmann elevators in the proximal portion should be avoided if possible (to ensure preservation of the deep branch of the radial nerve). Subperiosteal exposure is not required with fractures.

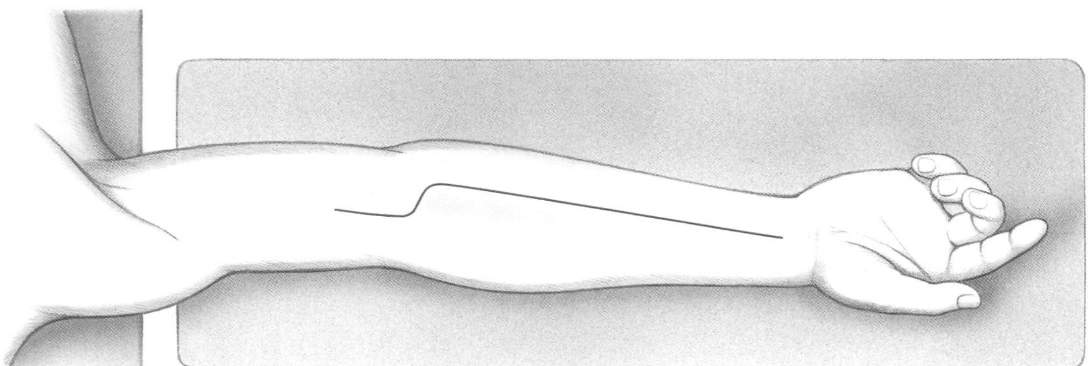

Fig. 18.1 Anterior approach to radius according to Henry (right side). Skin incision.

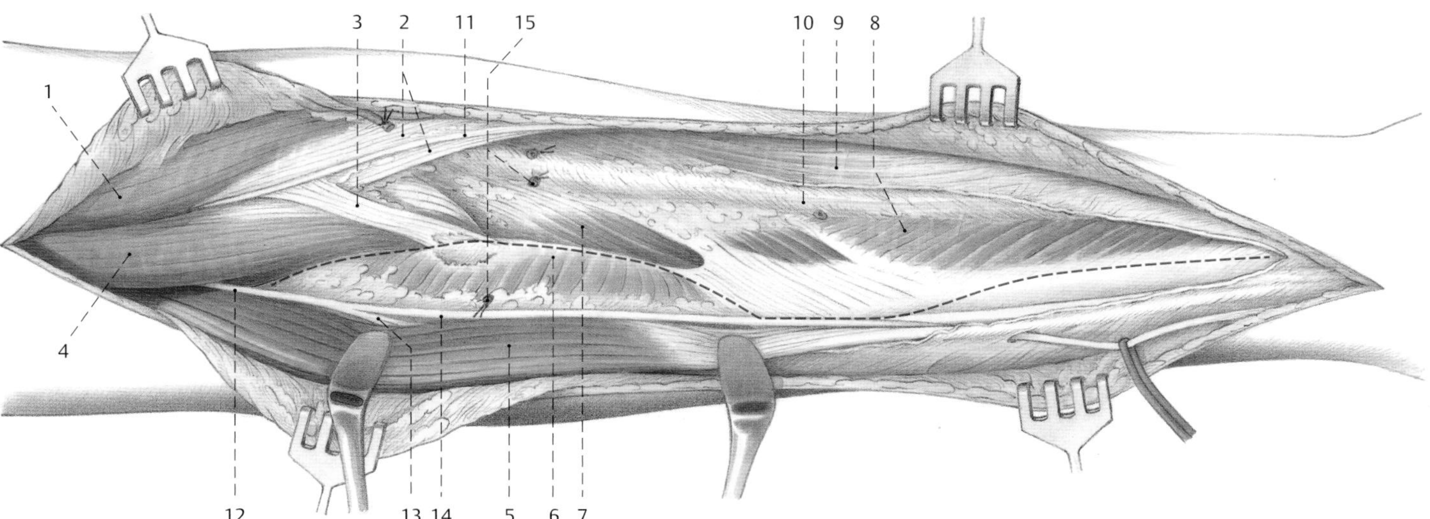

Fig. 18.2 After splitting of the fascia while sparing the lateral antebrachial cutaneous nerve, brachioradialis is retracted in a radial direction with the forearm supinated. The radial nerve is exposed, and the radial recurrent artery transected. The joint capsule is opened, and the radius exposed subperiosteally after stripping of the supinator (dashed line).

1 Biceps brachii
2 Aponeurosis of biceps brachii
3 Biceps brachii tendon
4 Brachialis
5 Brachioradialis
6 Supinator
7 Pronator teres
8 Flexor pollicis longus
9 Flexor carpi radialis
10 Radial vessels
11 Lateral cutaneous nerve of forearm
12 Radial nerve
13 Deep branch of the radial nerve
14 Superficial branch of the radial nerve
15 Radial recurrent artery

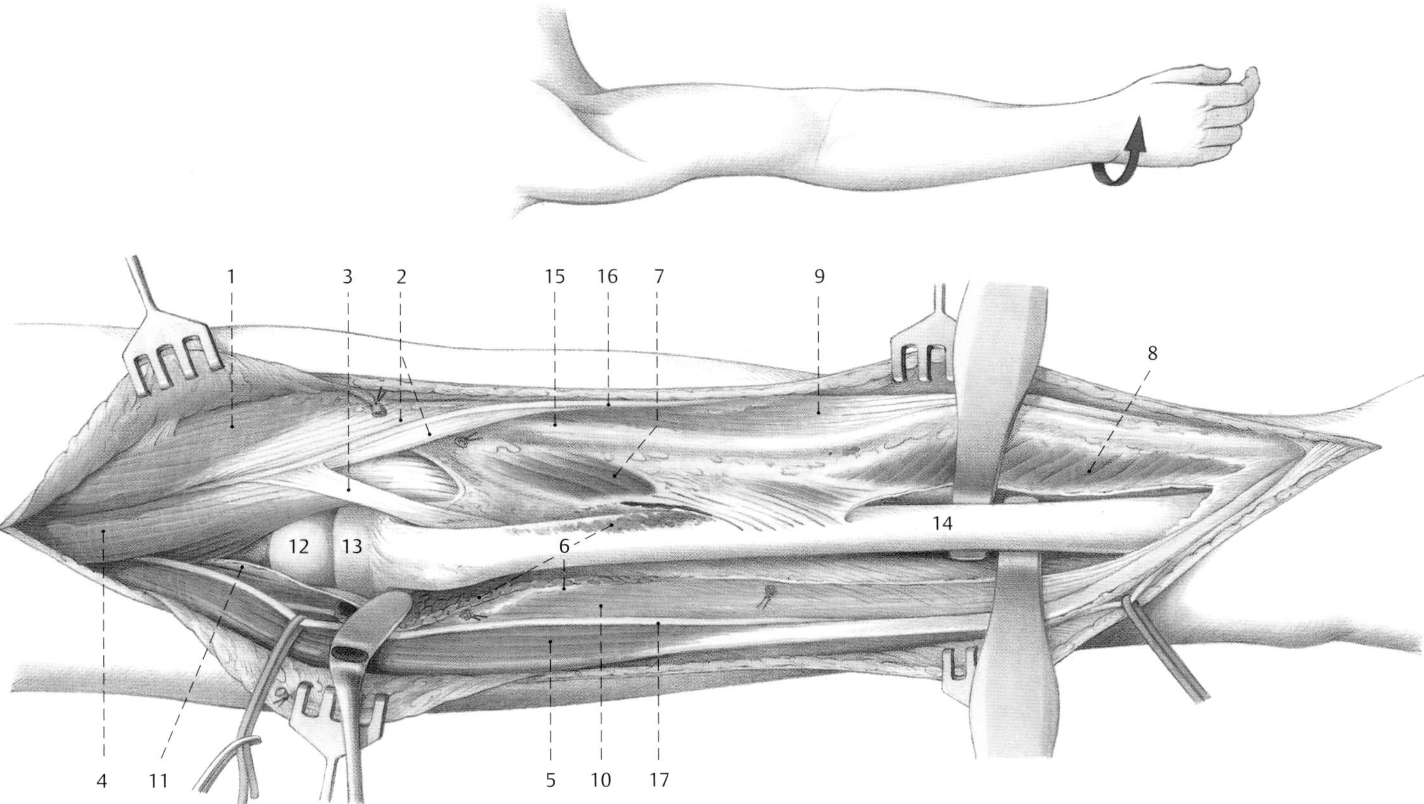

Fig. 18.3 By pronation of the forearm, the radius is exposed as far as the distal metaphysis. No detachment of pronator teres is necessary.

1 Biceps brachii
2 Aponeurosis of biceps brachii
3 Biceps brachii tendon
4 Brachialis
5 Brachioradialis
6 Supinator
7 Pronator teres
8 Flexor pollicis longus
9 Flexor carpi radialis
10 Extensor carpi radialis longus
11 Elbow joint capsule
12 Capitulum of the humerus
13 Head of the radius
14 Body of the radius
15 Radial vessels
16 Lateral cutaneous nerve of forearm
17 Superficial branch of the radial nerve

18.1.4 Anatomical Site

The cross-section of the proximal forearm in **Fig. 18.4** shows the approach to the radius between the radial extensors and the ulnar flexors. The same figure also shows the dorsoradial approach to the radius according to Thompson, as well as the Boyd approach to the proximal end of the ulna and the head of the radius (see Section 18.3). Note the position of the supinator and its relation to the deep branch of the radial nerve (see also **Fig. 18.9**).

18.1.5 Wound Closure

Of the deep layers, only the capsule needs to be sutured, and the supinator brought into apposition with the forearm supinated. No other muscle sutures are necessary. Further wound closure is performed in layers.

18.1.6 Dangers

During transection of the fascia in the proximal wound region, the terminal branch of the musculocutaneous nerve (lateral cutaneous nerve of the forearm) has to be spared. In the distal wound region, the main branch of the radial nerve passing through the fascia has to be spared (see **Fig. 18.3**). The supinator has to be stripped with the forearm supinated, close to the insertion of the biceps tendon, so that injury to the deep branch of the radial nerve may be prevented.

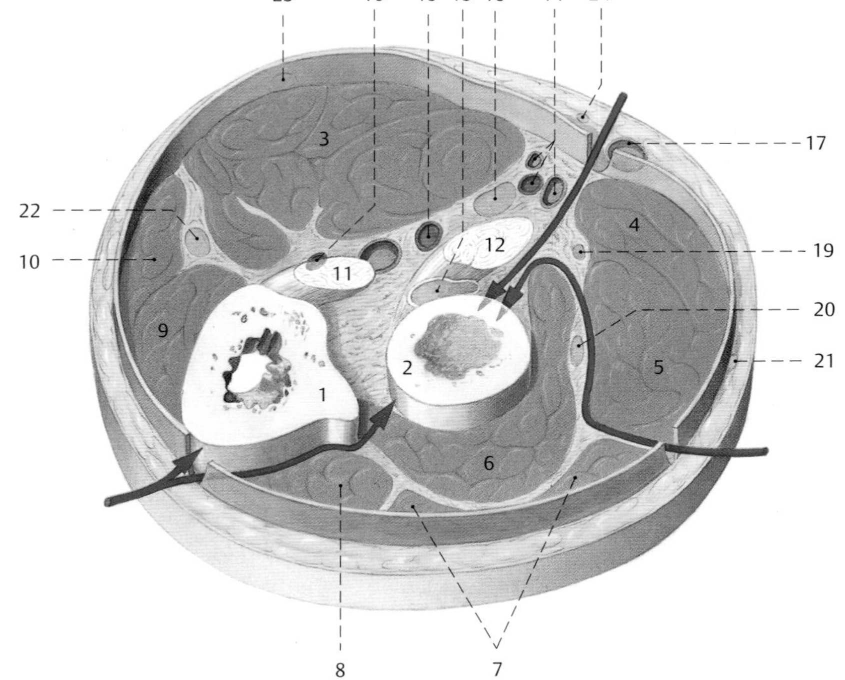

Fig. 18.4 Anatomical site. The schematic cross-section through the proximal forearm shows the approaches to the radius and ulna (arrows) (right arm, proximal view).

1 Ulna
2 Radius
3 Common head of the flexor muscles
4 Brachioradialis
5 Extensor carpi radialis
6 Supinator
7 Extensor digitorum
8 Extensor carpi ulnaris
9 Flexor digitorum profundus
10 Flexor carpi ulnaris
11 Brachialis tendon
12 Biceps brachii tendon
13 Bicipitoradial bursa
14 Radial artery and accompanying veins
15 Common interosseous artery
16 Ulnar artery
17 Cephalic vein
18 Median nerve
19 Superficial branch of the radial nerve
20 Deep branch of the radial nerve
21 Posterior cutaneous nerve of forearm
22 Ulnar nerve
23 Medial cutaneous nerve of forearm
24 Lateral cutaneous nerve of forearm

18.2 Dorsolateral Approach to the Radius According to Thompson

R. Bauer, F. Kerschbaumer, S. Poisel

Exposure of the radius from the posterior side except for parts close to the joint (elbow and wrist).

18.2.1 Principal Indications

- Fractures
- Pseudarthrosis
- Osteotomies
- Inflammation
- Tumors

18.2.2 Positioning and Incision

The patient is placed in the supine position with the arm abducted and resting on a side table, or laterally along the body. After application of a tourniquet, the arm is draped to allow free movement. The skin incision begins over the lateral epicondyle of the humerus and then curves anteriorly and continues in a straight line as far as the styloid process of the radius (**Fig. 18.5**).

After transection of the skin and subcutaneous tissue, the plane between the radial extensor group (brachioradialis, extensor carpi radialis longus and brevis) and the extensor digitorum is exposed by palpation. The fascia is split from distal to proximal, the incision starting over the readily visible muscle bellies of abductor pollicis longus and extensor pollicis brevis (**Fig. 18.6**). The proximad incision continues as far as the tendinous portion of the forearm extensors.

18.2.3 Exposure of the Radius

The supinator, at whose lower margin the deep branch of the radial nerve (posterior interosseous nerve) emerges, becomes visible in the depth of the operative field upon retraction of the muscle groups. If necessary, the distal third of the supinator may be subperiosteally detached from the radius as far anteriorly as possible, with the forearm supinated, and retracted laterally together with the radial nerve. The radius is exposed more distally along the dashed line shown in **Fig. 18.7**. Following subperiosteal dissection of the medial segment of the radial shaft, the forearm is pronated, and

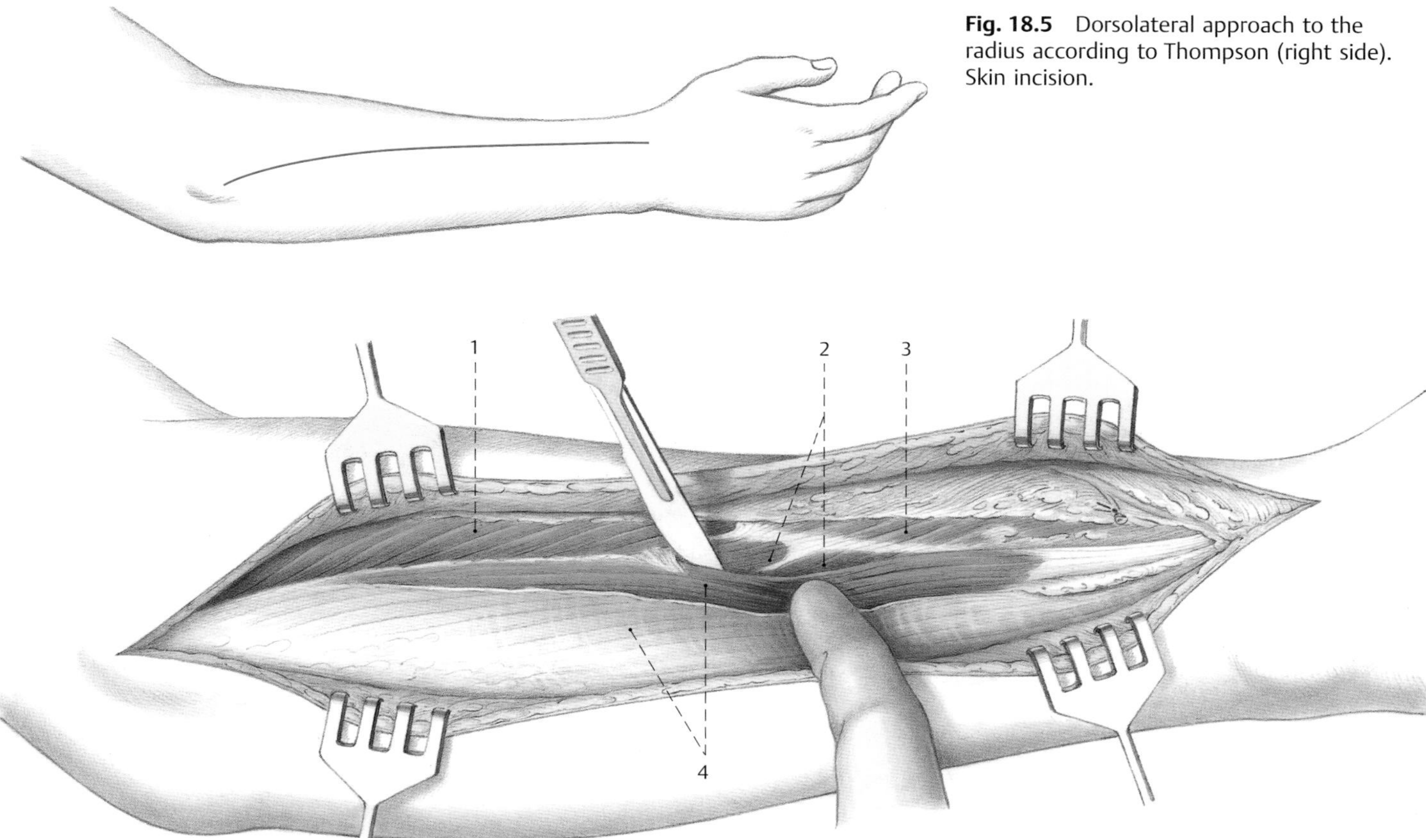

Fig. 18.5 Dorsolateral approach to the radius according to Thompson (right side). Skin incision.

Fig. 18.6 Division of the fascia, and incision between the radial extensors of the wrist and extensor digitorum. To spare the muscular branches of the radial nerve, the extensor of the fingers may be retracted.

1 Extensor carpi radialis brevis
2 Abductor pollicis longus
3 Extensor pollicis brevis
4 Extensor digitorum

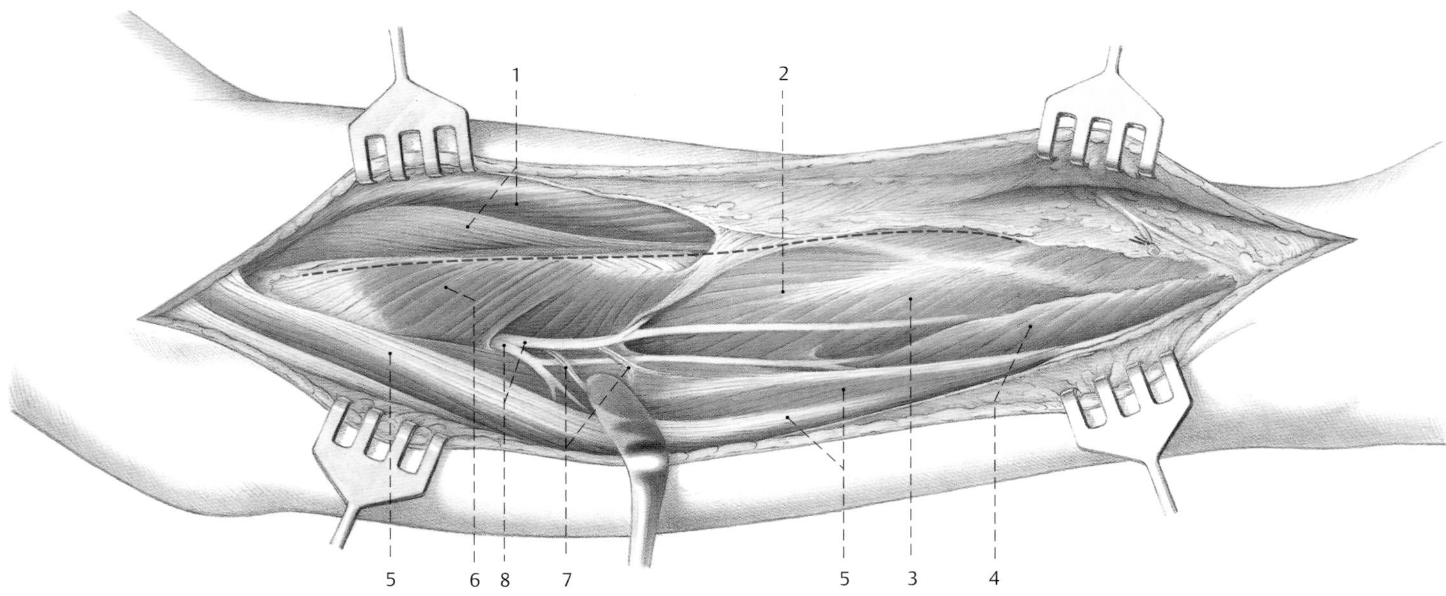

Fig. 18.7 Operative site after stripping of extensor digitorum as far as the lateral epicondyle of the humerus. For exposure of the radius, the distal parts of the supinator may be detached with the forearm supinated. The incision is then extended distally (dashed line).

1 Extensor carpi radialis brevis
2 Abductor pollicis longus
3 Extensor pollicis brevis
4 Extensor pollicis longus
5 Extensor digitorum
6 Supinator
7 Posterior interosseous artery (muscular branches)
8 Deep branch of the radial nerve

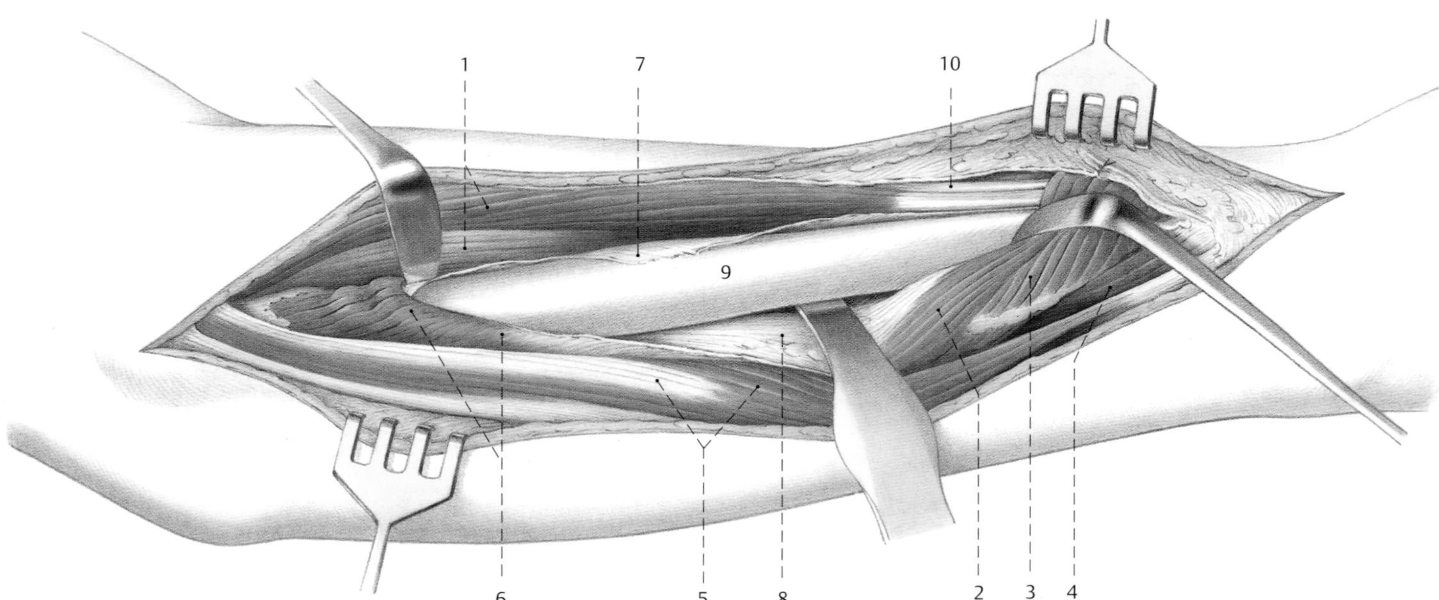

Fig. 18.8 Exposure of the mid shaft of the radius with the forearm pronated.

1 Extensor carpi radialis brevis
2 Abductor pollicis longus
3 Extensor pollicis brevis
4 Extensor pollicis longus
5 Extensor digitorum
6 Supinator
7 Pronator teres (insertion)
8 Periosteum
9 Body of the radius
10 Tendon of extensor carpi radialis longus

Hohmann elevators may then be introduced into the distal wound region (**Fig. 18.8**).

18.2.4 Extension of the Approach

The approach may be extended distally after retraction of abductor pollicis longus and extensor pollicis brevis in a proximal direction (see Section 18.5.3, **Figs. 18.19** and **18.20**).

18.2.5 Anatomical Site

(**Fig. 18.9**)

Figure 18.9 presents the dorsoradial side of the elbow and the forearm. Note the course of the deep branch of the radial nerve and its relation to the various muscles it innervates. The radial extensor group has been stripped off the humerus, the superficial portion of the supinator muscle has been split, and the extensor digitorum has been pulled out of the wound.

Compression syndromes of the radial nerve occur mostly between the superficial and deep portions of the supinator.

18.2.6 Wound Closure

Wound closure is effected by reapproximating the detached portions of the supinator while the forearm is supinated. No other muscle sutures are required.

18.2.7 Dangers

The supinator should be detached only in its distal third as mobilization in a proximal direction might cause damage to the deep branch of the radial nerve.

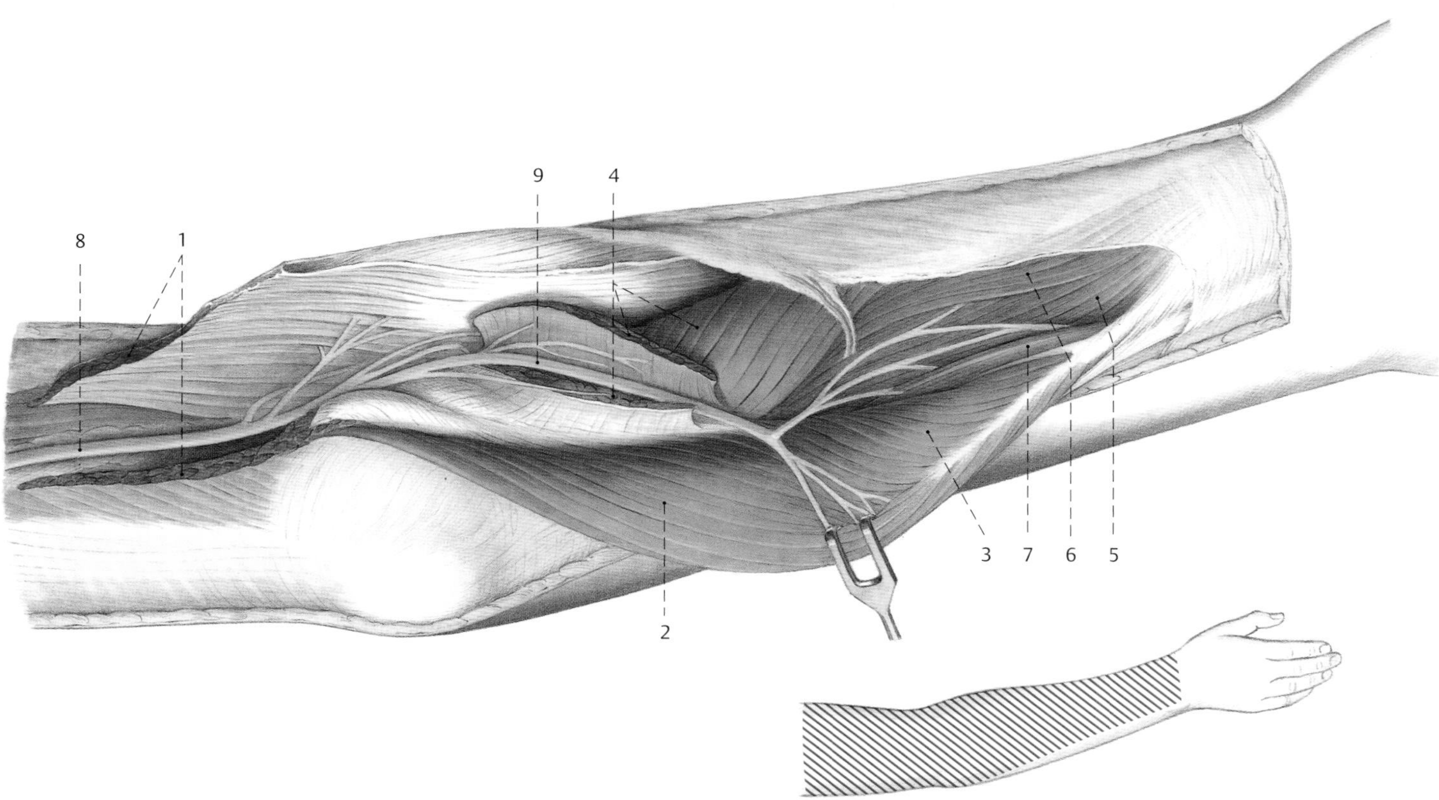

Fig. 18.9 Anatomical site. For exposure of the radial nerve, the brachioradialis has been detached from the humerus, and the superficial portion of the supinator transected.

1 Brachioradialis
2 Extensor digitorum
3 Extensor digitorum
4 Supinator
5 Extensor pollicis brevis
6 Abductor pollicis longus
7 Extensor pollicis longus
8 Radial nerve
9 Deep branch of the radial nerve

18.3 Approach to the Proximal Parts of the Radius and Ulna According to Boyd

R. Bauer, F. Kerschbaumer, S. Poisel

Posterior exposure of the proximal third of the radius and ulna.

18.3.1 Principal Indications

- Monteggia fracture
- Congenital radioulnar synostoses
- Dislocation of the head of the radius
- Removal of posttraumatic ossification
- Tumors
- Inflammation

18.3.2 Positioning and Incision

The patient is placed supine with a bolster under the shoulder and with the upper arm adducted. After application of a tourniquet, the arm is draped to allow free movement. The skin incision begins one fingerbreadth proximal to the tip of the olecranon between the lateral epicondyle of the humerus and the olecranon, and curves in a distal direction for approximately 10 cm along the posterior border of the ulna (**Fig. 18.10**). After transection of the skin and subcutaneous tissue, the fascia is split on the posterior ulnar border (**Fig. 18.11**).

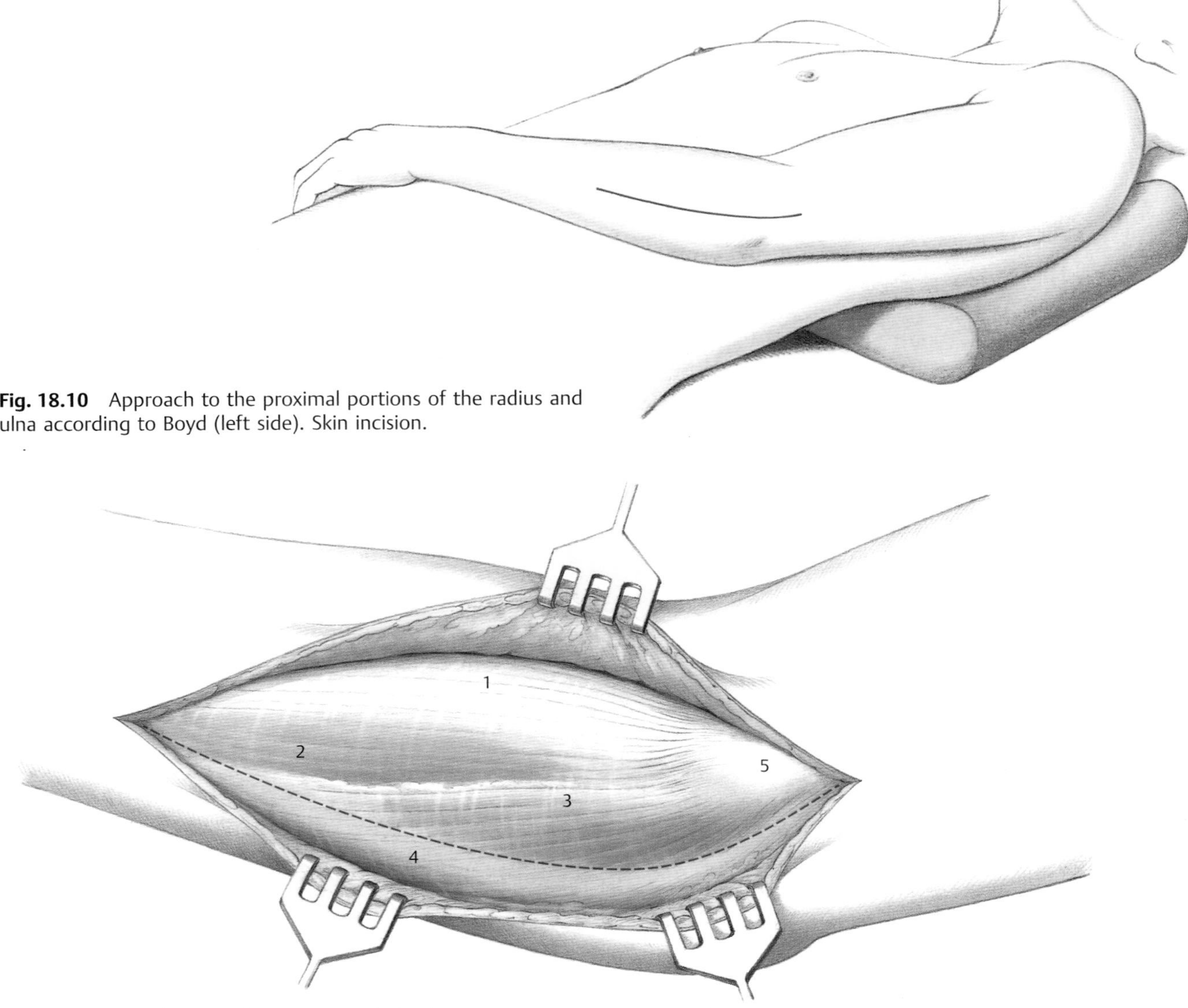

Fig. 18.10 Approach to the proximal portions of the radius and ulna according to Boyd (left side). Skin incision.

Fig. 18.11 Detachment of extensor carpi ulnaris and anconeus from the ulna (dashed line).

1 Extensor digitorum
2 Extensor carpi ulnaris
3 Anconeus
4 Ulna
5 Lateral epicondyle of humerus

18.3.3 Exposure of the Proximal Parts of the Radius and Ulna

The extensor carpi ulnaris and anconeus are detached from the ulna to a point beyond the tip of the olecranon and are retracted anteriorly. In the proximal portion of the wound, the joint capsule and the annular ligament of the radius may be split. More distally, the supinator is stripped off the ulna, with the forearm pronated, and the ulna is then dislocated anteriorly. The recurrent interosseous artery, seen in the distal portion of the wound, may be ligated and transected if necessary (**Fig. 18.12**).

18.3.4 Extension of the Approach

For exposure of the ulna and the interosseous membrane, the approach may be extended distally. Exposure of the radius in a distal direction is unsatisfactory for this approach. The approach may be extended as far as a handbreadth proximal to the lateral epicondyle of the humerus (see Section 17.2).

18.3.5 Wound Closure

After release of the tourniquet and hemostasis, the supinator and the annular ligament of the radius, as well as the anconeus and extensor carpi ulnaris, are reattached to the ulna.

18.3.6 Dangers

The detachment of the supinator should be performed close to the ulna with the forearm pronated so that injury to the deep branch of the radial nerve may be avoided.

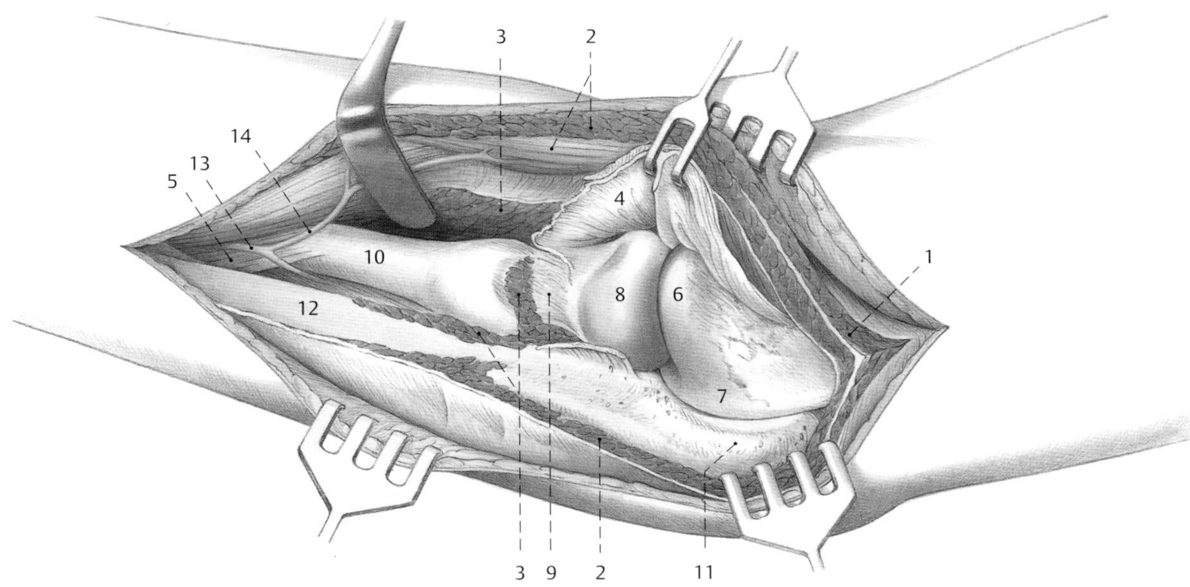

Fig. 18.12 Operative site after detaching the muscle and opening the joint capsule. The supinator muscle has been detached from the ulna. Exposure of the proximal portions of the interosseous membrane.

1 Triceps brachii
2 Anconeus
3 Supinator
4 Elbow joint capsule
5 Interosseous membrane
6 Capitulum of the humerus
7 Trochlea of the humerus
8 Head of the radius (articular circumference)
9 Neck of the radius
10 Body of the radius
11 Olecranon
12 Body of the ulna
13 Posterior interosseous artery
14 Recurrent interosseous artery

18.4 Lateral Approach to the Ulna

R. Bauer, F. Kerschbaumer, S. Poisel

18.4.1 Principal Indications

- Fractures
- Corrective osteotomies
- Inflammation
- Tumors

18.4.2 Positioning and Incision

The patient is placed in the supine position. After application of a tourniquet, the arm is draped to allow free movement and placed on a side table. The elbow is flexed, and the forearm pronated. The skin incision runs 1 cm posteriorly and parallel to the palpable posterior border of the ulna (**Fig. 18.13**).

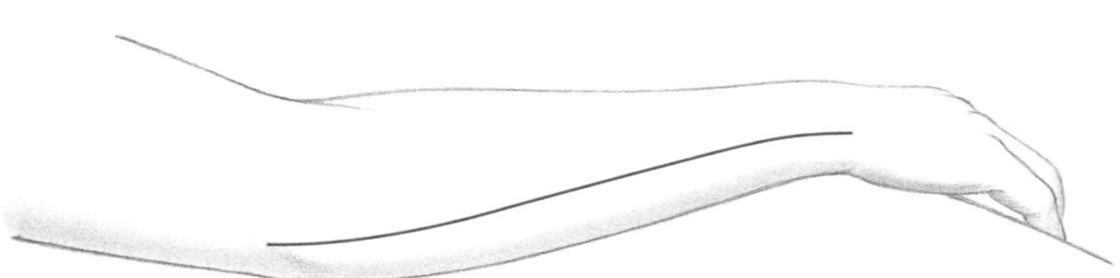

Fig. 18.13 Lateral approach to the ulna (right side). Skin incision.

18.4.3 Exposure of the Ulna

After division of the subcutaneous tissue, the fascia and the periosteum between extensor carpi ulnaris and flexor carpi ulnaris are split over the bone (**Fig. 18.14**). In the distal operative field, it is necessary to watch for the dorsal branch of the ulnar nerve. With the aid of a raspatory, the ulna is subperiosteally exposed for the desired length. Hohmann elevators may be inserted if necessary (**Fig. 18.15**). A circular subperiosteal denudation of the bone over a large distance should be avoided.

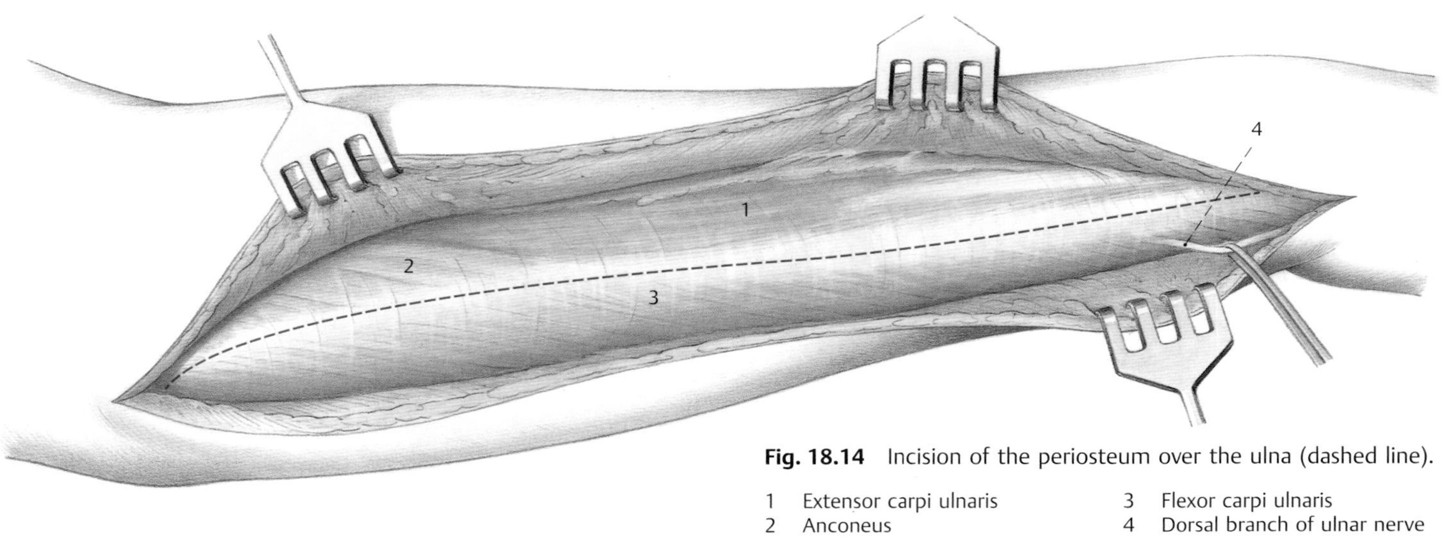

Fig. 18.14 Incision of the periosteum over the ulna (dashed line).

1 Extensor carpi ulnaris
2 Anconeus
3 Flexor carpi ulnaris
4 Dorsal branch of ulnar nerve

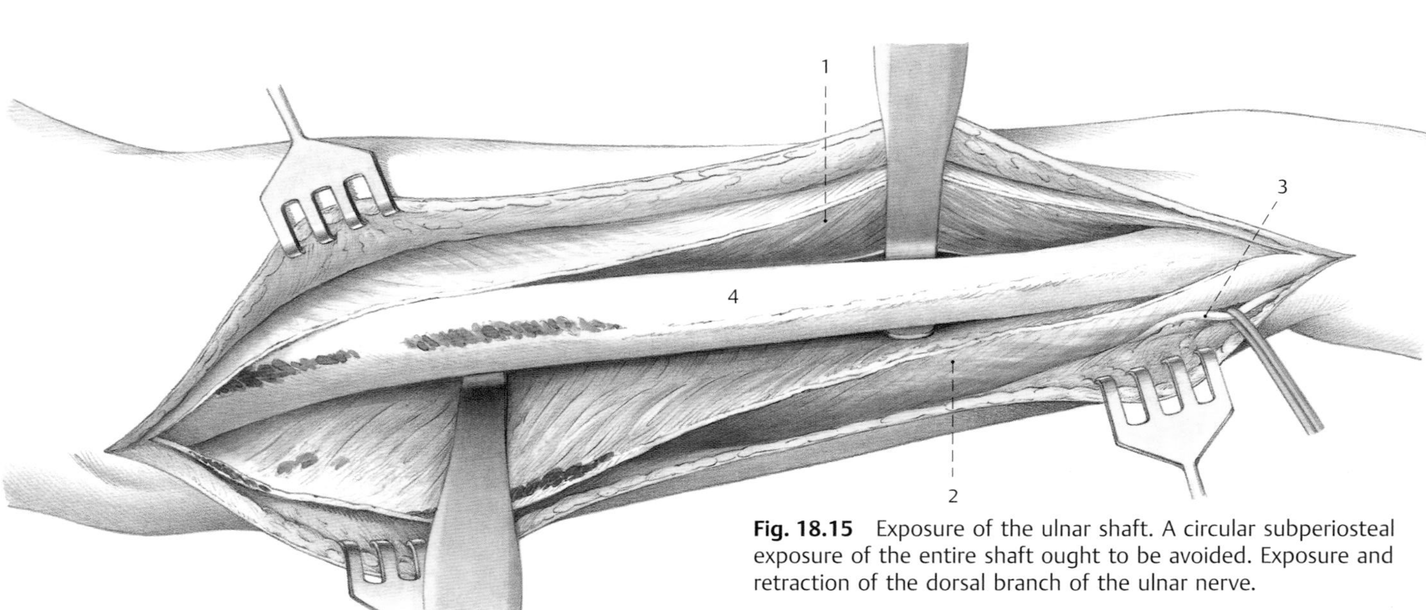

Fig. 18.15 Exposure of the ulnar shaft. A circular subperiosteal exposure of the entire shaft ought to be avoided. Exposure and retraction of the dorsal branch of the ulnar nerve.

1 Extensor carpi ulnaris
2 Flexor carpi ulnaris
3 Dorsal branch of the ulnar nerve
4 Body of ulna

18.4.4 Anatomical Site

Figure 18.16 provides a schematic cross-section through the distal forearm. The approaches to the ulna and radius are marked by arrows.

Note the position of the ulna and its relation to the flexor carpi ulnaris, flexor digitorum profundus, and extensor carpi ulnaris. In the distal third of the shaft, the flexor carpi radialis, instead of flexor digitorum profundus, adjoins the ulna on the flexor side.

18.4.5 Wound Closure

The fascia and the periosteum are sutured in single layers. The wound closure is otherwise performed in the usual fashion.

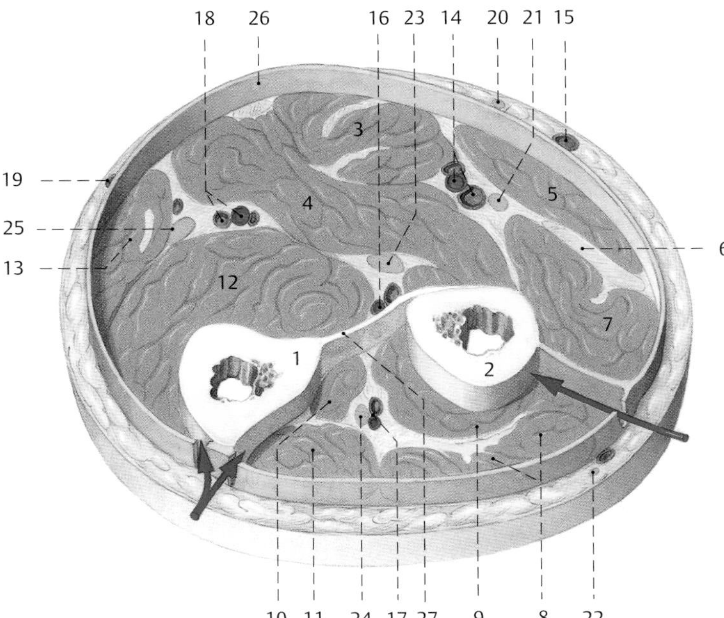

Fig. 18.16 Anatomical site. Schematic cross-section of the forearm between the middle and distal thirds. The approaches to the antebrachial bones are identified by arrows (right arm, proximal view).

1 Ulna
2 Radius
3 Flexor carpi radialis
4 Flexor digitorum superficialis
5 Brachioradialis
6 Extensor carpi radialis brevis
7 Extensor carpi radialis longus
8 Extensor digitorum
9 Abductor pollicis longus and extensor pollicis brevis
10 Extensor pollicis longus
11 Extensor carpi ulnaris
12 Flexor digitorum profundus
13 Flexor carpi ulnaris
14 Radial artery and accompanying veins
15 Cephalic vein
16 Anterior interosseous artery and vein
17 Posterior interosseous artery and vein
18 Ulnar artery and accompanying veins
19 Basilic vein
20 Lateral cutaneous nerve of forearm
21 Superficial branch of the radial nerve
22 Posterior cutaneous nerve of forearm
23 Median nerve
24 Posterior interosseous nerve of forearm
25 Ulnar nerve
26 Medial cutaneous nerve of forearm
27 Interosseous membrane

18.5 Posterior Approach to the Distal Part of the Radius

R. Bauer, F. Kerschbaumer, S. Poisel

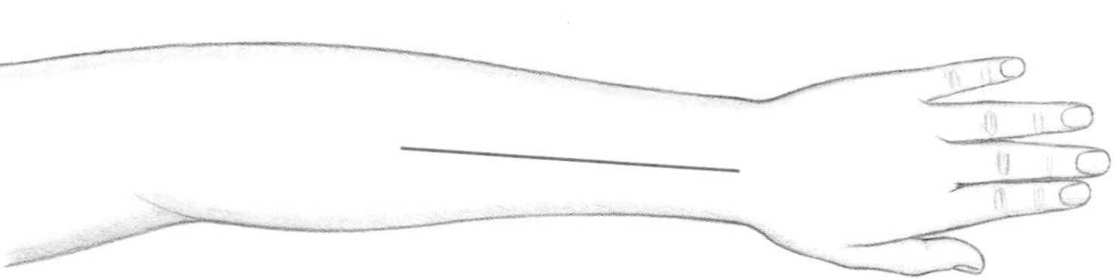

Fig. 18.17 Posterior approach to the distal part of the radius (left side). Skin incision.

18.5.1 Principal Indications

- Fractures
- Corrective osteotomies
- Inflammation
- Tumors

18.5.2 Positioning and Incision

The patient is placed in the supine position. After application of a tourniquet, the arm is draped to allow free movement and placed on a side table. The skin incision runs straight and posteriorly from the middle of the forearm to the wrist (**Fig. 18.17**). If conditions warrant, the skin incision may be displaced in a radial direction, while at the same time the ulna is exposed by a separate incision. After the subcutaneous tissue, the fascia, and the extensor retinaculum in the distal wound region have been split, the abductor pollicis longus and extensor pollicis brevis are revealed (**Fig. 18.18**).

18.5.3 Exposure of the Distal Part of the Radius

The abductor pollicis longus and extensor pollicis brevis, which cross the operative field obliquely, are isolated, undermined, and snared with a rubber band (**Fig. 18.19**). Alternate displacement of these muscles in a proximal and a distal direction provides a clear exposure of the distal metaphysis of the radius (**Fig. 18.20**). Subperiosteal exposure is not necessary with fractures.

18.5.4 Extension of the Approach

This approach may be extended proximally (see Section 18.2, **Figs. 18.5, 18.6, 18.7, 18.8**) as well as distally (see Section 19.2, **Figs. 19.5, 19.6, 19.7, 19.8**).

18.5.5 Wound Closure

The wound is closed in conventional fashion by suturing the fascia and the extensor retinaculum.

18.5.6 Dangers

Pay attention to the radially and subcutaneously coursing superficial branch of the radial nerve. In the distal wound region, note should be taken of the obliquely running tendon of extensor pollicis longus.

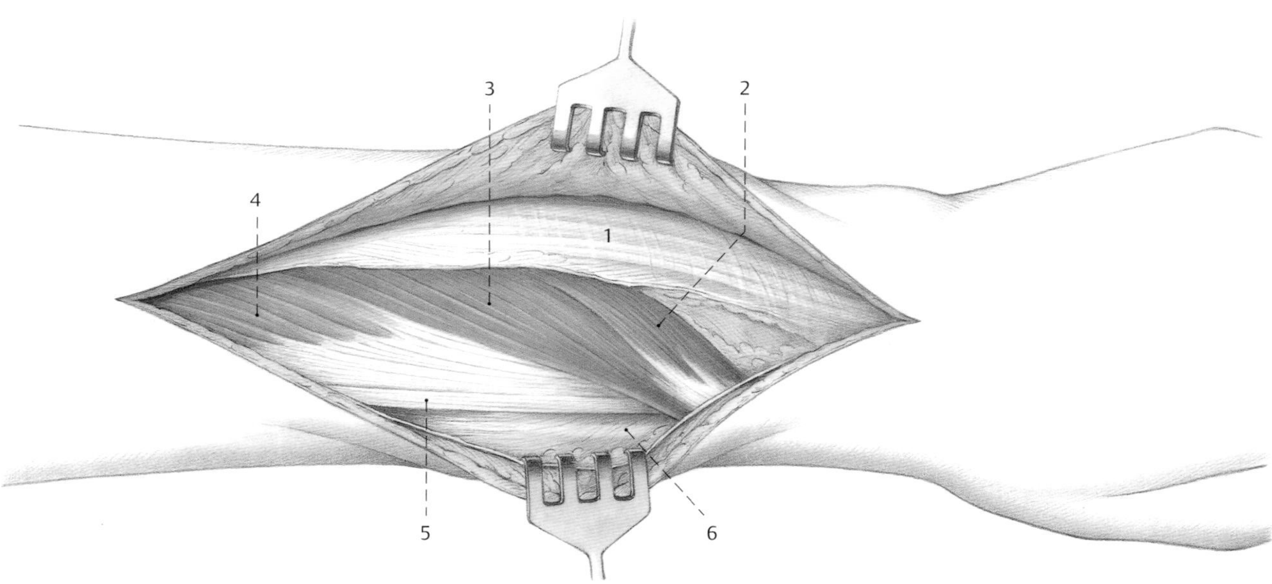

Fig. 18.18 Appearance after incision of the fascia. Exposure of abductor pollicis longus and extensor pollicis brevis.

1 Extensor digitorum
2 Extensor pollicis brevis
3 Abductor pollicis longus
4 Extensor carpi radialis brevis
5 Extensor carpi radialis longus
6 Superficial branch of the radial nerve

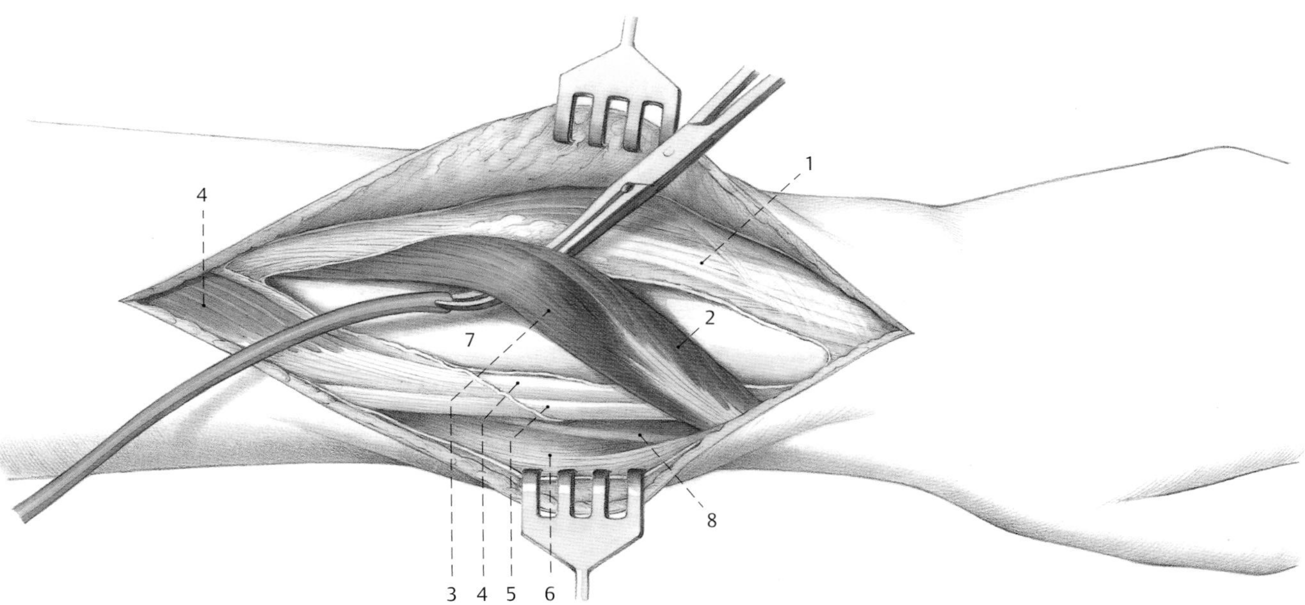

Fig. 18.19 Undermining and snaring of abductor pollicis longus and extensor pollicis brevis.

1 Extensor digitorum
2 Extensor pollicis brevis
3 Abductor pollicis longus
4 Extensor carpi radialis brevis
5 Extensor carpi radialis longus
6 Brachioradialis
7 Body of the radius
8 Superficial branch of the radial nerve

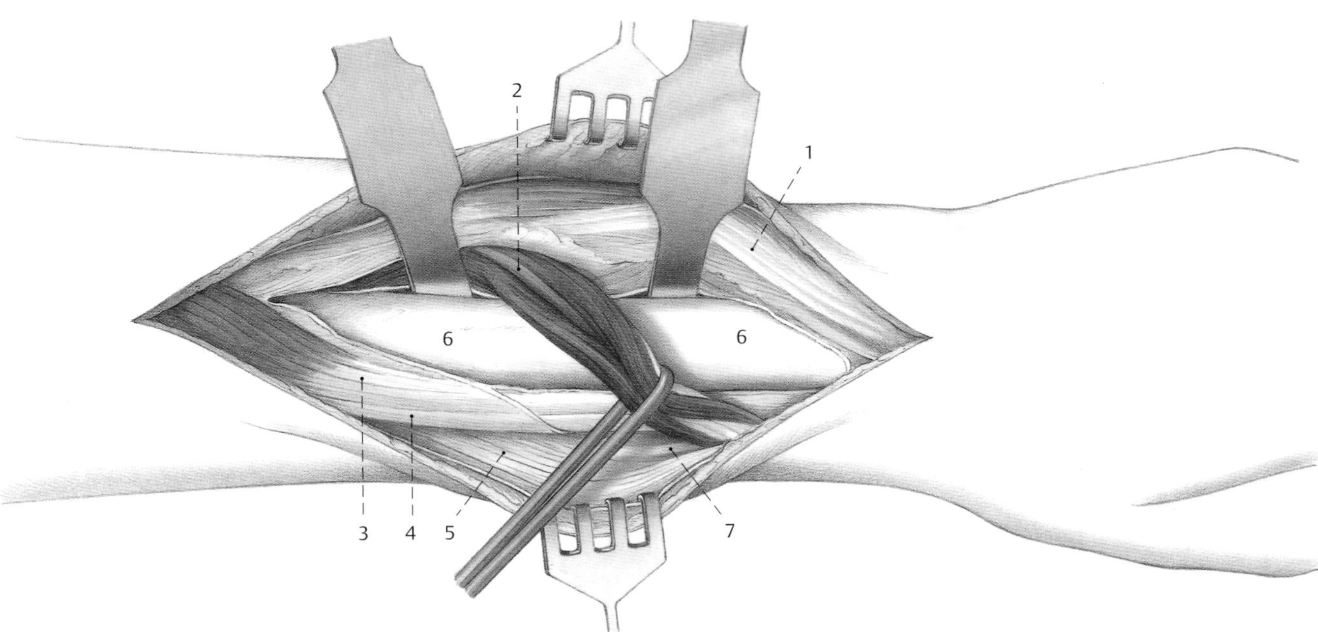

Fig. 18.20 Subperiosteal exposure of the distal shaft of the radius (not with fractures).

1 Extensor digitorum
2 Extensor pollicis brevis and abductor pollicis longus
3 Extensor carpi radialis brevis
4 Extensor carpi radialis longus
5 Brachioradialis
6 Body of the radius
7 Superficial branch of the radial nerve

18.6 Approach to the Distal Portion of the Ulna

R. Bauer, F. Kerschbaumer, S. Poisel

18.6.1 Principal Indications

- Corrective osteotomies after radial fractures with ulnar protrusion
- Madelung's deformity
- Head of ulna syndrome in rheumatoid arthritis
- Tenosynovitis of extensor carpi ulnaris

18.6.2 Positioning and Incision

After application of a tourniquet, the forearm is pronated and placed positioned on a side table. A roll is placed underneath the wrist. The skin incision is begun 2 cm distal to the styloid process of the ulna and continued proximally in a straight line (**Fig. 18.21**).

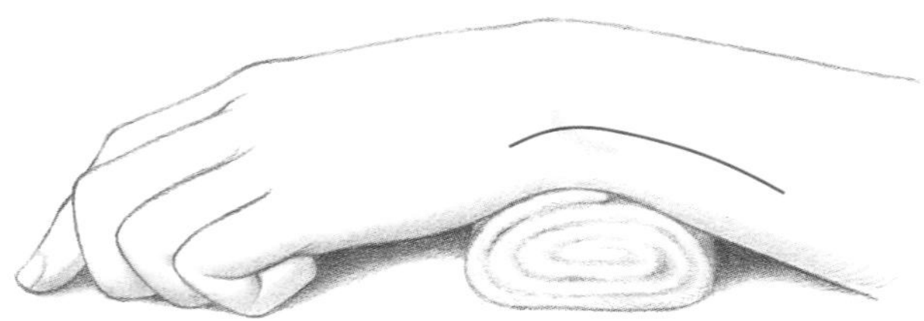

Fig. 18.21 Approach to the distal part of the ulna (left side). Skin incision.

18.6.3 Exposure of the Ulna

After splitting the subcutaneous tissue, the dorsal branch of the ulnar nerve is identified and snared (**Fig. 18.22**). The extensor retinaculum and the adjoining forearm fascia are split over the tendon of the extensor carpi ulnaris. Following radial displacement of the tendon of extensor carpi ulnaris, the ulna is exposed subperiosteally and raised by means of small Hohmann elevators (**Fig. 18.23**).

18.6.4 Wound Closure

If the head of the ulna is left intact, the capsule and the periosteum are sutured. After repositioning of extensor carpi ulnaris, its tendon sheath is closed. Following resection of the head of the ulna, the distal end of the ulna has to be carefully stabilized by means of capsular and periosteal sutures. If necessary, the capsule can be reinforced by the proximal portion of the extensor retinaculum.

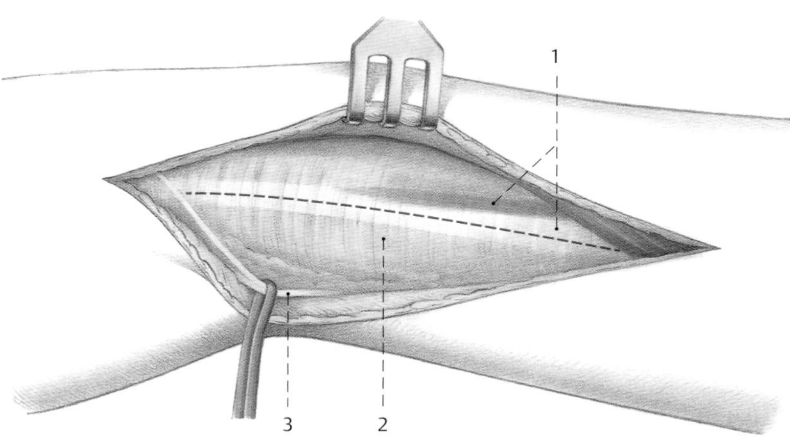

Fig. 18.22 Snaring of the dorsal branch of the ulnar nerve and tendon of extensor carpi ulnaris.

1 Extensor carpi ulnaris
2 Flexor carpi ulnaris
3 Dorsal branch of the ulnar nerve

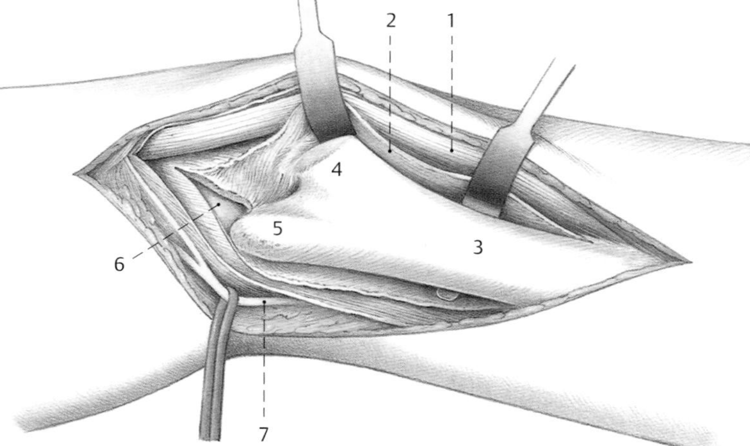

Fig. 18.23 After opening the tendon sheath over extensor carpi ulnaris, the ulna is subperiosteally exposed.

1 Extensor carpi ulnaris
2 Periosteum
3 Body of the ulna
4 Head of the ulna
5 Styloid process of the ulna
6 Triquetrum
7 Dorsal branch of the ulnar nerve

18.7 Palmar Approach to the Distal Part of the Radius

R. Bauer, F. Kerschbaumer, S. Poisel

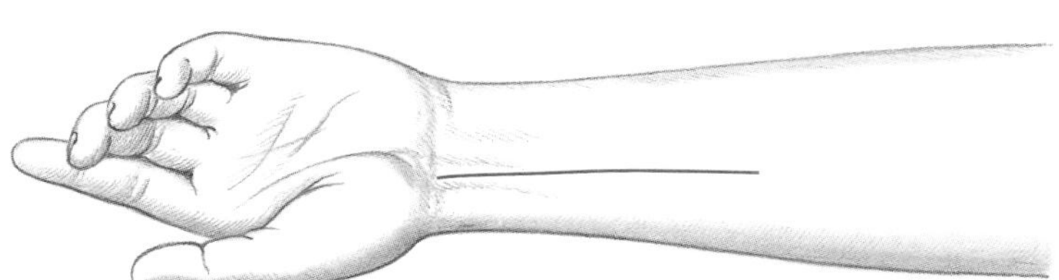

Fig. 18.24 Palmar approach to the distal portion of the radius (left side). Skin incision.

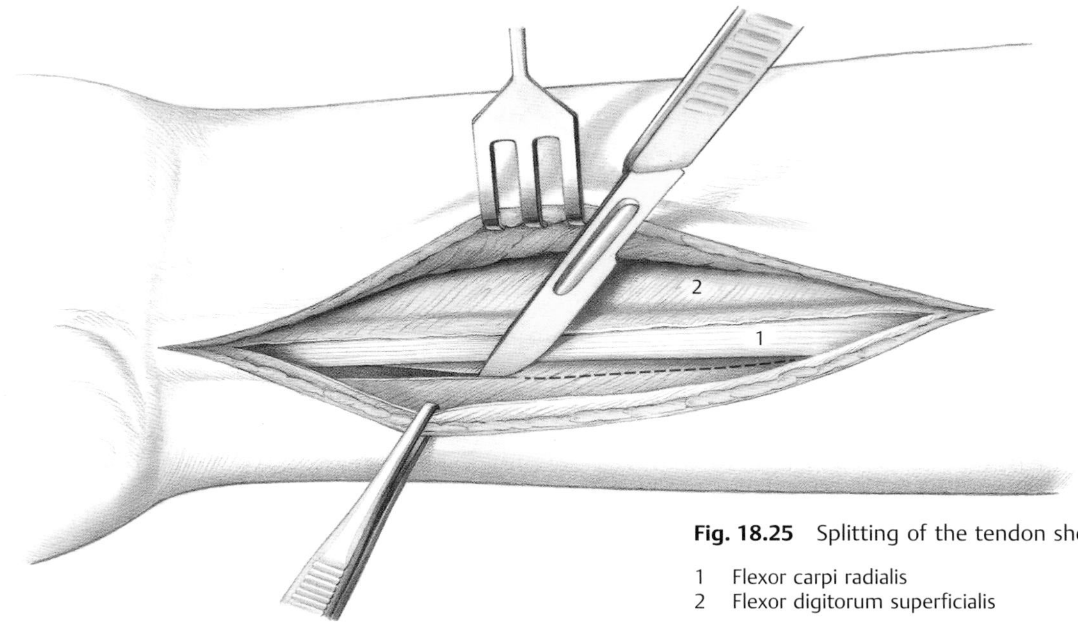

18.7.1 Principal Indications

- Fractures
- Corrective osteotomies
- Inflammation
- Tumors

18.7.2 Positioning and Incision

After application of a tourniquet, the forearm is supinated and placed on a side table. The skin incision runs from the distal flexion crease of the wrist approximately 10 cm proximally over the tendon of flexor carpi radialis (**Fig. 18.24**). The forearm fascia and the tendon sheath of flexor carpi radialis are split (**Fig. 18.25**). Retraction of the tendon of flexor carpi radialis brings the flexor digitorum superficialis and flexor pollicis longus into view (**Fig. 18.26**).

Fig. 18.25 Splitting of the tendon sheath of flexor carpi radialis.

1 Flexor carpi radialis
2 Flexor digitorum superficialis

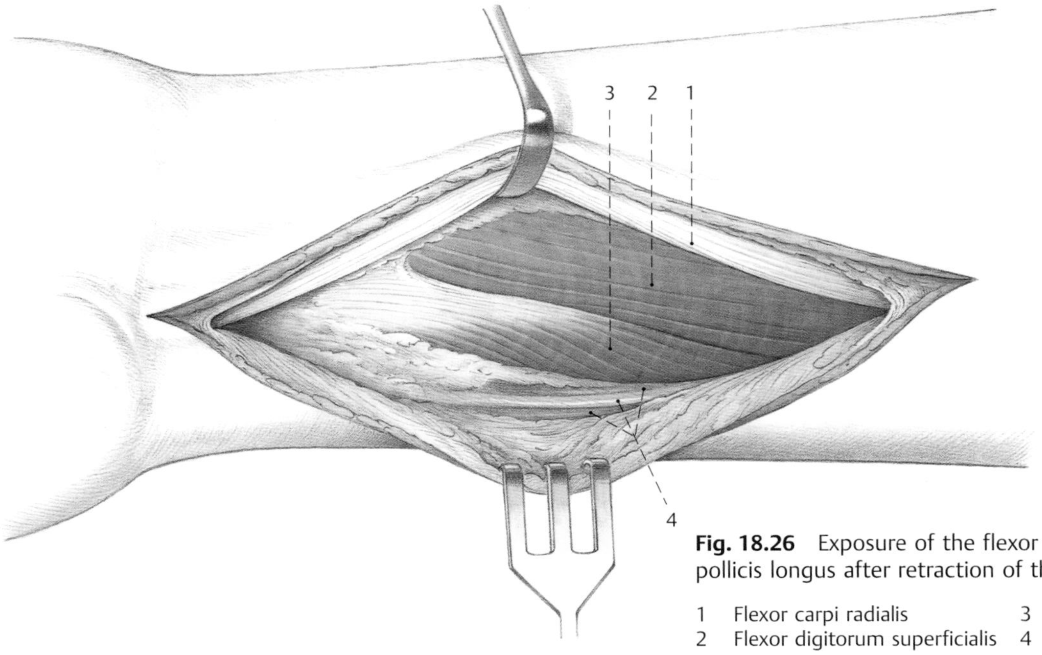

Fig. 18.26 Exposure of the flexor digitorum superficialis and flexor pollicis longus after retraction of the flexor carpi radialis.

1 Flexor carpi radialis
2 Flexor digitorum superficialis
3 Flexor pollicis longus
4 Radial artery, accompanying veins

18.7.3 Exposure of the Radius

The flexor digitorum superficialis and flexor pollicis longus are displaced toward the ulna. The pronator quadratus is stripped off the radius (**Fig. 18.27**), and retracted in an ulnar direction so that the distal and palmar portions of the radius are exposed (**Fig. 18.28**).

18.7.4 Extension of the Approach

This approach can be extended in a distal direction for palmar exposure of the scaphoid (see Section 20.1). It is possible to extend the incision in a proximal direction (see Section 18.1).

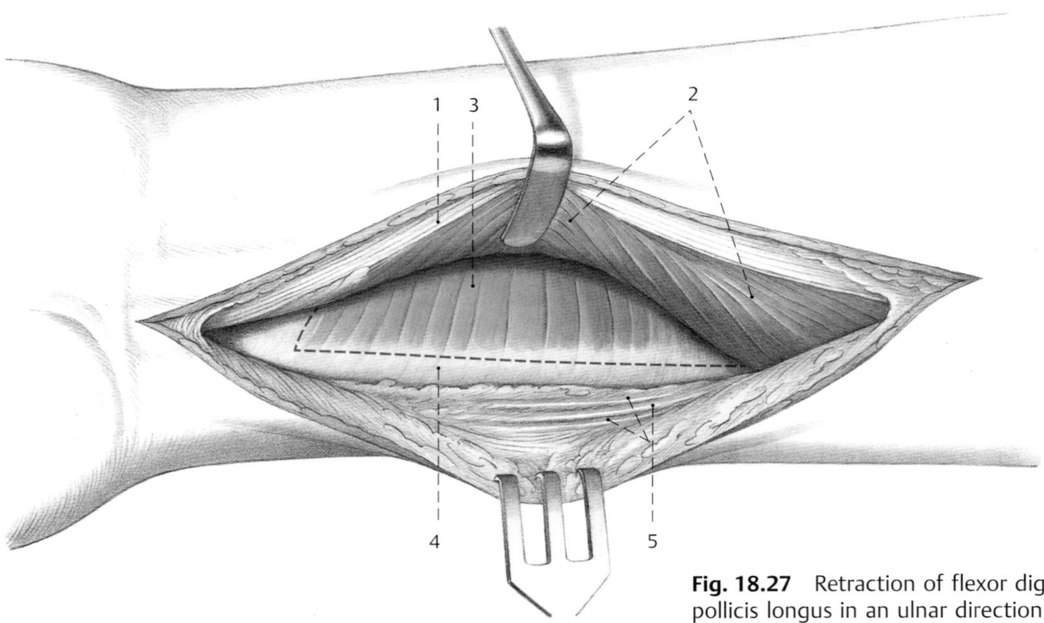

Fig. 18.27 Retraction of flexor digitorum superficialis and flexor pollicis longus in an ulnar direction, and detachment of pronator quadratus (dashed line).

1 Flexor carpi radialis
2 Flexor digitorum superficialis and flexor pollicis longus
3 Pronator quadratus
4 Body of the radius
5 Radial artery and accompanying veins

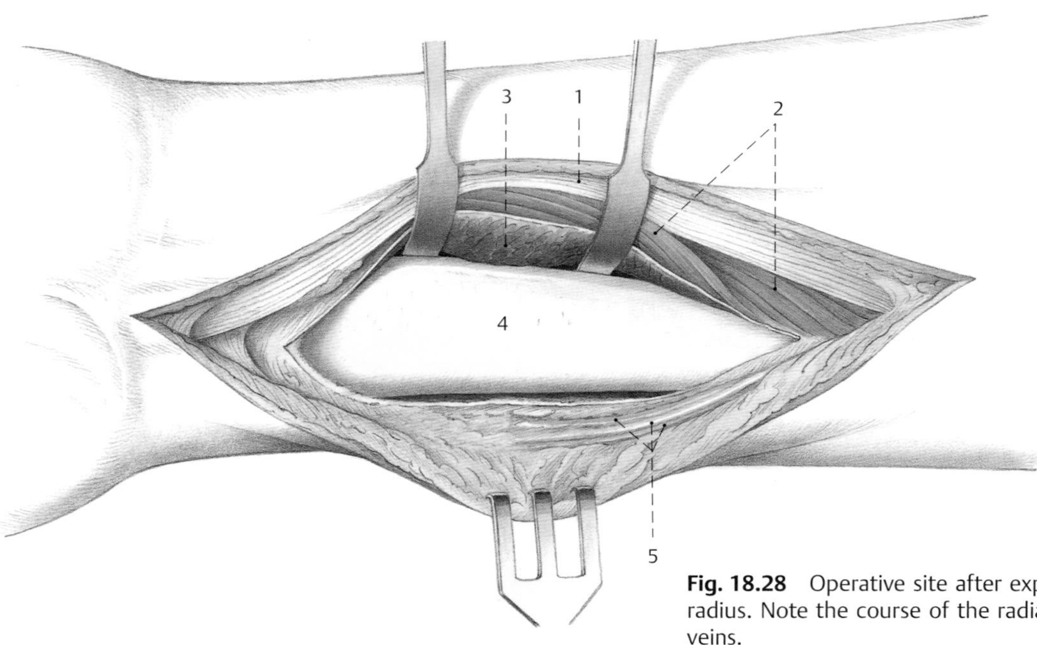

Fig. 18.28 Operative site after exposure of the distal shaft of the radius. Note the course of the radial artery with the accompanying veins.

1 Flexor carpi radialis
2 Flexor digitorum superficialis and flexor pollicis longus
3 Pronator quadratus
4 Body of the radius
5 Radial artery and accompanying veins

18.7.5 Anatomical Site

Figure 18.29 presents the superficial and deep flexor muscles of the forearm. For better exposure of the proximal ulnar nerve, the palmaris longus and flexor digitorum superficialis have been partly detached proximally. Note the position and course of the ulnar artery and the median nerve.

18.7.6 Wound Closure

The wound is closed by attaching the pronator quadratus to the periosteum of the radius and closing the forearm fascia.

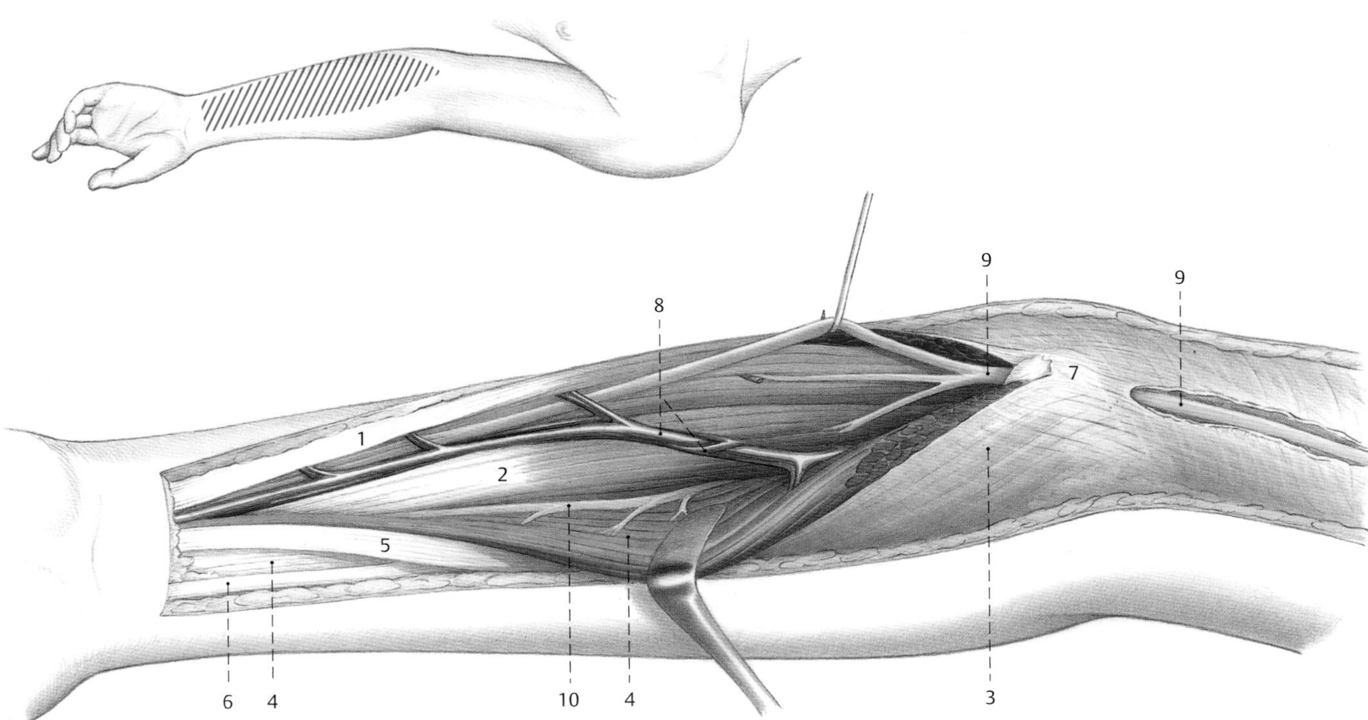

Fig. 18.29 Anatomical site. Exposure of the superficial and deep forearm flexor muscles, the median and ulnar nerves, and the ulnar artery.

1 Flexor carpi ulnaris
2 Flexor digitorum profundus
3 Common head of the flexor muscles
4 Flexor digitorum superficialis
5 Palmaris longus
6 Flexor carpi radialis
7 Medial epicondyle of the humerus
8 Ulnar artery and accompanying veins
9 Ulnar nerve
10 Median nerve

19 Wrist

19.1 Minimally Invasive Approach for Endoscopic Carpal Tunnel Division

F. Kerschbaumer

19.1.1 Principal Indications

- Carpal tunnel syndrome without motor deficit

19.1.2 Positioning and Incision

The two-incision technique described by Chow is presented.

After application of a tourniquet, the hand is supinated and an approximately 1 cm transverse incision is made at the level of the proximal wrist flexion crease on the ulnar side of the palmaris longus tendon. The subcutaneous tissue is undermined, the forearm fascia is exposed, and the fascia is then split with small mosquito forceps.

The mosquito forceps are now advanced distally under the flexor retinaculum into the carpal tunnel on the ulnar side of the median nerve. The wrist is then hyperextended approximately 30° until the tip of the mosquito forceps can be palpated subcutaneously. At this site, which is usually located at the intersection of a line along the distal border of the abducted thumb and a straight line between the middle and ring fingers, a 15 mm incision is made along the thenar palmar crease (**Fig. 19.1**). The mosquito forceps are removed, and the hand is then placed on a plastic splint that hyperextends the wrist and holds the hand in this position.

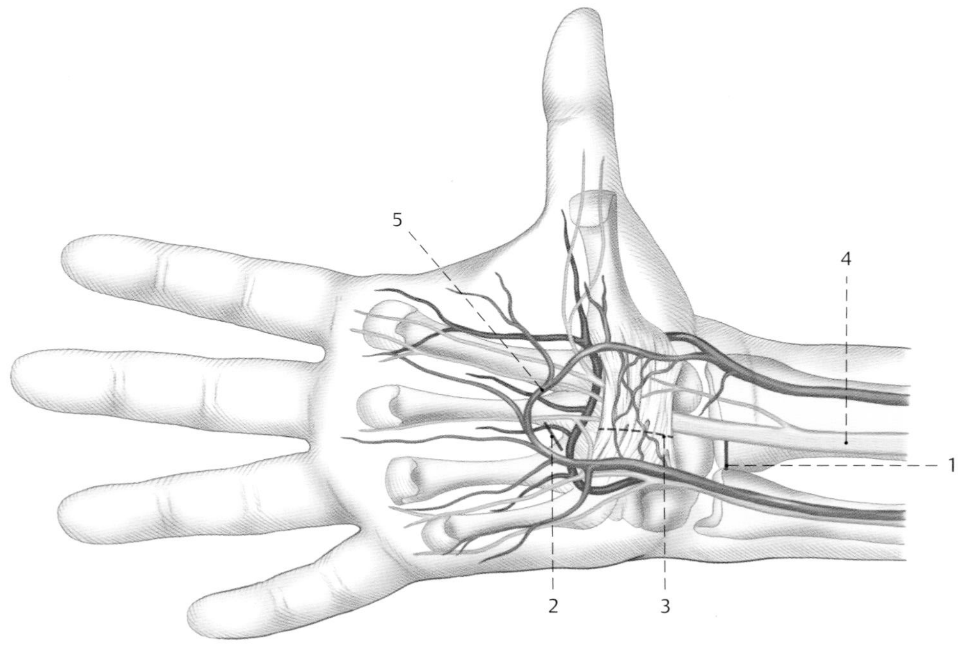

Fig. 19.1 Relations of the skin incisions, the planned direction of retinacular transection, and accessory lines for locating the distal incision.

1 Proximal incision (solid line)
2 Distal incision (solid line)
3 Incision of the flexor retinaculum (dashed line)
4 Median nerve
5 Superficial palmar arch

The slit trocar sleeve is now advanced cautiously from proximal to distal while the operator's thumb compresses the distal soft tissues to avoid damage to the nerves and superficial arterial palmar arch (**Fig. 19.2**). The skin and subcutaneous tissue can now be elevated with a small lid hook, and mosquito forceps or fine scissors are used to tunnel from the palmar aponeurosis to the proximal incision. It is advisable to tunnel on the ulnar side of the palmaris longus tendon to avoid injuring the palmar branch of the median nerve. **Fig. 19.2b** illustrates the cross-section of the carpal tunnel showing the relations of the flexor retinaculum, the median nerve, and the trocar sleeve for endoscopically assisted incision of the retinaculum.

19.1.3 Retinaculum Transection

The retinaculum is transected under endoscopic control. The optic is advanced from the proximal side, and the underside of the flexor retinaculum is inspected (**Fig. 19.3**). The transverse fibers can typically be seen over the tip of the trocar slit. If they are not visible, the optic is withdrawn and the synovial membrane is pushed away below the retinaculum with a dissector until the washboard-like resistance of the transverse fibers is encountered. The optic is now advanced again. The trocar can be rotated to right and left to ensure that there are no nerves in the planned incision region.

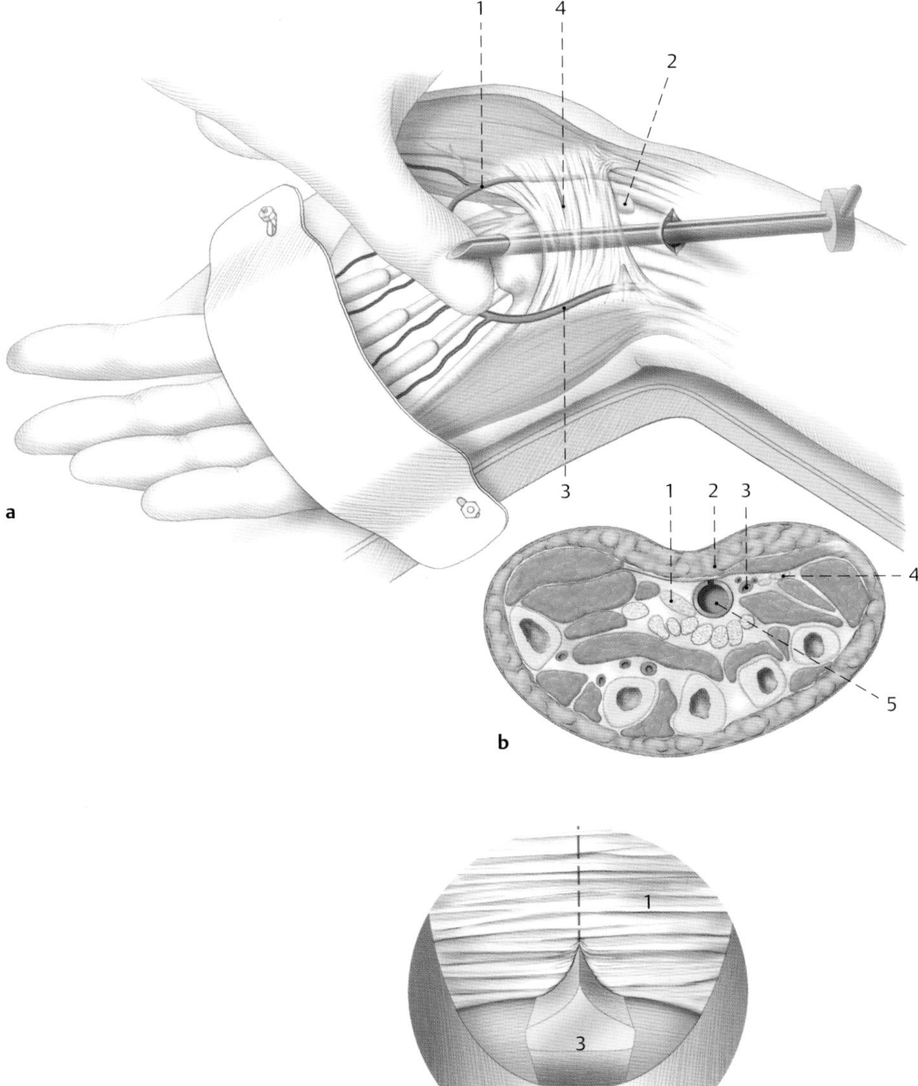

Fig. 19.2 a, b Positioning of the trocar sleeve.

a After making the two skin incisions, the hand is secured in a special plastic splint in hyperextension, and the trocar sleeve is advanced cautiously from proximal to distal. The operator's thumb pushes the soft tissues away.

1 Superficial palmar arch
2 Median nerve
3 Ulnar artery
4 Flexor retinaculum

b Anatomical cross-section of the carpal tunnel showing the relations between the trocar sleeve, the median nerve, and the flexor retinaculum. The slit in the trocar sleeve corresponds to the planned direction of incision of the flexor retinaculum.

1 Median nerve
2 Palmar aponeurosis
3 Ulnar artery
4 Ulnar nerve
5 Trocar

Fig. 19.3 View through the endoscope from proximal to distal, advancing the anterograde scalpel from distally to transect the flexor retinaculum.

1 Transverse fibers of the flexor retinaculum
2 Trocar
3 Anterograde scalpel

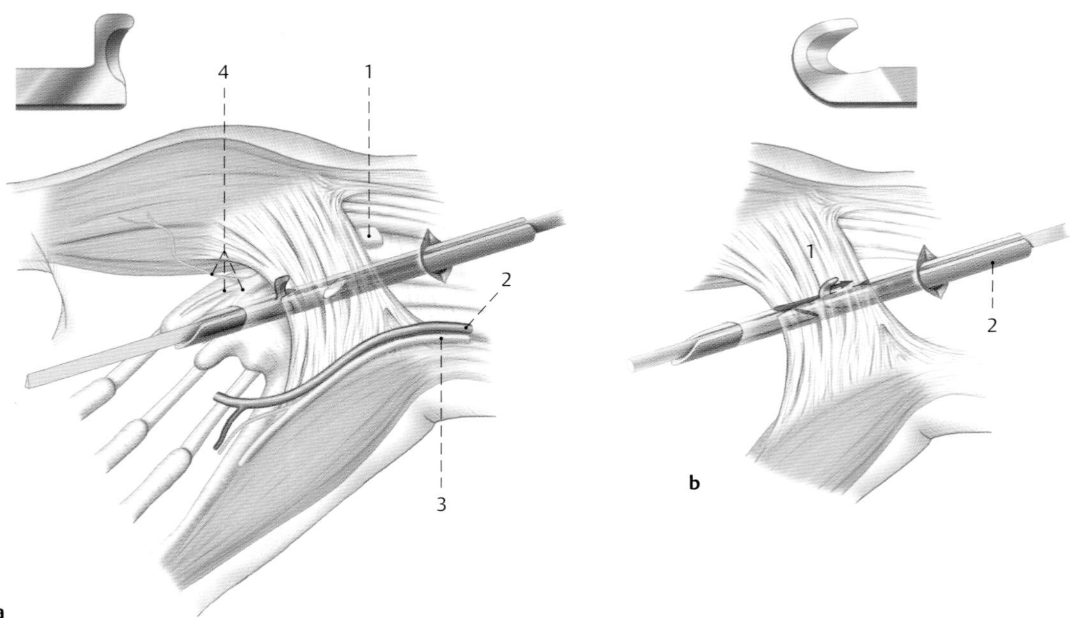

Fig. 19.4 a, b Transection of the distal and proximal parts of the retinaculum.

a Schematic representation of the optic inserted proximally, and the anterograde scalpel inserted distally.
1 Median nerve
2 Ulnar artery
3 Ulnar nerve
4 Common palmar digital nerves

b The optic is now inserted distally, and the retrograde scalpel is drawn proximally to complete the transection of the retinaculum.
1 Flexor retinaculum
2 Retrograde scalpel

The anterograde scalpel can now be introduced from distally (**Fig. 19.4a**). Again, it is advisable to elevate the skin and subcutaneous tissue with a small lid hook to ensure that the tip of the scalpel transects not only the retinaculum, but also the palmar aponeurosis. The scalpel is advanced as far as the proximal third of the retinaculum and is then removed, and the optic is then inserted distally. The anterograde or retrograde scalpel can now be inserted proximally to transect the remainder of the retinaculum (**Fig. 19.4b**).

19.1.4 Wound Closure

After irrigating both incisions, they are each closed with a single suture. The tourniquet is released only after a pressure dressing has been applied.

19.1.5 Dangers

The approach described here is usually less problematic than endoscopically assisted procedures with one portal. Nerve injury is possible, however, especially with variants of thenar motor innervation, for example a subligamentous, transligamentous, or ulnar origin of the motor thenar branch (see **Fig. 19.12**). In addition, a common palmar digital nerve may be injured if the median nerve divides more proximally (see **Fig. 20.4**). The superficial palmar arch is also vulnerable when the palmar incision is located too far distally. These complications can be minimized by subcutaneous undermining of skin and subcutaneous tissue as described, but cannot be excluded.

19.2 Posterior Approach to the Wrist

R. Bauer, F. Kerschbaumer, S. Poisel

19.2.1 Principal Indications

- Synovectomy of the extensor tendons and wrist
- Fractures of the distal segment of the radius
- Fractures and dislocations of the wrist
- Wrist fusion
- Wrist arthroplasty
- Inflammatory arthritis

19.2.2 Positioning and Incision

After application of a tourniquet, the forearm is pronated and placed on a side table. The skin incision is made in a straight line or in an S-shape on the dorsal aspect of the wrist. The straight skin incision is preferable in patients with rheumatoid arthritis (**Fig. 19.5**). The subcutaneous tissue is split and dissected free of the underlying fascia. Attention must be paid to the sensory branches of the radial and ulnar nerves (**Fig. 19.6**). The forearm fascia and the extensor retinaculum are split in a straight line over the fourth extensor tendon compartment. The tendons of extensor digitorum are retracted in an ulnar direction. On the ulnar side of the extensor pollicis longus and

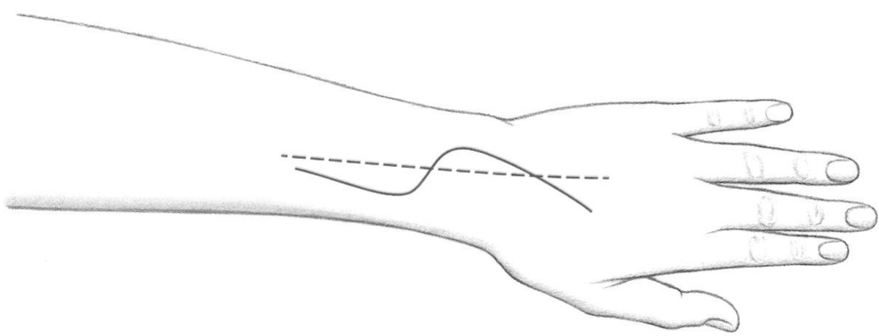

Fig. 19.5 Dorsal approach to the wrist joint (left side); possible skin incisions.

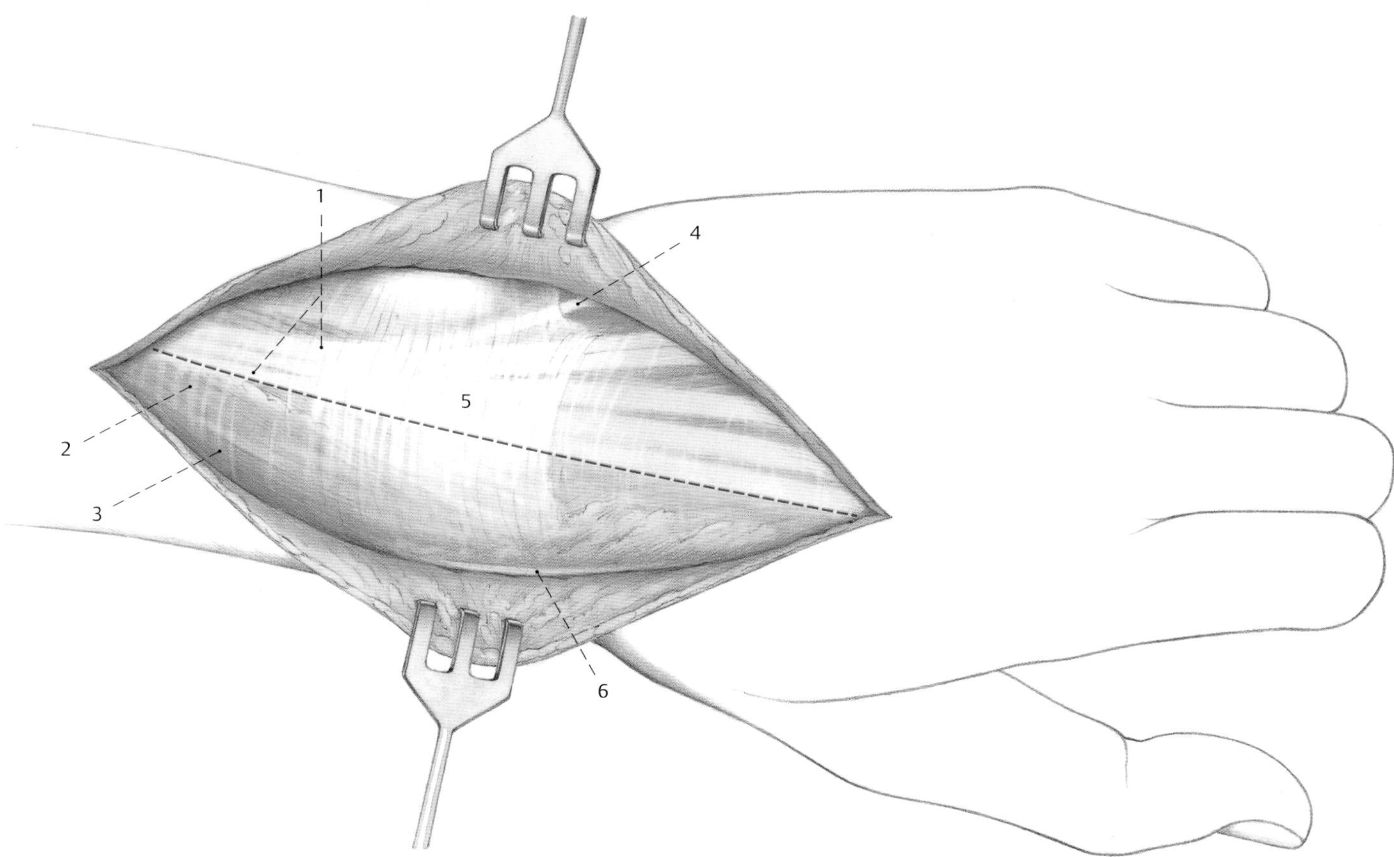

Fig. 19.6 Division of the forearm fascia and extensor retinaculum over the fourth tendon sheath compartment.

1 Extensor digitorum
2 Extensor pollicis brevis
3 Abductor pollicis longus
4 Extensor digiti minimi
5 Extensor retinaculum
6 Superficial branch of the radial nerve

the posterior interosseous nerve, the periosteum and the joint capsule are opened lengthwise over the radius and the wrist (**Fig. 19.7**). If the distal carpal bones need to be exposed, an additional transverse incision of the wrist joint capsule proximal to the dorsal carpal branch of the radial artery is recommended. In this case, the extensor retinaculum has to be split further distally, and the superficial branch of the radial nerve has to be exposed.

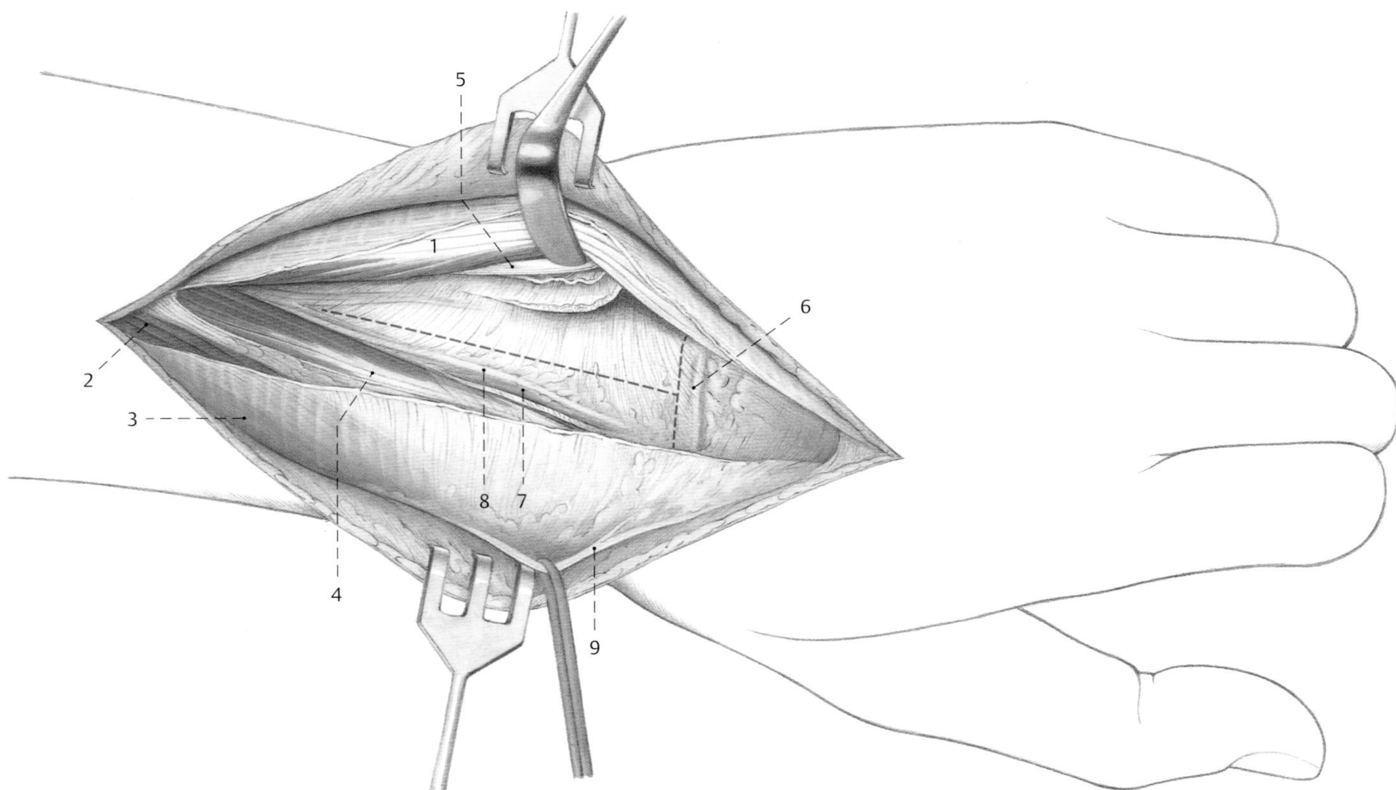

Fig. 19.7 Ulnar retraction of the finger extensor tendons. Incision of the periosteum and joint capsule (dashed line). Exposure of the superficial branch of the radial nerve is advisable.

1 Extensor digitorum
2 Extensor pollicis brevis
3 Abductor pollicis longus
4 Extensor pollicis longus
5 Extensor digiti minimi
6 Dorsal carpal branch of the radial artery
7 Posterior interosseous artery
8 Posterior interosseous nerve
9 Superficial branch of the radial nerve

19.2.3 Exposure of the Wrist Joint

The joint capsule and the periosteum are retracted in one layer in a radial and ulnar direction, the floors of the second and third extensor tendon compartments being displaced in a radial direction, and that of the fourth compartment in an ulnar direction (**Fig. 19.8**). In the case of fractures, the periosteum is preserved.

Thus, the distal radial metaphysis with Lister's tubercle (the dorsal tubercle), the lunate and scaphoid, and the proximal part of the capitate are clearly exposed (**Fig. 19.8**).

19.2.4 Extension of the Approach

The incision can be extended in a proximal (see Section 18.5, **Figs. 18.17**, **18.18**, **18.19**, **18.20**) as well as a distal direction for exposure of the metacarpal bones.

19.2.5 Wound Closure

The wrist joint capsule and the periosteum, as well as the extensor retinaculum, are closed in two layers with absorbable suture material.

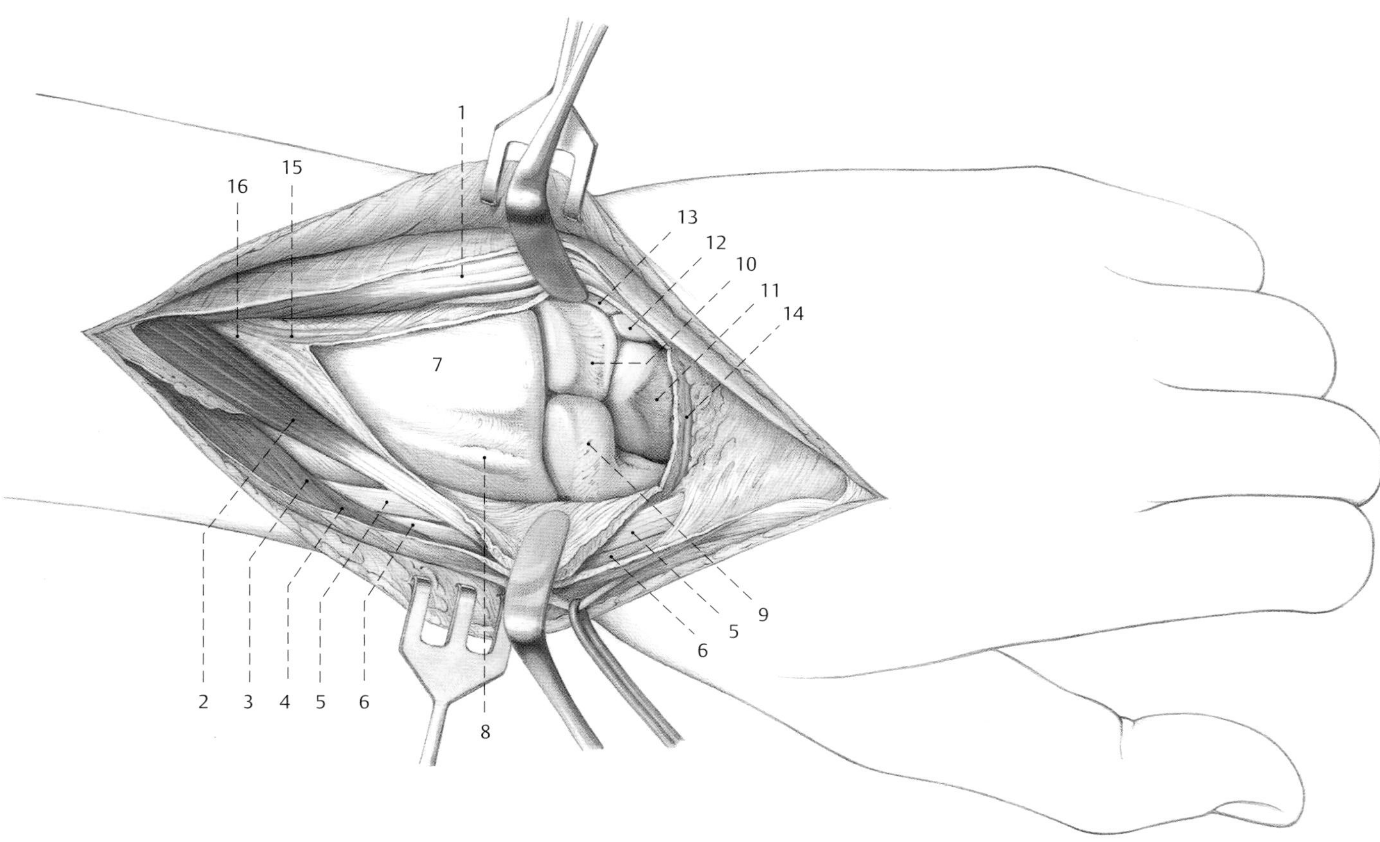

Fig. 19.8 Operative site after opening of the wrist joint capsule and subperiosteal exposure of the distal end of the radius (not with fractures).

1 Extensor digitorum
2 Extensor pollicis longus
3 Abductor pollicis longus
4 Extensor pollicis brevis
5 Extensor carpi radialis brevis
6 Long extensor carpi radialis
7 Radius
8 Dorsal tubercle
9 Scaphoid
10 Lunate
11 Capitate
12 Hamate
13 Triquetrum
14 Dorsal carpal branch of the radial artery
15 Posterior interosseous artery and vein
16 Posterior interosseous nerve

19.3 Palmar Approach to the Wrist

R. Bauer, F. Kerschbaumer, S. Poisel

19.3.1 Principal Indications

- Carpal tunnel syndrome
- Synovitis of the flexor tendons
- Fractures and dislocations of the carpal bones
- Inflammatory arthritis
- Aseptic necrosis of the carpal bones

19.3.2 Positioning and Incision

After application of a tourniquet, the hand is placed on a side table with the forearm supinated. A pad is placed under the dorsum of the hand. The skin incision runs a stepped course. The incision begins proximally between the tendons of flexor carpi ulnaris and palmaris longus, runs across to the middle of the distal flexion crease of the wrist, and then continues in a distal direction 1–2 mm ulnar to the thenar palmar crease as far as the proximal palmar flexion crease (**Fig. 19.9**). Splitting and dissection of the subcutaneous tissue are done sharply in part. Damage to the palmar branch of the median nerve on the side of the incision must be avoided. The forearm fascia and palmar aponeurosis are incised in a straight line on the ulnar side of the palmaris longus tendon (**Fig. 19.10**).

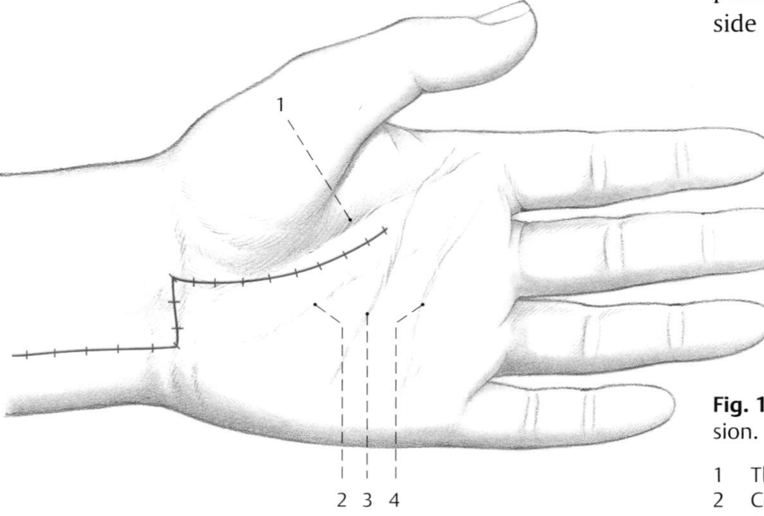

Fig. 19.9 Palmar approach to the wrist joint (left side). Skin incision.

1 Thenar palmar crease
2 Central palmar crease
3 Proximal palmar crease
4 Distal palmar crease

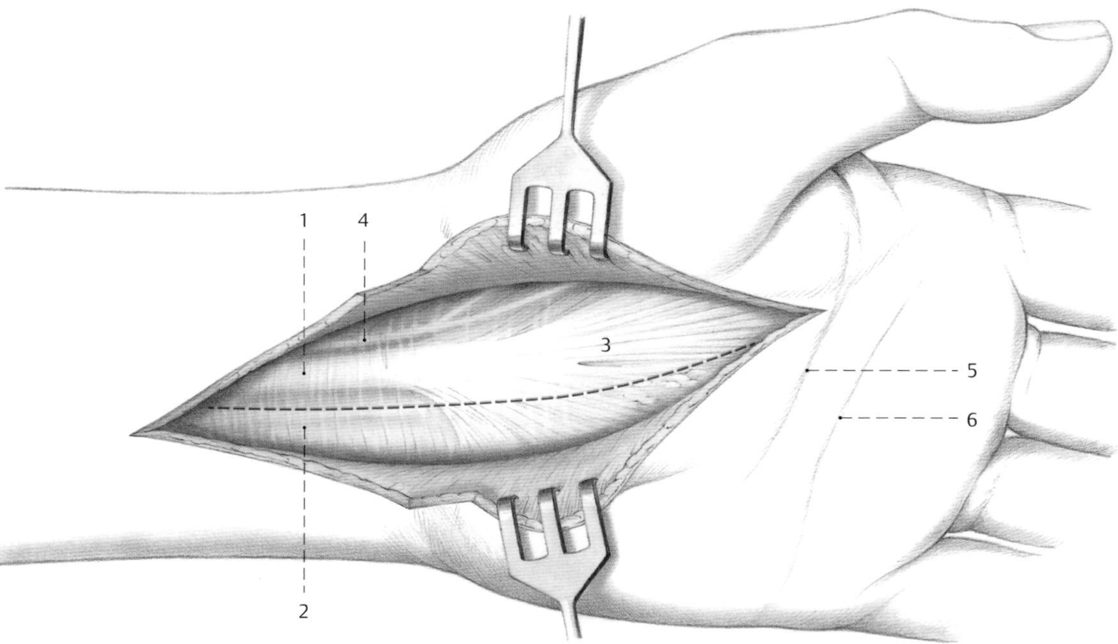

Fig. 19.10 Incision of the forearm fascia and palmar aponeurosis (dashed line); preservation of the palmar branch of the median nerve.

1 Palmaris longus
2 Flexor digitorum superficialis
3 Palmar aponeurosis
4 Palmar branch of median nerve
5 Proximal palmar crease
6 Distal palmar crease

19.3.3 Exposure of the Carpal Tunnel

Following transection of the forearm fascia and the palmar aponeurosis, the median nerve is identified and snared from underneath. The flexor retinaculum is transected with a scalpel under vision between the thenar and hypothenar muscles (**Fig. 19.11**). Attention should be paid to variations of the motor branch of the median nerve to the thenar muscles (**Fig. 19.12**). The retinaculum has to be divided as far as the superficial palmar arch. Now the median nerve as well as its thenar motor branch can be inspected. Lying directly below the median nerve are the superficial flexor tendons of the middle and ring fingers, which overlie those of the index and little fingers.

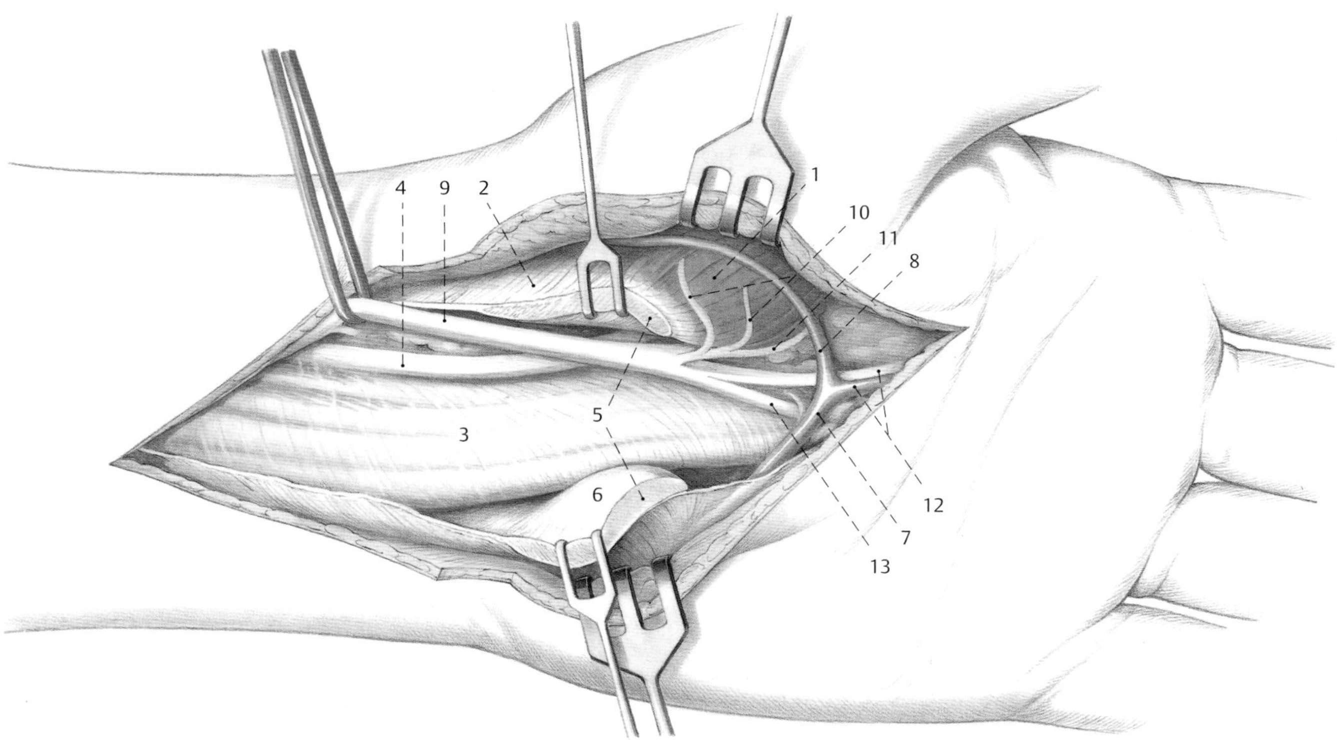

Fig. 19.11 Exposure of the median nerve and digital flexor tendons after transection of the flexor retinaculum.

1 Superficial head of flexor pollicis brevis
2 Abductor pollicis brevis
3 Flexor digitorum superficialis
4 Flexor pollicis longus
5 Flexor retinaculum
6 Hook of the hamate
7 Superficial palmar arterial arch
8 Superficial palmar branch of the radial artery
9 Median nerve
10 Muscular branches
11 Common palmar digital nerve of the thumb
12 Common palmar digital artery and nerve of the second finger
13 Common palmar digital nerve of the third finger

19.3.4 Variations of the Thenar Motor Supply

According to Poisel, three different courses of the thenar muscular branch of the median nerve can be distinguished:

- Type I, or the extraligamentous type, in which the muscular branch arises distal to the flexor retinaculum from the first common palmar digital nerve and runs toward the thenar muscles (46%).
- Type II, or subligamentous type, in which the muscular branch arises from the first common digital nerve in the carpal tunnel and continues in the carpal tunnel on its own up to its distal end to reach the thenar muscles (31%).
- Type III, or transligamentous type, in which the thenar muscular branch again arises in the carpal tunnel, but pierces the flexor retinaculum and reaches the thenar muscles by this route (23%) (**Fig. 19.12**, types I–III).

Another, rarely observed, variation is the ulnar origin of the thenar motor branch described by Mannerfelt and Hybinette (**Fig. 19.12**, type IV).

19.3.5 Exposure of the Wrist Joint

For exposure of the volar wrist joint capsule, the finger flexor tendons are retracted in an ulnar direction, and the flexor pollicis longus tendon is retracted radially (beware the median nerve). The wrist joint capsule may be opened along the dashed line shown in **Fig. 19.13**. The capsule and ligamentous structures are snared with stay sutures and sharply dissected free of the radius, lunate bone, and capitate bone (**Fig. 19.14**). Small Hohmann elevators may be inserted, giving clear exposure of the carpal articular surface of the radius, lunate, scaphoid, and capitate.

19.3.6 Wound Closure

The wrist joint capsule is closed with absorbable interrupted sutures. Following introduction of a drain, further wound closure is performed by means of skin sutures.

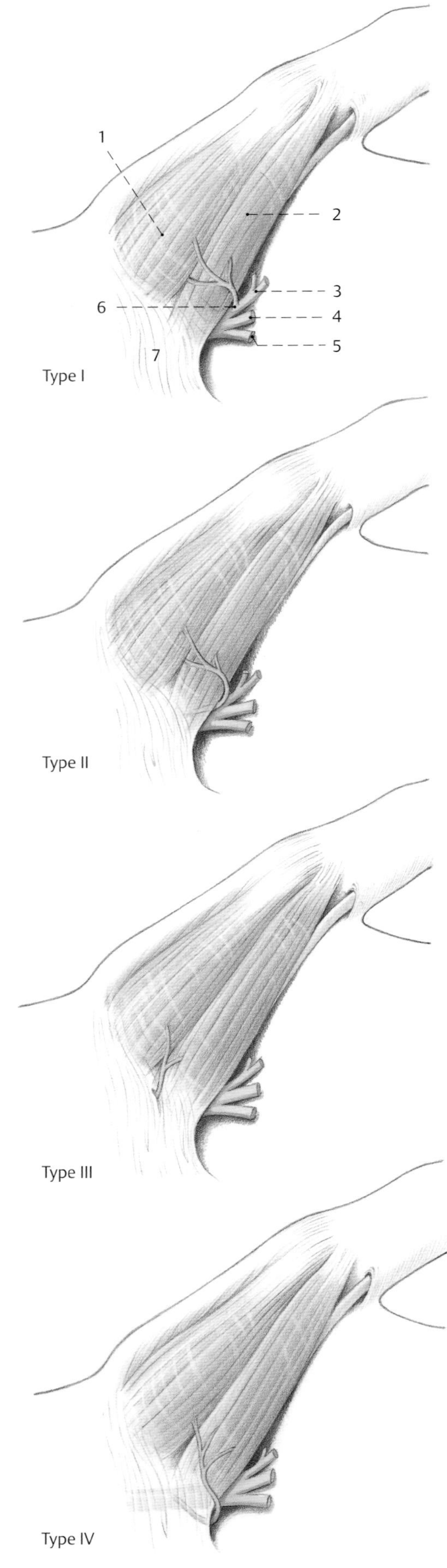

Fig. 19.12 Variants of thenar motor innervation.

Type I or extraligamentous type
Type II or subligamentous type
Type III or transligamentous type
(according to Poisel)
Type IV or ulnar origin of the thenar motor branch (according to Mannerfelt and Hybinette)

1 Abductor pollicis brevis
2 Superficial head of flexor pollicis brevis
3 Common palmar digital nerve of the thumb
4 Common palmar digital nerve of the second finger
5 Common palmar digital nerve of the third finger
6 Muscular branch
7 Flexor retinaculum

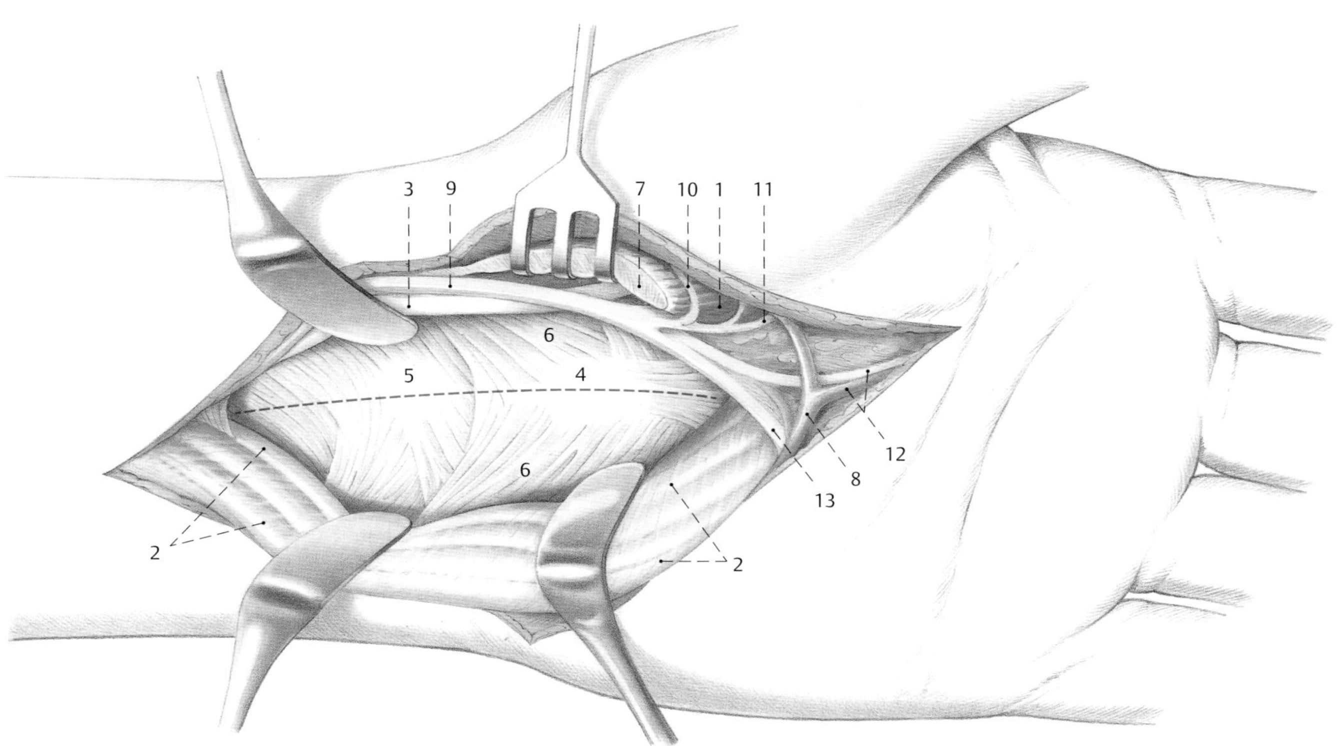

Fig. 19.13 Ulnar retraction of the flexor muscles of the fingers and opening of the wrist joint capsule.

1 Superficial head of flexor pollicis brevis
2 Flexor digitorum superficialis and profundus
3 Flexor pollicis longus
4 Capitate
5 Lunate
6 Radiate carpal ligament
7 Flexor retinaculum
8 Superficial palmar arterial arch
9 Median nerve
10 Muscular branch
11 Common palmar digital nerve of the thumb
12 Common palmar artery and nerve of the second finger
13 Common palmar digital nerve of the third finger

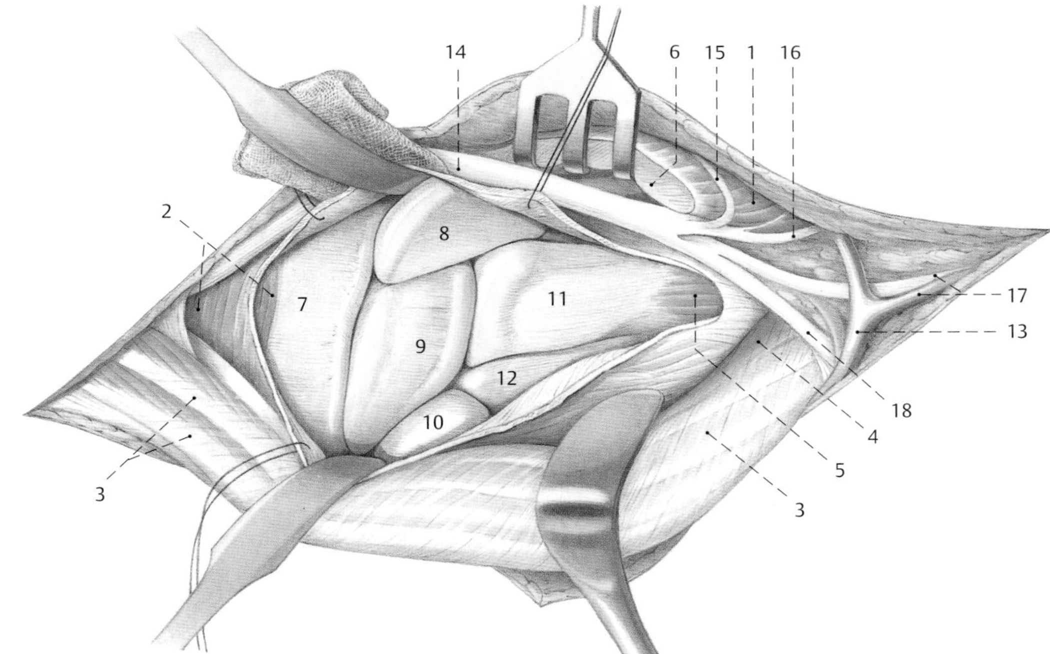

Fig. 19.14 Exposure of the wrist joint and carpal bones from the volar side.

1 Superficial head of flexor pollicis brevis
2 Pronator quadratus
3 Flexor digitorum superficialis and profundus
4 Lumbrical of the thumb
5 Palmar interosseous muscle of the second finger
6 Flexor retinaculum
7 Radius
8 Scaphoid
9 Lunate
10 Triquetrum
11 Capitate
12 Hamate
13 Superficial palmar arterial arch
14 Median nerve
15 Muscular branch
16 Common palmar digital nerve of the thumb
17 Common palmar digital artery and vein of the second finger
18 Common palmar digital nerve of the third finger

19.4 Approach for Arthroscopy

D. Kohn

19.4.1 Principal Indications

- Injury to the triangular disk
- Biopsy and synovectomy
- Chondroplasty

19.4.2 Positioning

The patient is placed in the supine position. Constant traction is required to widen the joint space. This is achieved by use of a sterilizable hand arthroscopy tower (**Fig. 19.15a**) but it can also be ensured at lower cost with the arm suspension employed for arthroscopy of the shoulder and elbow combined with finger traps and countertraction on the upper arm (**Fig. 19.15b**).

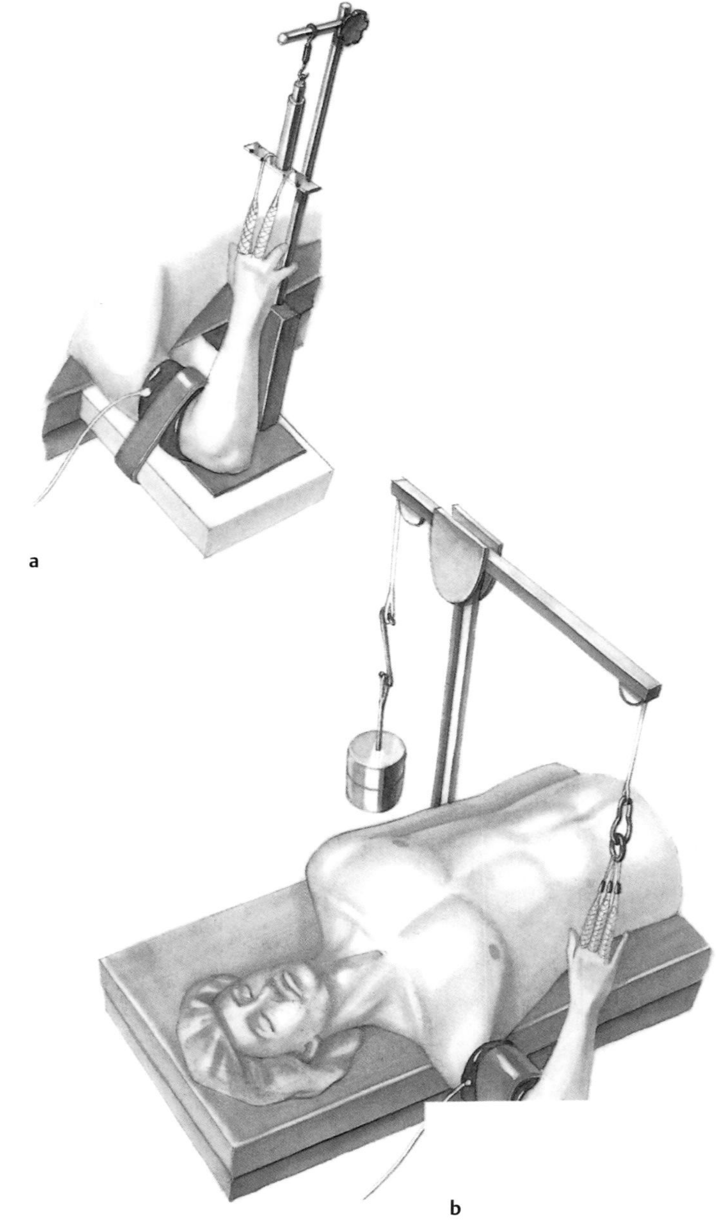

Fig. 19.15 a, b Positioning. (From: Bauer R, Kerschbaumer F, Poisel S. Schulter und obere Extremität. Stuttgart, Thieme; 1997. Orthopädische Operationslehre; Band 3.)

a Arm table and sterile hand arthroscopy tower (Tractiontower, Linvatec Germany)
b Suspending the arm from finger traps with countertraction on the upper arm.

19.4.3 Approaches

All approaches to the wrist are from the dorsal and dorsoulnar sides. All are located close to tendons, nerves, and vessels (**Fig. 19.16**). When obtaining the patient's informed consent, the possibility of injuring sensory nerve branches with the subsequent development of a neuroma must be pointed out.

19.4.4 Incision

The patient's hand and forearm are disinfected. Sterile finger traps are applied to the second, third, and fourth fingers, and countertraction is applied to the upper arm over the tourniquet. The required weight ranges from 2 kg in small and light patients to 5 kg in very muscular patients. The arm is suspended in the holder. The bony and tendon landmarks are

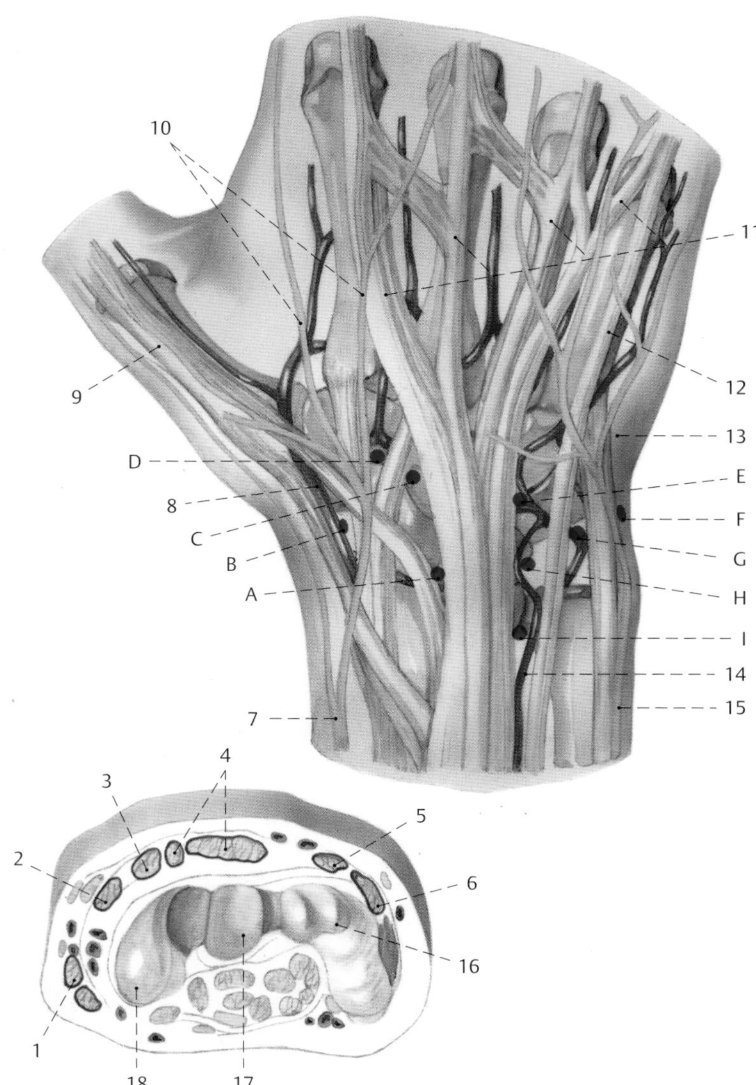

Fig. 19.16 Approaches to the wrist. (From: Bauer R, Kerschbaumer F, Poisel S. Schulter und obere Extremität. Stuttgart, Thieme; 1997. Orthopädische Operationslehre; Band 3.)

- A ¾ portal (extensor pollicis longus/extensor digitorum)
- B ½ portal (abductor pollicis longus/extensor carpi radialis)
- C MCR portal (midcarpal joint, radial)
- D STT portal (scapho-trapezio-trapezoid)
- E MCU portal (midcarpal joint, ulnar)
- F 6U portal (extensor carpi ulnaris/ulnar styloid process)
- G 6R portal (extensor digiti minimi/extensor carpi ulnaris)
- H ⅘ portal (extensor digitorum/extensor digiti minimi)
- I DRU portal (distal, radioulnar joint)

1–6 Tendon compartments:

1. Tendons of abductor pollicis longus and extensor pollicis brevis
2. Tendons of extensor carpi radialis longus and brevis
3. Tendon of extensor pollicis longus
4. Tendons of extensor digitorum and extensor indicis
5. Tendon of extensor digiti minimi
6. Tendon of extensor carpi ulnaris
7. Superficial branch of the radial nerve
8. Radial artery
9. Tendon of extensor pollicis longus
10. Dorsal digital nerves
11. Tendon of extensor digitorum communis
12. Tendon of extensor digiti minimi
13. Tendon of extensor carpi ulnaris
14. Posterior interosseous artery
15. Dorsal branch of the ulnar nerve
16. Triquetrum
17. Lunate
18. Scaphoid

marked (**Fig. 19.17**). General or regional anesthesia is required because of the tourniquet.

The first puncture is made at the ¾ portal (**Fig. 19.18**). The assistant fills the wrist with 5–10 mL Ringer solution. As the fluid enters the joint, it is distracted, the hand rotates approximately 10°, and the wrist moves into slight ulnar deviation so that the needle is finally more horizontal. Swelling of the distal radioulnar joint indicates a communication between the radiocarpal and distal radioulnar joints due to a defect in the disk complex. The midcarpal joint must also be observed closely during injection. If it fills, this indicates a leak between the radiocarpal and midcarpal joints. After the joint has been filled, the thumb of the nondominant hand is again placed on Lister's tubercle and the needle is withdrawn with slight pressure on the syringe.

The skin incision is made with a size 11 scalpel. It is held with the blade edge pointing toward the patient's fingers. To-and-fro movement of the scalpel is avoided so as not to damage the surfaces of the scaphoid and lunate. As soon as the blade has penetrated about half way, a decrease in resistance is felt. Holding the scalpel in a fixed position, the operator's thumb now draws the skin proximally against the scalpel blade to enlarge the skin incision without opening the joint capsule further. Abundant fluid now issues from the joint, and the scalpel is removed. The operator's thumb is not moved, thus immobilizing the tissue layers. Any movement will cause the

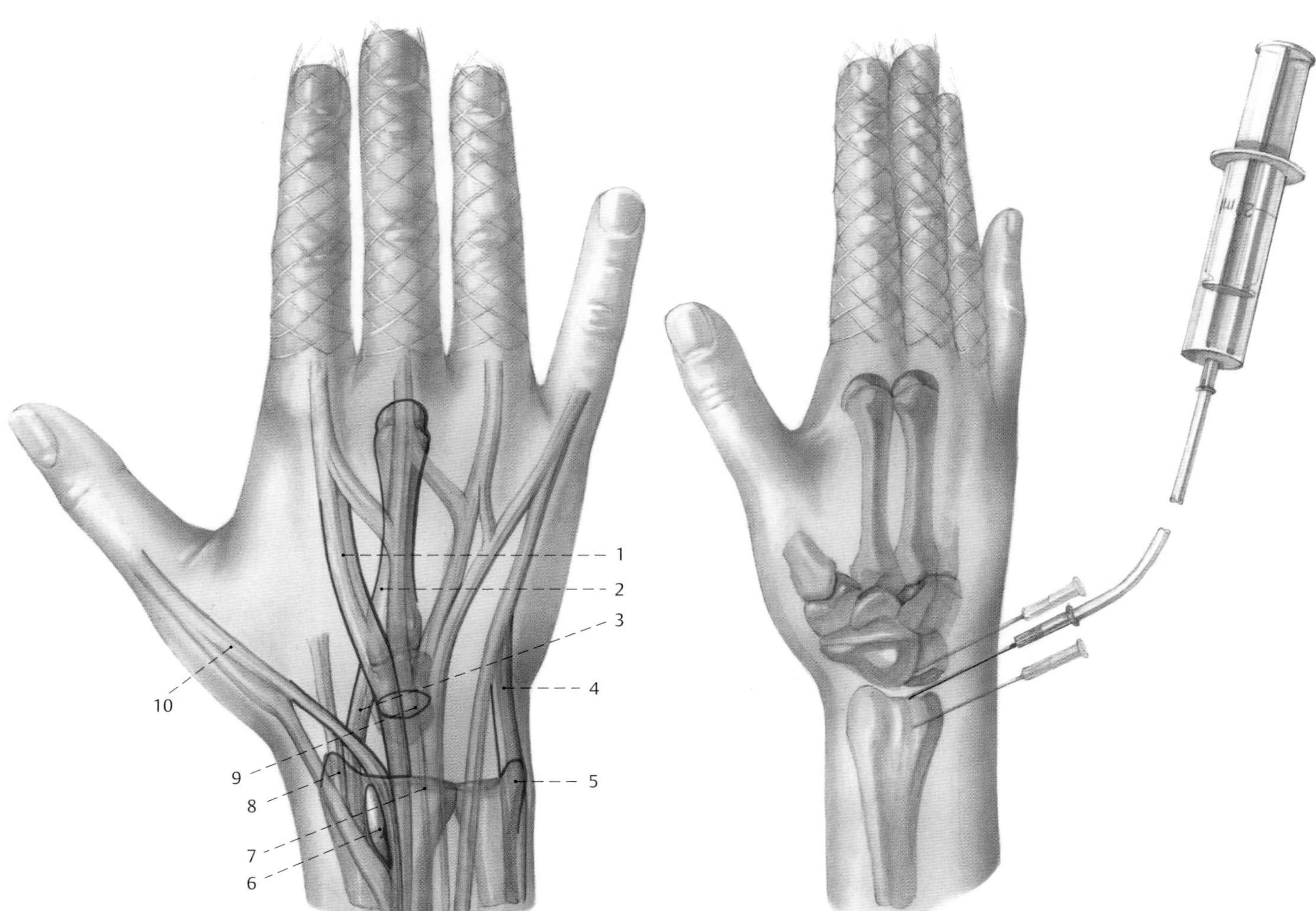

Fig. 19.17 Wrist landmarks. (From: Bauer R, Kerschbaumer F, Poisel S. Schulter und obere Extremität. Stuttgart, Thieme; 1997. Orthopädische Operationslehre; Band 3.)

1 Tendon of extensor digitorum to the index finger
2 Third metacarpal
3 Tendon of extensor carpi radialis brevis
4 Tendon of extensor carpi ulnaris
5 Ulnar styloid process
6 Lister's tubercle (dorsal tubercle of the radius)
7 Dorsal edge of the joint surface of the radius
8 Radial styloid process
9 Sulcus of the capitate
10 Tendon of extensor pollicis longus

Fig. 19.18 Puncture of the wrist over the ¾ portal. The thumb palpates first Lister's tubercle, and then the dorsal edge of the joint surface of the radius. The needle (22 G) follows the direction of the joint cavity. If the first puncture is unsuccessful, a second puncture in the same direction is attempted 2 mm further proximally or distally. (From: Bauer R, Kerschbaumer F, Poisel S. Schulter und obere Extremität. Stuttgart, Thieme; 1997. Orthopädische Operationslehre; Band 3.)

approach to close again. The trocar sleeve containing a blunt obturator is exchanged for the scalpel. The sleeve with obturator glides into the joint cavity under gentle pressure.

19.4.5 Wound Closure

Simple superficial skin suture.

19.4.6 Dangers

Forceful insertion must be avoided as the entire dorsal to palmar distance at the level of the ¾ portal is only approximately 2 cm, and the palmar joint capsule would be rapidly perforated (**Fig. 19.19**).

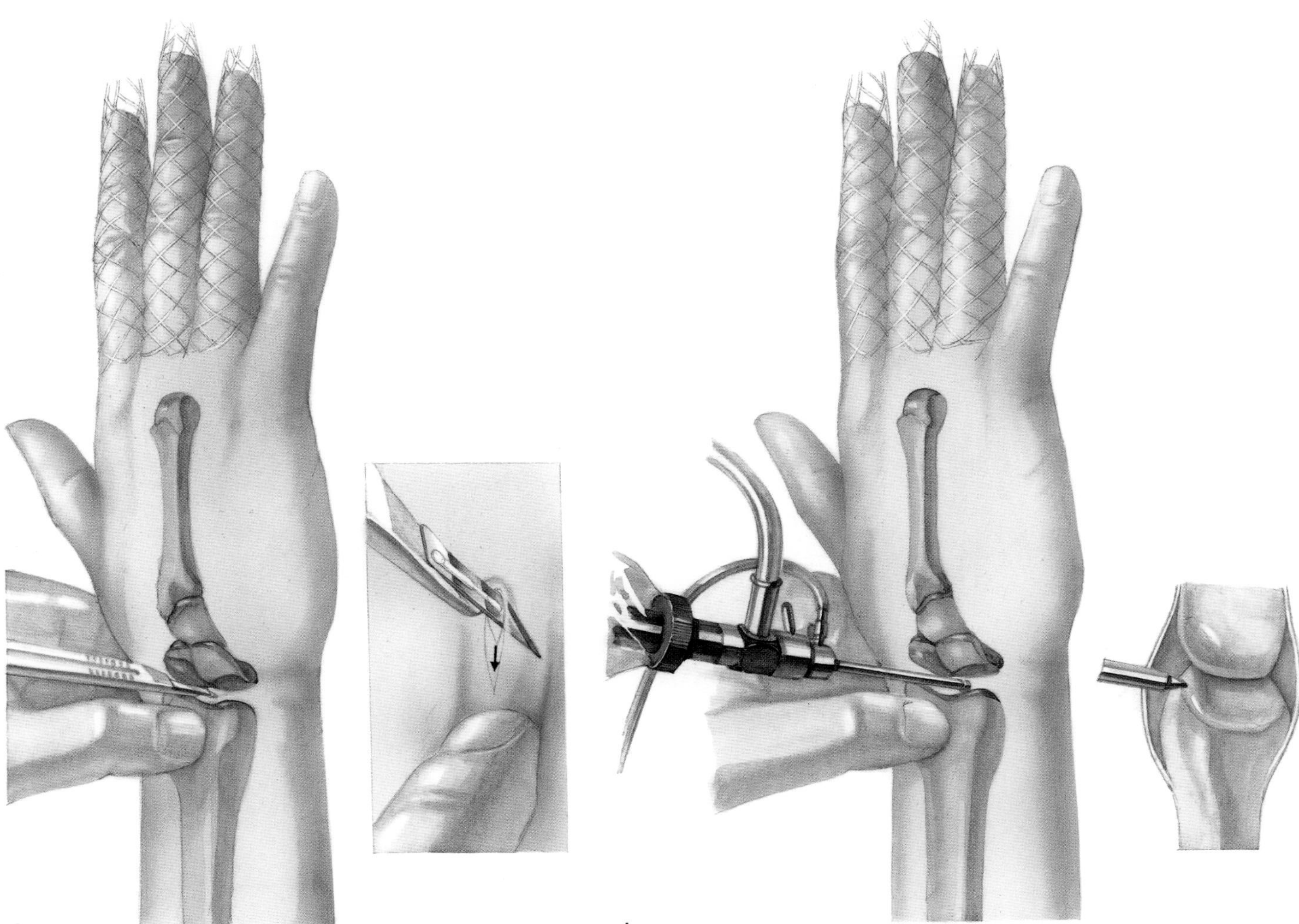

Fig. 19.19 a, b Opening of the ¾ portal and introduction of the arthroscope sleeve. (From: Bauer R, Kerschbaumer F, Poisel S. Schulter und obere Extremität. Stuttgart, Thieme; 1997. Orthopädische Operationslehre; Band 3.)

a Incision with a size 11 scalpel. The skin incision is enlarged by holding the scalpel and drawing the skin over it (detail).
b Introduction of the sleeve with a blunt trocar. The distance to the anterior capsule is only 2 cm (detail).

20 Hand

20.1 Approach to the Palm According to Skoog

R. Bauer, F. Kerschbaumer, S. Poisel

20.1.1 Principal Indications

- Dupuytren's contracture
- Inflammation
- Tenosynovitis
- Tendon rupture

20.1.2 Positioning and Incision

After application of a tourniquet, the forearm is supinated and the hand placed on a side table. Occasionally, immobilization of the fingers and the thumb by means of special positioning splints is advisable (see **Figs. 20.40** and **20.45**). A T-shaped skin incision is made between the third and the fourth metacarpal bones, the transverse cut lying in the area of the distal palmar flexion crease. If necessary, the incision may be extended distally (**Fig. 20.1**).

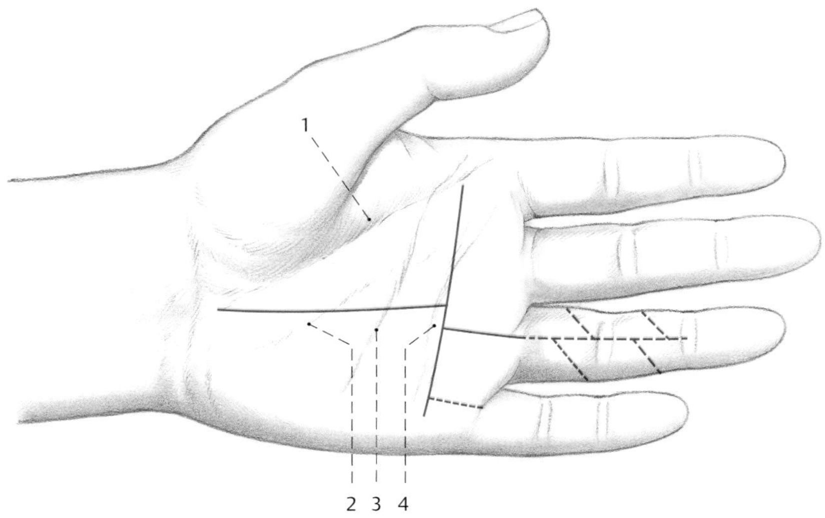

Fig. 20.1 Approach to the palm according to Skoog (left hand). Skin incision. If necessary (Dupuytren's contracture), the skin incision may be extended distally.

1 Thenar palmar crease
2 Central palmar crease
3 Proximal palmar crease
4 Distal palmar crease

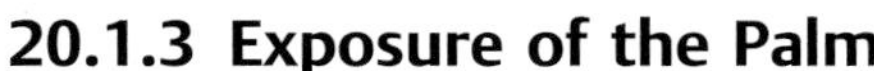

20.1.3 Exposure of the Palm

The skin flaps are sharply dissected free of the palmar aponeurosis and pulled up with the aid of stay sutures (**Fig. 20.2**).

Fig. 20.2 The skin is stripped from the palmar aponeurosis with a flat blade (detail). Incision of the palmar aponeurosis (dashed line).

1 Longitudinal fasciculi of the palmar aponeurosis
2 Transverse fasciculi of the palmar aponeurosis

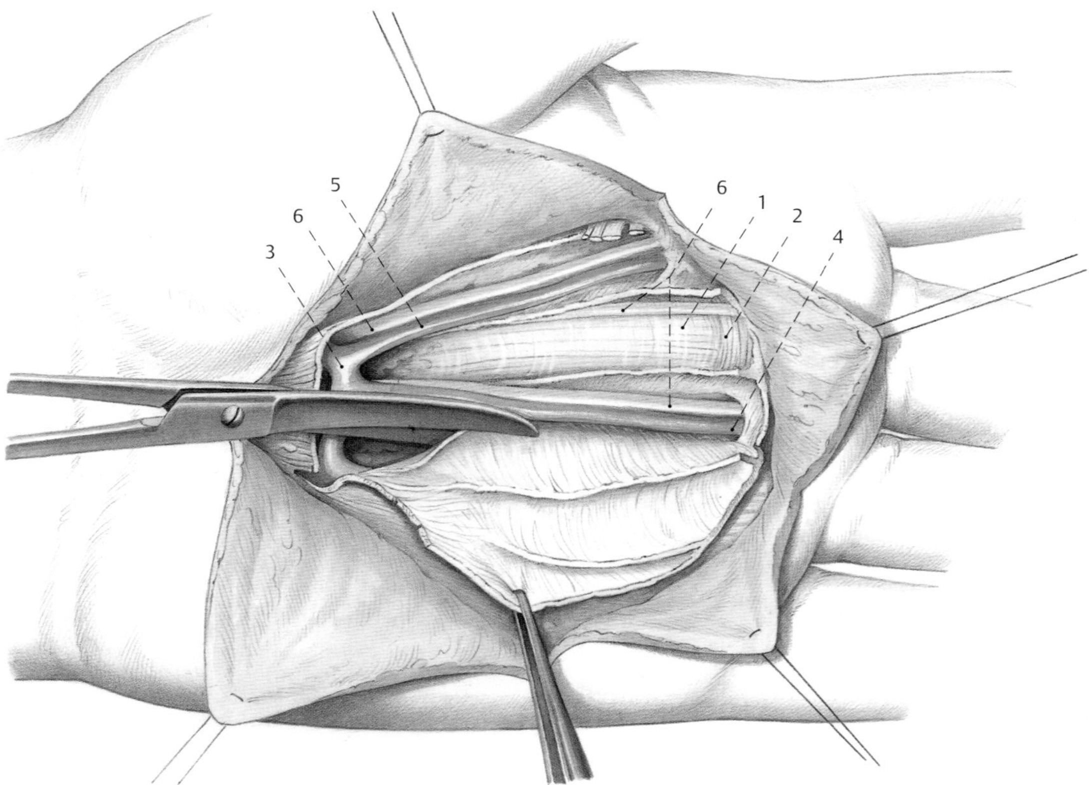

Fig. 20.3 Transection of the vertical septa of the palmar aponeurosis for exposure of the flexor tendons and neurovascular bundles.

1 Tendon of the superficial flexor muscle of the third finger
2 Annular ligaments
3 Superficial palmar arterial arch
4 Common palmar digital artery of the third finger
5 Common palmar digital artery of the second finger
6 Proper palmar digital nerve

In the proximal wound region, a probe is passed under the longitudinal fasciculi of the palmar aponeurosis, which are then transected. Next the septa coursing from the palmar aponeurosis to the deep palmar fascia are severed from proximal to distal with scissors (**Fig. 20.3**). By resection of the palmar aponeurosis, the palm with the superficial palmar arch, the branches of the median and ulnar nerves, the flexor tendons of the long fingers, and the lumbrical muscles is clearly exposed (**Fig. 20.4**).

20.1.4 Anatomical Site

In **Fig. 20.5**, the palmar aponeurosis has been removed, and the flexor retinaculum as well as the canal of Guyon split. Note the course and the relation of the common palmar digital arteries and nerves to the lumbrical muscles. The ulnar artery was retracted in a radial direction to expose the origin of the deep branch of the ulnar nerve (the motor branch to the interosseous muscles).

20.1.5 Wound Closure

After release of the tourniquet, hemostasis, and insertion of a drain, the wound is closed with skin sutures.

Fig. 20.5 Anatomical site. The palmar aponeurosis has been removed to achieve a clearer view. Note the position and course of the superficial palmar arterial arch, and of the ulnar and median nerves. The annular ligament of the tendon sheath is obliquely crossed by the radial digital nerve (median nerve). ▶

1 Abductor pollicis brevis
2 Superficial head of flexor pollicis brevis
3 Tendon of flexor pollicis longus
4 Oblique head of adductor pollicis
5 First dorsal interosseous muscle
6 Lumbrical
7 Tendons of flexor digitorum superficialis
8 Abductor digiti minimi
9 Flexor digiti minimi brevis
10 Annular ligaments of the tendon sheath of the fingers
11 Cruciate ligaments of the tendon sheath of the fingers
12 Ulnar artery
13 Superficial palmar arterial arch
14 Main artery to the thumb
15 Common palmar digital artery
16 Proper palmar digital artery
17 Cephalic vein of the thumb
18 Palmar branch of the median nerve
19 Common palmar digital nerves of the thumb and second finger
20 Common palmar digital nerve of the third finger
21 Ulnar nerve
22 Common palmar digital nerve of the fourth finger
23 Proper palmar digital nerve

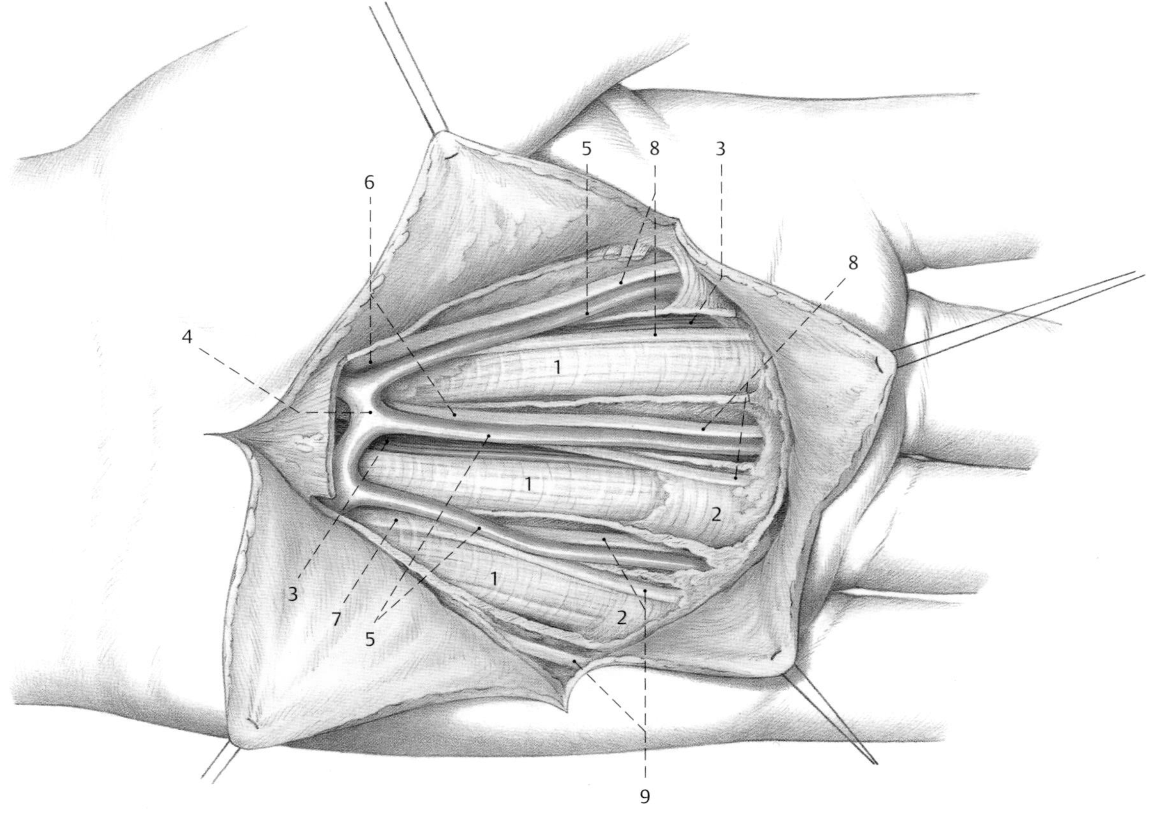

Fig. 20.4 Operative site after resection of the palmar aponeurosis.

1 Tendon of flexor digitorum superficialis
2 Annular ligaments of the tendon sheath of the fingers
3 Lumbrical
4 Superficial palmar arterial arch
5 Common palmar digital artery
6 Common palmar digital nerve (median nerve)
7 Common palmar digital nerve (ulnar nerve)
8 Proper palmar digital nerves (median nerve)
9 Proper palmar digital nerves (ulnar nerve)

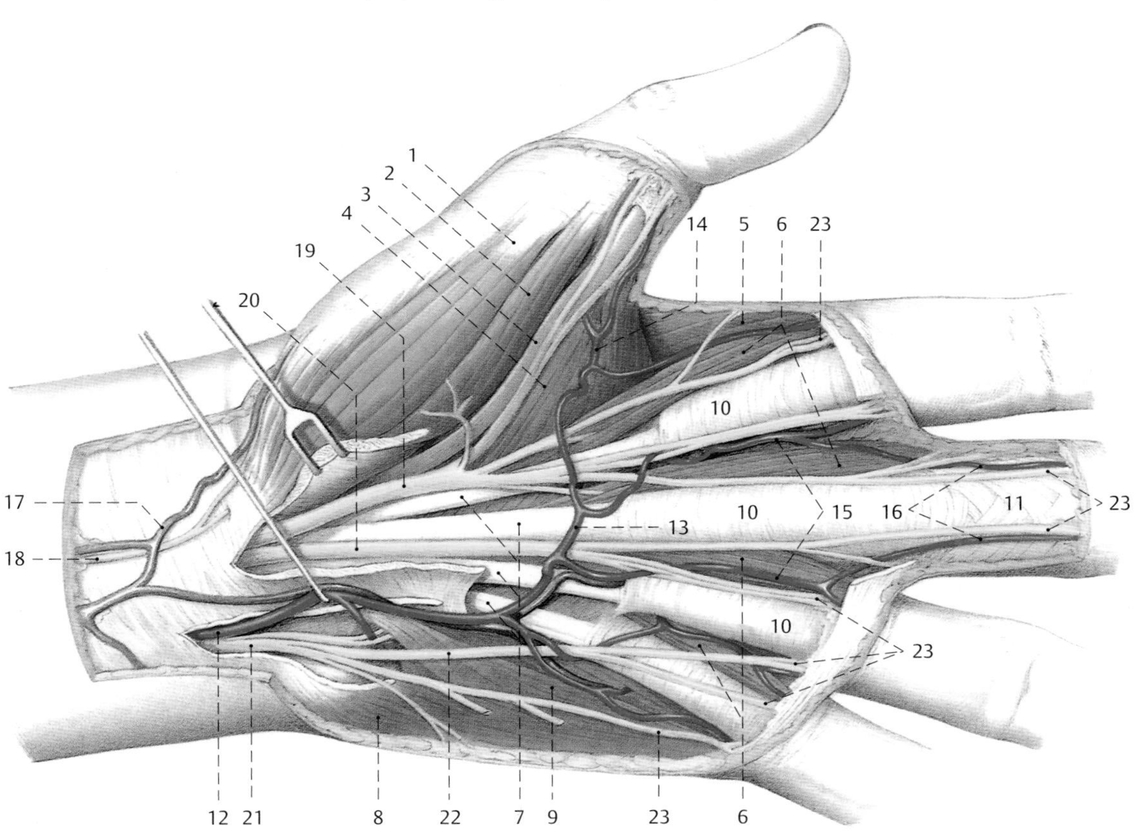

Fig. 20.5

20.2 Exposure of the Ulnar Nerve in the Canal of Guyon

R. Bauer, F. Kerschbaumer, S. Poisel

20.2.1 Principal Indication

- Ulnar nerve compression syndrome

20.2.2 Positioning and Incision

After application of a tourniquet, the hand rests on a side table with the forearm supinated. The S-shaped skin incision is made approximately 1 cm on the radial side of the flexor carpi ulnaris tendon (**Fig. 20.6**).

20.2.3 Exposure of the Ulnar Nerve

After incision of the subcutaneous tissue, the delicate forearm fascia in the proximal wound region is split, and the ulnar artery and nerve are identified and exposed (**Fig. 20.7**). The fibers between the palmar aponeurosis and the hypothenar eminence (palmar carpal ligament) with the irregularly occurring palmaris brevis, which form the roof of the canal of Guyon, are incised along the dashed line shown in **Fig. 20.7**. Cautious retraction of the ulnar artery in an ulnar direction exposes the division of the ulnar nerve into the superficial and deep branches (**Fig. 20.8**; see also **Fig. 20.5**). The deep branch penetrates in a distal direction between abductor digiti minimi and flexor digiti minimi brevis through a slit in the opponens digiti minimi, and ends in the adductor pollicis and flexor pollicis brevis (deep head). For exposure of the deep motor branch of the ulnar nerve, the insertion of the opponens digiti minimi at the base of the fifth metacarpal is partially incised (**Fig. 20.8**, dashed line). The superficial branch is passed under and snared, revealing the deep motor branch (**Fig. 20.9**). The floor of the canal of Guyon is formed by the pisohamate ligament.

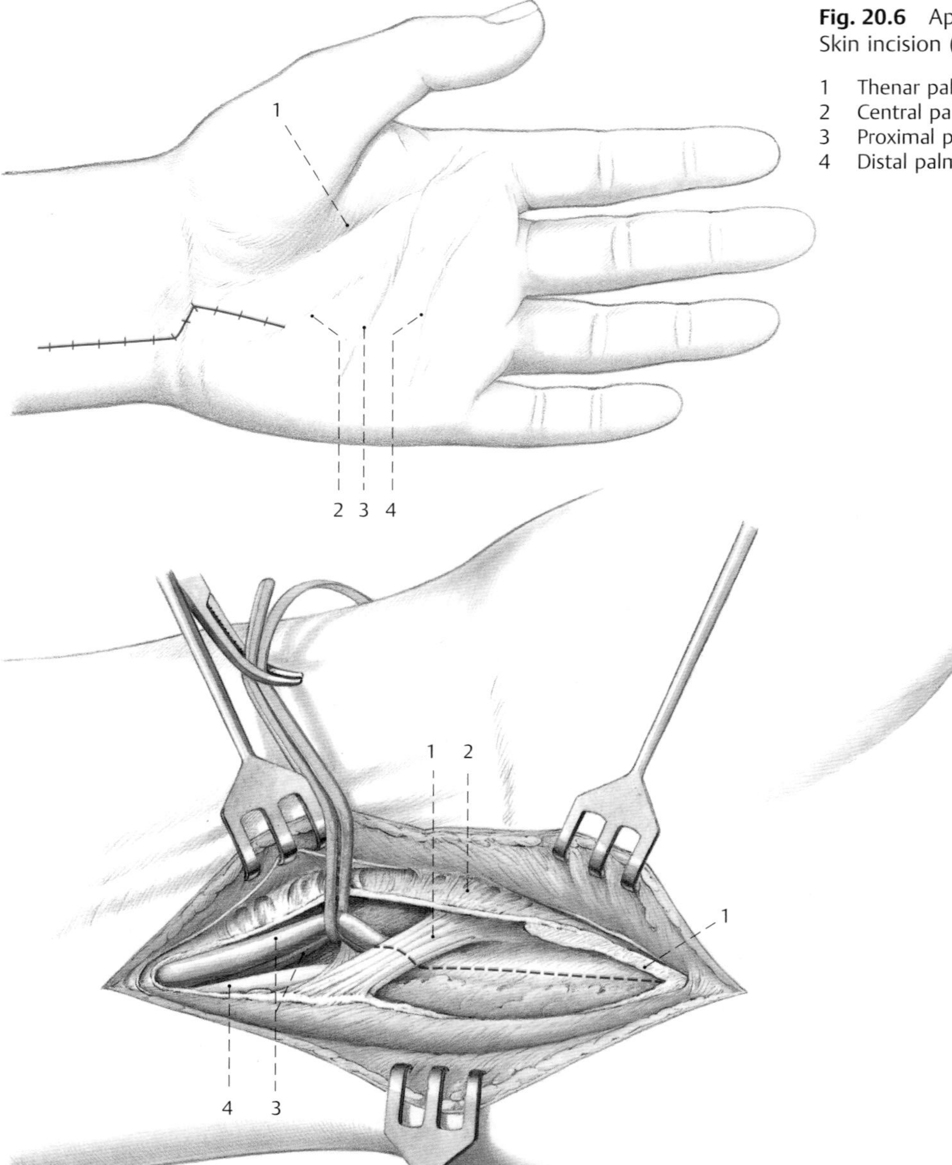

Fig. 20.6 Approach to the canal of Guyon (left side). Skin incision (solid line).

1 Thenar palmar crease
2 Central palmar crease
3 Proximal palmar crease
4 Distal palmar crease

Fig. 20.7 Transection of the forearm fascia and the fibrous tissue over the canal of Guyon. Exposure of the ulnar artery, vein, and nerve.

1 Palmar carpal ligament
2 Palmar aponeurosis
3 Ulnar artery and vein
4 Ulnar nerve

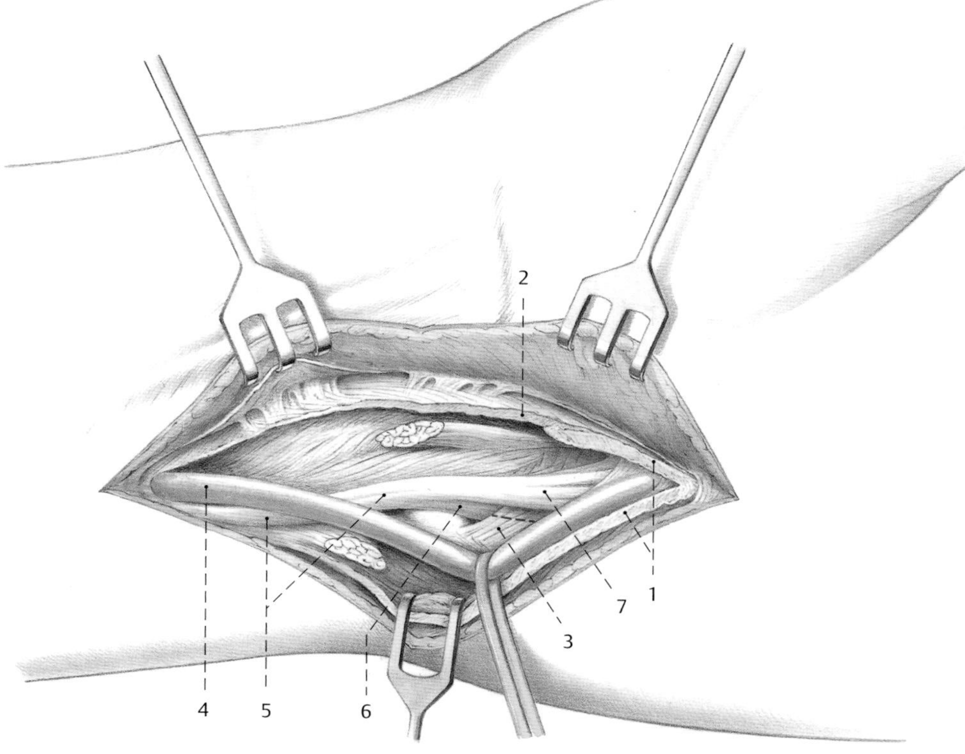

Fig. 20.8 Retraction of the ulnar artery and dissection of the bifurcation of the ulnar nerve. Partial incision of opponens digiti minimi.

1 Palmar carpal ligament
2 Palmar aponeurosis
3 Opponens digiti minimi
4 Ulnar artery
5 Ulnar nerve
6 Deep branch of the ulnar nerve
7 Superficial branch of the ulnar nerve

20.2.4 Wound Closure

After release of the tourniquet, hemostasis, and the introduction of a drain, the wound is closed with skin sutures.

20.2.5 Dangers

The course of the deep (motor) branch of the ulnar nerve after its origin in the canal of Guyon takes various forms. It may leave the canal of Guyon more distally than is normally the case, and may pass through a band-like structure that communicates with the opponens muscle and the pisohamate ligament. For visualization of this nerve branch, the use of magnifying glasses is recommended.

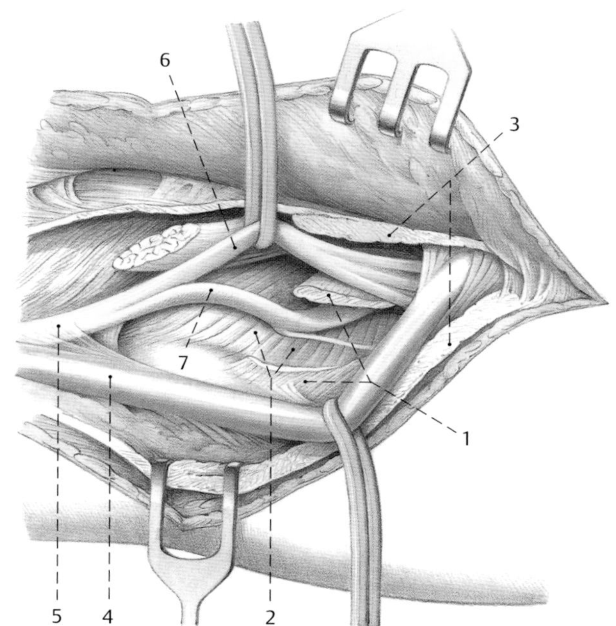

Fig. 20.9 Exposure of the deep branch of the ulnar nerve.

1 Opponens digiti minimi
2 Pisohamate ligament
3 Palmar carpal ligament
4 Ulnar artery
5 Ulnar nerve
6 Superficial branch of the ulnar nerve
7 Deep branch of the ulnar nerve

20.3 Palmar Approach to the Scaphoid

R. Bauer, F. Kerschbaumer, S. Poisel

20.3.1 Principal Indications

- Fractures
- Dislocations
- Pseudarthrosis

20.3.2 Positioning and Incision

After application of a tourniquet, the forearm is supinated, the wrist hyperextended, and the hand placed on a rolled pad (**Fig. 20.10**). The skin incision begins at the distal flexion crease of the wrist, and continues 4 cm in a proximal direction over the tendon of the flexor carpi radialis.

20.3.3 Exposure of the Scaphoid

After incision of the skin and subcutaneous tissue, the tendon sheath of flexor carpi radialis is split, and its tendon is retracted in an ulnar direction. The wrist joint capsule is incised along the dashed line shown in **Fig. 20.11** and is laterally retracted with the adherent periosteum (**Fig. 20.12**). The scaphoid and the distal end of the radius are thus clearly revealed from the palmar side.

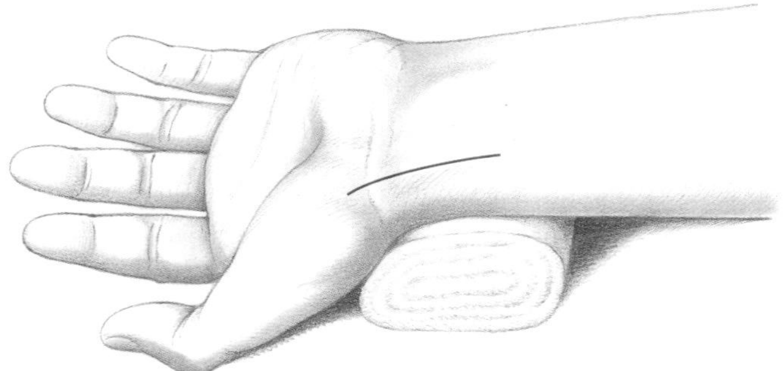

Fig. 20.10 Palmar approach to the scaphoid (left side). Skin incision.

20.3.4 Extension of the Approach

This approach can be extended proximally to expose the distal radius from the palmar side (see **Figs. 18.24, 18.25, 18.26, 18.27, 18.28**).

20.3.5 Wound Closure

The wound is closed by suturing the capsule and the tendon sheath of flexor carpi radialis.

20.3.6 Dangers

Damage to the radial artery can be avoided by correct positioning of the capsular incision, beneath the tendon of flexor carpi radialis. An excessive pull of retractors in the ulnar direction should be avoided to spare the median nerve.

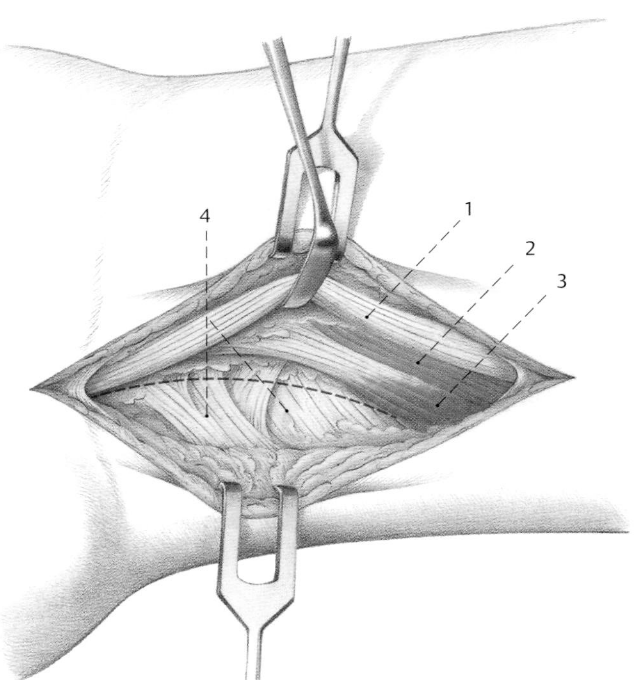

Fig. 20.11 After splitting of the tendon sheath, flexor carpi radialis is retracted in an ulnar direction, and the joint capsule is incised (dashed line).

1 Tendon of flexor carpi radialis
2 Flexor digitorum superficialis
3 Flexor pollicis longus
4 Palmar intercarpal ligaments

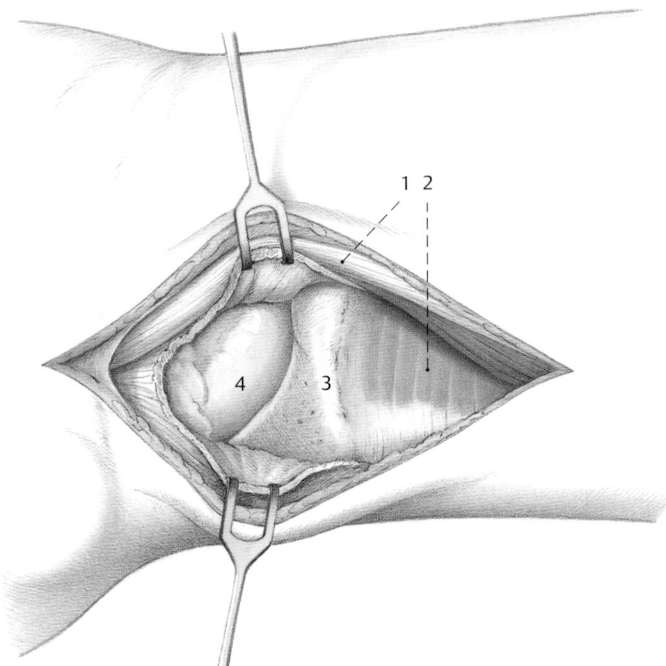

Fig. 20.12 Appearance after opening of the joint capsule. Exposure of the scaphoid and distal radius.

1 Tendon of flexor carpi radialis
2 Pronator teres
3 Distal end of the radius
4 Scaphoid

20.4 Approach to the Carpometacarpal Joint of the Thumb

R. Bauer, F. Kerschbaumer, S. Poisel

20.4.1 Principal Indications

- Osteoarthritis
- Fractures of the first metacarpal
- Dislocation fractures

20.4.2 Positioning and Incision

After application of a tourniquet, the hand is placed on a support in neutral rotation. An S-shaped skin incision approximately 5 cm long is made on the palmar radial side over the tendon of abductor pollicis longus (**Fig. 20.13**). After splitting the subcutaneous tissue, the sensory superficial branch of the radial nerve is identified and snared from underneath. The tendon sheath of the abductor pollicis longus and extensor pollicis brevis is divided (**Fig. 20.14**).

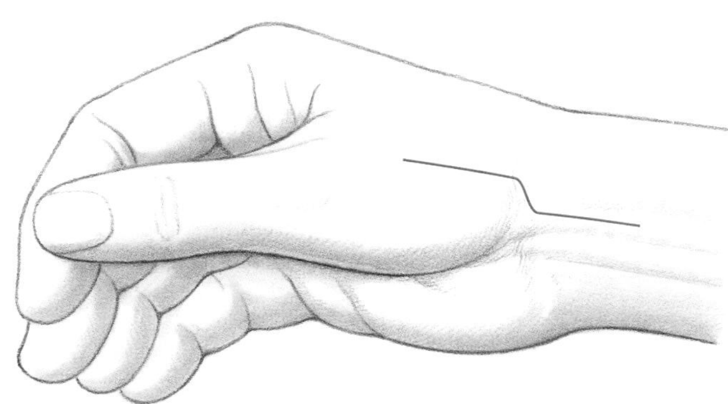

Fig. 20.13 Approach to the carpometacarpal joint of the thumb (right side). Skin incision (solid line).

20.4.3 Exposure of the Carpometacarpal Joint of the Thumb

The tendon of extensor pollicis brevis is retracted in a dorsal direction, and that of abductor pollicis longus is retracted toward the palmar side. The radial artery and the venae comitantes are identified, undermined, and snared (**Fig. 20.15**). Proximal retraction of the artery exposes the joint capsule; it should be opened along the dashed line shown in **Fig. 20.15**. The insertion of small Langenbeck retractors clearly reveals the saddle joint of the thumb (**Fig. 20.16**). If necessary, the capsular incision may be extended proximally to expose the joint between the scaphoid and trapezium.

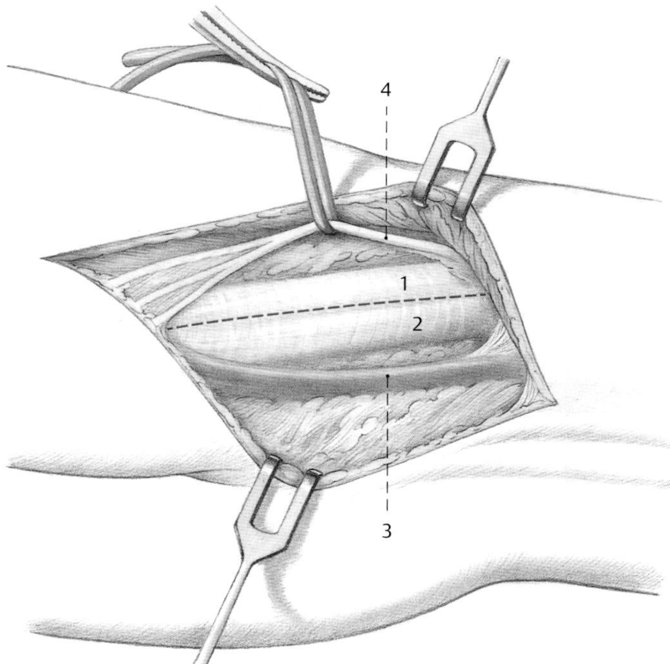

Fig. 20.14 Exposure of the superficial branch of the radial nerve; splitting of the tendon sheath over abductor pollicis longus and extensor pollicis brevis (dashed line).

1 Tendon of extensor pollicis brevis
2 Tendon of abductor pollicis longus
3 Cephalic vein of forearm
4 Superficial branch of the radial nerve

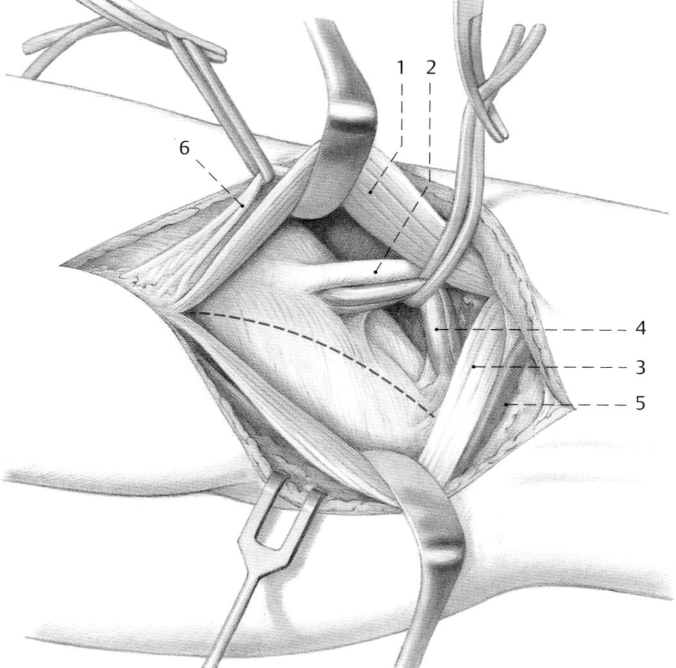

Fig. 20.15 After exposure and retraction of the radial artery, the joint capsule is opened over the carpometacarpal joint of the thumb (dashed line).

1 Extensor pollicis brevis
2 Extensor carpi radialis longus
3 Abductor pollicis longus
4 Radial artery and vein
5 Cephalic vein of forearm
6 Superficial branch of the radial nerve

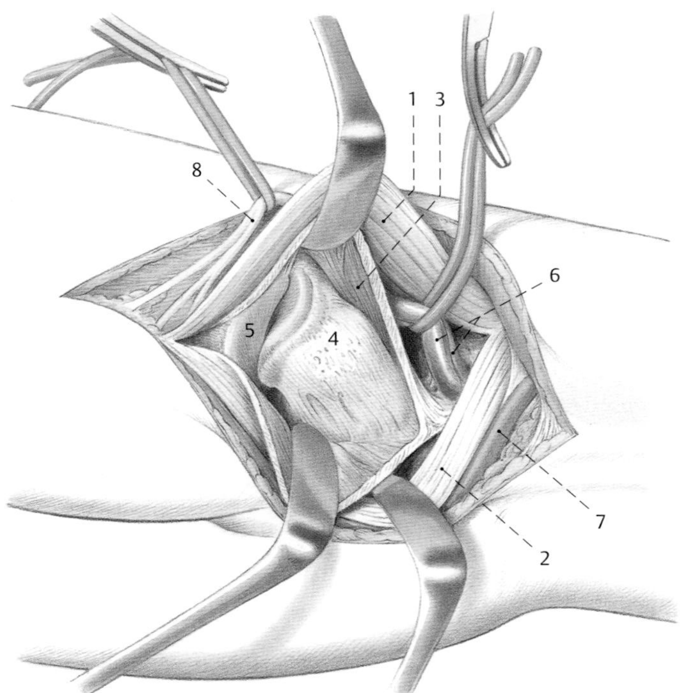

Fig. 20.16 Operative site after opening of the joint capsule over the carpometacarpal joint of the thumb.

1 Extensor pollicis brevis
2 Abductor pollicis longus
3 Capsule of the carpometacarpal joint of the thumb
4 Trapezium
5 Base of the first metacarpal
6 Radial artery and vein
7 Cephalic vein of forearm
8 Superficial branch of the radial nerve

20.4.4 Anatomical Site

Figure 20.17 shows the radial side of the wrist with the sensory branches of the superficial branch of the radial nerve and the underlying first extensor tendon compartment.

Note the duplicate tendon of abductor pollicis longus. The radial artery with the venae comitantes passes between these tendons and the carpal joint capsule, and runs in a dorsal direction into the first interosseous space.

20.4.5 Wound Closure

The capsule of the carpometacarpal joint of the thumb has to be closed with special care so that postoperative subluxation of the first metacarpal in a radial and palmar direction may be prevented.

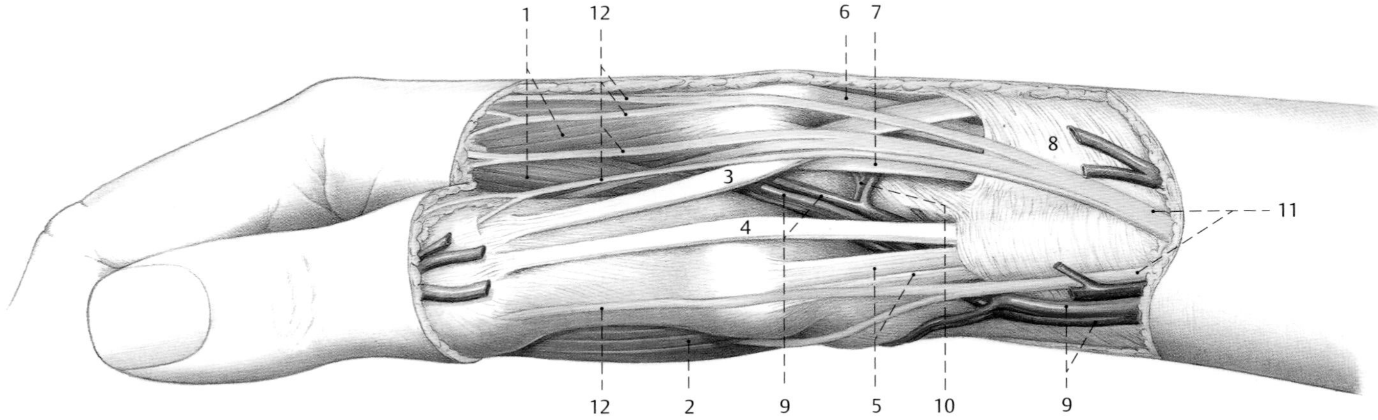

Fig. 20.17 Anatomical site of the radial side of the wrist.

1 First dorsal interosseous muscle
2 Abductor pollicis brevis
3 Extensor pollicis longus
4 Extensor pollicis brevis
5 Abductor pollicis longus
6 Extensor carpi radialis brevis
7 Extensor carpi radialis longus
8 Extensor retinaculum
9 Radial artery and vein
10 Dorsal carpal branch
11 Superficial branch of the radial nerve
12 Proper dorsal digital nerve

20.5 Approach to the First Extensor Tendon Compartment

R. Bauer, F. Kerschbaumer, S. Poisel

20.5.1 Principal Indications

- Stenosing tenosynovitis (De Quervain)
- Synovitis of the first extensor tendon compartment

20.5.2 Positioning and Incision

After application of a tourniquet, the hand is placed on a support in neutral rotation. The skin incision is made transversely over the first extensor tendon compartment, continuing the flexion crease of the wrist (**Fig. 20.18**).

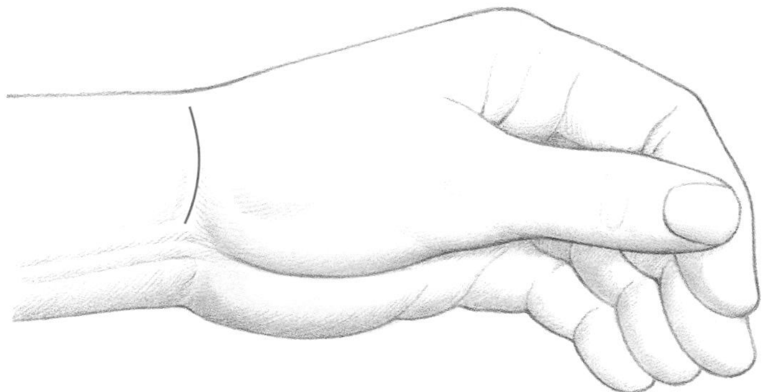

Fig. 20.18 Approach to the first extensor tendon compartment (left hand). Skin incision (solid line).

20.5.3 Exposure of the First Extensor Tendon Compartment

After splitting of the subcutaneous tissue, the superficial branch of the radial nerve is identified and snared from underneath. The tendon sheath is incised along the dashed line shown in **Fig. 20.19**. By undermining the subcutaneous tissue, it is possible to mobilize the skin edge proximally and distally, permitting complete division of the first extensor tendon compartment. In the presence of duplicate tendons of abductor pollicis longus (**Fig. 20.20**), a septum generally appears between these two tendons, and this too has to be split.

20.5.4 Wound Closure

The wound is closed with skin sutures.

20.5.5 Dangers

Longitudinal incisions over the first extensor tendon compartment lead to unsightly scarring. The superficial branch of the radial nerve has to be exposed and retracted.

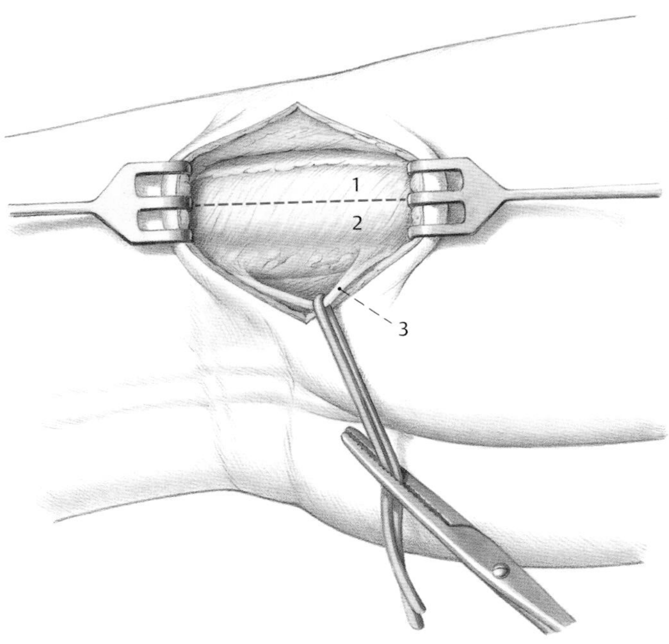

Fig. 20.19 Splitting of the first extensor tendon compartment after exposure of the superficial branch of the radial nerve (dashed line).

1 Extensor pollicis brevis
2 Abductor pollicis longus
3 Superficial branch of the radial nerve

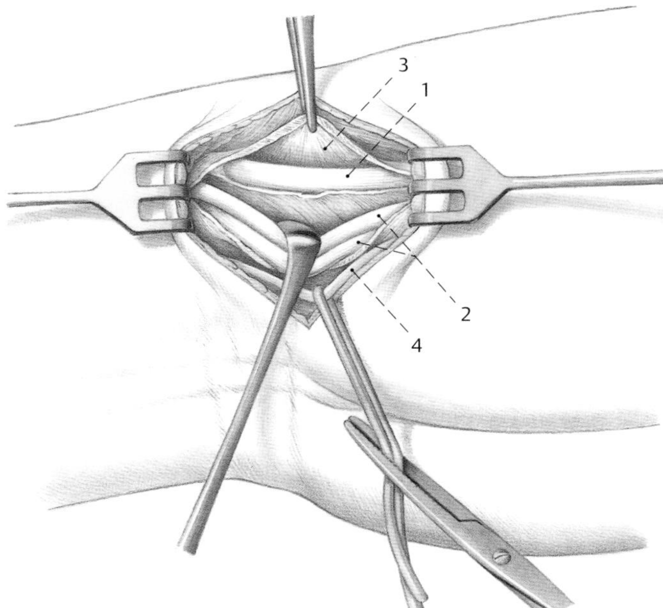

Fig. 20.20 Exposure of the tendons of extensor pollicis brevis and abductor pollicis longus (duplicate tendon).

1 Extensor pollicis brevis
2 Abductor pollicis longus
3 Tendon sheath
4 Superficial branch of the radial nerve

20.6 Dorsal Incisions Over the Dorsum of the Hand and Fingers

R. Bauer, F. Kerschbaumer, S. Poisel

20.6a Dorsal Incisions—General Points

Figure 20.21 shows dorsal incisions for exposure of the metacarpophalangeal joints.

The metacarpophalangeal joints may be exposed either by a transverse incision or by curved longitudinal incisions. A transverse incision is recommended when all four metacarpophalangeal joints of the fingers are to be exposed at the same time. Longitudinal incisions on the dorsum of the hand are used for exposure of the metacarpal bones.

20.6b Dorsal Approach to the Metacarpophalangeal Joint

20.6b.1 Principal Indications

- Synovectomy
- Arthroplasty
- Fractures
- Inflammation

20.6b.2 Positioning and Incision

After application of a tourniquet, the hand is placed on a side table, and a small roll is placed under the palm (**Fig. 20.22**). A curvilinear incision is recommended for exposure of an individual metacarpophalangeal joint (see **Fig. 20.21**).

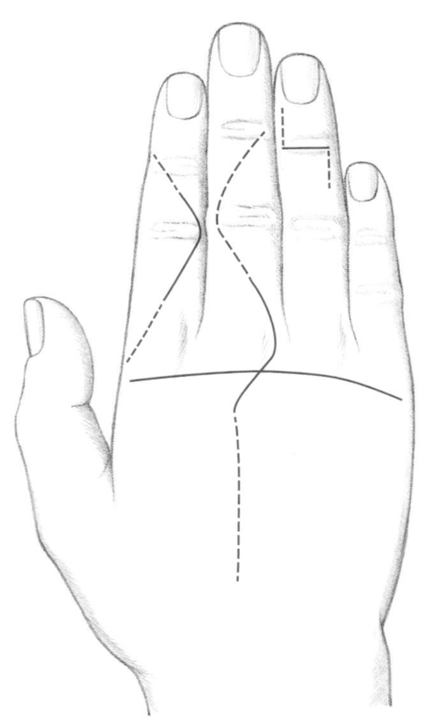

Fig. 20.21 Dorsal incisions for exposure of the metacarpophalangeal and proximal and distal
interphalangeal joints and metacarpal bones.

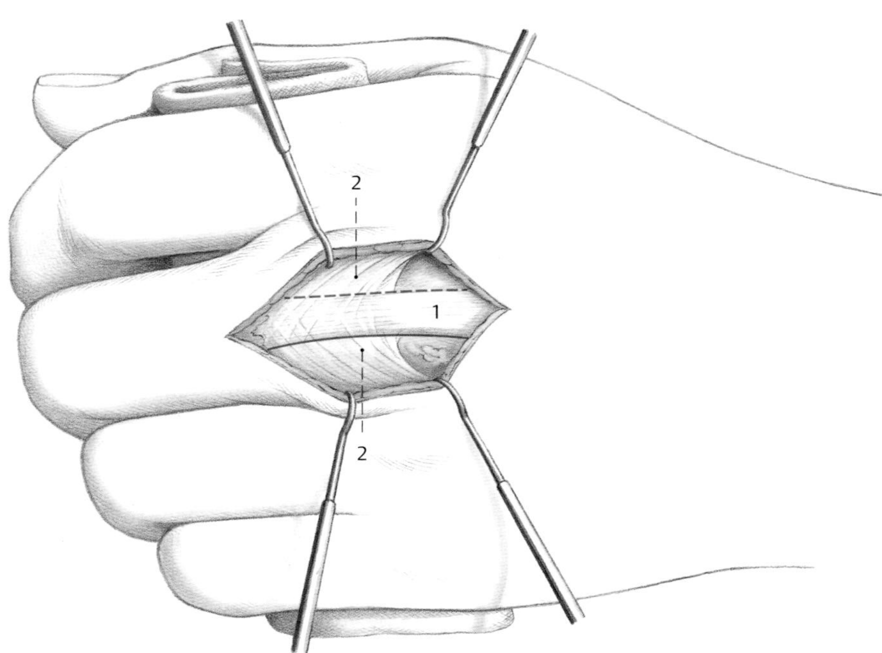

Fig. 20.22 Dorsal approach to the metacarpophalangeal joint (left hand). Status after skin incision. The dorsal aponeurosis may be incised in an ulnar (solid line) or radial (dashed line) position relative to the central extensor (intermediate tract).

1 Tendon of extensor digitorum
2 Dorsal aponeurosis

20.6b.3 Exposure of the Joint

The dorsal aponeurosis (transverse lamina according to Zancolli) may be incised on either the ulnar or the radial side of the central slip of the extensor tendons. In the presence of ulnar subluxation of the extensor tendon, splitting of the aponeurosis on the ulnar side is always required for later recentering of the extensor tendon over the metacarpal head. The dorsal aponeurosis is bluntly dissected free of the fibrous joint capsule, and retracted laterally.

The fibrous and synovial joint capsule is opened along the dashed line shown in **Fig. 20.23**. After retraction of the joint capsule and flexion of the finger, clear dorsal exposure of the metacarpal head and the base of the proximal phalanx is obtained (**Fig. 20.24**).

20.6b.4 Wound Closure

After release of the tourniquet and hemostasis, first the joint capsule and then the dorsal aponeurosis is closed with fine absorbable suture material.

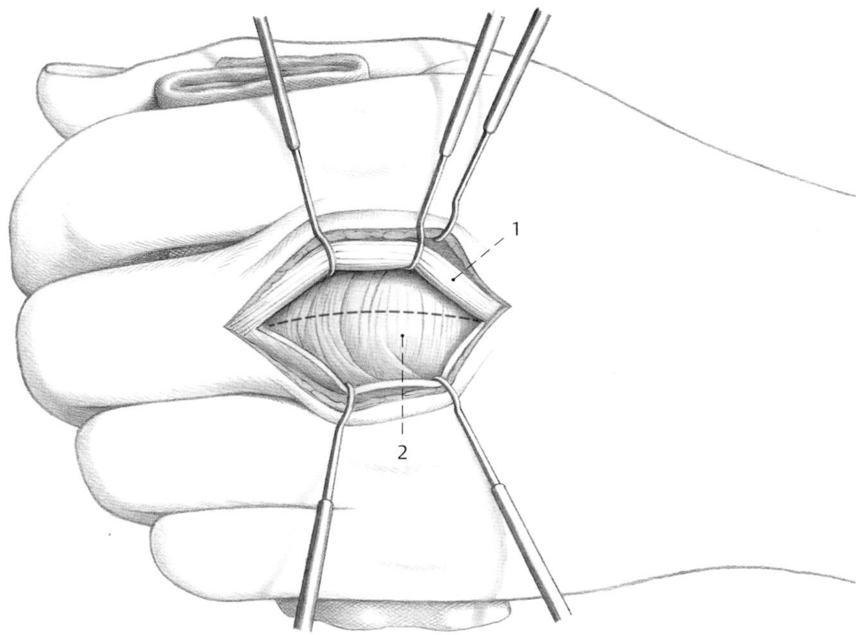

Fig. 20.23 Incision of the joint capsule after retraction of the extensor tendon.

1 Tendon of extensor digitorum
2 Metacarpophalangeal joint capsule

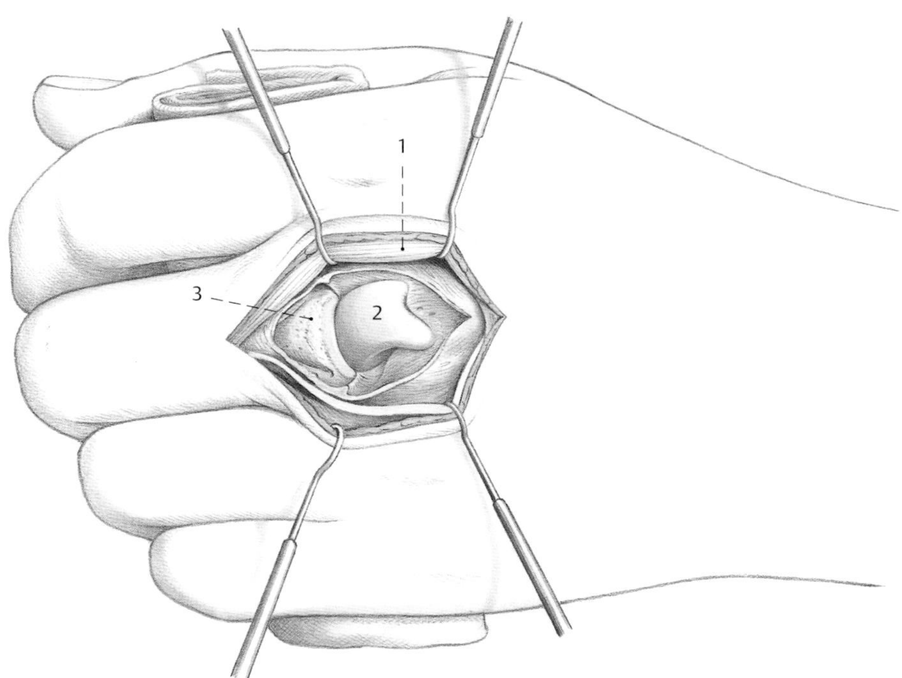

Fig. 20.24 Appearance after opening of the joint. Exposure of the head of the metacarpal with the finger flexed.

1 Tendon of extensor digitorum
2 Head of the third metacarpal
3 Base of the proximal phalanx

20.6c Dorsal Approach to the Proximal Interphalangeal Joint

R. Bauer, F. Kerschbaumer, S. Poisel

20.6c.1 Principal Indications

- Synovectomy
- Arthroplasty
- Fractures
- Inflammation

20.6c.2 Positioning and Incision

The skin incision follows the curvilinear course shown in **Fig. 20.21**.

20.6c.3 Exposure of the Joint

The skin and subcutaneous tissue together with the veins are dissected free of the dorsal aponeurosis and retracted. The central extensor (intermediate tract) may be split along the dashed line shown in **Fig. 20.25** together with the fibrous and synovial joint capsule. By flexion of the finger and simultaneous retraction of the capsule flaps, a clear dorsal exposure of the head of the proximal phalanx and the base of the middle phalanx is obtained (**Fig. 20.26**).

20.6c.4 Wound Closure

The capsule and the extensor apparatus can be closed in a single layer by means of fine absorbable interrupted sutures.

20.6c.5 Dangers

Too extensive stripping of the central extensor at the base of the middle phalanx should be avoided because this will result in a postoperative extension deficit in the proximal interphalangeal joint.

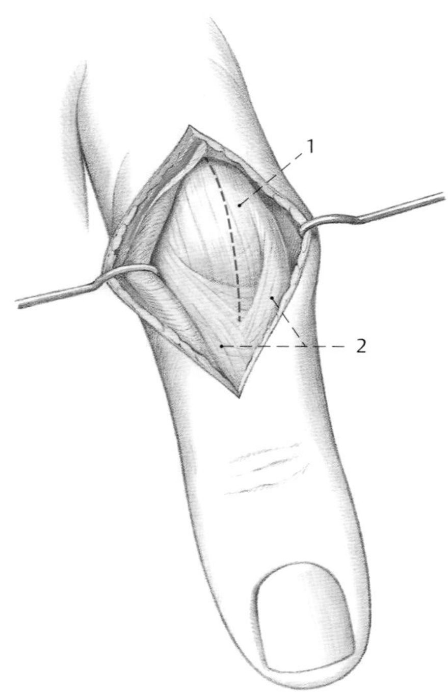

Fig. 20.25 Dorsal approach to the proximal interphalangeal joint after skin incision. Median cleavage of the central extensor and joint capsule.

1 Intermediate tract of the dorsal aponeurosis
2 Lateral tract of the dorsal aponeurosis

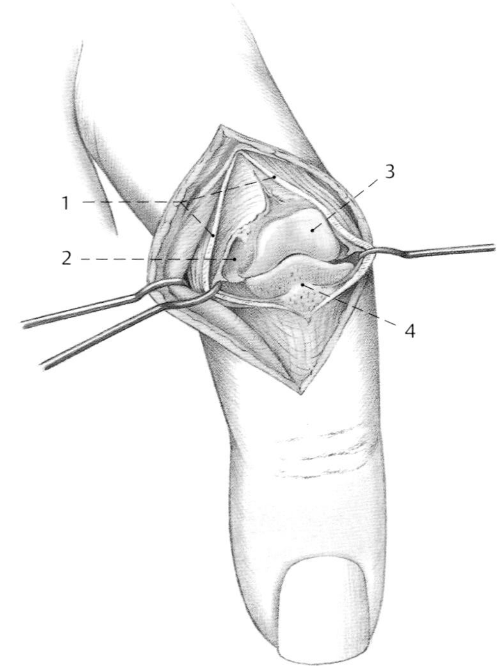

Fig. 20.26 Clear view of the proximal interphalangeal joint with the finger flexed after opening of the capsule.

1 Dorsal aponeurosis
2 Interphalangeal joint capsule
3 Head of the proximal phalanx
4 Base of the middle phalanx

20.6d Dorsal Approach to the Proximal Interphalangeal Joint Involving Transection of the Collateral Ligament

R. Bauer, F. Kerschbaumer, S. Poisel

20.6d.1 Principal Indications

- Synovectomy
- Arthroplasty
- Fractures

20.6d.2 Positioning and Incision

The skin incision is curved (see **Fig. 20.21**). The skin and subcutaneous tissue flaps are dissected free on both sides of the extensor apparatus.

20.6d.3 Exposure of the Joint

The dorsal aponeurosis may be transected either on both sides of the central extensor (**Fig. 20.27**) or, as shown in **Fig. 20.28**, lateral to the lateral bands. Parallel to the incisions of the dorsal aponeurosis, the fibrous and synovial joint capsules are now opened. The collateral ulnar ligament is snared with a nonabsorbable suture and transected proximally (**Fig. 20.29**). The site of resection of the collateral ulnar ligament is several millimeters distal to the origin of the collateral ligament at the head of the proximal phalanx (**Fig. 20.30**). Radial dislocation of the finger at the proximal interphalangeal joint reflects the joint far enough to bring into view not only the palmar portions of the joint capsule on the dorsal side, but also those on the ulnar side (**Fig. 20.31**).

20.6d.4 Wound Closure

Following suture of the collateral ulnar ligament, the joint capsule and the extensor aponeurosis are closed in two layers.

20.6d.5 Note

The dorsal approach to the proximal interphalangeal joint with transection of the collateral ligament is utilized particularly for synovectomies in rheumatoid arthritis. Dual incision of the dorsal aponeurosis lateral to the central extensor may be considered less invasive than its median incision. A single ulnar incision may suffice provided synovitis is not severe.

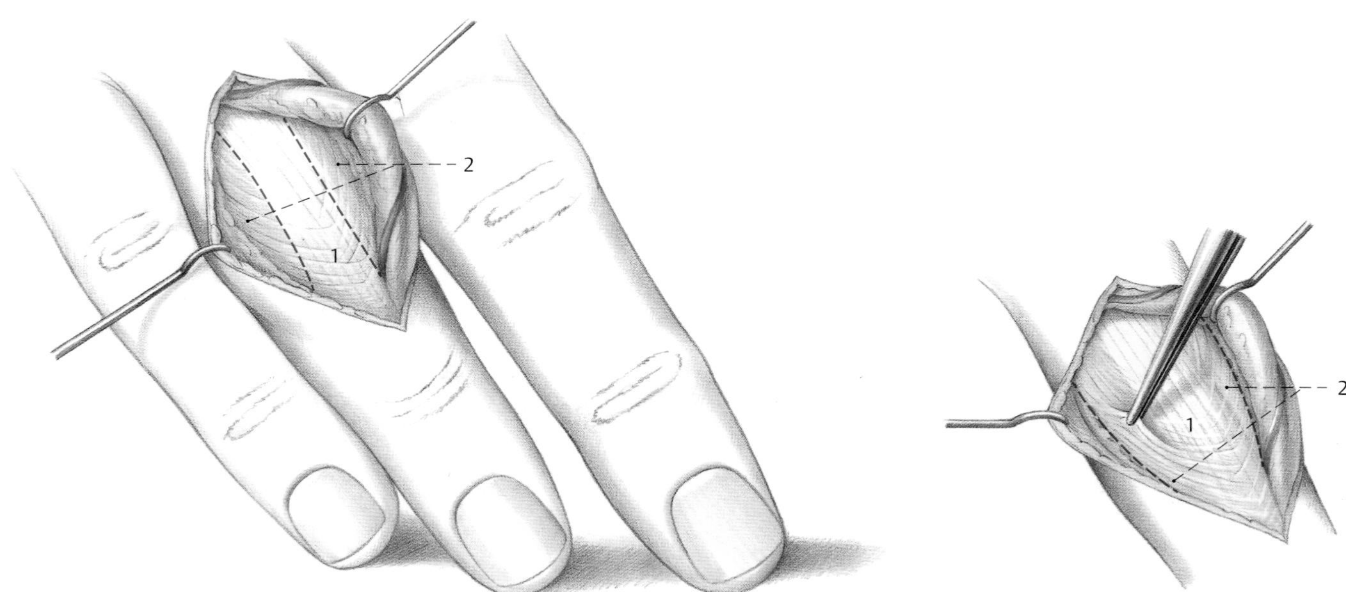

Fig. 20.27 First variant of the approach for exposure of the proximal interphalangeal joint from the dorsal side. Incisions are lateral to the central extensor.

1 Intermediate tract of the dorsal aponeurosis
2 Lateral tract of the dorsal aponeurosis

Fig. 20.28 Second variant of the approach for exposure of the proximal interphalangeal joint from the dorsal side. Incision of the extensor hood lateral to the lateral extensor band.

1 Intermediate tract of the dorsal aponeurosis
2 Lateral tract of the dorsal aponeurosis

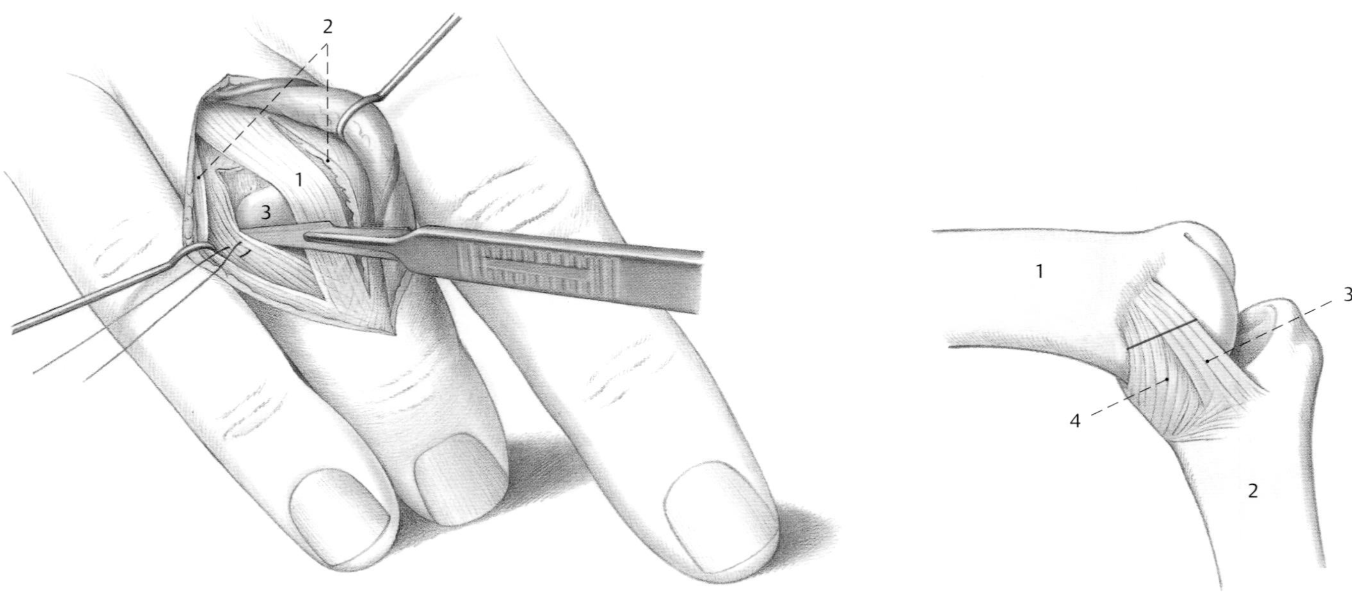

Fig. 20.29 After opening of the joint capsule, the ulnar collateral ligament is transected.

1 Intermediate tract of the dorsal aponeurosis
2 Lateral tract of the dorsal aponeurosis
3 Head of the proximal phalanx

Fig. 20.30 Schematic representation of the incision site on the ulnar collateral ligament (solid line).

1 Proximal phalanx
2 Middle phalanx
3 Collateral ligament
4 Accessory collateral ligament

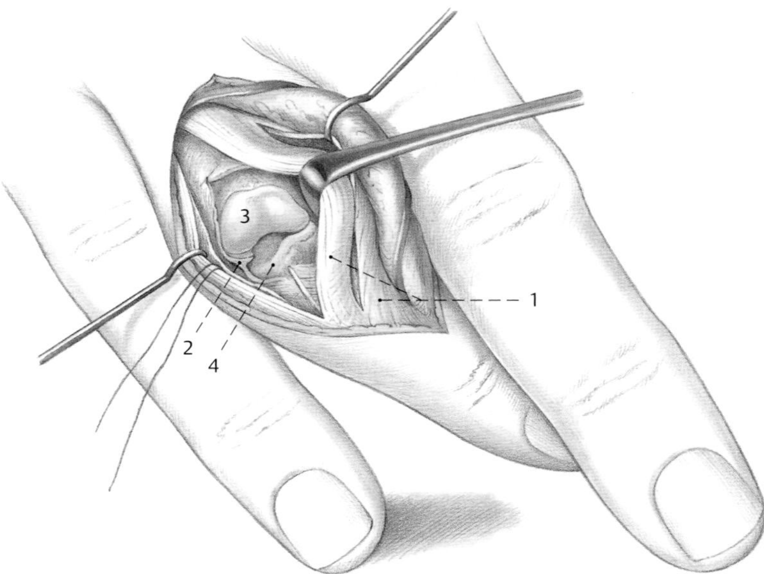

Fig. 20.31 The site after transection of the ulnar collateral ligament and reflection of the joint.

1 Dorsal aponeurosis
2 Capsule of the proximal interphalangeal joint
3 Head of the proximal phalanx
4 Base of the middle phalanx

20.6e Dorsal Approach to the Distal Interphalangeal Joint

R. Bauer, F. Kerschbaumer, S. Poisel

20.6e.1 Principal Indications

- Bony extensor tendon ruptures
- Fractures
- Arthrodesis

20.6e.2 Positioning and Incision

The skin incision may be transverse or step-shaped (see **Fig. 20.21**). Following dissection of the skin and subcutaneous tissue flaps, the extensor tendon is cut through transversely (**Fig. 20.32**).

20.6e.3 Exposure of the Joint

After transection of the extensor tendon, the joint capsule is opened in the same direction, and the distal joint is flexed. Thus, a clear exposure of the dorsal parts of the distal interphalangeal joint is obtained (**Fig. 20.33**).

20.6e.4 Wound Closure

The joint capsule and the extensors are sutured in a single layer with fine interrupted sutures. To secure the suture, the distal joint may be temporarily immobilized with a Kirschner wire. Alternatively, the extensor tendon is fixed with a pull-out wire (**Fig. 20.34**).

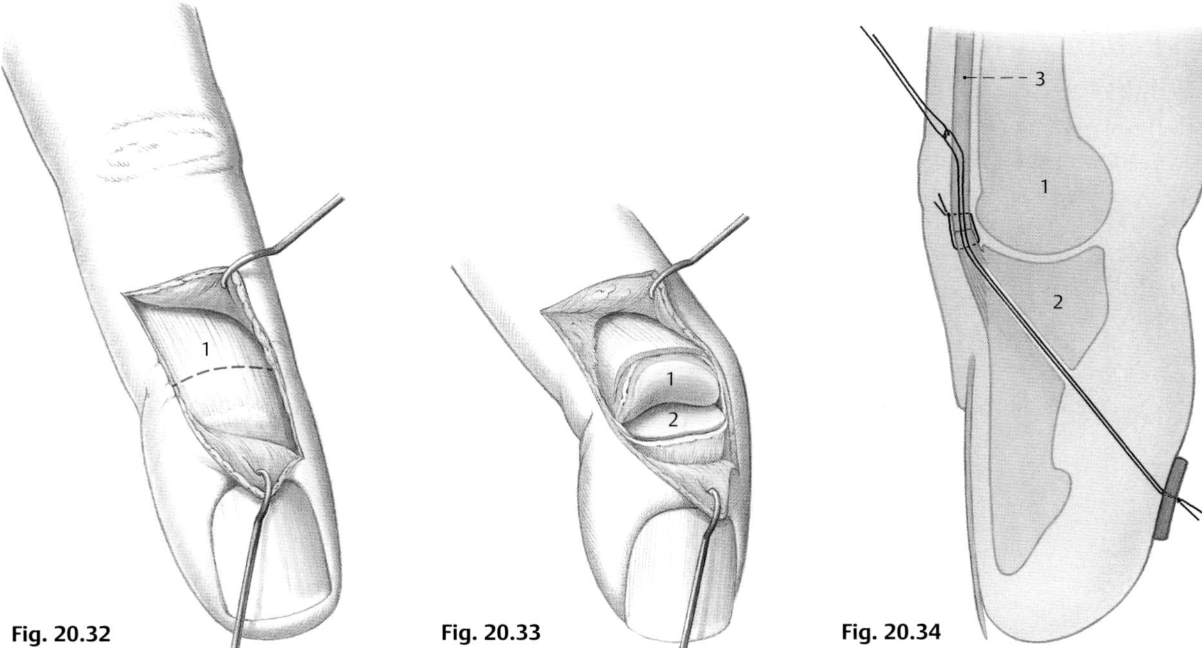

Fig. 20.32 Dorsal approach to the distal interphalangeal joint. Transection of the extensor tendon and joint capsule (dashed line).

1 Dorsal aponeurosis (extensor tendon)

Fig. 20.33 Exposure of the distal interphalangeal joint with the finger flexed.

1 Head of the middle phalanx
2 Base of the distal phalanx

Fig. 20.34 Suture of the extensor tendon and reinforcement of the suture using a pull-out wire.

1 Middle phalanx
2 Distal phalanx
3 Dorsal aponeurosis (extensor tendon)

20.7 Approach to the Finger Flexor Tendons

R. Bauer, F. Kerschbaumer, S. Poisel

20.7.1 Principal Indications

- Synovectomy
- Tendon rupture
- Tendon transfer
- Dupuytren's contracture
- Inflammation

20.7.2 Zigzag Incision According to Bruner

This incision is particularly suitable for flexor tendon synovectomy (**Fig. 20.35**).

20.7.3 Zigzag Incision According to Littler

Compared with the Bruner incision, this incision has the advantage that, if necessary, a V–Y reconstruction, and hence a skin extension, can be performed. This incision may find application in milder forms of Dupuytren's contracture (**Fig. 20.36**).

20.7.4 Midlateral Incision

Figures 20.37 and **20.38** present midlateral incisions for exposure of the flexor tendons of the thumb, index finger, and middle finger in addition to a transverse incision for exposure of the annular ligaments.

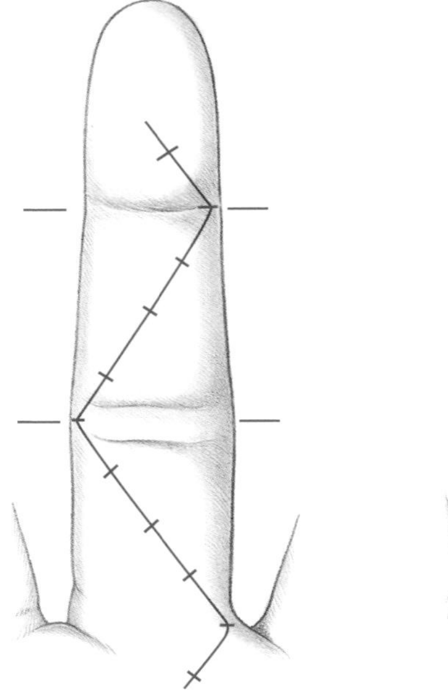

Fig. 20.35 Skin incision according to Bruner.

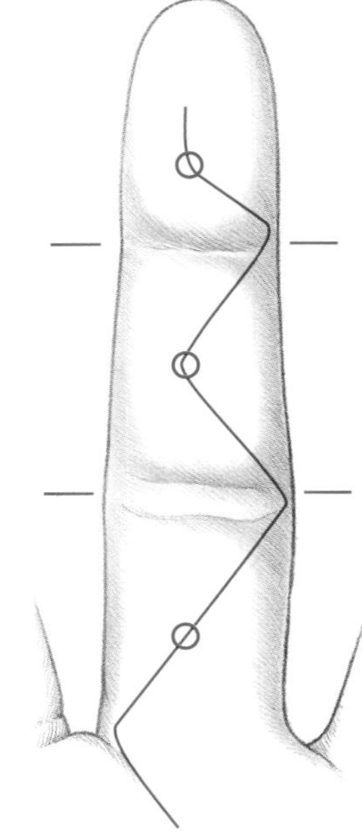

Fig. 20.36 Skin incision according to Littler.

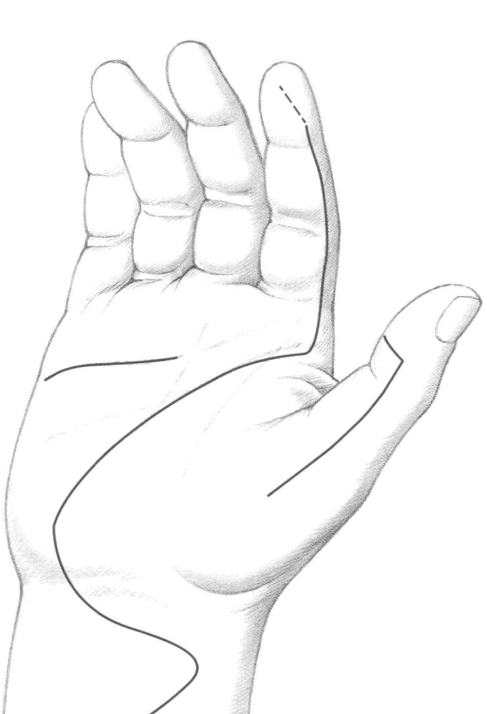

Fig. 20.37 Midlateral incision of the index finger with extension of the incision beyond the wrist joint. Incision over the flexor tendon of the thumb, and incision over the proximal palmar crease.

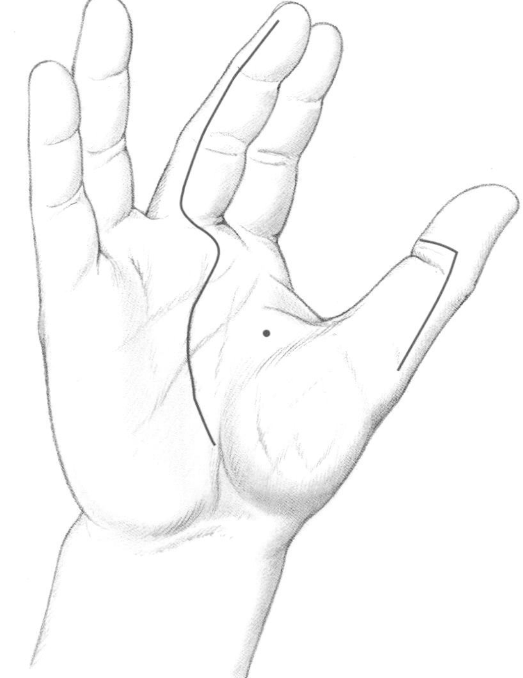

Fig. 20.38 Midlateral ulnar incision on the middle finger with extension to the palm. Palmar incision for exposure of the flexor tendon of the thumb.

20.7.5 Z-plasty

The incision shown in **Fig. 20.39** begins with a straight cut. After the skin and subcutaneous tissue have been dissected and undermined, Z-shaped incisions are made as outlined in **Fig. 20.39b**. After extension of the previously flexed finger, the triangular skin flaps are displaced (**Fig. 20.39c**). The wound is closed as indicated in **Fig. 20.39d**. The corner sutures are placed first.

This incision is utilized mainly in Dupuytren's disease with flexion contracture of the finger.

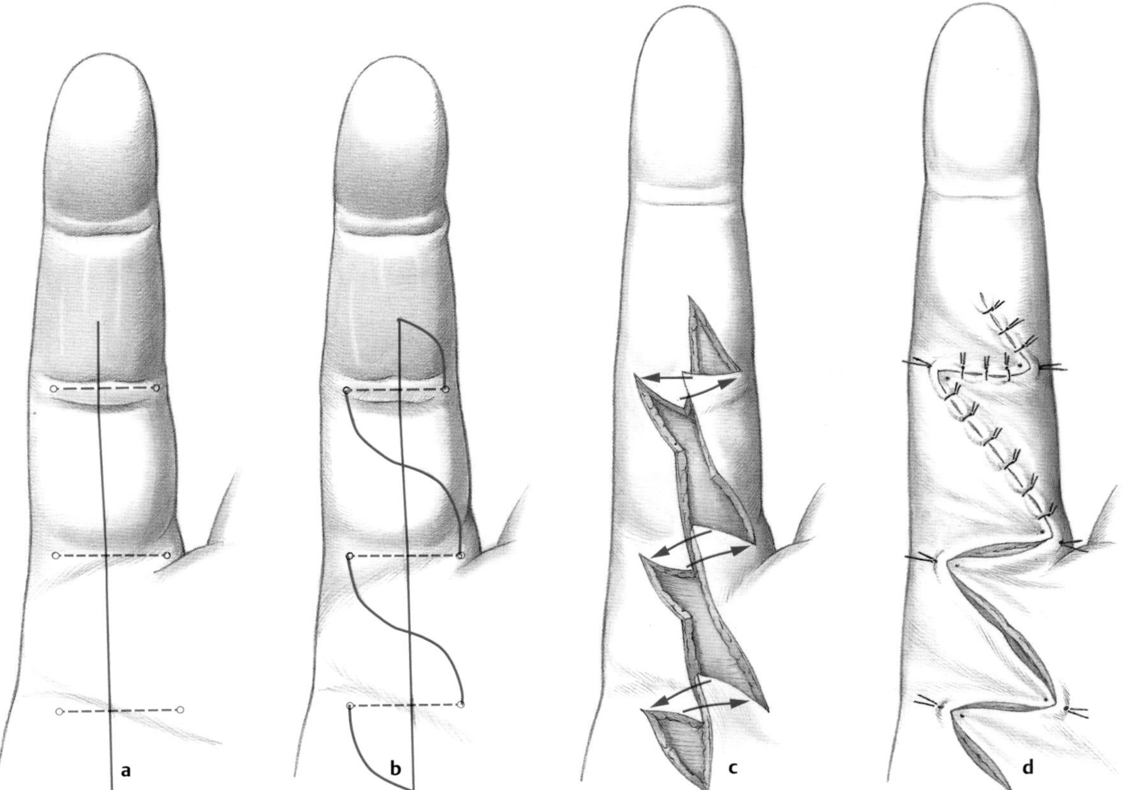

Fig. 20.39 a–d Z-plasty.

a Marking of the incision and of auxiliary points in the digital flexion creases.
b After straight division of the skin, Z-shaped flaps are cut at an angle of approximately 60°.
c Extension of the finger and displacement of skin flaps.
d Skin closure after placement of the corner sutures.

20.8 Palmar Exposure of the Flexor Tendon and Proximal Interphalangeal Joint

R. Bauer, F. Kerschbaumer, S. Poisel

20.8.1 Principal Indications

- Synovectomy
- Capsulotomy

20.8.2 Positioning and Incision

After application of a tourniquet, a pad is placed under the dorsum of the hand. The fingers and the thumb are mounted on a "lead hand." The skin incision is Z-shaped, as shown by the line in **Fig. 20.40**. After dissection of the skin and subcutaneous tissue flaps, these are snared with stay sutures, and are reflected (**Fig. 20.41**). The flexor tendon sheath as well as the radial and ulnar neurovascular bundle (covered by fascia, known as Grayson's ligament; see also **Fig. 20.50**) are thus clearly exposed.

20.8.3 Exposure of the Joint

If exposure of the proximal interphalangeal joint from the palmar side is required, the tendon sheath is split, and the superficial and deep flexor tendons are carefully elevated and retracted with a tendon hook (**Fig. 20.42**).

Under the vinculum breve of the digits of the hand, an H-shaped incision is made in the joint capsule. The vincula of the tendons should, if possible, escape injury in this capsulotomy. Retraction of the capsule flaps with small single-pronged hooks exposes the volar aspect of the joint (**Fig. 20.43**).

Figure 20.44 shows the flexor tendons with the corresponding vincula.

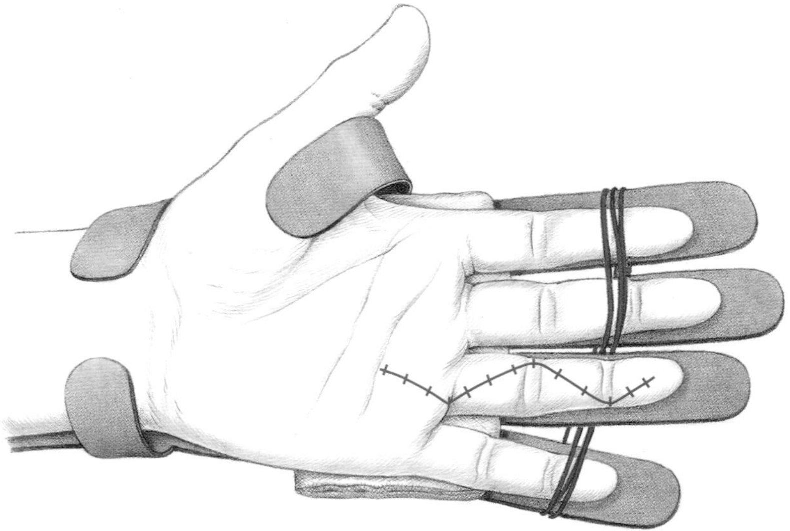

Fig. 20.40 Approach to the finger flexor tendon and to the proximal interphalangeal joint from the palm (left hand). Skin incision (solid line).

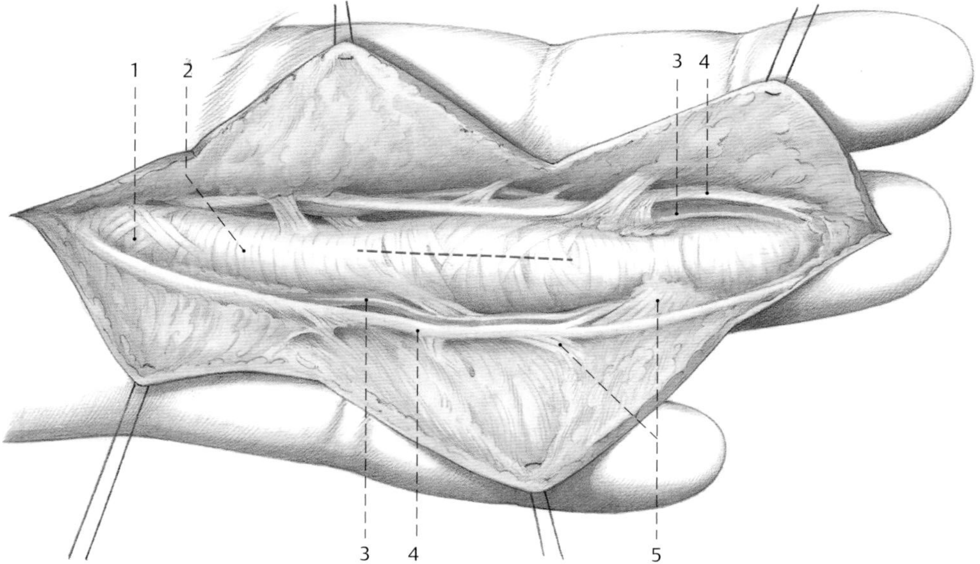

Fig. 20.41 Exposure of the neurovascular bundles after retraction of the skin flaps. Incision of the flexor tendon sheath (dashed line).

1 Cruciate ligament of the tendon sheath of the fingers
2 Annular ligament of the tendon sheath of the fingers
3 Proper palmar digital artery
4 Proper palmar digital nerve
5 Cleland's ligament

20.8.4 Wound Closure

Suturing of the palmar portions of the joint capsule and the flexor tendon sheath is not necessary. Closure of the wound with skin sutures is sufficient.

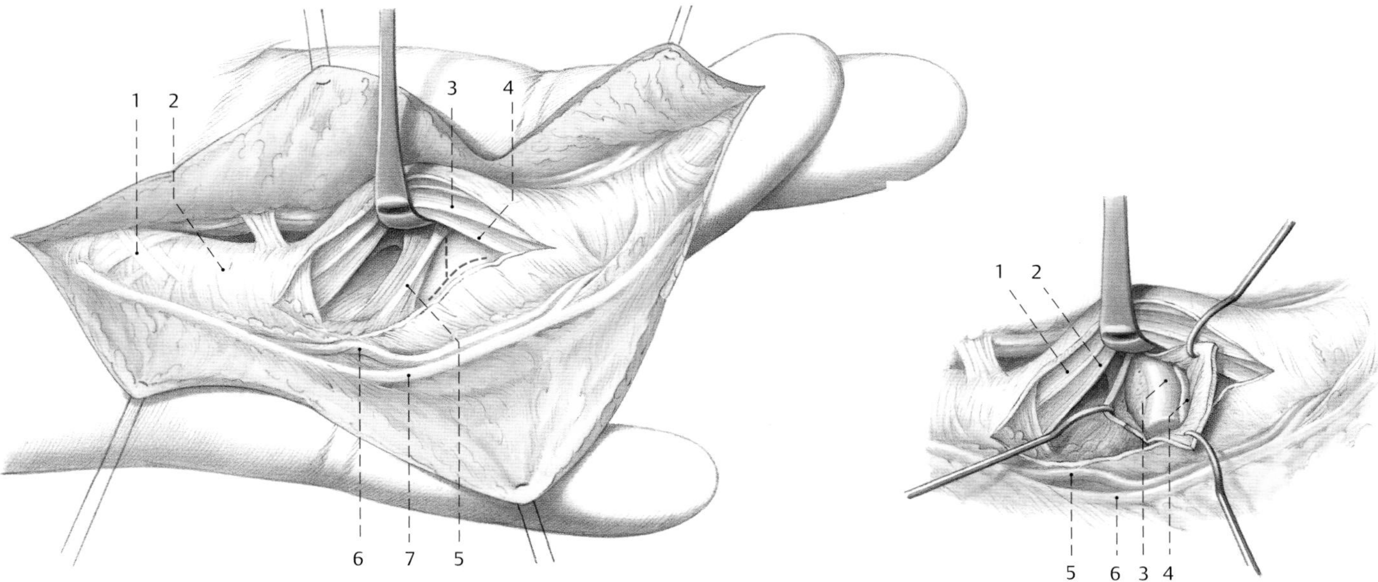

Fig. 20.42 Retraction of the superficial and deep flexor tendons while sparing the vinculum. Opening of the joint capsule (dashed lines).

1 Cruciate ligament of the tendon sheath of the fingers
2 Annular ligament of the tendon sheath of the fingers
3 Tendon of flexor digitorum profundus
4 Tendon of flexor digitorum superficialis
5 Vinculum tendinum
6 Proper palmar digital artery
7 Proper palmar digital nerve

Fig. 20.43 Appearance after the palmar opening of the joint capsule of the proximal interphalangeal joint.

1 Tendon of flexor digitorum profundus
2 Tendon of flexor digitorum superficialis
3 Head of the proximal phalanx
4 Base of the middle phalanx
5 Proper palmar digital artery
6 Proper palmar digital nerve

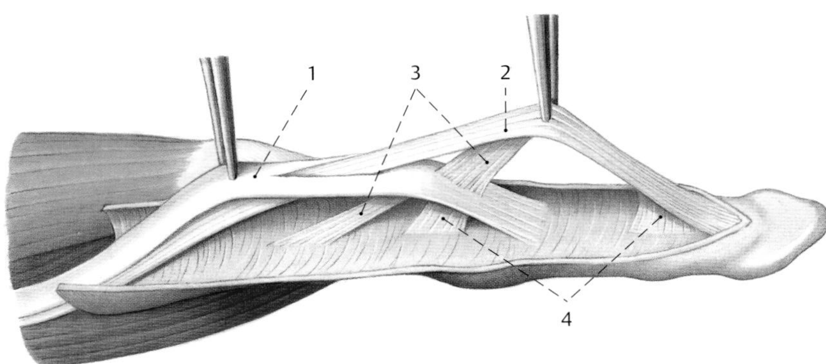

Fig. 20.44 Exposure of the flexor tendons with the vincula.

1 Tendon of flexor digitorum superficialis
2 Tendon of flexor digitorum profundus
3 Vincula longa
4 Vincula brevia

20.9 Approach to the Finger Flexor Tendon Via the Midlateral Incision

R. Bauer, F. Kerschbaumer, S. Poisel

20.9.1 Principal Indications

- Synovectomy of the flexor tendons
- Transplantation of the flexor tendons

20.9.2 Positioning and Incision

After application of a tourniquet, the dorsum of the hand is placed on a pad and the hand is secured with a positioning splint (**Fig. 20.45**). The splint illustrated in **Fig. 20.45** permits the use of small self-retaining retractors so that no assistant is needed (see also **Fig. 20.48**).

Before the line of incision is marked, the finger is deflected. Three points are marked off at the ends of the finger flexion creases (**Fig. 20.46**, detail). These points are connected, and the incision is subsequently extended into the palm along an S-shaped or step-shaped course (**Fig. 20.46**).

20.9.3 Exposure of the Flexor Tendon Sheath

After dissection of the skin flaps in the palm, the neurovascular bundle emerging distal to the transverse fasciculi of the palmar aponeurosis is exposed first (**Fig. 20.47**). The distal skin and subcutaneous tissue flap with the neurovascular bundle is elevated out of the wound with a fine single-pronged hook. The dissection is continued in a distal direction under vision so that the skin flap with the included neurovascular bundle can be reflected and retracted (**Fig. 20.48**). By this means, clear exposure of the flexor tendon sheath is obtained.

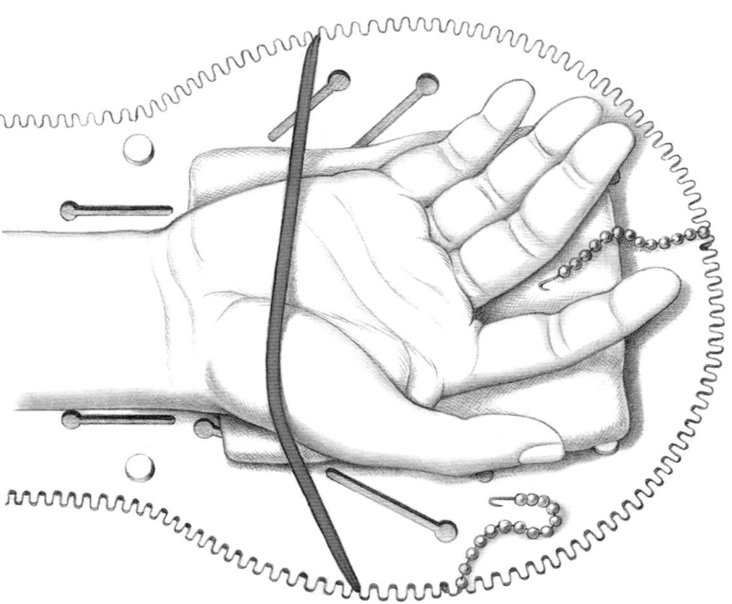

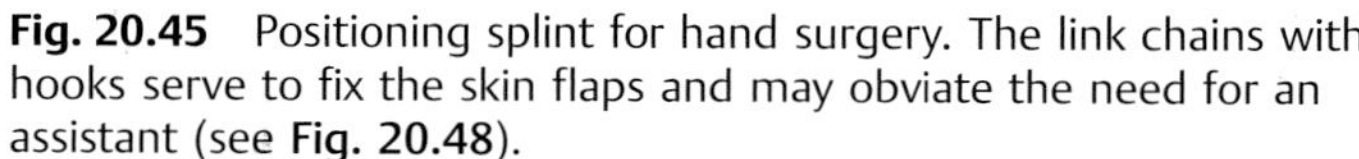

Fig. 20.45 Positioning splint for hand surgery. The link chains with hooks serve to fix the skin flaps and may obviate the need for an assistant (see **Fig. 20.48**).

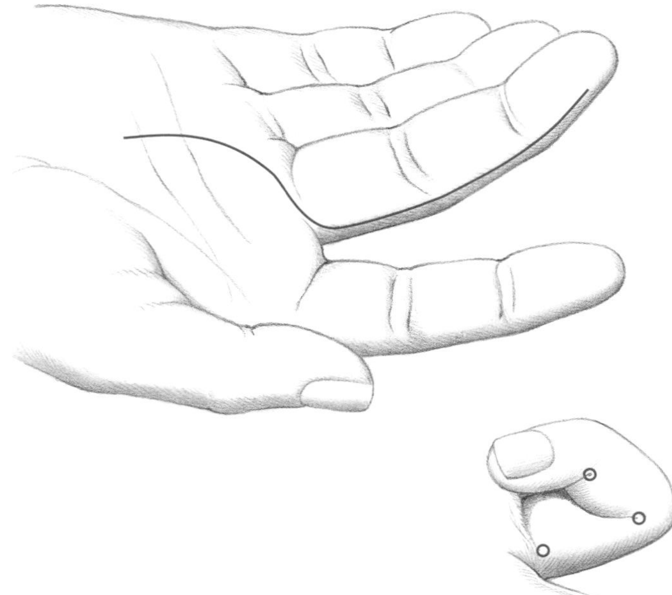

Fig. 20.46 After the designation of auxiliary points, the midlateral skin incision may be marked at the ends of the digital flexion creases while the finger is flexed (detail).

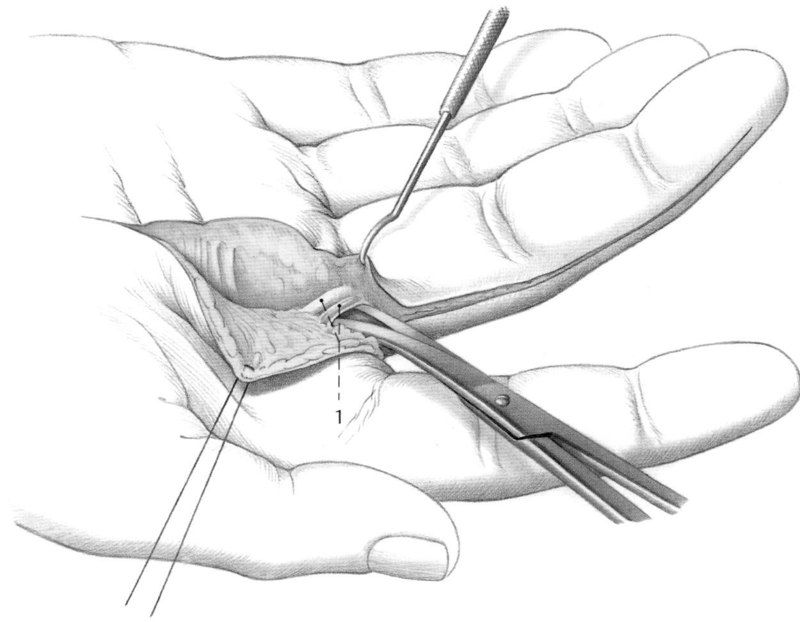

Fig. 20.47 Dissection of the neurovascular bundle distal to the palmar aponeurosis at the base of the finger.

1 Proper palmar digital artery and nerve

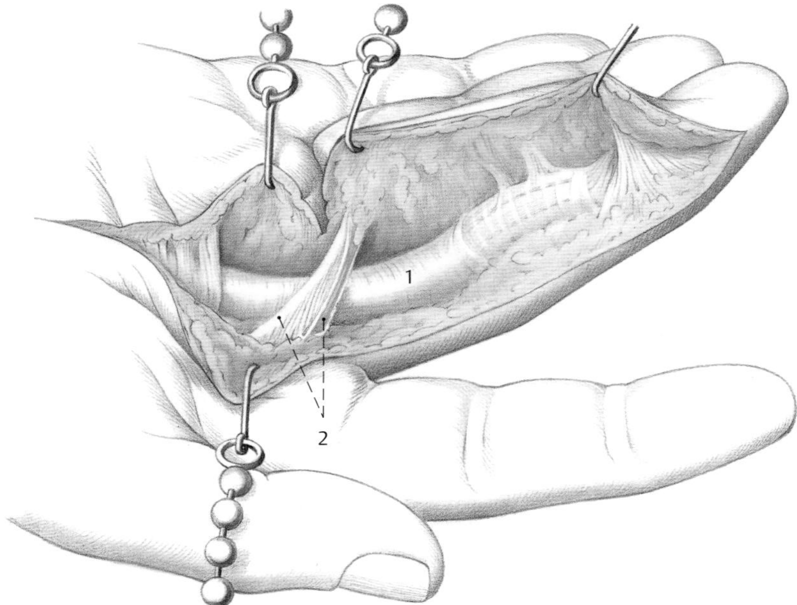

Fig. 20.48 Operative site after retraction of the skin and the subcutaneous tissue flap. The neurovascular bundle crosses the exposed flexor tendon sheath.

1 Synovial sheaths
2 Proper palmar digital nerve and artery

20.9.4 Anatomical Site

(**Figs. 20.49** and **20.50**)

Figure 20.49 shows the neural supply of the skin of the finger. Note that the dorsal cutaneous supply distal to the proximal interphalangeal joint is from the palmar side. **Figure 20.50** gives a schematic cross-section of the finger just proximal to the proximal interphalangeal joint.

20.9.5 Note

This incision is advantageous for operations in which major portions of the flexor tendon sheath have to be removed (flexor tendon synovectomy). Adhesions to the skin on the palmar side are observed less frequently than after Z-shaped incisions. A disadvantage of this approach is the more complicated dissection due to the oblique decussation of the neurovascular bundle at the base of the finger.

The unilateral transection of Cleland's ligament and of Landsmeer's retinacular ligament that is required with this incision does not entail any functional impairment.

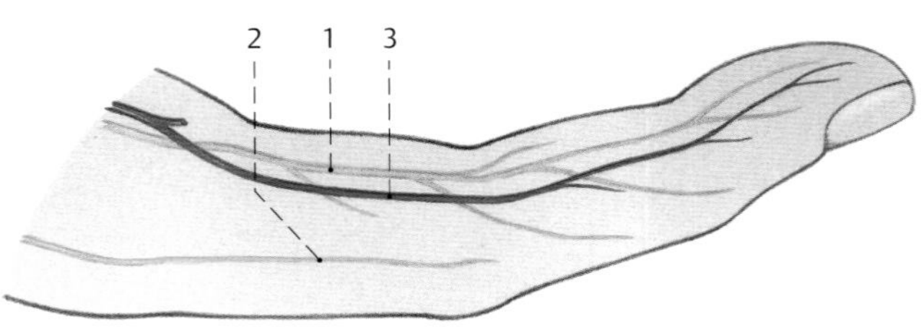

Fig. 20.49 Anatomical site. Schematic representation of the neural supply of skin of finger.

1 Proper palmar digital nerve
2 Dorsal digital nerve
3 Proper palmar digital artery

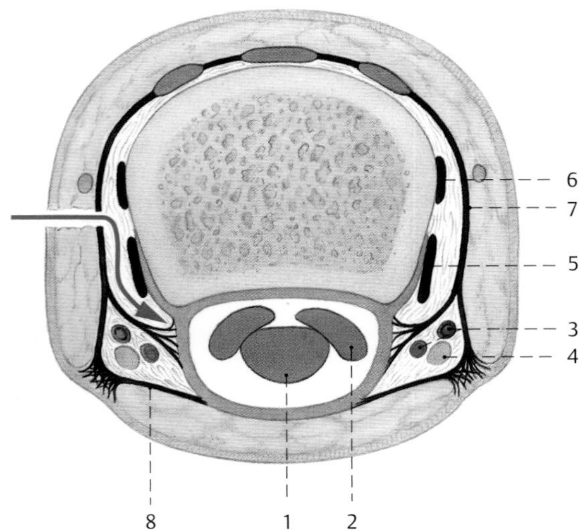

Fig. 20.50 Schematic cross-section of the finger just proximal to the middle joint; midlateral approach (arrow).

1 Tendon of flexor digitorum profundus
2 Tendon of flexor digitorum superficialis
3 Proper palmar digital artery and vein
4 Proper palmar digital nerve
5 Cleland's ligament
6 Oblique retinacular ligament (Landsmeer)
7 Transverse retinacular ligament (Landsmeer)
8 Grayson's ligament

20.10 Approach to the Annular Ligament on the Thumb

R. Bauer, F. Kerschbaumer, S. Poisel

20.10.1 Principal Indication

- Trigger thumb

20.10.2 Positioning and Incision

After application of a tourniquet, the skin in the area of the flexion crease is transversely incised. Following retraction of the skin, it is first necessary to expose the radial neurovascular bundle, which obliquely crosses the flexor tendon sheath (**Fig. 20.51**).

20.10.3 Exposure of the Flexor Tendon Sheath

After dissection of the radial neurovascular bundle, the skin flaps are slightly undermined, and the flexor tendon sheath may be exposed, possibly with the use of small cotton swabs. The annular ligament is split as shown by the dashed line in **Fig. 20.52**. The flexor tendon of the thumb is now clearly exposed (**Fig. 20.53**).

20.10.4 Dangers

Owing to its oblique course (from proximal ulnar to distal radial), the radial neurovascular bundle is susceptible to injury.

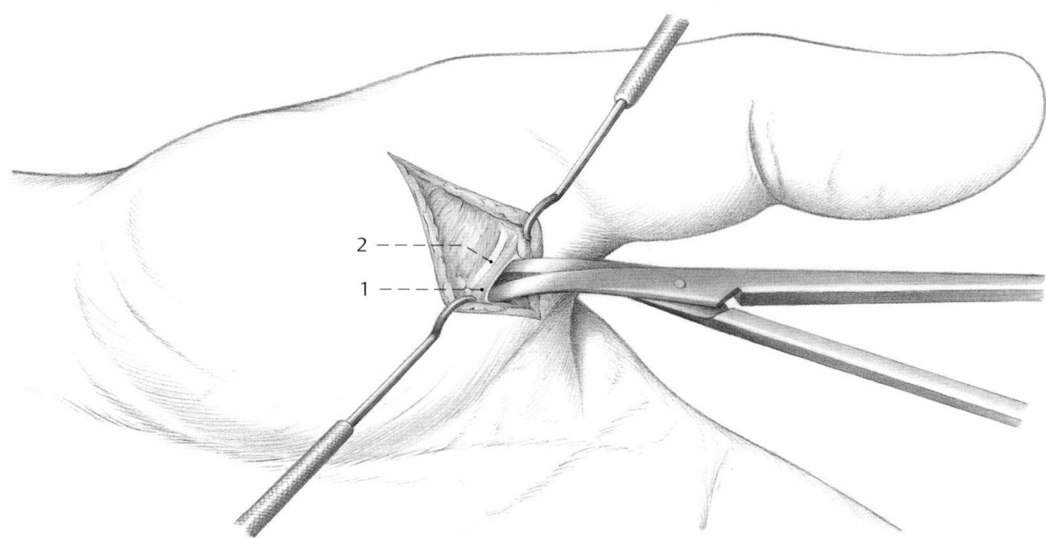

Fig. 20.51 Approach to the annular ligament on the thumb (left hand). After splitting the skin, the radial neurovascular bundle is first identified.

1 Proper palmar digital artery
2 Proper palmar digital nerve

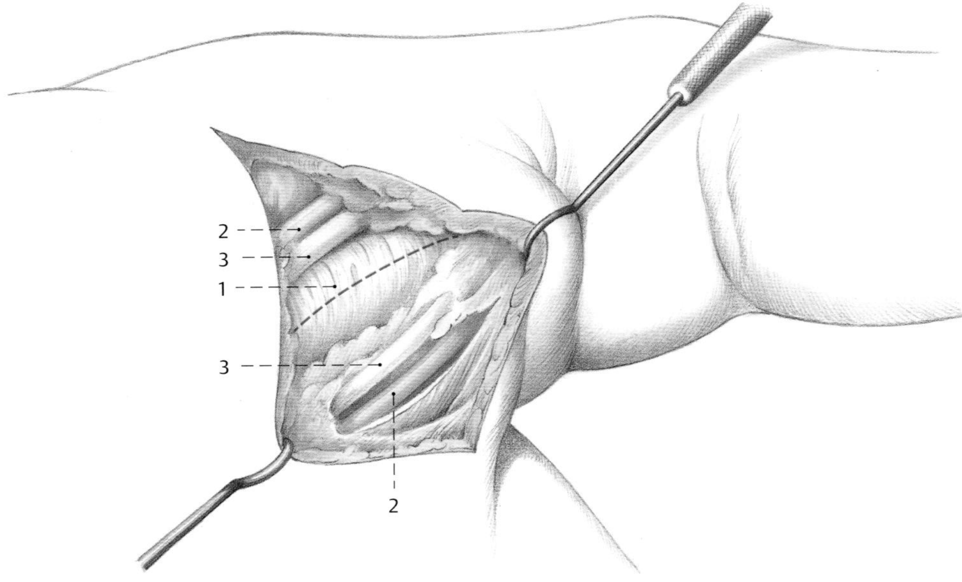

Fig. 20.52 After retraction of the skin and dissection of the ulnar neurovascular bundle, the annular ligament is incised (dashed line).

1 Tendon sheath (annular fibers)
2 Proper palmar digital artery
3 Proper palmar digital nerve

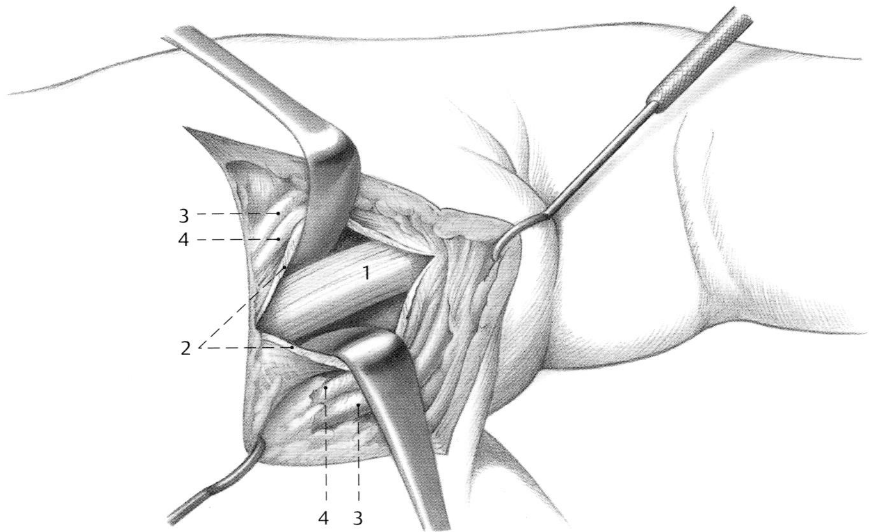

Fig. 20.53 Operative site after incision of the annular ligament and exposure of the flexor tendon of the thumb.

1 Tendon of flexor pollicis longus
2 Tendon sheath (annular fibers)
3 Proper palmar digital artery
4 Proper palmar digital nerve

Further Reading: Shoulder and Upper Extremity

[1] Alonso-Llames M. Bilaterotricipital approach to the elbow. Its application in the osteosynthesis of supracondylar fractures of the humerus in children. Acta Orthop Scand 1972;43(6):479–490

[2] Anson BJ, McVay CB. Surgical Anatomy. Vol 1. Philadelphia: Saunders; 1971

[3] Banks SW, Laufmann II. An Atlas of Surgical Exposures of the Extremities. Philadelphia: Saunders; 1968

[4] Bigliani LU, Morrison DS, April EW. The morphology of the acromion and its relationship to rotator cuff tears. Orthop Trans 1986;10:228

[5] Bigliani LU, Cordasco FA, McLlveen SJ, Musso ES. Operative repair of massive rotator cuff tears: long-term results. J Shoulder Elbow Surg 1992;1(3):120–130

[6] Bonnaire F, Bula P. Distale Humerusfrakturen. Trauma Berufskrankh 2010;12(Suppl. 2):96–103

[7] Brodsky JW, Tullos HS, Gartsman GM. Simplified posterior approach to the shoulder joint. A technical note. J Bone Joint Surg Am 1987;69(5):773–774

[8] Bryan RS, Morrey BF. Extensive posterior exposure of the elbow. A triceps-sparing approach. Clin Orthop Relat Res 1982;(166):188–192

[9] Consentino R. Atlas of Anatomy and Surgical Approaches in Orthopaedic Surgery; vol 1. Springfield, IL: Thomas; 1960

[10] Debeyre J, Patthie D, Elmelik E. Repair of ruptures of the rotator cuff of the shoulder: With a note of advancement of the supraspinatus muscle. J Bone Joint Surg 1965;47-B:36–42

[11] Ewerbeck V, Wentzensen A. Standardverfahren in der operativen Orthopädie und Unfallchirurgie. 2nd rev ed. Stuttgart: Thieme; 2004

[12] Fernandez DL, Jupiter JP. Fractures of the Distal Radius. Berlin: Springer; 1995

[13] Fernandez DL, Jupiter JP. Fractures of the Distal Radius. A Practical Approach to Management. Berlin: Springer; 1996

[14] Fucentese SF, Jost B. Posteriorer Zugang zum Schultergelenk. Operative Orthopädie und Traumatologie. Band 22. Berlin: Springer; 2010:188–195

[15] Geschwend N, Ivosevic-Radovanovic D, Brändli P. Die operative Behandlung der Rotatorenmanschettenruptur. In: Helbig B, Blauth W, eds. Schulterschmerzen und Rupturen der Rotatorenmanschette. Hefte zur Unfallheilkunde 180. Berlin: Springer: 1986:69–88

[16] Gohlke F, Hedtmann A. Schulter. In: Wirth CJ, Zichner L, eds. Orthopädie und orthopädische Chirurgie. Stuttgart: Thieme; 2002

[17] Habermeyer P, Brunner U, Wiedemann E, Wilhelm K. Kompressionssyndrome an der Schulter und deren Differentialdiagnose. Orthopade 1987;16(6):448–457

[18] Habermeyer P, Lichtenberg S, Magosch P. Schulterchirurgie. 4th ed. Munich: Urban & Fischer; 2008

[19] Hansis M, Schmidt HM. Unterarm und Handgelenk. In: Kremer K, Lierse W, Platzer W, Schreiber HW, Weller S, eds. Chirurgische Operationslehre—Schultergürtel, obere Extremität. Stuttgart: Thieme; 1995

[20] Hepp P, Theopold J, Voigt C, Engel T, Josten C, Lill H. The surgical approach for locking plate osteosynthesis of displaced proximal humeral fractures influences the functional outcome. J Shoulder Elbow Surg 2008;17(1):21–28

[21] Hirner A, Weise K. Chirurgie. 2nd rev ed. Stuttgart: Thieme; 2008

[22] Höntzsch D, Maurer H. Schultergürtel. In: Kremer K, Lierse W, Platzer W, Schreiber HW, Weller S, eds. Chirurgische Operationslehre – Schultergürtel, obere Extremität. Stuttgart: Thieme; 1995

[23] Hoppenfeld S, de Boer P. Surgical Exposures in Orthopaedics. Philadelphia: Lippincott; 1984

[24] Iannotti JP, Williams GR. Disorders of the Shoulder: Diagnosis and Management. Vols 1 and 2. Philadelphia: Lippincott Williams & Wilkins; 2007

[25] Kaplan E. Functional and Surgical Anatomy of the Hand. Philadelphia: Lippincott; 1965

[26] Kremer K, Lierse W, Platzer W, Schreiber HW, Weller S. Schultergürtel und obere Extremität. Stuttgart: Thieme; 1995. Chirurgische Operationslehre; Band 9

[27] Krettek C, Wiebking U. Proximale Humerusfraktur: Ist die winkelstabile Plattenosteosynthese der konservativen Behandlung überlegen? Unfallchirurg 2011;114(12):1059–1067

[28] von Laer L. Frakturen und Luxationen im Wachstumsalter. Stuttgart: Thieme; 1996

[29] Landsmeer LM. Atlas of Anatomy of the Hand. Edinburgh: Churchill-Livingstone; 1976

[30] Matsen FA III, Thomas SC, Rockwood CA. Anterior Glenohumeral Instability. In: Rockwood CA, Matsen FA III, eds. The Shoulder. Philadelphia: Saunders; 1990:526

[31] Matsen FA III, Thomas SC, Rockwood CA, Wirth MA. Glenohumeral Instability. In: Rockwood CA, Matsen FA. The Shoulder. 2nd ed. Philadelphia: Saunders; 1998:611–754

[32] Morrey DF. The Elbow and its Disorders. Philadelphia: Saunders; 2000

[33] Müller ME, Allgöwer M, Schneider R, Willenegger H. Manual der Osteosynthese. Berlin: Springer; 1992

[34] Neer CS II. Anterior acromioplasty for the chronic impingement syndrome in the shoulder: a preliminary report. J Bone Joint Surg Am 1972;54(1):41–50

[35] Neer CS. Shoulder Reconstruction. Philadelphia: Saunders; 1990: 202–207

[36] Neviaser JS. Surgical approaches to the shoulder. Clin Orthop Relat Res 1973; (91):34–40

[37] Nicola T. Atlas operativer Zugangswege in der Orthopädie. Munich: Urban & Schwarzenberg; 1971

[38] Oestern HJ, Tscherne H. Ergebnisse der AO-Sammelstudie über Unterarmschaftfrakturen. Unfallheilkunde 1983;86(3):136–142

[39] Platzer W. Atlas der topografischen Anatomie. Stuttgart: Thieme; 1982

[40] Platzer W. Bewegungsapparat. In: Kahle E, Leonhardt H, Platzer W. Taschenatlas der Anatomie. Band 1. 4th ed. Stuttgart: Thieme; 1984

[41] Rauber/Kopsch. Anatomie des Menschen. Band 1–4. Stuttgart: Thieme; 1988

[42] Resch H, Beck E. Praktische Chirurgie des Schultergelenks. Innsbruck: Bronweiler; 1989

[43] Resch H, Maurer H. Schultergelenk. In: Kremer K, Lierse W, Platzer W, Schreiber HW, Weller S, eds. Chirurgische Operationslehre – Schultergürtel, obere Extremität. Stuttgart: Thieme; 1995

[44] Resch H, Povacz P, Ritter E, Matschi W. Transfer of the pectoralis major muscle for the treatment of irreparable rupture of the subscapularis tendon. J Bone Joint Surg Am 2000;82(3):372–382

[45] Rockwood CA, Green ADP, Buchholtz RW. Fractures in Adults. 3rd ed. Philadelphia: Lippincott; 1991

[46] Rüedi T, von Hochstetter AHC, Schlumpf R. Operative Zugänge zur Osteosynthese. Berlin: Springer; 1984

[47] Schünke M, Schulte E, Schumacher U. Prometheus—Lernatlas der Anatomie. Stuttgart: Thieme; 2005

[48] Putz R, Pabst R, eds. Sobotta: Anatomie des Menschen. Munich: Urban & Fischer; 2006

[49] Tscherne H, Blauth M, Kasperczyk W. Indikationen zur konservativ-funktionellen und operativen Therapie von Frakturen am Schultergürtel. In: Rahmanzadeh R, Meißner A, eds. Unfall- und Wiederherstellungschirurgie des Schultergürtels. Berlin: Springer; 1992

[50] Tubiana R, Valentin P. The anatomy of the extensor apparatus of the fingers. Surg Clin North Am 1964;44:897–906

[51] Tubiana R, McCullough CJ, Masquelet AD. An Atlas of Surgical Exposure of the Upper Extremity. London: Martin Dunitz; 1990

[52] Weise K, Firbas W. Ellbogen. In: Kremer K, Lierse W, Platzer W, Schreiber HW, Weller S, eds. Chirurgische Operationslehre—Schultergürtel, obere Extremität. Stuttgart: Thieme; 1995

[53] Weise K. Verletzungen des Oberarms, Ellenbogens, Unterarms und Handgelenks. In: Mutschler W, Haas NP, eds. Praxis der Unfallchirurgie. 2nd rev ed. Stuttgart: Thieme; 2004

[54] Wiedemann E. Scapulafraktur. In: Habermeyer P, ed. Schulterchirurgie. 2nd ed. Munich: Urban & Schwarzenberg; 2002

[55] Wiedemann E. Frakturen der Skapula. Unfallchirurg 2004;107 (12):1124–1133

[56] Winker KH, Maurer H. Oberarm. In: Kremer K, Lierse W, Platzer W, Schreiber HW, Weller S, eds. Chirurgische Operationslehre—Schultergürtel, obere Extremität. Stuttgart: Thieme; 1995

Index

Note: Page numbers followed by *f* indicate figures.

D

E

F

G

H

I

J

K